THE CALORIEKING®
Calorie, Fat & Carbohydrate Counter
Contents

BONUS DIET GUIDES & COUNTERS

D0026995

Weight Control Tips

✔ Eat & Drink Sensibly

- Avoid fad diets. Eat 3 sensible portion-controlled meals daily.
- Limit fats, high-fat foods/snacks and sugar. Eat adequate fresh fruit & vegetables.
- Limit soft drinks, energy drinks, fruit juice and alcohol. Quench your thirst on water. (See Sample Meal Plan ~ Page 11)

✔ Exercise Daily

- Aim for at least 30 minutes daily – even in 5-10 minute lots. For motivation, find an exercise buddy, personal trainer or join a gym. *(Extra Notes ~ Page 12)*

✔ Reshape Eating Behaviors

- Be aware of eating and shopping behaviors that lead to overeating.
- Also focus on social and emotional situations that may trigger compulsive eating. *(Extra Notes ~ Page 14)*

✔ Keep a Food & Exercise Journal

- A journal helps you see exactly what you eat and drink, and how much you exercise. *(Extra Notes ~ Page 15)*
- An excellent motivator and proven weight loss aid. Keeps you honest!

✔ Arrange Moral Support

- Gain the support of family and friends.
- Get extra professional help if required, from your doctor, dietitian, psychologist, exercise trainer, or slimming group.
- Beware of family saboteurs who may discourage you from adopting a healthier diet and lifestyle!

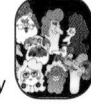

DOCTOR CHECK-UP

Ask your doctor to check your blood pressure, blood sugar and blood cholesterol levels.

HEALTHY WEIGHTS
~ MEN & WOMEN ~
(Over 18 Years)

Based on weights with least risk of disease or death from heart disease, diabetes, stroke and cancer.

Based on Body Mass Index of 20-25

BMI calculated as: $\dfrac{\text{Weight (kg)}}{\text{Height (m)}^2}$

Height (No Shoes) Ft Ins ▼		Healthy Weight Range (Pounds) ▼
4'7"	~	86-108
4'8"	~	88-110
4'9"	~	92-114
4'10"	~	97-121
4'11"	~	99-123
5'0"	~	101-127
5'1"	~	105-132
5'2"	~	110-136
5'3"	~	112-140
5'4"	~	114-145
5'5"	~	119-149
5'6"	~	123-156
5'7"	~	127-158
5'8"	~	129-162
5'9"	~	134-167
5'10"	~	138-173
5'11"	~	143-178
6'0"	~	145-182
6'1"	~	149-187
6'2"	~	156-193
6'3"	~	158-198
6'4"	~	162-202
6'5"	~	170-211
6'6"	~	172-215
6'7"	~	175-220

Body Fat Distribution & Health

Moderate amounts of body fat do not compromise health. However, excess fat above the hips carries a far greater health risk than fat on or below the hips - better to be a 'pear-shape' than an 'apple-shape'.

Abdominal obesity greatly increases the risk of developing diabetes, heart disease, high blood fats, hypertension, stroke, sleep apnea, arthritis and some cancers. So-called 'cellulite' carries no extra health risk.

Waist Circumference directly reflects the increased health risk of abdominal obesity. Waist size associated with a high health risk:

Men ~ Over 40 inches   **Women** ~ Over 35 inches

Body Mass Index (BMI)

BMI is a general (but not specific) indicator of body fatness. Although BMI alone is not diagnostic, the higher the BMI, the greater the health risk of developing diabetes, high blood pressure and heart disease. BMI does not apply to heavily muscled persons. BMI is used in a different way for children.

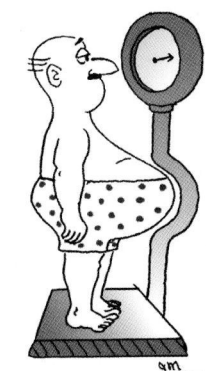

Abdominal obesity greatly increases the risk of ill-health and earlier death.

Check Your BMI: Find your height (no shoes) - look across the row to the weight nearest your own. Then track down to BMI.

Ht	WEIGHT (LBS) ~ ADULTS													
5'1"	100	106	111	116	122	127	132	137	143	148	153	158	185	211
5'2"	104	109	115	120	126	131	136	142	147	153	158	164	191	218
5'3"	107	113	118	124	130	135	141	146	152	158	163	169	197	225
5'4"	110	116	122	128	134	140	145	151	157	163	169	174	204	232
5'5"	114	120	126	132	138	144	150	156	162	168	174	180	210	240
5'6"	118	124	130	136	142	148	155	161	167	173	179	186	216	247
5'7"	121	127	134	140	146	153	159	166	172	178	185	191	223	255
5'8"	125	131	138	144	151	158	164	171	177	184	190	197	230	262
5'9"	128	135	142	149	155	162	169	176	182	189	196	206	236	270
5'10"	132	139	146	153	160	167	174	181	188	195	202	207	243	278
5'11"	136	143	150	157	165	172	179	186	193	200	208	215	250	286
6'0"	140	147	154	162	169	177	184	191	199	206	213	221	258	294
6'1"	144	151	159	166	174	182	189	197	204	212	219	227	265	302
6'2"	148	155	163	171	179	186	194	202	210	218	225	233	272	311
6'3"	152	160	168	176	184	192	200	208	216	224	232	240	279	319
6'4"	156	164	172	180	189	197	205	213	221	230	238	246	287	328
BMI	19	20	21	22	23	24	25	26	27	28	29	30	35	40

BMI Classification:

BMI Below 19
Underweight

BMI 19-24.9
Healthy Weight
(Low Health Risk)

BMI 25-29.9
Overweight
(Moderate Health Risk)

BMI 30-40
Obese (High Health Risk)

BMI Over 40
Morbid Obesity
(Very High Risk)

Interactive BMI Calculator
www.calorieking.com

Calories in Food

Calories in food are derived from protein, fat and carbohydrate. Alcohol also provides calories. Vitamins, minerals and water provide no calories.

Calorie Values Per Gram

Fat/Oil	~ 9 Calories
Carbohydrate	~ 4 Calories
Protein	~ 4 Calories
Alcohol	~ 7 Calories

Note that fats have over double the calories of protein and carbohydrate. The higher the fat content of food, the higher the calories.

Sample Calculation

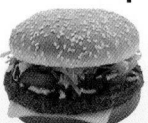

**QUARTER POUNDER®
WITH CHEESE**
has 510 calories
derived from:

26g Fat (x 9 cals/gram)	= 234
40g Carbohyd.(x 4 cals/gram)	= 160
29g Protein (x 4 cals/gram)	= 116
Total Calories	= 510

Calorie Levels for Weight Loss

Start with a calorie-controlled diet that allows a moderate weight loss of ½ - 1 pound per week. Weight loss is usually much greater in the first few weeks due to extra fluid losses.

Note: It is better to increase exercise rather than lessen food calories too drastically.

Suggested Calories for Weight Loss

Women:	Non-active	1000 - 1200
	Active	1200 - 1500
Men:	Non-active	1200 - 1500
	Active	1500 - 1800
Teenagers:		1200 - 1800

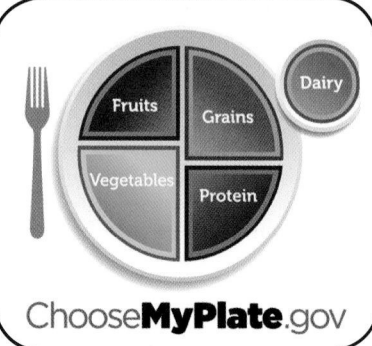

Choose**MyPlate**.gov

The MyPlate symbol represents the recommended proportion of foods from each food group. It focuses on the importance of making smart food choices in every food group, every day. Daily physical activity is also important. *(More info: www.ChooseMyPlate.gov)*

Examples of Single Serving Sizes

Grains (Eat 6 servings per day):
- 1 slice wholegrain bread (1 oz)
- ½ bun, small bagel or English muffin
- 4 small crackers or 1 tortilla
- 1 oz ready-to-eat wholegrain cereal
- ½ cup cooked cereal, rice or pasta

Vegetables (Eat 3-5 servings per day):
- 1 cup raw leafy vegetables
- 1½ cups raw chopped vegetables
- ½ cup cooked vegetables
- ½ - ¾ cup vegetable juice

Fruit (Eat 3-5 servings per day):
- 1 medium apple, orange, banana
- ½ cup canned fruit (in own juice)
- ¼ cup dried fruit
- ½ cup fruit juice (unsweetened)
- ¼ medium avocado

Protein (2-3 servings per day):
- 2-3 oz (cooked) lean meat/poultry/fish
- 2 eggs **or** 6 oz tofu **or** ¼ cup nuts
- 1 cup (cooked) dried beans **or** chickpeas

Dairy (2-3 servings per day):
- 1 cup (8 fl.oz) milk/soy (enriched)/yogurt
- 1½oz cheese or ½ cup cottage cheese

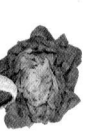

Portion Size Counts!

Food portion size is critical to controlling calorie intake for weight control.

Super-sized food servings have become more common when eating out and in the home. This can mean a day's worth of calories being consumed in one meal; or a snack being equivalent to a full meal.

It is easy to underestimate portion size of foods and drinks, and unwittingly consume excess calories – even if the fat content is low or even zero!

To more accurately estimate portion size of different foods, weigh and measure your food with food scales, measuring spoons and cups. Better control of calories will result.

For a visual idea of portion sizes, **visit www.CalorieKing.com** See examples (fries and cola) on this page.

Allow for Extra Calories in Packaged Food

The actual weight of packaged foods is usually 5-10% more than the label net weight (the minimum legal weight) – and in some cases up to 50% more. However, manufacturers calculate the calories based on the net weight. For actual calories, weigh the product and calculate the extra calories.

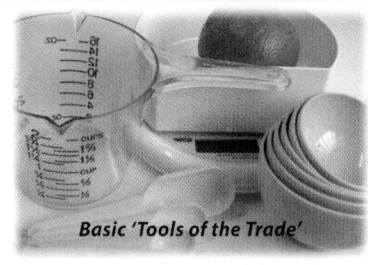

Basic 'Tools of the Trade'

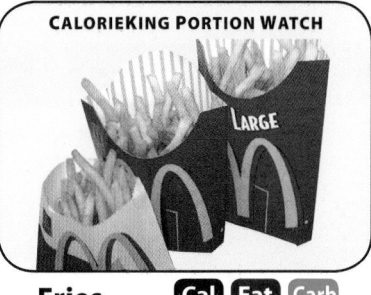

CALORIEKING PORTION WATCH

Fries	Cal	Fat	Carb
Small	230	11	29
Medium	380	19	48
Large	500	25	63

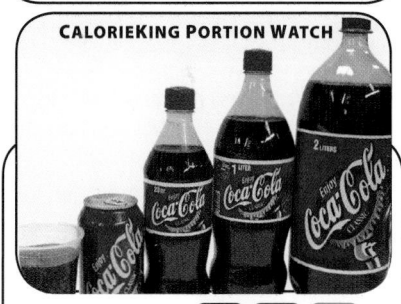

CALORIEKING PORTION WATCH

Cola	Cal	Fat	Carb
8 fl.oz Cup	100	0	25
12 fl.oz	Can	150	0 37
20 fl.oz Bottle	250	0	63
1 Liter Bottle	400	0	100
2 Liter Bottle	800	0	200

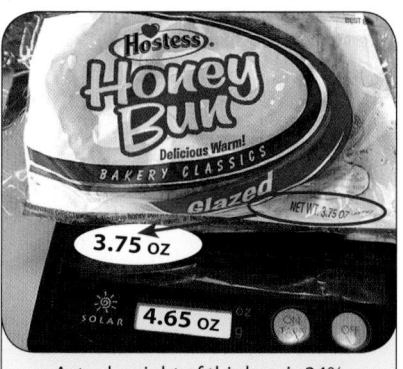

Actual weight of this bun is 24% more than the stated net weight.

Recommended Fat Intake

▶ Fat in the Diet

Fats in the diet are essential for good health. However, too much fat can contribute to obesity and a higher risk of heart disease, high blood pressure, diabetes, gallstone and certain cancers.

Dietary fat and oils have over double the calories of carbohydrates and protein. (Example: Changing from whole-milk to non-fat milk halves the calories.)

Calories	Fat
MAXIMUM DESIRABLE FAT INTAKE (DAILY)	
1200 cals	30g fat
1500 cals	40g fat
1800 cals	50g fat
2000 cals	60g fat
2200 cals	70g fat
2500 cals	80g fat
3000 cals	110g fat

ZERO GRAMS TRANS FAT

*Don't be fooled by **Zero Grams Trans Fat** boldly displayed on some high-fat snacks. They are still high in fat and calories.*

Examples: Cheetos 99c pkg ~ 24g fat, 380 cals Lay's Chips (2¾ oz pkg) ~ 27g fat, 430 calories

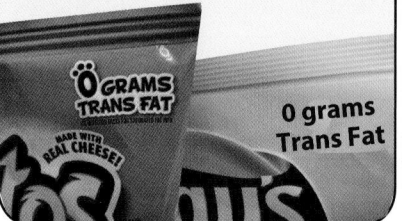

0 grams Trans Fat

▶ Beware low-fat foods

It is a mistake to think that eating low-fat or fat-free foods allows you to eat double the quantity. You can end up with even more calories than eating smaller amounts of regular-fat products.

Food products which are fat-free but high in calories include soda drinks, fruit juices, beer, alcoholic spirits, sugar and candy. Bread, rice and pasta also have negligible fat but need to be eaten in controlled amounts.

Ultimately, **it is food portion size as well as total calories that count** whether from fat, carbohydrate or protein. Remember, cows get fat on grass!

Reduced fat and fat-free foods are not necessarily low calorie. Portion size is still important.

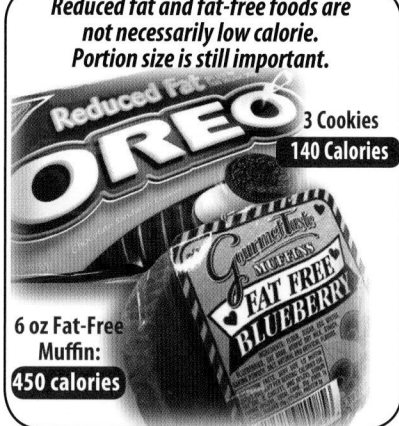

3 Cookies
140 Calories

6 oz Fat-Free Muffin:
450 calories

FOOD LABEL MEANINGS

FDA Nutrition Claim Definitions
(All are on a Per Serving Basis)

Low Calorie: **40 Calories or less**

Light or Lite: **One third fewer calories or, 50% or less fat than regular product**

Fat-Free: **Less than half a gram of fat**

Low-Fat: **3 grams or less of fat**

Reduced Fat: **25% less fat than regular product**

Fewer or Less Calories: **At least 25% fewer calories than regular product**

▶ Meats, Poultry, Fish

- **Choose lean cuts** of meat with little marbling. **Trim all visible fat** from meat and remove the skin from poultry. Removal of fat after cooking, is okay (to prevent dryness). Choose 'extra lean' ground beef.
- **Avoid high-fat meat products** such as salami, bacon, sausage and franks.
- **Broil or bake. Avoid frying in oil.** Allow casseroles to cool and skim off surface fat.
- **Avoid fried fish,** frozen fish in batter and canned fish in oil.

▶ Fats & Oils

- **Use minimal amounts** of all types of fat and oil. All are high in calories.
- **Choose** 'light' and 'reduced fat' spreads but still use sparingly.
- Use minimal amounts of oil when stir-frying. Use no-stick sprays like Pam.

▶ Salad Dressings & Sauces

- **Avoid regular mayonnaise and oil dressings.** Choose 'light', 'reduced fat' or 'fat-free' brands.
- **Choose low-fat or fat-free sauces** (mainly tomato-based). Avoid 'pesto', 'alfredo', 'cheese' and 'creamy' sauces.

▶ Milk, Cheese

- **Choose low-fat or nonfat milks and yogurts.** Avoid full-cream milk, cream, Half & Half.
- **Cheese:** Choose fat-free, and low-fat cheese. Part-skim ricotta is still high in fat. Low-fat cottage cheese is a good choice. Cheese substitutes can still be high in fat.

▶ Snacks, Cookies, Candy

- **Avoid** high-fat snacks such as potato chips, corn/tortilla chips, cheese puffs, buttered popcorn, chocolate and carob bars.

▶ Desserts/Sweets

- **Avoid high-fat desserts,** such as cake, pie, pastries, cheesecake, full-fat puddings.
- **Choose** fresh fruits, fresh fruit salad, canned fruit in water pack, low-fat ice cream. Use low-fat yogurt in place of cream.

▶ Fast-Foods & Take-Out

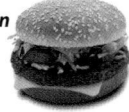

Check the Fast-Foods Section of this book for actual fat and calorie counts.

- **Avoid deep-fried foods such as** chicken, french fries and onion rings.
- **Pizzas:** Avoid sausage/pepperoni. Choose vegetarian topping and modest quantity of cheese. Eat a moderate serving. Eat extra salad and fresh fruit.
- **Hamburgers:** Choose medium size, lower fat burgers. Avoid bacon. Have a side salad (with fat-free dressing).
- **Delis:** Choose sandwiches/bread rolls, pitas with low-fat fillings and plain salad. Limit meat/cheese to small portions.
- **Coffees:** Avoid large sizes of latte and frappuccino. Request nonfat milk and no whipped cream. Avoid cookies and pastries.

Extra Information: www.CalorieKing.com

FRYING ADDS FAT!

The greater the surface area of potato exposed to fat or oil, the higher the fat content and calories.

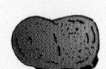 **Whole Potato (3 oz)**
`0g Fat` 65 Cals

 Roasted Potato (3 oz)
`5g Fat` 155 Cals

 Fries (Large cut, 3 oz)
`12g Fat` 220 Cals

 Fries (Small, 3 oz)
`15g Fat` 265 Cals

 Potato Chips (3 oz)
`30g Fat` 450 Cals

Carbohydrates ~ Friend or Foe?

Naturally-Friendly Carbs

- **Carbohydrate foods in their more natural forms** (not overly processed) are essential to good health. They are the main source of fuel for the body, and also provide important vitamins, minerals, antioxidants and fiber – all of which help protect against heart disease, diabetes, hypertension, constipation-related ailments and many other diseases.

- Carbohydrates even help the body produce serotonin, the 'feel good' brain chemical that helps control appetite and overeating. Too little serotonin can lead to mood swings and depression.

Carbohydrates are found in different forms in food as:

- Sugars in fruit, sugar cane, milk
- Starches in whole grains, legumes, nuts, seeds and vegetables
- Dietary fiber (See Fiber Guide ~ Page 264)

Glycemic Index & Diabetes ~ Page 21

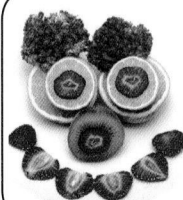

Carbohydrate foods (minimally processed) are essential to good health.

Be sure to eat adequate fruit and vegetables (5 - 7 servings) every day.

RECOMMENDED CARBOHYDRATE INTAKE		
Calories (Daily)	Carbohydrate (Grams)	Percent Carbohydrate Calories
1200 cals	100-120g	35-40%
1500 cals	140-170g	40-45%
1800 cals	180-200g	40-45%
2000 cals	200-250g	40-50%
2500 cals	310-350g	50-55%
3000 cals	410-450g	55-65%

How Much Do We Need?

- As shown in the chart, well-balanced diets above 2000 calories contain 50-60% of total calories from carbohydrates.

- At lower calorie levels used for weight control (1200-1500 calories), carbohydrates account for as little as 40% of total calories. This is because protein calories have nutritional priority.

- Carbohydrates & Diabetes ~ See Page 21

Low-Carbohydrate Diets

- Popular low-carbohydrate diets are extreme in their recommendations to initially cut carb intake to as little as 20 grams per day – the amount in 1 thick slice of bread, or 1 medium apple, or 1 small potato.

  This greatly increases the risk of nutritional deficiencies and compromises health, particularly if fat intake is excessive through fatty meats, high-fat dairy products, and fried foods.

- While overweight Americans do need to reduce carbohydrate intake, it should be done **sensibly as part of reducing portion size and total calories.**

- Simply eating 'low-carb' food products without regard to portion size, calories or fats, will do little to promote weight loss or good health.

- **Low-carb diets (and indeed any diet) only work if total calories are reduced.**

- Refined sugars should be one of the first targets in reducing carb intake.

FAT MATTERS CARBS COUNT **BUT** CALORIES **ARE** **KING!**

Extra Info ~ www.CalorieKing.com

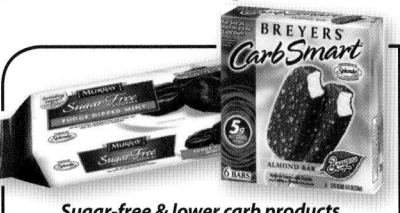

Sugar-free & lower carb products may still be high in calories and fat.

- **Excess Sugar:** Many overweight, inactive people consume over 500 calories of refined sugars per day, either self-added or as part of food products. This is equivalent to over 30 level teaspoons – a significant amount in weight control terms. Halving this amount would be reasonable and worthwhile.

Note: Naturally occurring sugars in fruits, vegetables and milk are fine when consumed in normal recommended amounts. These foods are also rich in other nutrients.

Refined sugar is referred to as having **'empty calories'**. Sugar supplies calories but negligible nutrients and no fiber.

- **Most sugar in our diet is 'hidden'** in processed foods such as soft drinks, fruit drinks, candy, cookies, cake, jam, sauces, ice cream, desserts, canned foods, and processed breakfast cereals.

For serious weight control, severely limit these foods and substitute healthier higher fiber wholefoods.

Note: Be careful not to substitute sugar-rich foods with high-fat foods which might boost calories even more!

- **Be aware that sugar comes in different forms** such as sucrose, glucose, fructose, malt, high-fructose corn syrup, molasses, honey and maple syrup. Check the label.

- **Sugar alcohols** such as sorbitol, mannitol and maltitol are carb-based and have ½ - ¾ the calories of regular sugar. While not counted as sugar on food labels, they do add to the carb count. Excess amounts can cause bloating, gas and diarrhea.

- **Sugar-free sweeteners** make it easy to reduce sugar in drinks and recipes. However, use minimally since research suggests possible ill-effects of some artificial sweeteners on friendly gut microbes. This may increase the risk of glucose intolerance and an increase in appetite.

Note: Most recipes can be adapted to contain less sugar with little effect on taste.

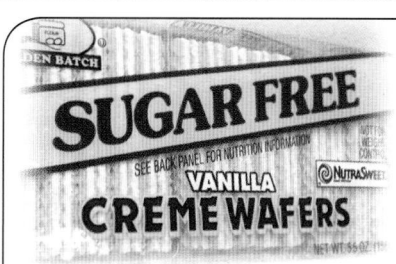

Sugar-free snacks and foods may be higher in fat and calories than the regular product.

Example	~ Creme Wafers (3):
Regular	~ 115 cals, 6g fat
Sugar-Free	~ 160 cals, 10g fat

SUGAR CONTENT OF SOME COMMON FOODS

Teaspoons of Sugar

Coca Cola or *Pepsi*, 12 fl.oz	10
20 fl.oz size	17
Iced Tea, sweetened, 12 fl.oz	8
Chocolate Milk, 12 fl.oz	6
Honey Smacks Cereal, ¾ cup, 1 oz	4
Popcorn, caramel, 1 cup	3.5
Chocolate Bar, 1.5 oz	6
M&M's 1.7 oz pkg	7
Muffin, large, 4 oz	6
Choc Chip Cookie, 1 oz	2
Donut, iced	6
Apple Pie, 1 piece	7
Jell-O, ½ cup	4.5
Jam, 1 Tbsp, ¾ oz	2.5
Syrup, maple, 1 Tbsp	3

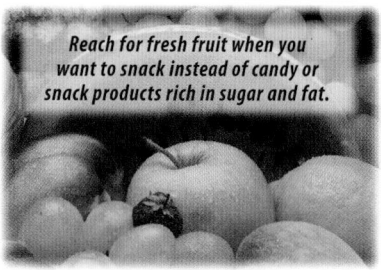

Reach for fresh fruit when you want to snack instead of candy or snack products rich in sugar and fat.

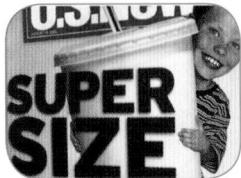

The XL Generation

Some 15% of American kids and adolescents are overweight; and childhood obesity has doubled over the last 20 years. Diabetes, high blood pressure and high cholesterol are major problem areas for overweight children and adolescents, as are depression, low self-esteem, sleep apnea and bone joint problems.

To address this problem, cooperation is required between kids, parents, schools and government. Weight control is a family and community affair.

Five Simple Tips To Get Started:

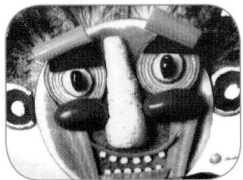

❶ Watch Soda Intake

Limit soda and sugary drinks to one serving on the weekends. Soda should not be an everyday beverage – water should be. When at restaurants or using a soda fountain, choose small servings with ice or choose diet soda instead. Schools should provide water and restrict access to soda as should parents when eating out or in the home!

❷ Cut back on Fast-Foods and Eating Out

Many more calories are consumed when you eat out. Healthy meals prepared at home are best for the whole family.

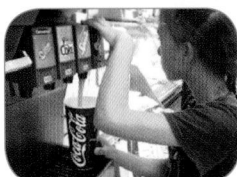

❸ Say "No" to Super-Sizing

When meals are upsized, loads more calories are consumed. Choose sensible portion sizes when eating out and at home. Use smaller plates and choose smaller packages.

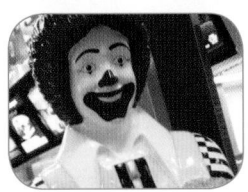

❹ Limit Between-Meal Snacking

Watch out for high-fat and high-calorie snacks – they can have more calories than a meal! Keep your eye on portion sizes and limit salty snack foods and candy to parties and special occasions. Choose fresh fruit, vegetables, nuts and low-fat milk instead.

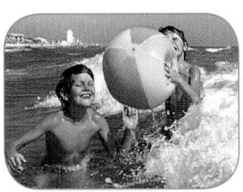

❺ Get Moving ~ Watch Less TV

Kids need at least 60 minutes of physical activity every day. It's critical for their fitness, and greatly lessens the risk of obesity.

Encourage kids to be active out of school hours. Wearing a pedometer can be highly motivational for kids to move more – as can playing dance video games such as *Dance Dance Revolution. Dance Central* (XBox360) and *Wii Fit (Nintendo)* are also excellent fitness motivators.

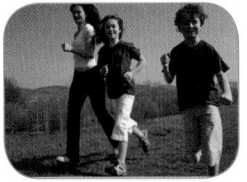

Limit TV and non-active computer games to just one hour per day. Also limit the accompanying snacks! Include exercise in family activities.

Extra information and tips ~ www.CalorieKing.com

Sample Meal Plan ~ 1400 Calories

**For Healthy, Overweight Persons ~ Not for Persons With Any Medical Condition
~ Please Check With Your Doctor & Dietitian ~**

Breakfast (approx. 300 cal)

	1 Small Fruit or ½ oz Dried Fruit
Plus	Cereal: 1½ oz Dry (high fiber)
	or 1 cup cooked Oatmeal
Plus	½ oz Almonds/Seeds
Plus	Milk (from daily allowance) or Yogurt (low-fat)

Daily Milk Allowance (approx.160 calories)
2 cups Non-Fat Milk or 1½ cups Low-fat (1%) Milk
or equivalent Soy Drink, Yogurt, Cheese, Tofu

Fat Allowance (140 calories; 15g Fat)
4 tsp Fat or 6-8 tsp Diet Margarine or 3 tsp Oil
or 1½ Tbsp Mayonnaise or ½ medium Avocado
or 1½ Tbsp Peanut Butter or 30g Nuts/Seeds

Breakfast ~ Choice 2

	1 Small Fruit
Plus	2 Eggs (no added fat)
	or 2 oz Cheese (low-fat)
	or 4 oz Cottage Cheese (low-fat)
	or 2 oz Lean/Canadian Bacon
Plus	1 Tomato
Plus	1 Slice Wholegrain Toast

Between Meals

Water, Coffee, Tea, Diet drinks,
Fruit from main meals; Raw Vegetable
Pieces, Milk from Daily Allowance

Lunch (approx. 440 calories)

	2 slices Wholegrain Bread (2 oz)
	or 4 Crispbreads/Crackers or 6" Pita
Plus	2 oz lean Meat, Chicken or Turkey
	or 3½ oz Tuna (in water) or 2½ oz Salmon
	or 1 oz Cheese or ½ cup (4 oz) Cottage Cheese
	or ½ cup (4 oz) Ricotta Cheese (low-fat)
	or ½ cup (4 oz) Fruit Yogurt (low-fat)
	or ½ cup (4 oz) Bean Salad
Plus	Large Salad (Oil-free dressing)
Plus	1 small Fruit or ½ oz Dried Fruit

Dinner (approx. 360 calories)

	Soup (fat-free)
Plus	3 oz lean Meat (cooked weight)
	or 4 oz Chicken Breast (no skin)
	or 3 oz Chicken Thigh/Leg (no skin)
	or 5 oz Fish (grilled, no fat)
	or ¾ cup (6 oz) Beans (Soy, Kidney, Pinto etc)/Lentils
	or Low-fat Entree (e.g. Lean Cuisine)
Plus	1 small Potato
	or ½ cup Rice/Pasta/Sweet Corn
	or 1 slice Wholegrain Bread
Plus	2-3 servings Vegetables/Salad
Plus	1 small Fruit + Diet Gelatin Dessert

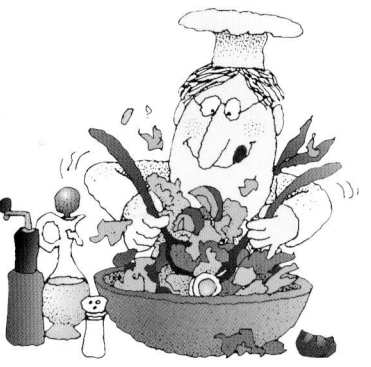

- **Persons who exercise regularly lose more weight** and keep it off longer than non-exercisers. Blood glucose control also improves; as do beneficial gut microbes.
- **Exercise also improves general health and well-being.** Mood, confidence and self-esteem are also enhanced.
- **Exercise** is a good way to 'wake up' a sluggish metabolism and burn excess body fat.
- **Aerobic (huff and puff) exercise most days** is great for burning calories and for cardiovascular fitness. But, it is strength training that mainly builds the muscles that burn calories.
- **Strength training is the key to retaining or rebuilding muscles.** As we age, we lose some 6 pounds of muscle per decade. This results in a lower metabolism and fewer calories burnt.

  Muscles are the furnaces that burn calories. The more muscle you have, the more calories burnt – and as a bonus, the more food you can eat.

- **Regular strength training (2-3 times weekly)** can increase our metabolic rate for several days following exercise – with up to an extra 100 calories per day being burnt.

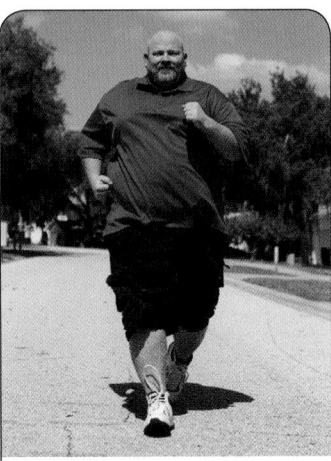

Brisk walking each day is a safe and effective way to burn calories and keep fit.
Try it – you'll like it!
Be sure to wear sun-protective clothing.

  While 2-3 pounds of muscle may be gained in the first 8-10 weeks, weight from exercised muscles is ok. It is excess fat (particularly abdominal fat) that is a potential health hazard.

- **Body reshaping** is enhanced by gaining muscle and losing fat - even if the scales don't show it.
- **Avoid injury** by beginning with walking, low impact aerobics, or weight-supported exercise (e.g. swimming, cycling). Avoid competitive sports. Allow 2-3 days of recovery between strength training sessions. Get professional advice.
- **How Much?** Start with 10-20 minutes per day and progress to 30-60 minutes per day. Also walk up stairs instead of using elevators. Take a brisk walk at lunch. Use an exercise bike, treadmill or stair machine while watching TV. Walk the dog.
- **How Often?** While aerobic fitness may require only 3-4 sessions weekly, **weight control is a daily event which requires daily exercise to burn calories.** Also add in strength training 2-3 times weekly.

Note: Persons on cholesterol-lowering statin drugs may experience muscle pains and weakness (as well as damage to muscle microfibrils). Supplementing with coenzyme Q10, magnesium, selenium, vitamins D and K2, may be beneficial. Check with your healthcare provider.

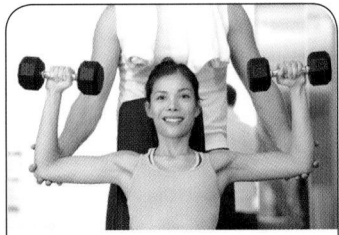

Strength training is the key to retain or rebuild muscles.
Exercized muscles burn extra calories even while you sleep.
For extra guidance and motivation, seek a qualified trainer or join a gym.

Calories Used in Exercise

LIGHT	MODERATE	HEAVY
130 lbs ~ 3 Cals/Min	130 lbs ~ 5 Cals/Min	130 lbs ~ 8 Cals/Min
170 lbs ~ 4 Cals/Min	170 lbs ~ 6 Cals/Min	170 lbs ~ 10 Cals/Min
220 lbs ~ 5 Cals/Min	220 lbs ~ 7 Cals/Min	220 lbs ~ 12 Cals/Min

LIGHT
- Walking, slow
- Cycling, light
- Frisbee playing
- Gardening, light
- Golf, social
- Tennis, doubles
- Housework, cleaning
- Calisthenics, light
- Bowling
- Ping-pong, social
- Ice Skating, light
- Aquarobics, light
- Skate Boarding
- Line/Square Dancing
- Tai Chi, Yoga
- Volleyball

MODERATE
- Walking, brisk
- Cycling, moderate
- Swimming, crawl
- Weight-training, light
- Tennis, moderate
- Racquetball, beginners
- Aerobics, light
- Football, touch
- Basketball, Baseball
- Walking Downstairs
- Snow Skiing (downhill)
- Shovelling snow
- Dancing (ballroom)
- Rowing, moderate
- Volleyball, competitive

HEAVY
- Walking (power), Jogging
- Cycling (vigorous)
- Swimming, strenuous
- Weight-training, heavy
- Wrestling/Judo, advanced
- Racquetball, advanced
- Tae Bo, Kick Boxing
- Football, training
- Basketball (Pro)
- Climbing Stairs
- Skipping Rope
- Skiing (cross country)
- Aquarobics, advanced
- Dancing (strenuous), Zumba
- Rowing, vigorous
- Martial Arts

Note: Only those sports or activities that are sustained over a period of time (e.g running) qualify for heavy exercise. Stop-start sports such as tennis are considered 'moderate'.

WALKING PROGRAM

USE DISTANCE, STEPS OR TIME

Weeks	Distance	Steps Pedometer	Time
1-2	1 mile	2000	20 mins
3-5	1.5 miles	3000	28 mins
6-8	2 miles	3500	35 mins
9-10	2.5 miles	4500	45 mins
11+	3.5 miles	6000	60 mins

10,000 STEPS PER DAY

A pedometer can motivate you to be more active. It clips to your belt or waist band and registers each step.

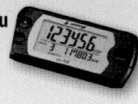

Alternatively, use a *Fitbit*, *Garmin* or *Striiv* activity tracker, or your smartphone inbuilt accelerometer.

Aim for 8,000 - 10,000 steps per day, insead of an average of only 3,000 - 4,000 steps.

Reshaping Eating Behaviors

- Eating is a behavior that is largely controlled by people with whom we live or socialize, places in which we carry out our lives, and our emotions. Become aware of those situations that commonly lead to extra food being eaten.

- We may also be unaware of 'bad' eating habits that can lead to excess calorie intake; e.g. eating quickly, large mouthfuls, eating when tense or bored, finishing a large serving of food when not hungry.

Tips to help uncover and correct those 'bad' or problem eating habits:

- **Don't eat while engaged in other activities;** for example, watching TV, reading. Eat only at the table, not at the fridge or while standing.

- **Don't eat quickly.** Chewing slowly allows time to register a feeling of fullness. Don't use fingers, only utensils. Cut food into smaller pieces. Don't load your fork until the previous mouthful is finished.

- **Don't purchase problem high calorie foods.** Shop from a set list to prevent impulse buying. Avoid shopping with children.

- **Buy snack foods** in the smallest package. The larger the serving size or package, the more you are likely to eat or drink.

- **Plan meals in advance. Stick to a set menu.**

- **Plan a strategy to avoid uncontrolled eating** and drinking at social events, or when your emotions urge you to binge.

  Rehearse repeatedly in your mind exactly what you will do in such situations. Remind yourself several times each day that you are in charge of your actions and that you can be strong-willed. Seek counseling or coaching on various strategies.

- **Distract yourself** when you feel the urge to snack impulsively. Engage in some activity that will distract you from thinking about food. Examples: go for a walk, brush your teeth, phone a friend.

  If you eat out of boredom, find some new hobby or interest that gets you out of the house. Even enrol in an adult education class.

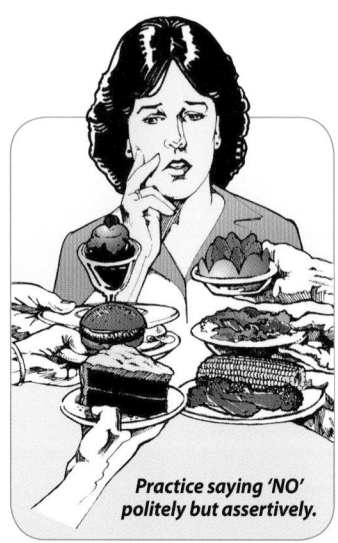

Practice saying 'NO' politely but assertively.

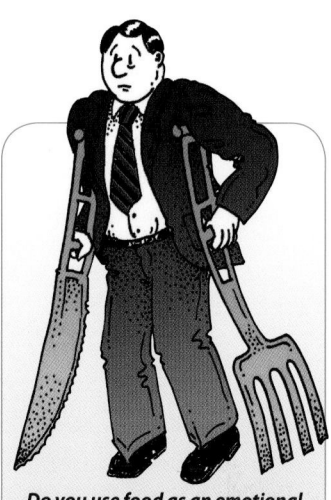

Do you use food as an emotional crutch? If so, professional counseling may be helpful.

The food journal is the most powerful proven aid for dieters. Persons who keep a food and exercise journal not only lose more weight, they also keep it off. Here are some of the reasons:

- **Recording your eating and exercise habits** jolts you into realizing just what you do eat and drink each day; and also whether you exercise sufficiently.

- **Helps you identify problem foods** and drinks with excessive calories and fat.

- **Helps identify moods**, situations and events that lead to excessive eating of unwanted calories. You can then plan to overcome or avoid them.

- **Prevents 'calorie amnesia'**, the forgetfulness that leads to rebound weight gain after successful weight loss. Recording puts you back on the right track.

- **Helps you develop greater self-discipline.** You will think twice about overindulging if you have to record it - especially if someone checks your journal regularly. It certainly keeps you honest!

- **Motivates you** to carefully plan your meals and to exercise each day.

- **Serves as a check system** for your doctor, dietitian or counselor to assess your progress and make recommendations.

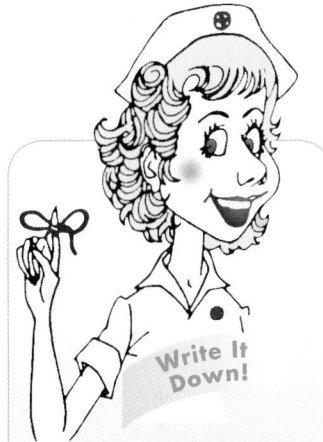

Write It Down!

"Keeping a journal gives me feedback on exactly what I eat and drink each day.

It helps prevent 'calorie amnesia' and reminds me to exercise each day.

It's a 'must' for successful weight control!"

3 Easy Ways to Track Your Food & Exercise Calories!

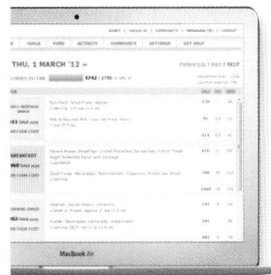

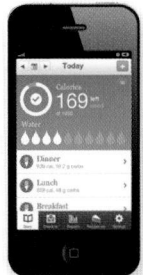

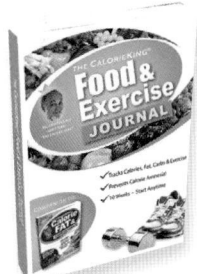

CalorieKing Online
Part of a comprehensive personalized program that includes tools, reports and a supportive community.

CalorieKing App
ControlMyWeight
Make smart food choices wherever you are! Easy to use.

Book
A 10-week journal that fits in your pocket. Includes Weekly Summary page and Progress Checklist.

Extra Information ~ www.CalorieKing.com

What is Diabetes?

Diabetes occurs when the body has difficulty processing glucose sugar in the blood.

- **After digestion**, sugar and starches are changed into **glucose** – the simplest form of sugar vital for body energy and growth.

- Insulin is the hormone which acts like a key that opens the door to body cells and allows glucose to enter.

- **Without enough insulin**, glucose builds up in the blood and passes into the urine. High blood glucose levels lead to frequent urination, extreme thirst, and tiredness.

- **Untreated diabetes increases the risk of damage to nerves and blood vessels.** This, in turn, increases the risk of heart disease, stroke, blindness, kidney damage, foot ulcers and gangrene (with amputation), impotence, Alzheimer's Disease and other prolems.

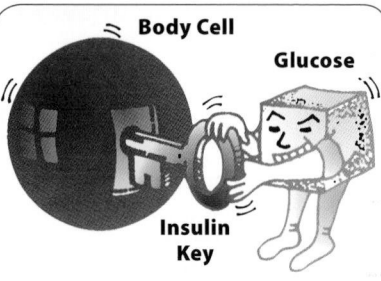

Body Cell

Glucose

Insulin Key

Insulin acts like a key.
It opens the door to body cells and allows glucose to enter.

People with type 1 diabetes and some with type 2 have too few or no keys and require insulin injections.

Others (primarily type 2) make enough insulin but the body doesn't use it as well as it should – particularly if obese and inactive.

SYMPTOMS OF DIABETES

- Frequent urination
- Extreme thirst
- Unusual hunger
- Rapid weight loss
- Extreme fatigue
- Blurred vision
- Skin infections that are slow to heal
- Tingling/numbness in feet

Note: Diabetes can be present even with no symptoms.

DON'T IGNORE DIABETES

IT'S A SERIOUS DISEASE!

TYPE 2 DIABETES

- Occurs in 90% of diabetes cases
- Occurs mainly in adults - particularly in overweight and inactive persons
- Insulin is produced but body cells resist its action and glucose   cannot enter cells
- Usually treated with meal planning and physical activity. Sometimes requires medication (pills or insulin)

TYPE 1 DIABETES

- Occurs in 10% of diabetes cases
- Usually in children and young adults
- Pancreas produces little or no insulin. Daily insulin injections (or use of an insulin pump) are necessary, as well as:
  - matching pre-meal insulin to the amount of carbohydrate eaten
  - weight control and regular physical activity

GESTATIONAL DIABETES

- Occurs in some women during pregnancy. It usually disappears after the baby's birth.
- Women who have had gestational diabetes still have a high risk of developing type 2 diabetes within 5 to 10 years. One in 3 do.
- Requires weight control, a healthy lifestyle and regular medical checks during and after pregnancy.

Are You At Risk for Diabetes?

Pre-Diabetes ~ An Early Warning!

Pre-diabetes means your blood glucose levels are higher than normal, but not high enough to be called diabetes.

If you have pre-diabetes, you have a higher risk for getting diabetes later on.

The good news is that you can start taking steps to prevent diabetes by making healthy lifestyle changes – such as losing weight if overweight, and being more physically active.

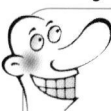

WHAT'S YOUR RISK?

Find out if you're at risk for diabetes by answering the following questions:

☐ I have been told I have pre-diabetes

☐ I have a family history of diabetes

☐ I am African American, Latino American, Asian American, Native American or a Pacific Islander

☐ I have had gestational diabetes (diabetes during pregnancy)

☐ I am over age 45

☐ I am overweight

☐ My waist is larger than: 35 inches (for a woman) or 40 inches (for a man)

☐ I get little or no physical activity

☐ My blood pressure is higher than 130 over 85

☐ My HDL (good cholesterol) is too low

☐ My triglycerides (blood fats) are too high

✔ CHECK YOUR RESULT

• If you've put a check mark in two or more of the boxes, you may be more likely to develop type 2 diabetes.

• Talk with your healthcare provider to see if you should have a blood test for diabetes.

BLOOD GLUCOSE CLASSIFICATION OF DIABETES

Normal:	**Below 100 mg/dl***
Pre-Diabetes:	**100-125 mg/dl***
Diabetes:	**Over 125 mg/dl***

(*Fasting Blood Glucose)

KNOW YOUR BGL

(Blood Glucose Level)
Everyone over the age of 45 should have a blood glucose test every three years.

Importance of Weight Control

• **Type 2 diabetes** is more common in people who are overweight.

• **Being overweight** means that your insulin doesn't work as well to control blood glucose levels.

• **Losing just 10 to 20 pounds** can help you better manage your diabetes and lower your risk for heart disease.

Keys to weight control include:

• Follow a healthy eating plan

• Control food portions

• Be physically active every day. Track your daily activity.

• Keep food records ~ *See Page 15*

• Get the support of family and friends.

• **Work with a registered dietitian** who can help you reach a weight that's ideal for you.

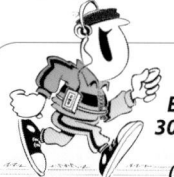

KEEP MOVING!

Every day, do at least 30 minutes of moderate intensity exercise.
(even in 5-minute sets)

It's the key to improving insulin action.
Add muscle strength training 3-4 times a week to double the benefits.

Managing Diabetes

Don't battle diabetes alone. Establish a partnership with your doctor, dietitian, certified diabetes educator, and pharmacist.

Extra Support:
• *American Association of Diabetes Educators*
• *American Diabetes Association*
• *BeyondType1.org*
• *Joslin Diabetes Center*
• *Juvenile Diabetes Research Foundation*
• *National Diabetes Education Program*

Tips to keep blood glucose within safe limits:

• **Control your food intake.** Know what and when you will eat. Seek referral to a dietitian for expert advice.

• **Exercise regularly.** It assists weight control and can improve sensitivity of body cells to insulin. Plan physical activity into your daily routine.

• **Monitor your blood glucose** at home and work with a blood glucose meter. It will help you become familiar with your blood glucose patterns, and the effects of food, activity and medication.

• **Take insulin or oral medication as prescribed.** If on insulin, know what action to take if hypoglycemia (low blood glucose) occurs. Also educate your family and friends.

Be Heart Smart ~ Know Your ABCs

If you have diabetes, you are at a higher risk for heart attack and stroke than someone without diabetes. But you can fight back!

Be smart about your heart!

Take control of the ABCs of diabetes and live a long and healthy life. Talk to your healthcare provider about your ABC targets.

Ⓐ is for A1C
The A1C (A-one-C) test – short for hemoglobin A1C. It reflects your average blood glucose (sugar) over the last 3 months.
Suggested Target: Below 7%

Ⓑ is for Blood Pressure
High blood pressure makes your heart work too hard.
Suggested Target: Below 130/80

Ⓒ is for Cholesterol
Bad cholesterol, or LDL, can build up and clog your arteries. **Suggested Target: Below 100**

Blood glucose meters and insulin pumps can greatly improve control of diabetes

BLOOD GLUCOSE METERS (EXAMPLES)

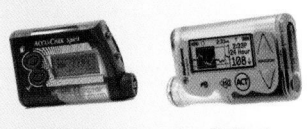

INSULIN PUMPS (EXAMPLES)

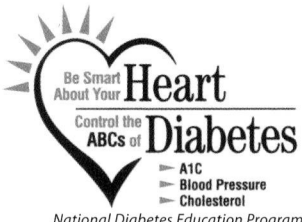

| Roche Accu-Chek | Medtronic MiniMed |

Be Smart About Your **Heart**
Control the **ABCs** of **Diabetes**
➤ A1C
➤ Blood Pressure
➤ Cholesterol
National Diabetes Education Program

Be smart about your heart!
Take control of the ABC's of diabetes and live a long and healthy life.

Talk to your healthcare provider about your ABC targets.

Take action now to lower your risk for heart attack, stroke and other diabetes problems.

◄ *Note: These targets are suggested by the National Institutes for Health and the American Diabetes Association*

Guidelines for choosing a healthy diet apply equally to people with or without diabetes. Eating a wide variety of foods that are mainly low in fat, low in refined sugars, and high in fiber, is recommended.

However, actual food quantities, as well as when you eat, will also influence control of blood glucose. Your dietitian will individualize a meal plan to suit your food preferences, lifestyle and medical status.

Here are a few tips:

- **Maintain a healthy weight.** If overweight, even a modest weight loss plus daily physical activity can help manage blood glucose in type 2 diabetes.

- **Don't skip meals.** If you take insulin or an oral hypoglycemic agent, regular meals are important.

  If on insulin, eat meals at the same time each day. Eat a similar amount of food at each meal. Eating about the same amount of carbohydrate over the day will make best use of insulin and prevent wide variations in blood glucose levels.

- **Know which foods contain carbohydrate;** and learn how to check the *Nutrition Facts Label* on foods. Check the serving size, total fat and total carbohydrate – not just the sugar content. All carbohydrate breaks down to sugars after digestion.

- **Choose wholegrain breads, cereals and pasta.** Eat fresh fruits, vegetables and legumes. These foods contain more fiber and slow the release of glucose into your blood after a meal.

- **Limit foods high in saturated fat, trans fat and cholesterol.** Enjoy fish, soy foods, and other foods rich in omega-3 fats. *(Extra Notes: Page 259)*

- **Limit sugars and foods high in added sugar** particularly if overweight. Small amounts of sugar as part of a meal may occasionally be okay. Check with your dietitian. *(Extra Notes: Page 9)*

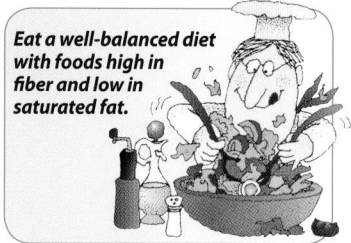

Eat a well-balanced diet with foods high in fiber and low in saturated fat.

A fiber-rich diet assists the growth of friendly gut microbes that can benefit our metabolism, weight and blood glucose levels – as well as hunger, mood and our immune system.
(Also see Fiber Guide ~ Page 264)

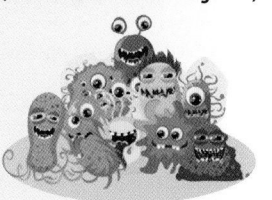

ALCOHOL TIPS

- **If you drink alcohol, have only moderate amounts:**
  Men ~ 1-2 drinks/day
  Women ~ 1 drink/day
  For some people, safe drinking will mean no alcoholic drinks at all.
  (Also see Alcohol Guide ~ Page 23)

- **Drink along with your food –** especially if you use insulin or diabetes medication pills.

- **Do not omit any carb food** in exchange for an alcoholic drink. However, non-alcoholic beers (12 fl oz) count as one carb exchange.

- **Alcohol increases the risk of hypoglycemia** (low blood sugar) and drug interactions if you take insulin and certain types of diabetes pills.

- **Check with your doctor and dietitian.**

The Plate Method – An Easy Way to Eat Healthfully

The plate method is a helpful tool to guide your food choices until you see a dietitian for your own meal plan.

For a healthy meal:

- Fill half of your plate with non-starchy vegetables (broccoli, green beans, carrots).
- Fill a quarter of your plate with carbohydrate (wholegrain bread, pasta, potato, brown rice).
- Fill the other quarter of your plate with 3-4 ounces of lean meat, poultry, or fish.
- Use 1-2 teaspoons of tub margarine or a heart-healthy vegetable oil.
- Add a small piece of fruit or 8 ounces of skim/low-fat milk or yogurt.

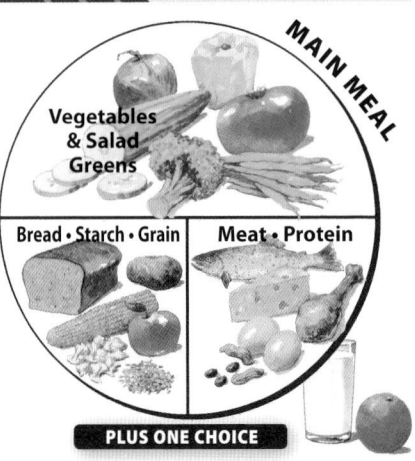

MAIN MEAL

Vegetables & Salad Greens

Bread · Starch · Grain | Meat · Protein

PLUS ONE CHOICE

Milk, Fruit, Dessert or other Carb Food

How Much Carbohydrate Should You Eat?

A dietitian can best determine how much carbohydrate you need at each of your meals, based on your lifestyle, food preferences, and overall diabetes control.

Until you see a dietitian, aim to keep the amount of carbohydrate you eat the same at each of your meals.

CARB CHOICES MEAL PLAN
One Carb Choice = 15 Grams of Carb

The amount in: 1 slice Bread **or** ¾ cup Cereal (unsweetened) **or** 1 small Potato **or** 1 small Fruit

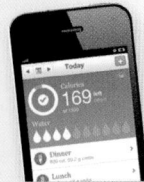 **Breakfast**
- Eat 2-3 carb choices (30-45 grams)
- Include a low-fat protein source such as egg whites or skim milk.

Lunch and Dinner
- Eat 3-4 carb choices (45-60 grams carb)
- Include fruit and non-starchy vegetables. Choose small portions of low-fat protein foods.

Snacks: If needed, eat 1-2 carb choices (15-30 grams carb).

Note: Above plan is for adults. Carbohydrate amounts will vary with physical activity level.

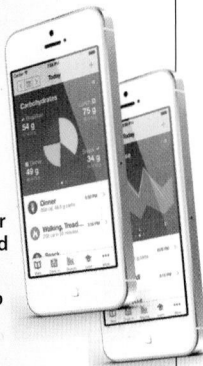

Carb Type Affects Blood Glucose

The various forms of carbohydrate affect blood glucose levels in different ways. It is difficult to predict the effect of particular foods, sugars, or meals, simply by their carbohydrate content.

Thus the same amount of carbohydrate from different foods may affect blood sugar levels very differently. **Many factors affect the rate of digestion and absorption such as:**

- the type of sugar, starch, and fiber
- the degree of processing and cooking (which increases digestion rate)
- the amount of protein and fat (which slow stomach emptying and digestion).

Glycemic Index (GI)

The GI is a method of ranking carbo-hydrate foods on a scale (0-100) according to how they affect blood glucose levels. (See next column).

The higher the GI value, the greater the food's ability to rapidly raise blood glucose levels; and the more insulin that is needed by the body (not desirable).

Eating low-GI foods may lead to better control of blood glucose and insulin levels (which in turn lowers the risk of damage to blood vessels and nerves). The slower digestion of low-GI foods may also help to delay hunger pangs and benefit weight control.

Cautionary Notes on GI

Choosing low-GI foods is not a license to eat unlimited amounts. Calorie restriction and portion control for weight control is of prime importance.

Also remember, **low-GI foods are carbo-hydrate foods** and must still be counted as part of any dietetic carbohydrate plan.

GI is not meant to be used by itself without regard to portion size, and other dietary recommendations for healthy eating. Foods are not good or bad on the basis of their GI.

While GI may be a helpful tool for some people with diabetes, what is most important is to control the total amount of carbohydrate that you eat.

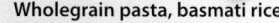

LOWER-GLYCEMIC FOODS

Slower-Acting Carbohydrates

These foods are more slowly digested and absorbed. They help maintain more even blood glucose levels, as long as excessive amounts are not eaten. Use these foods regularly but still limit portion size for weight control.

Examples:

- Dried beans, peas, lentils
- Nuts and seeds
- Wholegrain breads
- Bran cereals, oats
- Sweet corn, barley, quinoa buckwheat
- Wholegrain pasta, basmati rice
- Fresh fruit: apples, avocados, bananas (firm), berries, cherries, grapefruit, grapes, olives, oranges, pears, plums. Fresh juices.
- Vegetables: broccoli, yam, nopales, salad greens
- Milk, yogurt, soy drinks
- Dark chocolate, cacao
- Sugar alcohols (sorbitol, maltitol)

HIGHER-GLYCEMIC FOODS

Quicker-Acting Carbohydrates

These foods more rapidly raise blood glucose levels. Eat only in moderation.

- White bread, rice cakes, bagels, croissants, doughnuts
- Low-fiber cereals: Cornflakes, *Rice Krispies, Froot Loops*
- White potatoes, white rice
- Watermelon, ripe bananas, cantaloupe, pineapple
- Soda, sugar-sweetened sports and energy drinks
- Sugar, candy, popcorn (plain)
- Ice cream (low-fat), frozen yogurt

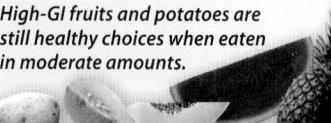

High-GI fruits and potatoes are still healthy choices when eaten in moderate amounts.

» **Calorie and fat values have been rounded off.**
Calories ~ to the nearest 5 or 10 calories.
Fat ~ to nearest half gram. **Note:** Trace amounts of fat (less than 0.3 grams) have been treated as zero.

» **Carbohydrate figures** in this book are for total carbohydrate, and not **Net Carbs** (which deducts fiber, polydextrose and sugar alcohols from total carbs).

» Because manufacturers' figures on labels are rounded off, figures in this book may differ slightly from the label. Serving sizes may also vary.

IMPORTANT DISCLAIMER

* The authors and publishers of this book are not physicians and are not licensed to give medical advice. This book is not a substitute for professional advice. Users should consult their medical professional before making any health, medical or other decisions based on the material contained herein.

* This book is a compilation of original material from other sources intended for educational purposes only. Because food manufacturers constantly change their products, only they are the authoritative source for food's most current nutritional information.

* Persons using the information herein for any medical purposes, such as matching insulin dosage to carbohydrate intake, should not rely solely on the accuracy of figures herein and should independently check food labels or contact the food manufacturer for the latest data.

Canadian Readers:

Please note that figures in this book are based on U.S. food products and restaurants. Equivalent Canadian foods may vary and should be checked independently.

* WARRANTY DISCLAIMER:

THE AUTHOR AND PUBLISHER DISCLAIM ANY LIABILITY ARISING DIRECTLY OR INDIRECTLY FROM THE USE OF THIS BOOK. THE INFORMATION HEREIN IS PROVIDED "AS IS" AND WITHOUT ANY WARRANTY EXPRESSED OR IMPLIED. ALL DIRECT, INDIRECT, SPECIAL, INCIDENTAL, CONSEQUENTIAL OR PUNITIVE DAMAGES ARISING FROM ANY USE OF THIS INFORMATION IS DISCLAIMED AND EXCLUDED.

This information is also provided subject to Family Health Publications' Terms and Conditions found at the website, www.calorieking.com/terms and incorporated herein.

C ~ Calories
F ~ Fat (grams)
Cb ~ Carbohydrate (grams)

Abbreviations

tsp	= teaspoon
Tbsp or T	= Tablespoon
oz	= ounce(s)
c	= cup
fl.oz	= fluid ounce(s)
g	= gram(s)
avg	= average
pkg	= package

Volume Measures

(All measures are level)
3 tsp = 1 Tbsp
2 Tbsp = 1 fl.oz
½ cup = 4 fl.oz
1 cup = 8 fl.oz
2 cups = 1 Pint
2 Pints = 1 Quart
Note: 8 oz weight is not the same as 8 fl oz volume (space occupied). Dense foods weigh more per set volume. Examples:
1 cup popcorn weighs ½ oz
1 cup milk weighs 8½ oz
1 cup pudding weighs 10 oz

Metric Conversion

½ oz = 14 grams
1 oz = 28.4 grams
2 oz = 57 grams
3½ oz = 100 grams
1 fl.oz = 30 mls
1 cup (8 fl.oz) = 240 mls
33 fl.oz = 1 liter (volume)

INFORMATION SOURCES

• U.S. Dept. of Agriculture
• U.S. Food Manufacturers
• Food Industry Boards & Councils
• Author extrapolations

FEEDBACK WELCOME!

Please contact the author with your queries and suggestions.
feedback@calorieking.com

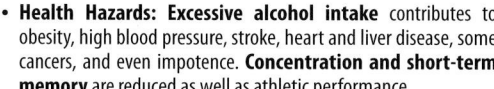
- **Health Hazards: Excessive alcohol intake** contributes to obesity, high blood pressure, stroke, heart and liver disease, some cancers, and even impotence. **Concentration and short-term memory** are reduced as well as athletic performance.

  Other alcohol hazards include: Fetal Alcohol Syndrome, stomach upsets, gut dysbiosis, menstrual and menopausal problems, depression, snoring, sleep problems, work absenteeism, impaired judgement, risky behaviors and social/family problems.

- **Alcohol contributes to obesity** through its high calories and by lessening the body's ability to burn fat. Fat storage is promoted, particularly in the belly – a health danger zone. Alcohol can also stimulate the appetite; and weaken the dieter's resolve!

- **Alcohol is potentially more harmful while dieting:** Blood sugar levels may drop with resultant fatigue and further impairment of concentration, reflexes and driving skills.

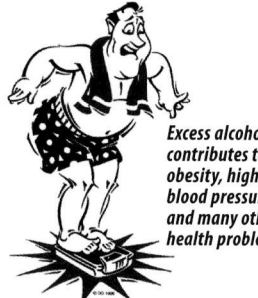

Excess alcohol contributes to obesity, high blood pressure and many other health problems

LOWER RISK ALCOHOL LIMITS

WOMEN:
No more than
1 drink per day

MEN:
No more than
2 drinks per day
(1 drink if over 65 y.o.)

(At least 2 days a week should be alcohol-free)

1 DRINK CONTAINS 14 GRAMS ALCOHOL
- 12 fl.oz Regular Beer (5% Alc.)
- OR 14 fl.oz Light Beer (4.2% Alc.)
- OR 5 fl.oz Wine (12% Alc.)
- OR 1½ fl.oz Spirits (80 Proof)

**Note: You cannot save daily drinks for one occasion.
Binge drinking is particularly harmful:
4 drinks for males or 3 drinks for females (within 2 hours).**

For some people, safe drinking means no alcohol at all. Even one drink may impair driving skills, particularly if tired. For women who drink frequently, breast cancer risk is increased by 9% for each drink after the first drink. In men, just 2 drinks a day doubles the risk of cancers of the mouth and throat.

It is advisable not to drink at all if you are:
- pregnant, trying to conceive or breastfeeding
- taking medication or have liver or heart disease (unless approved by your doctor or pharmacist)
- planning to drive, use machinery or play sports
- studying or needing to concentrate
- a child or adolescent

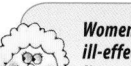

Women and adolescents are more prone to alcohol's ill-effects due to their lower body weight, smaller livers and lesser capacity to metabolize alcohol. As we age, our ability to handle alcohol decreases.

HOW TO CALCULATE ALCOHOL CONTENT

Percent alcohol on label refers to alcohol volume (ml alcohol/100ml). Note: 100ml = 3½ fl.oz

To convert to grams (weight) of alcohol, multiply the alcohol volume by 0.8 – since 1 ml of alcohol weighs only 0.8 grams.

*EXAMPLE:
12 fl.oz Can Beer
(5% alcohol)*
5% alc. volume
= 5% of 12 fl.oz = 0.6 fl.oz
= 18ml alcohol (Note: 1 fl.oz = 30ml)
Weight (18ml x 0.8) = 14.4g alcohol

GOVERNMENT WARNINGS!

(1) According to the Surgeon General, women should not drink alcoholic beverages during pregnancy because of the risk of birth defects.

(2) Consumption of alcoholic beverages impairs your ability to drive a car or operate machinery, and may cause health problems.

EXTRA INFORMATION
Alcohol & Diabetes ~ See Page 19
Alcohol & The Heart ~ See Page 18
Tips to Avoid Harmful Drinking ~ Page 19

Quick Guide
Alc ~ Alcohol (Grams)

Beer:
Cb ~ Carbohydrate

Beer Contains Zero Fat:	C	Alc	Cb
Regular Beer (5% Alc. Vol.):			
7 fl.oz Glass	80	8.5	4
12 fl.oz Bottle/Can/Glass	140	14	10
16 fl.oz/Pint	185	19	13
22 fl.oz Bottle	260	26	18
24 fl.oz Can	280	28	20
32 fl.oz / ½ Yard	370	38	28
40 fl.oz Bottle	470	47	35
50 fl.oz Football	590	59	50
Light Beer (4.2% Alc. Vol.):			
7 fl.oz Glass	65	7	4
12 fl.oz Bottle/Can/Glass	110	12	7
16 fl.oz/Pint	145	16	9
22 fl.oz Bottle	200	22	13
24 fl.oz Can	220	24	14

Non-Alcoholic Brews:
(Less than 0.5% alcohol by volume)

Average all Brands, 12 fl.oz	70	1	14

Beer ~ Brands

Note: Figure shown are for the United States except for the states of Utah, Colorado, Kansas and Oklahoma who have certain restrictions limiting the alcohol content to not more than 4% by volume (3.2% by weight).

Percentage alcohol listed is by volume - not by weight.
Per 12 fl.oz Serving

Amstel, Light (3.5%)	95	10	5
Anchor: Porter (5.6%)	210	15	23
Steam (4.9%)	160	14	14
Asahi: Kuronama (5.3%)	165	14	14
Select (4.7%)	140	13	11
Super Dry (4.9%)	150	14	11
Bass, Pale Ale (5.1%)	155	14	12
Beck's: Original (5%)	145	14	11
Premier Light (2.3%)	65	7	4
Sapphire (6%)	160	17	9
Big Sky: Original IPA (6.2%)	195	18	17
Moose Drool (5.3%)	175	15	16
Scape Goat (4.7%)	155	14	14
Trout Slayer Ale (4.7%)	145	14	12
Blatz: Original (4.6%)	145	13	13
Light (3.9%)	110	11	8
Blue Moon:			
Belgian White (5.4%)	170	15	14
Cinnamon Horchata (5.5%)	175	15	16
Mango Wheat (5.4%)	175	15	16
Bohemia (4.73%)	140	14	12
Bud Ice (5.5%)	120	16	4

Brands (Cont)
Alc ~ Alcohol (Grams)

Per 12 fl.oz Serving

	C	Alc	Cb
Bud Light: Regular (4.2%)	110	12	7
Clamato Chelada (4.2%)	150	12	16
Extra Lime (4.2%)	160	12	17
Lime (4%)	115	12	8
Orange (4.2%)	145	12	15
Budweiser: Lager (5%)	145	14	11
Clamato Chelado (5%)	185	14	21
Clamato Picante Chelada (5%)	200	14	23
Copper Lager (6.2%)	195	17	16
Freedom Reserve (5.4%)	170	15	15
Platinum (6%)	140	17	5
Select (4.3%)	100	12	3
Select 55 (2.4%)	55	7	2
Busch: Original (4.3%)	115	12	7
Ice (5.9%)	135	17	4
Light (4.1%)	95	12	3
NA (0.4%)	60	1	13
Carlsberg, Pilsner (5%)	135	14	10
Carta Blanca (4.6%)	145	13	11
Cerveza, Aguila (4%)	125	11	11
Colt 45, Malt Liquor (5.6%)	155	16	11
Coors: Banquet (5%)	145	14	11
Extra Gold (5%)	150	14	12
Light (4.2%)	100	12	5
Corona: Extra (4.5%)	150	13	13
Light (4.1%)	100	12	5
Premier (4%)	90	11	11
Dos Equis XX: Ambar (4.7%)	145	14	12
Lager (4.5%)	140	13	11
Fosters: Lager (5%)	145	14	11
Premium Ale (5.5%)	160	16	13
Genesee: Lager (4.5%)	150	13	14
Genny Light Lager (4%)	100	10	4
George Killian's, Irish Red (5.4%)	170	16	15
Grolsch: Blonde (2.8%)	120	8	16
Light (3.6%)	95	11	6
Premium (5%)	145	14	10
Guinness: Draught (4%)	125	12	10
Extra Stout (6%)	175	17	14
Blonde American (5%)	150	14	11
Nitro IPA (5.8%), 11.2oz	155	19	5
Hamm's: Original (4.7%)	145	13	12
Special Light (3.9%)	110	12	8
Heineken: Lager (5%)	140	14	10
Special Dark (5%)	165	14	15
Premium Light (3.5%)	100	10	7
Hurricane: Malt Liquor (6%)	140	17	4
High Gravity (8.1%)	185	23	6
Icehouse: Original (5.5%)	150	16	10
Light (5%)	125	14	7
Keystone: Ice (5.9%)	145	17	7
Light (4.1%)	100	12	5

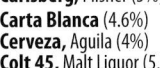
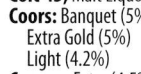
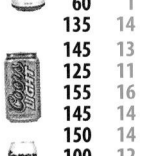
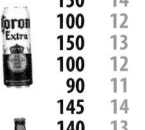
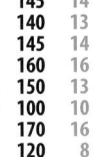
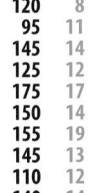
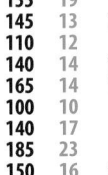

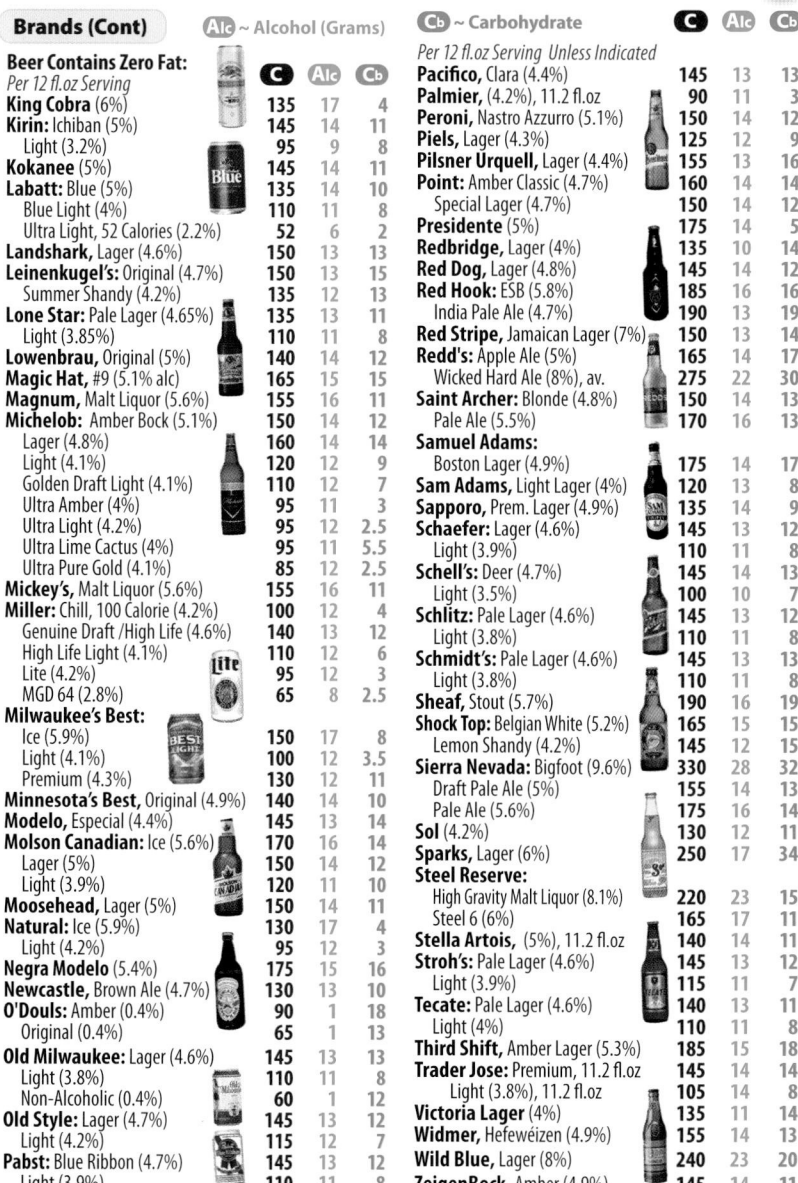

Brands (Cont) — Alc ~ Alcohol (Grams) | Cb ~ Carbohydrate

	C	Alc	Cb
Beer Contains Zero Fat:			
Per 12 fl.oz Serving			
King Cobra (6%)	135	17	4
Kirin: Ichiban (5%)	145	14	11
Light (3.2%)	95	9	8
Kokanee (5%)	145	14	11
Labatt: Blue (5%)	135	14	10
Blue Light (4%)	110	11	8
Ultra Light, 52 Calories (2.2%)	52	6	2
Landshark, Lager (4.6%)	150	13	13
Leinenkugel's: Original (4.7%)	150	13	15
Summer Shandy (4.2%)	135	12	13
Lone Star: Pale Lager (4.65%)	135	13	11
Light (3.85%)	110	11	8
Lowenbrau, Original (5%)	140	14	12
Magic Hat, #9 (5.1% alc)	165	15	15
Magnum, Malt Liquor (5.6%)	155	16	11
Michelob: Amber Bock (5.1%)	150	14	12
Lager (4.8%)	160	14	14
Light (4.1%)	120	12	9
Golden Draft Light (4.1%)	110	12	7
Ultra Amber (4%)	95	11	3
Ultra Light (4.2%)	95	12	2.5
Ultra Lime Cactus (4%)	95	11	5.5
Ultra Pure Gold (4.1%)	85	12	2.5
Mickey's, Malt Liquor (5.6%)	155	16	11
Miller: Chill, 100 Calorie (4.2%)	100	12	4
Genuine Draft /High Life (4.6%)	140	13	12
High Life Light (4.1%)	110	12	6
Lite (4.2%)	95	12	3
MGD 64 (2.8%)	65	8	2.5
Milwaukee's Best:			
Ice (5.9%)	150	17	8
Light (4.1%)	100	12	3.5
Premium (4.3%)	130	12	11
Minnesota's Best, Original (4.9%)	140	14	10
Modelo, Especial (4.4%)	145	13	14
Molson Canadian: Ice (5.6%)	170	16	14
Lager (5%)	150	14	12
Light (3.9%)	120	11	10
Moosehead, Lager (5%)	150	14	11
Natural: Ice (5.9%)	130	17	4
Light (4.2%)	95	12	3
Negra Modelo (5.4%)	175	15	16
Newcastle, Brown Ale (4.7%)	130	13	10
O'Douls: Amber (0.4%)	90	1	18
Original (0.4%)	65	1	13
Old Milwaukee: Lager (4.6%)	145	13	13
Light (3.8%)	110	11	8
Non-Alcoholic (0.4%)	60	1	12
Old Style: Lager (4.7%)	145	13	12
Light (4.2%)	115	12	7
Pabst: Blue Ribbon (4.7%)	145	13	12
Light (3.9%)	110	11	8
Per 12 fl.oz Serving Unless Indicated			
Pacifico, Clara (4.4%)	145	13	13
Palmier, (4.2%), 11.2 fl.oz	90	11	3
Peroni, Nastro Azzurro (5.1%)	150	14	12
Piels, Lager (4.3%)	125	12	9
Pilsner Urquell, Lager (4.4%)	155	13	16
Point: Amber Classic (4.7%)	160	14	14
Special Lager (4.7%)	150	14	12
Presidente (5%)	175	14	5
Redbridge, Lager (4%)	135	10	14
Red Dog, Lager (4.8%)	145	14	12
Red Hook: ESB (5.8%)	185	16	16
India Pale Ale (4.7%)	190	13	19
Red Stripe, Jamaican Lager (7%)	150	13	14
Redd's: Apple Ale (5%)	165	14	17
Wicked Hard Ale (8%), av.	275	22	30
Saint Archer: Blonde (4.8%)	150	14	13
Pale Ale (5.5%)	170	16	13
Samuel Adams:			
Boston Lager (4.9%)	175	14	17
Sam Adams, Light Lager (4%)	120	13	8
Sapporo, Prem. Lager (4.9%)	135	14	9
Schaefer: Lager (4.6%)	145	13	12
Light (3.9%)	110	11	8
Schell's: Deer (4.7%)	145	14	13
Light (3.5%)	100	10	7
Schlitz: Pale Lager (4.6%)	145	13	12
Light (3.8%)	110	11	8
Schmidt's: Pale Lager (4.6%)	145	13	13
Light (3.8%)	110	11	8
Sheaf, Stout (5.7%)	190	16	19
Shock Top: Belgian White (5.2%)	165	15	15
Lemon Shandy (4.2%)	145	12	15
Sierra Nevada: Bigfoot (9.6%)	330	28	32
Draft Pale Ale (5%)	155	14	13
Pale Ale (5.6%)	175	16	14
Sol (4.2%)	130	12	11
Sparks, Lager (6%)	250	17	34
Steel Reserve:			
High Gravity Malt Liquor (8.1%)	220	23	15
Steel 6 (6%)	165	17	11
Stella Artois, (5%), 11.2 fl.oz	140	14	11
Stroh's: Pale Lager (4.6%)	145	13	12
Light (3.9%)	115	11	7
Tecate: Pale Lager (4.6%)	140	13	11
Light (4%)	110	11	8
Third Shift, Amber Lager (5.3%)	185	15	18
Trader Jose: Premium, 11.2 fl.oz	145	14	14
Light (3.8%), 11.2 fl.oz	105	14	8
Victoria Lager (4%)	135	11	14
Widmer, Hefeweizen (4.9%)	155	14	13
Wild Blue, Lager (8%)	240	23	20
ZeigenBock, Amber (4.9%)	145	14	11

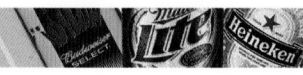

Alc ~ Alcohol (Grams)   Cb ~ Carbohydrate

Cider ~ Alcoholic/Hard

Per 12 fl.oz Unless Indicated

	C	Alc	Cb
Ace: Cider (5%), average all flavors	155	14	12
Joker (6.9%)	135	20	12
Angry Orchard: Crisp Apple (5%)	190	14	25
Easy Apple (4.2%)	150	12	19
Green Apple (5.5%)	210	14	31
Crispin: Original (5%), 12 fl.oz	160	14	15
Blackberry (5%), 12 fl.oz	170	14	16
Brut (5.5%), 12 fl.oz	170	16	13
Pacific Pear (4.5%), 12 fl.oz	160	13	17
Hornsby's: Amber (5.5%)	180	16	19
Crisp (5.5%), 12 fl.oz	190	16	26
Johnny Appleseed, (5.5%)	210	16	26
Magners, (4.5%)	125	13	9
Michelob, Ultra Light Cider (4%)	120	10	10
Saint Archer, Hard Cider (6.1%)	170	17	11
Smith & Forge, (6%)	220	17	26
Stella Artois Cidre, (4.5%)	180	13	22
Strongbow: *Per 11.2 fl oz*			
Cherry/Or. Blossom, (4.5%), av.	180	12	24
Gold Apple (5%)	170	13	20
Rose Apple (5%)	140	13	11
Woodchuck: Amber (5%)	200	14	21
Granny Smith (5%), 12 fl.oz	160	14	11
Pear (4%), 12 fl.oz	150	12	18
Raspberry (4%), 12 fl.oz	170	12	22
Semi-Dry (5.5%), 12 fl.oz	160	14	13
Wyder's: Dry Pear (4%)	140	12	22
Dry Raspberry (4%), 12 fl.oz	120	12	17
Prickly Pear (5%), 12 fl.oz	180	14	22
Reposado (6.9%), 12 fl.oz	250	19	30

Quick Guide

Table Wines:
Average all Varieties (11.5% Alc.)
(Wine Contains Zero Fat)

	C	Alc	Cb
4 fl.oz, 1 small wine glass OR ½ large wine glass	100	12	3
6 fl.oz, (¾ large wine glass)	145	18	5
8 fl.oz, (1 large wine glass)	195	25	7
½ Carafe/Bottle, 12 fl.oz	295	37	10
1 Bottle, 750ml, 25.4 fl.oz	620	78	21

Table Wines

Red: *Per 4 fl.oz*

	C	Alc	Cb
Burgundy/Cabernet/Merlot, av.	100	11	4

White: *Per 4 fl.oz*

	C	Alc	Cb
Dry (Chenin; Fume Blanc; Chardonnay)	95	11	4
Sparkling, 4 fl.oz	95	11	4
Zinfandel Sweet, (Moselle/Sauterne), 4 fl.oz	85	11	2

Table Wines (Cont)

	C	Alc	Cb
Champagne: *Per 4 fl.oz*			
Average all types, 1 glass	85	11	2
with Orange Jce (3:1 orange)	75	8	4
with Orange Jce (1:1 orange)	65	5	7
Mulled Wine (Gluhwein), 4 fl.oz	180	14	20
Non-Alcoholic Wine: *Less than 0.5% Alcohol*			
Ariel: White varieties, average, 4 fl.oz	35	0.5	8
Red varieties, average, 4 fl.oz	25	0.5	5
Reduced Alcohol Wine:			
Average all types, (6%), 4 fl.oz	80	6	10
Skinnygirl, Red/White, (8.5%), 5 fl.oz	100	10	5
Sake (Gekkeikan), (16%), 4 fl.oz	120	15	5
Sangria (Skinnygirl), (4%), 5 fl.oz	130	5	23

Flavored Wines

Average All Brands (6% alcohol)
(Arbor Mist, Wild Vines, Boone's Farm):

	C	Alc	Cb
1 small wine glass, 4 fl.oz	80	6	10
1 large wine glass, 8 fl.oz	160	11	20
1 bottle, 750 ml (25.4 fl.oz)	510	35	64

Dessert Wines

	C	Alc	Cb
Madeira (18%), 2 oz	85	9	5
Marsala (18%), 2 oz	110	9	11
Port, Muscatel (18%), 2 oz	85	9	5
Sherry (15%), 2 oz:			
Dry, 1 Sherry glass	90	7	7
Sweet/Cream, average	90	7	8
Vermouth (Martini & Rossi):			
Extra Dry (18%), 2 oz	65	9	2
Martini Rosso (16%), 2 oz	90	8	8

Cooking Wines

	C	Alc	Cb
Holland House:			
Marsala, (14%), 2 T., 1 fl.oz	45	4	4
Red/White, (10%): 2 T., 1 fl.oz	20	2	1
1 cup, 8 fl.oz	160	24	8
Sherry, (17%), 2 Tbsp, 1 fl.oz	45	5	2

Cooking with Wine:

For alcohol to evaporate, sufficient heat and cooking time (at least 30 minutes) is required.
Red and white table wines;
   Negligible residual calories.
Sweetened wines (Marsala/Sherry)
   Approx. 10 calories per 1 fl.oz.
Flambé Desserts: Only surface alcohol is burned off, so negligible reduction in alcohol or calories.

Quick Guide   Alc ~ Alcohol (Grams)

Spirits/Liquors:
Includes Bourbon, Brandy, Gin, Rum, Scotch, Tequila, Vodka, Whiskey.
Note: All spirits with same alcohol proof have similar calories and zero fat.

Average All Brands	C	Alc	Cb
80 Proof (40% Alcohol by Volume):			
1 fl.oz	65	9.5	0
1.5 fl.oz (1 shot)	100	14	0
3 fl.oz (Double shot)	195	28	0
½ Bottle, 350 ml (12 fl.oz)	770	113	0
1 Bottle, 700 ml (24 fl.oz)	1540	227	0
86 Proof (43% Alc):			
1 fl.oz	70	10	0
1.5 fl.oz (1 shot)	105	15	0
1 Bottle (24 fl.oz)	1670	247	0
100 Proof (50% Alc),			
1.5 fl.oz	125	18	0
Shochu (Soju),			
average all types (25% alc), 2 fl.oz	65	12	0

Flavored Spirits

	C	Alc	Cb
Captain Morgan: *Per 1.5 fl.oz*			
Original (35%)	85	12	0.5
Black Spiced (47.3%)	115	14	1
Parrot Bay (21%), average	90	7.5	10
Silver Spiced (35%)	95	12	2
Malibu Rum,			
Original/Fruit Flavors (21%), 1.5 fl.oz	80	8	8
Southern Comfort (35%), 1.5 fl.oz	100	13	3

Hard Lemonade, Sodas & Tea

	C	Alc	Cb
Henry's Hard Soda:			
Grape (4.2%), 12 fl.oz	225	12	35
Orange (4.2%)	190	12	28
Sparkling Water, av., (4.2%)	90	12	3
Margaritaville: *Per 12 fl.oz*			
Lime Margarita (8%)	310	23	30
Paradise Punch (8%)	340	23	46
Mike's Hard Lemonade:			
Black Cherry (5%), 11.2 fl.oz	220	13	33
Lite (5%), 11.2 fl.oz	150	13	15
Lemonade (5%), 11.2 fl.oz	220	13	33
Lite (5%), 11.2 fl.oz	100	13	4
Harder (8%), 16 fl.oz	395	31	44
Sparks: *Per 16 fl.oz Can*			
Blackberry (8%)	385	31	44
Original (6%)	335	23	45
Twisted Tea: Original (5%)	220	14	31
Half & Half (5%)	260	14	34
Zumbida Mango, (4.2%), 12 fl.oz	150	12	17

Coolers & Premix Cocktails

Ready-To-Drink: *Zero Fat Unless Indicated*	C	Alc	Cb
Bacardi: *Per 4 fl.oz*			
Party Drinks (Ready To Pour):			
Bahama Mama; Mai Tai (10%)	130	9	16
Mojito (15%)	160	14	16
Rum Island Ice Tea (12.5%)	150	12	16
Bacardi Silver: *Per 12 fl.oz*			
Lemonade/Sangria (6%), av.	270	17	41
Raz/Strawberry (5%)	240	14	36
Mojito (5%)	240	14	36
Bartles & Jaymes: *Per 11.2 fl.oz*			
Malt Based Coolers (3.2%):			
Exotic Berry	195	9	31
Fuzzy Navel	215	9	36
Margarita	245	9	43
Pina Colada	250	9	45
Pomegranate Raspberry	205	9	35
Sangria	240	9	40
Strawberry Daiquiri	205	9	34
Captain Morgan's,			
Parrot Bay (4.1%), all var. av., 11.2 fl.oz	210	10	35
Chi Chi's: Long Is. Iced Tea, 4 fl.oz	145	12	17
Mexican Mudslide, 4 fl.oz (8g fat)	240	1.5	42
Mojito, 4 fl.oz	160	11	21
Pina Colada, 4 fl.oz (6g fat)	240	4	42
White Russian, 4 fl.oz (7g fat)	245	1.5	43
Daily's, Frozen Pouches (5%),			
average all flavors, 10 fl.oz	285	12	47
Jack Daniels, Country Cocktails (4.8%),			
average all varieties, 10 fl.oz	200	9	30
Jose Cuervo:			
Margaritas:			
Classic Lime (10%), 6 fl.oz	210	14	29
Golden (12.7%), 4.7 fl.oz	170	14	19
Seagram's:			
Escapes Coolers (3.2%):			
Bahama Mama, 11.2 fl.oz	200	9	36
Strawb. Daiquiri, 11.2 fl.oz	225	9	41
Skinnygirl:			
Vodka with flavors (30%), 1.5 fl.oz	75	11	0
Cocktails (10%), av., 3 fl.oz	70	8	4
Smirnoff:			
Ice (4.5%): Original, 11.2 fl.oz	220	13	33
Mango; Pineapple, av., 11.2 fl.oz	230	13	35
Spiked Sparkling Seltzer,			
(4.5%), all flav., 12 fl.oz can	90	13	1
TGI Friday's:			
On The Rocks: *Per 6 fl.oz*			
Long Island Ice Tea (15%)	250	21	28
Margarita (7.5%)	185	11	29
Mudslide (10%)	365	14	31
Blenders (12.5%), Mudslide, 6 fl.oz	365	18	31

Coolers & Premix Cocktails (Cont)

Ready-To-Drink:

The Club Premix Cocktails: *Per 3.4 oz Serving (½ can)*

	C	Alc	Cb
Censored on Beach; Margarita (7.5%)	105	6	17
Gin/Vodka Martini (21%), average	155	17	0.2
Ice Tea (15%)	145	12	17
Manhattan (17%)	115	13	5
Mudslide/Pina Colada (10%), average	200	8	16
Screwdriver (7.5%)	95	6	14
Whiskey Sour (10%)	95	8	11

Shooters — Alc ~ Alcohol (Grams)

	C	Alc	Cb
Alabama Slammer	110	14	2
Amaretto Sour	120	6	19
B52	145	14	11
Beam Me Up Scotty	145	13	13
Blue Tequila	160	18	6
Jager Bomb	205	8	30
Jager Bomb, w/ Sugar-Free Red Bull	155	8	18
Jell-O Shot: 3 oz, with 1.5 oz Vodka	180	14	19
with Diet Jell-O	110	14	0
Kamikaze	75	8	3
Kool-Aid	160	15	14
Orgasm	100	12	6
Peppermint Patty	195	8	11
Stinger	170	18	12
Surfer on Acid	90	7	11

Cocktail Mixers ~ Non-Alcoholic

Bacardi: *Per 8 fl.oz, Prepared from 2 fl.oz Concentrate*

	C	Alc	Cb
Daiquiris; Rum Runner	120	0	32
Margarita	90	0	25
Mojito	110	0	30
Pina Colada	170	0	36

Baja Bob's: *Per 4 fl.oz*

	C	Alc	Cb
Cranberry Cosmo Martini	10	0	2
Pina Colada	30	0	4

Jose Cuervo:

	C	Alc	Cb
Margaritas: Av. all flav., 4 fl.oz	85	0	21
Light (Sugar Free), Lime, 4 fl.oz	5	0	1

Mr & Mrs T:

	C	Alc	Cb
Bloody Mary: Original, 5 oz	30	0	7
Bold & Spicy, 4 oz	35	0	7
Mai Tai	130	0	32
Margarita	100	0	26
Pina Colada	170	0	44
Strawberry Daiquiri	180	0	46

TGI Friday's:

	C	Alc	Cb
Mudslide, 2.3 fl.oz	110	0	23
Cosmo; Berrytini, 2 fl.oz	80	0	20
Strawb. Daiquiri; Marg., 4 fl.oz	190	0	46

Cocktails — Alc ~ Alcohol (Grams)

Made to Standard Recipes (Standard Size):

(Main Reference: The New American Bartender's Guide)

Zero Fat Unless Indicated

	C	Alc	Cb
Adios Mother F.	260	23	23
Bacardi & Coke (with 1.5 oz Bacardi)	160	14	17
Bellini, 4.5 fl.oz	95	11	7
Bloody Mary (with 1.5 oz Vodka)	125	10	7
Blushin' Russian (20g fat)	405	14	23
Bourbon & Soda (with 2 oz Bourbon)	130	19	0
Brandy Alexander (10g fat)	300	20	15
Chupa Naranjas (with 1.5 oz Tequila)	150	16	8
Cosmopolitan	215	24	12
Daiquiri (w/ 2 oz Rum), av. all types	140	19	4
Frozen Daiquiri (with 2 oz Rum):			
without fruit	155	19	6
with fruit (with 1.5 oz Rum)	145	14	11
Grasshopper	260	17	28
Harvey Wallbanger (2 oz)	200	19	17
Highball (1.5 oz Whiskey)	100	14	0
Irish Coffee (10g fat)	205	14	2
Kahlua Mudslide: with milk (3g fat)	145	11	12
with cream (12g fat)	230	11	10
Lemon Drop, 4 fl.oz	130	14	10
Long Island Iced Tea (with 3 oz Cola)	270	19	32
with 3 oz Diet Cola	235	19	22
Mai Tai (with 2 oz Rum)	290	24	33
Manhattan	130	17	5
Margarita	160	18	7
Martini: Dry, with 1.5 oz gin	100	14	0
Sour Apple, w/ 2 oz Vodka/1 oz Schnapps	250	31	10
Mint Julep (with 2½ oz Bourbon)	180	24	4
Mojito (with 2 oz rum)	170	19	9
Moscow Mule (with 1.5 oz Vodka)	180	14	20
Pina Colada (10g fat), 6 oz	250	15	18
Red Bull & Vodka (with 1.5 oz vodka)	210	14	28
with Sugar Free Red Bull	105	14	3
Rum & Coke (with 1.5 oz Rum)	160	14	17
Sake Bomb (1.5 oz Sake & 5 oz Beer)	105	12	7
Sangria: with 1 oz Fruit Juice, 5 oz	120	12	9
with 0.5 oz Brandy, 5.5 oz	150	17	9
Screwdriver	160	14	15
Sex On The Beach	235	19	25
Spritzer (with 3 oz Wine)	65	8	2
Tequila Sunrise	200	14	25
Tom Collins (with 2 oz Gin)	210	19	18
Vodka Soda (with 1.5 oz Vodka)	100	14	0
Vodka Tonic (with 1.5 oz Vodka)	165	14	18
Whiskey Sour (w/ 2 oz Whiskey)	155	19	7
White Russian (10g fat)	240	19	7
Non-Alcoholic:			
Cinderella	45	0	11
Shirley Temple (with 6 oz Ginger Ale)	140	0	34

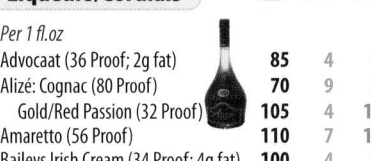
Liqueurs/Cordials

	C	**Alc**	**Cb**

Per 1 fl.oz

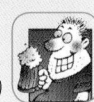

	C	Alc	Cb
Advocaat (36 Proof; 2g fat)	85	4	9
Alizé: Cognac (80 Proof)	70	9	2
Gold/Red Passion (32 Proof)	105	4	11
Amaretto (56 Proof)	110	7	17
Baileys Irish Cream (34 Proof; 4g fat)	100	4	8
Benedictine (80 Proof)	90	9	5
Chambord (33 Proof)	105	4	11
Chartreuse (80 Proof)	100	9	9
Cherry Brandy (48 Proof)	80	6	9
Coffee Liqueur (53 Proof)	115	7	16
Cointreau (80 Proof)	95	9	7
Creme de Cacao (54 Proof)	100	6	15
Creme de Menthe (72 Proof)	125	9	14
Curacao (70 Proof)	95	8	6
Drambuie (80 Proof)	105	9	9
Frangelico (40 Proof)	65	5	12
Galliano (86 Proof)	100	10	8
Grand Marnier (80 Proof)	100	9	7
(40 Proof)	85	5	14
Kirsch (68 Proof)	80	8	6
Midori (42 Proof)	80	5	11
Ouzo (80 Proof)	105	9	11
Pernod (80 Proof)	75	9	11
Sambuca (84 Proof)	100	10	11
Schnapps (100 Proof)	115	12	9
Southern Comfort (70 Proof)	65	8	3
Tia Maria (40% Proof)	90	7	10

Liqueur Coffee & Hot Drinks

Per Standard Drink

	C	Alc	Cb
Liqueur Coffee: Av. all types	200	10	10
Irish, 1.5 oz Whiskey & 1 oz whip	205	9	4
Hot Toddy, with 1½ oz liquor, av. all	170	9	19
Mulled Wine (Glühwein), 4 fl.oz, av	195	14	25

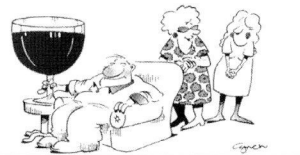

"The doctor told him to cut down to just one glass a day."

TEN TIPS TO AVOID HARMFUL DRINKING

1. **Add up the alcohol** you typically drink each day and on social occasions. How does this compare with 'low risk' amounts? (*See page 23*)

2. **Compare the alcohol content** of different drinks and select the lowest. Request half shots of alcohol in cocktails and mixed drinks. Dilute them and keep topping off with non-alcoholic drinks.

3. **Go easy on 'Light' beers.** At 4% alcohol, on average, they are still high in alcohol compared to regular beer (5% alcohol).

4. **Try low alcohol or non-alcohol** alternatives such as fruit juices and mineral water. Take your own to parties.

5. **Before drinking alcohol,** quench your thirst with water and non-alcoholic drinks – particularly after vigorous exercise or sports.

6. **Slow the rate of drinking.** Chugging or drinking fast is the major cause of illness and death from alcohol poisoning.

7. **Avoid drinking in 'rounds'.**

8. **Have a non-alcoholic 'spacer'** between drinks (e.g. mineral water, orange juice).

9. **Don't drink on an empty stomach.** Food slows the rate of alcohol absorption.

10. **Keep track of the number of drinks** and know when to stop. Stick to a set limit.

Note: Alcohol can be very dangerous when taken with prescription or street drugs, or when you are very tired.

Extra Info: www.CalorieKing.com

Cocktail Mixers & Extracts

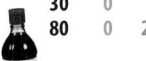
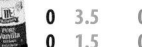

	C	Alc	Cb
Angostura Bitters, ¼ tsp	2	0	0.5
Grenadine, ½ tsp	6	0	2
Lime/Lemon Juice, 2 Tbsp, 1 oz	10	0	2
Maraschino Cherry, 1 small	8	0	2
Simple Syrup, 1 Tbsp, av.	50	0	14
Sweet & Sour Mix, 2 Tbsp, 1 oz	30	0	7
Tonic Water, 8 fl.oz	80	0	22
Flavor Extracts (McCormick):			
Pure Lemon (83%), 1 tsp	0	3.5	0
Pure Vanilla (35%), 1tsp	0	1.5	0

Baking Ingredients	C	F	Cb
Almond Paste,			
(Marzipan), 2 Tbsp	170	7	24
Apple Pie Filling,			
Sweetened, 9.4 oz	290	0	69
(Bean Water), 1/4 c., 2 oz	10	0	2
Baking Powder: Regular, 1 tsp	5	0	1
Cream of Tartar, 1 tsp	10	0	2
Baking Mix (*Bisquick*):			
Original, 1/3 cup, 1.5 oz	160	5	26
Batter Mix (*Golden Dipt*),			
All Purpose, 1/4 cup	100	0	20
Butter/Margarine, 1/2 cup, 4 oz	800	88	1
Stick (*Land O' Lakes*), 0.5 oz	100	11	0
Cacao Butter, 2 Tbsp, 1 oz	240	28	0
Cacao Nibs, raw, 3 Tbsp, 1 oz	180	14	8
Cacao Powder, raw: 1 Tbsp, 0.3 oz	35	2	3
1/4 cup, 1 oz	150	9	11
Carob Flour, 1/2 cup	115	0.5	46
Chocolate Baking Bars: *Average all Brands*			
Sweet (*Baker's*):			
1 oz portion	120	7	16
4 oz bar	470	28	64
Semi-sweet, 1 oz	140	9	16
White Baking, 1 oz	160	9	16
Unsweetened: 1 oz	140	14	8
Grated, 1 cup, 4.5 oz	660	69	39
Chocolate Baking Chips: *Average all Brands*			
Milk Choc./Semi Sweet, 1 oz	140	8	18
1/2 cup, 3 oz	420	24	54
1 cup, 6 oz	840	48	108
Dark, 1 Tbsp, 0.5 oz	70	5	3
Mini Kisses (*Hershey*), 1 piece	5	0.5	1
Cocoa Powder, unsweetened:			
1 Tbsp, 0.2 oz	15	0.5	3
1/3 cup, 1 oz	60	4	17
Coconut, dried:			
Sweetened/Flaked:			
1 oz	130	8	15
1/2 cup, 1.3 oz	195	12	22
Toasted (*Baker's*), 1 oz	170	13	13
Unsweetened, 1 oz	190	18	7
Coconut Cream/Milk ~ *See Page 89*			
Coconut Manna (*Nutiva*), 1 Tbsp	100	9	3
Cornstarch, 1 Tbsp	30	0	7
Eggs: Large (1)	75	5	0
Jumbo (1)	90	6	0.5
Egg White: 1 Egg White	15	0	0
1/2 cup (4 egg whites), 4 oz	60	0	1
Flour: Whole Wheat, 1 cup, 4.2 oz	400	2	84
White: 1 Tbsp, 0.3 oz	25	0	5.5
1 cup, 4.2 oz	400	1	88

Flavor Extracts: *Av. all Brands*	C	F	Cb
Imitation, 1 tsp	10	0	2
Pure Extract, 1 tsp	10	0	0.5
Almond; Vanilla, 1 tsp	10	0	0.5
Fruit Pectin: Swtnd, 1/4 tsp	5	0	1
Unsweetened, 1/4 tsp	0	0	0
Gelatin, dry, unsweetened, 0.3 oz	20	0	0
Glaze (*Duncan Hines*): Choc., 2 T.	150	7	21
Vanilla, 2 Tbsp	140	6	22
Golden Dipt, Batter Mix			
1/4 cup, 1 oz	100	0	23
Honey, 1/2 cup, 6 oz	515	0	145
Lemon/Orange Peel, 1/4 cup	25	0	6
Lighter Bake (*Sunsweet*):			
(Butter & Oil replacement)			
1 Tbsp, 1/2 oz	35	0	9
1/4 Cup, 2.7 oz	140	0	36
Milk: Whole, 1 cup, 8 fl.oz	150	8	12
2%, 1 cup, 8 fl.oz	120	5	12
1%, 1 cup, 8 fl.oz	100	2.5	12
Fat-Free, 1 cup, 8 fl.oz	90	0.5	13
Pastry ~ *See Page 134*			
Pie Crusts ~ *See Page 134*			
Pie Fillings, Fruits ~ *See Page 134*			
Lemon Creme, 1/3 cup	130	1.5	28
Mincemeat, 3.5 oz	190	5	45
Pumpkin, 1 cup, 9.3 oz	270	1.5	60
Prune Puree, 1/4 cup, 3 oz	220	0	55
Raisins, 1/2 cup, 2.8 oz	240	0.5	63
Rennin, 0.4 oz pkt	10	0	2
Soy Milk ~ *See Pages 49-50*			
Sprinkles, all types, 1 tsp	20	1	3
Sugar: 1 Tbsp, 0.5 oz	55	0	14
1 oz	110	0	28
1 cup, 7 oz	775	0	195
16 oz (1 lb)	1760	0	454
Sweeteners & Sugar Substitutes ~ *See Page 156*			
Vinegar, average all types, 1 oz	5	0	1
Whey, sweet, dry, 1 oz	100	0.5	21
Yeast:			
Active, dry, 0.3 oz pkg	25	0.5	3
Bakers, compressed, 1 oz	30	0.5	5
Fleischmann's, 0.6 oz pkg	0	0	0

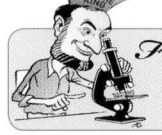

For Full Nutritional Data & Product Updates
~ *See Author's Website*
www.CalorieKing.com

Note: Actual weight of bars is usually 5-10% more than label Net Weight. Weigh bar and allow extra calories.

Bars ~ Brands   C   F   Cb

Per Bar

	C	F	Cb
AdvantEdge ~ *See EAS*			
Annie's Homegrown:			
Gluten Free, all varieties, 1 oz	110	3	20
Organic Chewy Granola Bars: *Per 0.9 oz Bar*			
Chocolate Chip	100	2.5	18
Oatmeal Raisin	90	1.5	19
PB Chocolate Chip	100	3.5	16
Atkins:			
Harvest Trail Bars: *Per 1.34 oz Bar*			
Coconut Almond	160	11	16
Dark Chocolate:			
Peanut Butter	170	13	13
Sea Salt Caramel	180	14	13
Meal Bars: *Per 1.7 oz Unless Indicated*			
Blueb. Greek Yogurt	200	9	21
Choc. Chip Cookie Dough, 2 oz	220	10	32
Chocolate Chip Granola	200	9	18
Chocolate Peanut Butter, 2 oz	250	14	23
Choc. Peanut Butter Pretzel	210	10	19
Cookies 'n Crème,1.76 oz	200	11	22
Peanut Butter Granola	210	11	19
Vanilla Pecan Crisp	200	0	17
Snack Bars: *Per 1.55 oz Bar Unless Indicated*			
Caramel Chocolate Nut Roll	190	13	19
Caramel Chocolate Peanut Nougat	170	11	20
Caramel Double Chocolate Crunch	160	9	22
Cashew Trail Mix, 1.4 oz	170	11	19
Choc. Chip Crisp, 1.23 oz	140	6	16
Classic Trail Mix, 1.34 oz	190	15	13
Coconut Almond Delight	200	15	18
Dark Chocolate Decadence	150	6	23
Lemon Bar, Triple Choc., av., 1.4 oz	160	8	16
Sweet & Salty Trail Mix, 1.34 oz	190	14	15
Note: Snack Bars Carb figures includes 4-15g sugar alcohol			
Balance:			
Original Bars:			
Average, 1.8 oz	200	7	21
Dark Chocolate var., av., 1.6 oz	180	7	22
Duo-licious: *Per 2 Pieces*			
Choc. C'rml P'nut Nougat, 1.55 oz	190	10	22
Choc. Pepeprmint Patty, 1.4 oz	160	4	27
Dulce de Leche & Caramel, 1.4 oz	150	5	24

Per Bar   C   F   Cb

	C	F	Cb
Cascadian Farms *(General Mills):*			
Chewy Granola: Av. all var., 0.77 oz	85	2	16
1.23 oz Bars: Peanut varieties	160	7	22
Chocolate Chip	140	3	26
Crunchy Granola, av., 2 bars, 1.4 oz	185	8	27
Protein Granola Bars, av.1.76 oz	250	15	20
Soft Baked Squares, av., 1.23 oz	150	5.5	23
Clif:			
Blueberry Crisp, 2.4 oz	250	5	44
Builder's, average, 2.4 oz	275	9	30
Crunch, average, 1.48 oz	200	9	26
Energy: Av. all varieties., 2.4 oz	260	6	43
Mini size, average, 1.2 oz	100	2.5	17
Fruit Smoothie Filled, 1.76 oz	230	11	29
Mojo, average, 1.6 oz	205	10	22
Nut Butter Filled, av., 1.76 oz	230	11	27
Whey, P'B & Chocolate, 2 oz	260	13	24
Corazonas:			
Heartbar Oatmeal Squares: *Per 1.8 oz Bar*			
White Chocolate Macadamia	200	7	29
Average other varieties	185	7	28
Detour:			
Lean Muscle:			
Cookie Dough Caramel Crisp, 3.2 oz	370	12	33
P'nut Butter Choc. Crunch, 3.2 oz	420	18	33
Lower Sugar, average all varieties:			
1.4 oz Bar	170	6	16
2.8 oz Bar	340	13	33
Note: Low Sugar Bars Carb figures include 12-28g sugar alcohol			
Simple:			
Full size, 20g Protein, av., 2 oz	225	7	24
Snack size, 10g Protein, av., 1 oz	110	4	11
Smart: Coconut Almond, 1.3 oz	150	5	16
Fruit varieties, 1.3 oz	130	2.5	18
Peanut Butter Chocolate, 1.3 oz	160	6	16
dotFIT:			
dotBAR:			
Double Choc. Brownie, 3.3 oz	370	13	38
Peanut Butter Cup, 3.3 oz	370	13	38
Note: dotBARS Carb figures includes 21g sugar alcohol			
dotSTICK, Iced, all varieties, 2 oz	190	6	26
Note: dotSTICK Bars Carb figures includes 8g sugar alcohol			
EAS:			
AdvantEDGE, Protein Bars, average all varieties,1.76 oz	190	7	20
Extend Bar: Yogurt, av., 1.4 oz	150	5.5	23
Anytime, av. all varieties, 1.4 oz	150	3	20
Note: Extend Bars Carb figure includes 3-10g sugar alcohol			

Bars ~ Brands (Cont)

	C	**F**	**Cb**
Per Bar			
Fiber One:			
90-Calorie Bar, av., 0.8 oz	90	2	17
Chewy: Layered, Dble Choc. Almond,			
1.27 oz	140	4	25
Oat varieties, average, 1.4 oz	140	4	29
Protein: Av. all varieties: 1.2 oz	140	6	18
Nut, Chocolate Pretzel, 1.4 oz	180	11	15
General Mills: *Per 1.6 oz Bar*			
Milk 'n Cereal Bar,			
Honey Nut Cheerios	160	4	28
Glucerna:			
Snack Bars,			
Peanut/Choc. Chip, av., 1.4 oz	155	5.5	20
Note: Carbohydrate figure includes 7g sugar alcohol			
Mini Snack Bar, average, 0.7 oz	80	3.5	11
Note: Carbohydrate figure includes 3g sugar alcohol			
Great Value *(Walmart):*			
Chewy Granola: 90 calorie, 0.8 oz	90	1.5	18
Other varieties, 0.8 oz	100	2.5	18
Dipped, Peanut Butter, 1.1 oz	150	7	20
Protein, average, 1.4 oz	190	12	14
Sweet & Salty, Almond, 1.23 oz	170	8	20
Crunchy Granola,			
Oats & Honey, 2 bars, 1.48 oz	200	7	29
Fiber, Oats & Chocolate, 1.4 oz	140	4	30
Fruit & Grains, Cereal, av., 1.3 oz	130	3	25
Health Valley,			
Multigrain, Cobbler Cereal Bars,			
average all flavors, 3 oz	130	2.5	25
HMR, Benefit Bars, av. all, 1.4 oz	160	5	22
Init: *Per 1.4 oz Bar*			
Dark Choc., average	180	10	23
Mixed Nut & Sweet Berries	180	9	24
Roasted Nuts & Honey Chipotle	190	13	18
Jenny Craig, all var., 1.2 oz	110	3	14
Kashi:			
Cereal Bars, 1.3 oz	130	3	25
GoLean, Plant Based Bars, av., 1.6 oz	195	10	21
Granola Bars:			
Chewy, average all varieties, 1.3 oz	135	5	23
Chewy Nut Butter, av., 1.23 oz	150	7	21
Crunchy, all varieties,			
2 bars, 1.4 oz	175	6	26
Layered, av. all, 1.1 oz	125	4	21
Kellogg's:			
Nutrigrain ~ *See page 33*			
Special K ~ *See page 34*			

Per Bar	**C**	**F**	**Cb**
Kind Bars: *Per 1.4 oz Bar*			
Breakfast: Peanut Butter (2), 1.76 oz	230	11	28
Blueb. Alm; Honey Oat (2), 1.76 oz	220	8	33
Other varieties (2),1.76 oz	215	10	26
Almond & Apricot	180	11	21
Almond & Coconut	190	12	21
Caramel Almond & Sea Salt	200	16	15
Dark Choc. Almond	200	12	21
Dark Choc. Cherry Cashew	170	10	22
Honey Roasted Nuts & Sea Salt	210	15	15
Peanut Butter Dark Choc	200	13	16
Healthy Grain, av. all varieties, 1.2oz	145	5	24
Kind Kids:			
Chewy Choc. Chip	90	3	19
Chewy Honey Oat	90	2.5	16
Peanut Butter	100	4	15
Pressed, Strawberry Apple Chia	110	0.5	25
Protein, average, 1.76 oz	250	17	18
Kudos, av. all varieties, 0.9 oz	100	3	17
Labrada:			
Cookie Roll, average, 2.8 oz	315	10	34
Lean Body Protein Bar: *Per 2.54 oz*			
Cookie Dough; Fudge Brownie	290	9	32
PB Chocolate Chip	310	11	32
Lean Body Gold, all var., 2.96 oz	330	8	32
Rockin' Roll, Nutty Peanut, 2.47 oz	290	16	25
Larabar:			
Original Fruit & Nut, av.	200	9	26
Fruits & Greens, av.	130	3	23
Nuts & Seeds, average	195	15	13
Lindora Bars:			
Protein Bars:			
Caramel Cocoa,1.6 oz	160	5	18
Chocolate Mint, 1.45 oz	150	4.5	21
Oatmeal Cinn. Raisin, 1.5 oz	150	5	19
Peanut Butter Crunch, 1.5 oz	150	5	18
Sweet & Salty Crunch. 1.4 oz	160	5	21
Zesty Lemon Crunch, 1.5 oz	160	7	16
Luna Bars:			
Regular, av., 1.7 oz	195	7	26
Rica, average, 1.4 oz	165	9	22
5G Sugar, average, 1.48 oz	175	9	20
Protein, av. all varieties, 1.6 oz	175	5	21
Marathon *(Snickers):*			
Energy: Chewy, av. all var., 2 oz	210	8	26
Crunchy, Dark Chocolate, 1.6 oz	150	4.5	22
Protein, average all var., 2.8 oz	285	9	40

Bars ~ Brands (Cont) | C | F | Cb

Per Bar

	C	F	Cb
Mars, Protein Bar, 2 oz	200	4.5	22
Medifast:			
Chewy, all varieties, 1.3 oz	110	3	15
Crunch, av. all varieties, 1.2 oz	110	3	13
Note: Crunch Bars Carb figure includes 2-3g sugar alcohol			
Maintenance, Cararmel Nut, 1.5 oz	170	5	22
Met-Rx:			
Big 100: *Per 3.52 oz*			
Crispy Apple Pie	400	10	48
Chocolate Caramel Coconut	400	10	46
Peanut Butter Pretzel	410	12	47
Peanut Butter Caramel Crunch	410	13	44
Super Cookie Crunch	410	14	42
Protein Plus: Choc. Choc. Chunk, 3 oz	310	10	29
Choc. Roasted Peanut w/ Crml, 3oz	320	10	33
Peanut Butter Crisp, 3 oz	310	10	33
Mojo Bars ~ *See Clif*			
Muscle Milk *(Cytosport):*			
Protein Bars:			
Almond Cookie Flav.; Choc PB, 2.25 oz	250	9	28
B'Day Cake; Cookies 'N Crm, 1.76 oz	185	6	23
Blueberry Waffle, 2.18 oz	230	6	27
Double Fudge Brownie, 2.22 oz	240	7	28
Peanut Butter Cookie, 1.76 oz	190	6	22
Note: Protein Bars Carb figures include 6-14g sugar alcohol			
Nature's Path:			
Chewy Breakfast, av., 1.2 oz	140	4	25
Love Crunch, av., 1.1 oz	150	7	19
Superfood, av., 1.34 oz	185	10	20
Nature Valley:			
Chewy, XL Protein, average, 2 oz	290	19	21
Crunchy, 2 bars, average, 1.5 oz	190	8	29
Nut Crunch, av. all var, 1.23 oz	190	14	14
Nut Crisp, average, 0.9 oz	135	9	10
Protein, all var., 1.4 oz	190	12	14
Sweet & Salty, average, 1.3 oz	160	7	22
NuGo:			
Dark, average all varieties, 1.76 oz	200	6	27
Family:			
Choc. Banana, 1.76 oz	190	3.5	23
Av. other var., 1.76 oz	170	3	26
Fiber d'Lish: Orange Cranb., 1.58 oz	130	3	32
Coc. Macaroon; P'nut Choc. Chip, 1.58 oz	160	6	28
Average other varieties, 1.58 oz	135	4	31
Gluten Free, av. all varieties, 1.58 oz	180	4	27
Organic, all varieties, 1.58 oz	190	5	26
Slim: Espresso, 1.58 oz	170	5	20
Average other varieties	185	5	19

Per Bar

	C	F	Cb
NuGo (Cont):			
Smarte Carb: Choc. Black Berry, 1.76 oz	150	3	22
Peanut Butter Crunch, 1.76 oz	160	4	19
Note: Smarte Carb Carb figures include 12-14 g sugar alcohol			
Stronger: *Per 2.8 oz Bar*			
Cookies 'N Crm; Caramel Pretzel, av.	290	10	37
Dark Choc C'rml.; Peanut Cluster, av.	315	13	35
Nutri-Grain *(Kellogg's):*			
Bakery Delights,			
average, 1.4 oz	160	5	27
Soft Baked B'fast Cereal Bars,			
all varieties, 1.3 oz	130	3.5	25
NutriSystem:			
Breakfast: Cinnamon Bun	150	3.5	26
Harvest Nut	160	6	22
Lunch: Choc. P'nut Butter; Trail Mix	200	8	24
Double Chocolate Caramel	180	6	28
Snacks: Dark Chocolate & Sea Salt Nut	200	13	16
Average other varieties	150	4	23
Oh Yeah! (ISS):			
Original: *Per 3 oz Bar*			
Almond Fudge Brownie			
Choc. Caramel Candies	350	17	36
Cookie Caramel Crunch	340	13	32
Peanut Butter & Caramel	380	19	30
Good Grab, average, 1.6 oz	190	10	19
Optifast:			
800 Bars:			
Apple Cinnamon, 1.52 oz	160	4	18
Chocolate, 1.65 oz	160	4.5	18
Peanut Butter Chocolate, 1.52 oz	160	5	18
Note: 800 Bars Carb figures include 1-4g sugar alcohol			
PowerBar:			
Performance Energy, average	230	4	45
Protein: Clean Way, average, 2.1 oz	190	5	25
Note: Protein Bars Carb figures include 8g sugar alcohol			
Protein Plus, average, 2.1 oz	205	7	25
Note: Protein Plus Bars Carb figures include 16-18g sugar alcohol			
Snack, average	230	13	23
Power Crunch *(BNRG):*			
Orig. Protein Bar, av. all var., 1.4 oz	205	12	10
Power Crunch, Choklat, av., 0.75 oz	105	6	8
PR:			
Protein: Chocolate Mint, 2.1 oz	200	6	22
Chocolate Peanut, 1.8 oz	200	7	21
Oatmeal Raisin Granola, 1.8 oz	210	7	22
Premier Protein *(Premier Nutrition):*			
Chocolate Peanut Butter, 2.54 oz	290	8	25
Dark Chocolate Mint, 2.54 oz	280	7	24
Yogurt Peanut Crunch, 2.54 oz	290	8	25

Note: Actual weight of bars is usually 5-10% more than label Net Weight. Weigh bar and allow extra calories.

Bars ~ Brands (Cont)

Per Bar **C** **F** **Cb**

Promax:

	C	F	Cb
Original, av. all varieties, 2.6 oz	285	6	39
Lower Sugar, av. all varieties, 2.4 oz	215	7	32

Note: Lower Sugar Carbohydrate figures include 5-6g Sugar Alcohol

	C	F	Cb
Proti Bars *(Bariatrix),* av. all var.	160	5.5	16
PureFit, av. all varieties, 2 oz	220	7	25

Pure Protein:

Hi Protein, average all varieties:

	C	F	Cb
1.76 oz bar	190	5	18
2.1 oz	195	7	24
2.75 oz bar	300	8	27

Note: Carbohydrate figures include 5-8g Sugar Alcohol

Quaker:

	C	F	Cb
B'fast Squares: P'nut Butter, 2.1 oz	250	10	35
Other flavors, 2.1 oz	210	4.5	41

Note: Carbohydrate figures include 2-6g Sugar Alcohol

	C	F	Cb
B'fast Flats: Banana Honey Nut (3)	180	7	27
Av. other varieties (3)	175	6.5	28

Granola Bars:

	C	F	Cb
Chewy: 25% Less Sugar, average, 0.8 oz	95	3	17
Big, average all varieties, 1.9 oz	175	6	30
Bites, average, 8 pieces	135	5	21
Dipps, average, 1.2 oz	140	6	22
Snackwich, av., 1.4 oz	165	6	29
Yogurt, all varieties, 1.2 oz	150	4.5	25

Quest Bar:

	C	F	Cb
Hero: Choc. Caramel Pecan, 2.1 oz	200	11	27
Average other varieties, 2.1 oz	175	8	30

Note: Carbohydrate figure include 1-4g Sugar Alcohol

	C	F	Cb
Protein,, av., 2.1 oz	195	9	22

Note: Carbohydrate figures includs 1-6g Sugar Alcohol

RX Bar:

Protein Bars:

	C	F	Cb
Blueberry/Mixed Berry	210	7	25
Chocolate Sea Salt	210	9	24
Peanut Butter Chocolate	210	10	22

Skratch Bars:

Anytime Energy: *Per 1.76 oz Bar*

	C	F	Cb
Cherries & Pistachios; Ginger & Miso	210	10	27
Chocolate Chips & Almonds	200	8	30

Slim-Fast:

	C	F	Cb
Bake Shop Bars, average all, 1.6 oz	180	6.5	17

Note: Carbohydrate figures include 12-13g Sugar Alcohol

	C	F	Cb
Snickers, Protein Bar, 1.8 oz	200	7	18
Solo, Gi, average all varieties 1.8 oz	200	7	26

Per Bar **C** **F** **Cb**

Special K:

Chewy Snack Bars,

	C	F	Cb
av. all varieties, 0.88 oz	100	2	19

Nourish:

	C	F	Cb
Bites, all varieties, 6 pieces	180	9	20
Chewy Nut Bars, av. all var., 1.3 oz	170	10	16
Protein Snack, av. all var., 1.23 oz	155	7	17

Supreme Protein:

High Protein:

	C	F	Cb
Caramel Nut Chocolate, 3.4 oz	390	15	26
PB Crunch, 3 oz	390	18	26
PB Jelly, 3.4 oz	390	15	35

Note: Carbohydrate figures include 14-15g sugar alcohol

thinkThin: *Per Bar*

	C	F	Cb
High Protein: Average all var.	230	9	24

Note: Carbohydrate figure includes 5-22g sugar alcohol

	C	F	Cb
Prot. & Fiber, average all var., 1.4 oz	150	5	20
Prot & Superfruit, av. all varieties	244	9	32
Protein Nut, average all var., 1.4 oz	190	12	16

Tiger's Milk:

	C	F	Cb
Protein Rich, 1.2 oz	140	5	19
Peanut Butter Crunch, 1.2 oz	150	6	18
King Size, average all varieties, 2 oz	225	9	28

Trader Joe's:

Chewy Coated Granola Bars, 6-Packs:

	C	F	Cb
Chocolate Chip, 1.3 oz	150	4	26
Raises the Bar, av., 1.2 oz	140	4	23
Fruit Bars: Fig 1.5 oz	120	2	24
Average other varieties, 1.5 oz	140	2.5	27

Granola Bars, 6-packs:

	C	F	Cb
Fiberful, average,1.2 oz	125	5	21
Trail Mix, 1.3 oz	150	5	23

Tri-O-Plex *(Chef Jay's):*

High Protein,

	C	F	Cb
Ban. Walnut, 4.2 oz	405	14	40
Duo, Bursting Peanut Butter	395	17	35

Vega:

	C	F	Cb
Protein Bars: Choc. P'Nut Butter, 2.5 oz	290	10	27
Sport, Choc. P'nut Butter, 2.1 oz	260	11	27
Snack Bar, Choc. Caramel, 1.6 oz	1280	8	21

Wickedly Prime: *Per 1.4 oz Bar*

	C	F	Cb
Banana Nut	180	11	21
Cashews & Cranberry	170	9	24
Cherry Nut Crunch	190	14	15
Nuts & Sea Salt	200	16	14
Peanut & Almond	200	15	14

Zone Perfect:

	C	F	Cb
High Protein Bars, average, 2 oz	235	9	22

Nutrition Bars:

	C	F	Cb
Chocolate Peanut Butter, 1.76 oz	210	7	24
Dark Choc. Almond, 1.58 oz	190	6	22
Salted Caramel Brownie, 1.58 oz	200	9	19

Cocoa & Hot Chocolate C F Cb

	C	F	Cb
Cocoa:			
Small (8 fl.oz):			
with Whole Milk	205	8.5	22
with Nonfat Milk	145	1	23
Tall (12 fl.oz): with Whole Milk	280	12	26
with Nonfat Milk	185	1	28
Hot Chocolate:			
Small (8 fl.oz): with Whole Milk	180	7	26
with Nonfat Milk	140	2	27
Tall (12 fl.oz): with Whole Milk	260	10	36
with Nonfat Milk	190	2	37
Cinnabon, Mochalatta Chill, 16 oz	420	17	63
Swiss Miss, Mixes, av., 1 packet	120	2.5	22

Cocoa - Chocolate Mixes

Add extra cals/fat/carbohydrate for milk
Carnation Breakfast Drinks ~ *See Page 38*

	C	F	Cb
Carnation: *Per 3 Tbsp*			
Malted Milk: Original	90	2	15
Chocolate	90	1	18
Ghirardelli:			
Premium Hot Cocoa: Caramel, 0.8 oz	90	1	20
Chocolate Mocha, 3 Tbsp	120	1.5	29
Double Chocolate, 3 Tbsp	120	1.5	30
Hershey's, Cocoa,			
Natural, unsweetened,			
1 Tbsp, 0.2 oz	10	0.5	3
Land O Lakes:			
Arctic White Coccoa, 1.3 oz	160	6	26
Other varieties, 1.3 oz	140	3.5	26
Nestle: *Per Per Single Serve Envelope*			
Chocolate Caramel	100	3	19
Dark Chocolate	100	3	19
Rich Milk Chocolate:			
Regular	80	3	14
Fat Free	20	0	4
No Sugar Added Fat Free	20	0	5
Nesquik Powder: *Per 2 Tbsp*			
Chocolate; Strawberry	50	0.5	12
Chocolate No Added Sugar	35	1	7
Ovaltine, All Natural Cocoa Mixes,			
average all varieties, 2 Tbsp	40	0	10
Swiss Miss: *Per Single Serve Envelope*			
Breakfast Blends: Great Start	60	1	11
Pick Me Up	110	2	23
Classics, Milk Chocolate:			
Hot Cocoa Mix	90	2	16
No Added Sugar	60	1	11
with Marshmallow	90	2	16
Rich Chocolate	120	2	23

Instant Coffee C F Cb

	C	F	Cb
Powder/Granules: *Regular or Decaffeinated,*			
1 level tsp	2	0	0.5
1 rounded tsp	4	0	1
Ground, 3 tsp	7	0	2
Brewed/Percolated, 1 cup, 8 fl.oz	4	0	1
Coffee with Milk/Cream/Creamers: *Per 8 oz Cup*			
Black:	4	0	1
with Whole Milk: Dash, 1 Tbsp	15	0.5	2
2 Tbsp, 1 fl.oz	25	1	2.5
with 2% Milk, 2 Tbsp	20	0.5	2.5
with 1% Milk, 2 Tbsp	20	0.5	2.5
with Fat Free Milk, 2 Tbsp	15	0	2.5
with Soy Milk: 1 Tbsp	10	0	1.5
2 Tbsp, 1 oz	15	0.5	2
with Half & Half: 2 Tbsp	50	3	3
¼ cup, 2 fl.oz	90	6	4
with Cream (light coffee), 2 Tbsp	65	6	2
with Coffee Mate: Liquid, reg., 1 T.	20	1	3
Liquid Fat Free, 1 Tbsp	25	0	2
Powder, 1 heaping tsp	15	1	2
Sugar ~ Add Extra: 1 heaping tsp	25	0	6
Single portion, 1 package	25	0	6
Sweeteners, *(Equal/Splenda/Sweet N Low),*			
Powder, 1 package	0	0	0

Flavored Coffee Mixes

	C	F	Cb
Chicory:			
Instant Coffee, 1 tsp	5	0	1
Coffee Essence, 1 tsp	15	0	4
Caffé D'Vita:			
Hot Cocoa, 1 oz	110	1.5	24
Hot Cocoa, Sugar Free, 0.5 oz	70	4.5	7
General Foods International:			
Average all varieties, 0.5 oz	60	3	10
Sugar-free, av. all varieties, 1 tsp	30	2.5	2
Cappuccino Coolers, all varieties, 0.5 oz	60	0	15
Hills Bros: *Per 3 Tbsp, 1 oz*			
Cappuccino: French Vanilla	120	4.5	19
Chocolate Hazelnut	110	3.5	19
Classic Cappuccino	120	5	17
Dark Chocolate	110	4	19
Mocha Mint	120	4	20
Nescafe, Memento, 1 stick,			
average all varieties	100	2.5	19
Starbucks, VIA, Iced Coffee,			
all varieties, 1 stick/packet	100	0	24

Coffee Shops/Restaurants

Per 8 fl.oz Cup (Unless Indicated) **C** **F** **Cb**

	C	F	Cb
Coffee, Regular/Percolated/Filtered	5	0	0
Americano Drip Coffee, 1 cup	7.5	0	1
Cafe Au Lait: 1 cup, 8 fl.oz	60	3.5	5
Nonfat Milk, 1 cup, 8 fl.oz	35	0	5
Caffe Latté:			
8 fl.oz cup: with Whole Milk	110	6	9
with 2% Milk	100	3.5	9
with Nonfat Milk	70	0	10
12 fl.oz: with Whole Milk	180	9	14
with Nonfat Milk	100	0	15
16 fl.oz: with Whole Milk	220	11	18
with Nonfat Milk	130	0	19
Cafe Mocha (Mochaccino): 8 fl.oz	150	6	20
12 fl.oz	230	9	31
16 fl.oz	290	12	41
Cappuccino:			
8 fl.oz cup: with Whole Milk	90	3.5	7
with 2% Milk	80	3	8
with Nonfat Milk	50	0	8
12 fl.oz: with Whole Milk	110	6	9
with 2% Milk	90	3.5	9
with Nonfat Milk	60	0	9
16 fl.oz: with Whole Milk	140	7	11
with 2% Milk	120	3.5	11
with Nonfat Milk	80	0	12
Mocha: *With Cream*			
8 fl.oz: with Whole Milk	200	11	22
with Nonfat Milk	160	6	22
12 fl.oz: Whole Milk	290	15	33
with Nonfat Milk	230	8	34
Iced Mocha: *Without Cream*			
12 fl.oz: with Whole Milk	170	6	26
with Nonfat Milk	130	2	27
Espresso: Single (Solo), 1 fl.oz	5	0	1
Double (Doppio), 2 fl.oz	10	0	2
Espresso con Panna,			
(w/ dollop wh. cream), solo, 1 fl.oz	30	2.5	2
Espresso Macchiato, solo, 1 fl.oz	5	0	1
Frappuccino: Tall, 12 fl.oz	180	2.5	37
Grande, 16 fl.oz	240	3	48
Frappuccino Mocha:			
(with Cream): Tall, 12 fl.oz	280	11	43
Grande, 16 fl.oz	380	15	57
Iced Latte, Similar to Caffe Latte			

McCafe (McDonald's) ~ See Fast Food, Page 216
Starbucks ~ See Fast-Foods Section , Page 243

Coffee Substitute Mixes **C** **F** **Cb**

Roasted Cereal Beverages ~ *(No Caffeine)*

	C	F	Cb
Cafix, Instant Beverage, 1 tsp	5	0	1
Kaffree Roma, Instant Beverage, 1 tsp	10	0	2
Teeccino, Herbal Coffees, 1 tsp	10	0	2

Irish & Liqueur Coffees

	C	F	Cb
Irish Coffee, without sugar	175	10	0
Liqueur Coffee, with cream,			
all varieties, av., 1 fl.oz	100	5	7

Coffee Extras

	C	F	Cb
Chocolate (Cocoa) Topping, $\frac{1}{2}$ tsp	5	0	1
Flavored Syrups: Regular, 2 Tbsp	80	0	20
Sugar-free, 2 Tbsp	0	0	0
Half & Half Cream: 2 Tbsp	40	3.5	1
Single serve pkg, $\frac{3}{8}$ fl.oz	15	1.5	0.5
Light whipped cream, 2 Tbsp	15	1.5	1
Marshmallows, miniature (2)	5	0	1
Sugar:			
1 single portion package	20	0	5
1 level tsp	15	0	4
1 heaping tsp	25	0	6
Equal/Splenda/Sweet 'N Low	0	0	0

Coffee Shop ~ Cakes, Cookies

Cookies:

	C	F	Cb
Biscotti, 1 oz	140	6.5	18
Chocolate Chip, 3 oz	350	15	54
Oatmeal Raisin, 3 oz	350	12	56
Peanut Butter, 3 oz	410	25	39
White Choc. Macadamia, 3.33 oz	420	20	55
Cakes/Pastries:			
Almond Croissant, 5 oz	620	35	67
Apple Danish, 5 oz	450	18	67
Banana Walnut, 4.5 oz	410	17	60
Brownie, 3 oz	390	24	42
Bundt, Chocolate, 4 oz	440	21	61
Carrot Cake, 4 oz	400	22	45
Chocolate Cake, 5 oz	530	28	65
Crumble Coffee Cake, 4.5 oz	500	25	65
Cupcake, 3 oz	330	16	43
Pound Cake, av., 3 oz	330	17	40
Cinnamon Roll, 6 oz	500	15	83
Donuts:			
Sugared, 1.8 oz	220	11	27
Glazed, 2 oz	250	12	34
Pretzel, large, 4 oz	290	5	52

Starbucks Bakery Items ~ See Page 244

READY TO DRINK COFFEE **C** **F** **Cb**

Bottled & Chilled:

Califia Farms: *With Almond Milk*

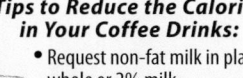

	C	F	Cb
Cold Brew Coffee, av., 10.5 fl.oz	115	4.5	18
Dunkin Donuts,			
Iced Coffee, av., 13.7 fl.oz	290	6	47
International Delight:			
Iced, all flavors, 8 fl.oz	150	2.5	29
Light varieties, 8 fl.oz	90	2.5	14
Kahlua, Cappuccino Shake, 10.5 fl.oz	130	2	24
Starbucks:			
Cold Brew: *Per 11 fl.oz*			
Regular	50	0	13
Unsweetened	15	0	3
Cocoa & Honey, w/ Cream	150	5	24
Vanilla & Fig, w/ Cream	150	4	24
Doubleshot Energy: *Per 15 fl.oz Can*			
Coffee Drink	210	2.5	36
Hazelnut Drink	210	3	31
Mocha/Vanilla Drink	205	2.5	34
White Chocolate Drink	210	3	31
Doubleshot Espresso: *Per 6.5 fl.oz Can*			
Espresso & Cream	140	6	18
Espresso & Cream Light	70	4	5
Frappuccino Coffee Drink: *Per 9.5 fl.oz Bottle*			
Mocha	180	3	33
Light Mocha	100	3	12
Vanilla	200	3	37
Iced Coffee: *Per 11 fl.oz Bottle*			
Coffee: with Milk, sweetened	110	0.5	23
Light, sweetened	50	0	11
Caramel; Vanilla, swtnd, av.	110	0.5	23
Vanilla	120	0.5	22
Iced Espresso Classics (Chilled): *Per 8 fl.oz Bottle*			
Caffe Mocha	140	2.5	23
Caramel Macchiato; Van. Latte	130	2.5	21
Skinny, Caramel Macchiato, Van. Latte	70	0	10
Starbucks Refreshers ~ *See Page 40*			
TruMoo:			
Coffee Milk:			
Low-Fat (1%), 8 fl.oz	130	2.5	20
Fat-Free, 8 fl.oz	110	0	20

Tips to Reduce the Calories in Your Coffee Drinks:

- Request non-fat milk in place of whole or 2% milk
- Downsize to 8 fl.oz or 12 fl.oz
- Avoid cream on frappuccinos
- Replace sugar with *Equal, Splenda, Stevia* or *Sweet 'N Low*
- Avoid syrup add-ons

CAFFEINE COUNTER

Moderate caffeine intake is not harmful to healthy adults. However, frequent large amounts (over 350mg/day) may cause dependency ('caffeinism') and adversely affect health. **To be safe, limit caffeine to 200mg/day.** Avoid if pregnant, breastfeeding, a child under 8, have sleep problems, an overactive bladder or heart arrhythmia.

	Caffeine (mg)
Coffee: Instant: Weak, 1 level teaspoon	30
Medium, 1 rounded teaspoon	60
Strong, 1 heaping teaspoon	100
Decaffeinated, 1 rounded teaspoon	2
Bags (Folgers), 1 bag (6-8 fl.oz)	115
Ground, 1 Tbsp, 0.2 oz	60
Bottled (Ready-To-Drink), 9.5 fl.oz	70
Coffee Shop: Brewed, 8 fl.oz	110-150
Cappuccino/Latte: 1 cup, 8 fl.oz	75
Tall, 12 fl.oz	110
Large, 16 fl.oz	150
Decappuccino, decaffeinated	5
Espresso: Regular/Single/Solo	75
Double/Doppio	150
Iced Coffee w/o Milk, 12 fl.oz	140
Latte, 1 cup, 8 fl.oz	75
Mocha, 1 cup, 8 fl.oz	90
Hot Chocolate, 8 fl.oz	15
Black Tea: Weak, 1 cup	20
Medium Strength, 1 cup	40
Strong, 1 cup	70
Decaffeinated Tea, 1 cup	0-5
Herbal Tea, 1 cup	0
Green Tea, 1 cup	20
Iced Tea, tall glass/can, 12 fl.oz	20-30
Soft Drinks: *Per 12 fl.oz Can*	
Coca-Cola; Pepsi (Regular/Diet)	35
Diet Coke; TAB; RC Cola (Regular)	45
Dr. Pepper; Sunkist Orange	40
Pepsi One; Mountain Dew; Mellow Yellow; Surge	55
Pepsi Max (Regular/Diet) Sun Drop (Reg/Diet)	70
7-Up, Fanta, Sprite, Fresca, Diet Rite Cola	0
Energy Drinks (with added caffeine):	
(AMP, Adrenaline Rush, Full Throttle Monster, No Fear, Red Bull, Rockstar)	
Average all brands: 8 fl.oz	80
16 fl.oz	160
NOS Energy, 16 fl.oz	260
Chocolate Bars: Milk Chocolate, 2 oz	20
Dark Chocolate, 2 oz	30
Choc Chip Cookies, 2 medium, 2 oz	6
Chocolate Syrup, 2 Tbsp, 1.4 oz	5
Guarana, *GNC*, 1 tablet	90
Medicinals: *Excedrin Extra*/Migraine, 1 tab.	65
Jet Alert/NoDoz, 1 tablet	200
Stay Awake (Walgreens), Vivarin, 1 tab.	200

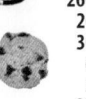

Energy/Protein Drinks	C	F	Cb
5-hour Energy, 2 fl.oz	4	0	1
A.B.B:			
Energy: Speed Shot, 8.5 fl.oz	0	0	0
Ripped Force, 18 fl.oz	90	0	23
Pure-Pro:			
Pure Pro 35 Shake, all flav., 12 fl.oz	160	0.5	5
Pure Pro 50, all flavors, 14.5 fl.oz	240	1.5	7
Maxx Recovery, all flavors, 18 fl.oz	400	0.5	60
AdvantEDGE (EAS),			
RTD Shakes, av., 11 fl.oz	100	2.5	5
AllSport Hydration:			
Regular, all flavors, 20 fl.oz	150	0	40
Zero, 20 fl.oz	0	0	0
AMP Energy: Per 16 fl.oz Can			
Orig.; Strawb. Limeade; P'Fruit	220	0	58
Cherry Blast	120	0	31
Tropical Punch	100	0	26
Boosted, Wild Berry Cherry	100	0	26
Arbonne:			
Protein Shakes, 2 scoops, 1.5 oz	160	3	14
Arizona: Per 11.5 fl.oz Can			
Nat. Energy: Arnold Palmer	70	0	20
Other Fruit Flavors	100	0	26
Atkins, Shakes, av., 11 fl.oz	155	9	4
Bariatrix, Proti-Max,			
Anytime Shakes, av., 11 fl.oz	160	9	3
Bawls Guarana: Per 10 fl.oz Bottle			
Original; Cherry, average	120	0	31
Ginger; Orange; Root Beer	135	0	33
Blue Sky,			
Blue Energy Drink, 8 fl.oz	120	0	29
BodyArmor, SuperDrinks,			
all flavors, 16 fl.oz	140	0	36
Bolthouse: Per 8 fl.oz			
Breakfast Smoothies,			
Peach/Strawb. Parfait, average	190	2.5	35
Protein Plus: Chocolate	210	3	29
Mango	200	0.5	33
Vanilla Bean	170	3	21
Boost (Nestle Health Care): Per 8 fl.oz			
Original, all flavors	240	4	41
Glucose Control, all flavors	190	7	16
High Protein, all flavors	240	6	33
Plus, all flavors	360	14	45
Carnation:			
B'Fast Essentials, Powder:			
Av. all flav., 1 env., 1.3 oz	130	0	27
Light Start, av., 0.7 oz	60	0	12
Ready To Drink: Reg., all flav., 8 fl.oz	240	4	41
High Protein, average, 8 fl.oz	220	6	28
Celestial Seasoning,			
Kombucha, all flavors, 2 oz shot	30	0	8

	C	F	Cb
CeraSport,			
EX1, Lime Flavor, 8.5 fl.oz	20	0	1
Champion Lyte, Sports Drink, 8 fl.oz	0	0	0
Champion Performance:			
Heavyweight Gainer 900,			
av. all flavors, 4 scps, 5.4 oz	600	7	102
Metabolol II, 2 scoops, 2.3 oz	260	3	40
Pure Whey Plus, av., 1 scoop, 1.2 oz	130	2	5
UltraMet, 2.7 oz pkt	280	4	20
Clif: Protein Mix, Chocolate, 1.6 oz	160	0	31
Shot, Energy Gel, av., 1.2 oz pkt	100	0	24
Cocaine, Energy, 8.4 fl.oz can	70	0	18
Core Power:			
26g, av. all flavors, 11.5 fl.oz	240	3.5	27
Elite, 42g, av. all flav., 14 fl.oz	240	3.5	12
Light, 20g, av. all flavors, 11.5 fl.oz	150	3.5	12
Curves, Protein Drink,			
Choc.; Vanilla, 2 scoops, 1 oz	120	1	12
EAS ~ See AdvantEdge & Myoplex			
Ensure: Per Bottle			
Original, all flavors, 8 fl.oz	220	6	33
Clear, all flavors, 10 fl.oz	180	0	37
Enlive, av. all flavors, 8 fl.oz	350	11	44
High Protein , all flav., 8 fl.oz	160	2	19
Plus, all flavors, 8 fl.oz	350	11	50
Enterex, Diabetic, all flavors, 8 fl.oz	240	9	27
Enu, Nutritional Shakes, av., 11 fl.oz	450	17	53
FRS, Energy & Endurance, all flav., 11.5 fl.oz	80	0	22
Fruit₂O (Veryfine): Classic 20 fl.oz	0	0	0
Sparkling, 20 fl.oz	0	0	1
Full Throttle: Per 16 fl.oz			
Energy: Citrus; Blue Agave	220	0	58
Orange	220	0	52
Fuze:			
Blends, average, 16.9 fl.oz	185	0.5	43
Juice: Berry Punch, 8 fl.oz	80	0	21
Strawb. Lemonade, 8 fl.oz	100	0	26
Gatorade G Series:			
Endurance: Carb Energy Drink, 4 fl.oz	120	0	30
Thirst Quencher: 12 fl oz	90	0	22
Flow, Thirst Quencher, 20 fl.oz	140	0	35
Prime, Sports Fuel, 4 fl.oz	100	0	25
Recover, Protein Shake,			
Chocolate, 11.2 fl.oz	280	1	46
Whey Protein Powder Shakes:			
Chocolate, ⅓ cup, 1.1 oz	120	2	6
Other Flavors, ⅓ cup, 1 oz	110	1.5	4
Genisoy, Prot. Pdr, Choc.; Van., 1.3 oz	125	0	18

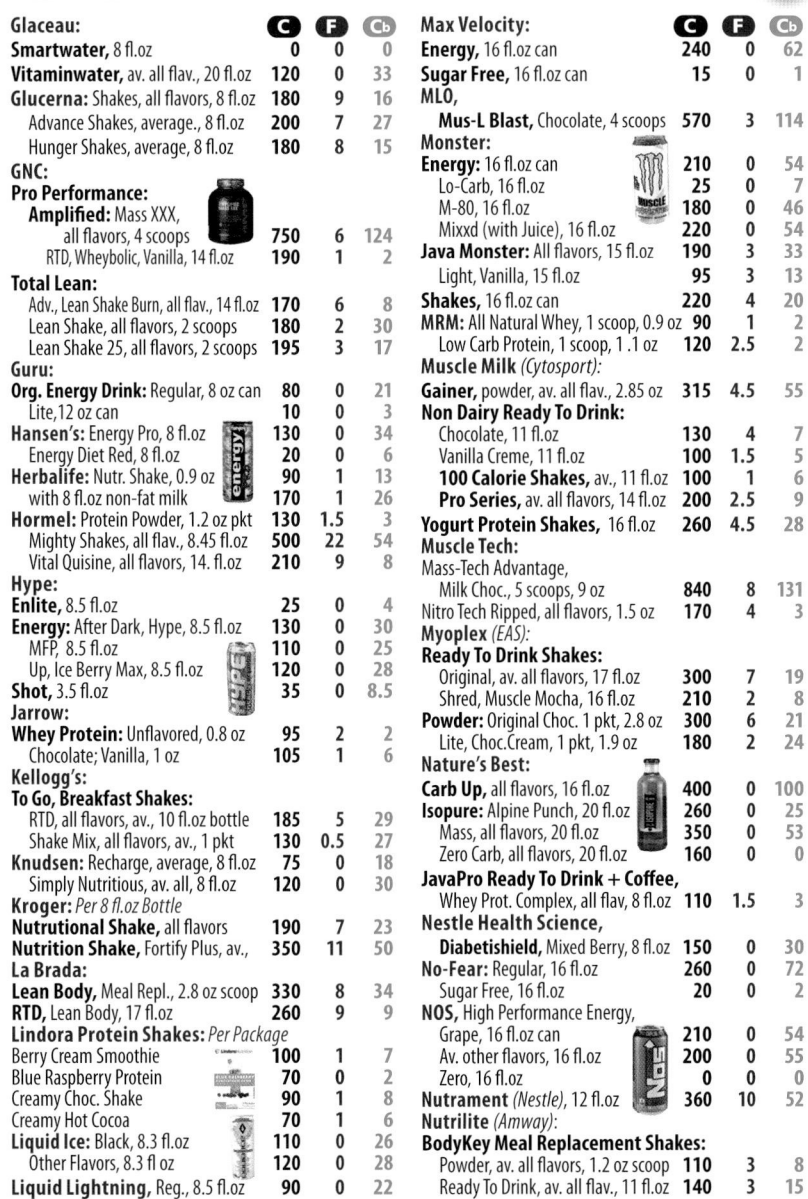

	C	F	Cb
Glaceau:			
Smartwater, 8 fl.oz	0	0	0
Vitaminwater, av. all flav., 20 fl.oz	120	0	33
Glucerna: Shakes, all flavors, 8 fl.oz	180	9	16
Advance Shakes, average., 8 fl.oz	200	7	27
Hunger Shakes, average, 8 fl.oz	180	8	15
GNC:			
Pro Performance:			
Amplified: Mass XXX,			
all flavors, 4 scoops	750	6	124
RTD, Wheybolic, Vanilla, 14 fl.oz	190	1	2
Total Lean:			
Adv., Lean Shake Burn, all flav., 14 fl.oz	170	6	8
Lean Shake, all flavors, 2 scoops	180	2	30
Lean Shake 25, all flavors, 2 scoops	195	3	17
Guru:			
Org. Energy Drink: Regular, 8 oz can	80	0	21
Lite,12 oz can	10	0	3
Hansen's: Energy Pro, 8 fl.oz	130	0	34
Energy Diet Red, 8 fl.oz	20	0	6
Herbalife: Nutr. Shake, 0.9 oz	90	1	13
with 8 fl.oz non-fat milk	170	1	26
Hormel: Protein Powder, 1.2 oz pkt	130	1.5	3
Mighty Shakes, all flav., 8.45 fl.oz	500	22	54
Vital Quisine, all flavors, 14. fl.oz	210	9	8
Hype:			
Enlite, 8.5 fl.oz	25	0	4
Energy: After Dark, Hype, 8.5 fl.oz	130	0	30
MFP, 8.5 fl.oz	110	0	25
Up, Ice Berry Max, 8.5 fl.oz	120	0	28
Shot, 3.5 fl.oz	35	0	8.5
Jarrow:			
Whey Protein: Unflavored, 0.8 oz	95	2	2
Chocolate; Vanilla, 1 oz	105	1	6
Kellogg's:			
To Go, Breakfast Shakes:			
RTD, all flavors, av., 10 fl.oz bottle	185	5	29
Shake Mix, all flavors, av., 1 pkt	130	0.5	27
Knudsen: Recharge, average, 8 fl.oz	75	0	18
Simply Nutritious, av. all, 8 fl.oz	120	0	30
Kroger: *Per 8 fl.oz Bottle*			
Nutrutional Shake, all flavors	190	7	23
Nutrition Shake, Fortify Plus, av.,	350	11	50
La Brada:			
Lean Body, Meal Repl., 2.8 oz scoop	330	8	34
RTD, Lean Body, 17 fl.oz	260	9	9
Lindora Protein Shakes: *Per Package*			
Berry Cream Smoothie	100	1	7
Blue Raspberry Protein	70	0	2
Creamy Choc. Shake	90	1	8
Creamy Hot Cocoa	70	1	6
Liquid Ice: Black, 8.3 fl.oz	110	0	26
Other Flavors, 8.3 fl oz	120	0	28
Liquid Lightning, Reg., 8.5 fl.oz	90	0	22

	C	F	Cb
Max Velocity:			
Energy, 16 fl.oz can	240	0	62
Sugar Free, 16 fl.oz can	15	0	1
MLO,			
Mus-L Blast, Chocolate, 4 scoops	570	3	114
Monster:			
Energy: 16 fl.oz can	210	0	54
Lo-Carb, 16 fl.oz	25	0	7
M-80, 16 fl.oz	180	0	46
Mixxd (with Juice), 16 fl.oz	220	0	54
Java Monster: All flavors, 15 fl.oz	190	3	33
Light, Vanilla, 15 fl.oz	95	3	13
Shakes, 16 fl.oz can	220	4	20
MRM: All Natural Whey, 1 scoop, 0.9 oz	90	1	2
Low Carb Protein, 1 scoop, 1.1 oz	120	2.5	2
Muscle Milk *(Cytosport):*			
Gainer, powder, av. all flav., 2.85 oz	315	4.5	55
Non Dairy Ready To Drink:			
Chocolate, 11 fl.oz	130	4	7
Vanilla Creme, 11 fl.oz	100	1.5	5
100 Calorie Shakes, av., 11 fl.oz	100	1	6
Pro Series, av. all flavors, 14 fl.oz	200	2.5	9
Yogurt Protein Shakes, 16 fl.oz	260	4.5	28
Muscle Tech:			
Mass-Tech Advantage,			
Milk Choc., 5 scoops, 9 oz	840	8	131
Nitro Tech Ripped, all flavors, 1.5 oz	170	4	3
Myoplex *(EAS):*			
Ready To Drink Shakes:			
Original, av. all flavors, 17 fl.oz	300	7	19
Shred, Muscle Mocha, 16 fl.oz	210	2	8
Powder: Original Choc. 1 pkt, 2.8 oz	300	6	21
Lite, Choc.Cream, 1 pkt, 1.9 oz	180	2	24
Nature's Best:			
Carb Up, all flavors, 16 fl.oz	400	0	100
Isopure: Alpine Punch, 20 fl.oz	260	0	25
Mass, all flavors, 20 fl.oz	350	0	53
Zero Carb, all flavors, 20 fl.oz	160	0	0
JavaPro Ready To Drink + Coffee,			
Whey Prot. Complex, all flav, 8 fl.oz	110	1.5	3
Nestle Health Science,			
Diabetishield, Mixed Berry, 8 fl.oz	150	0	30
No-Fear: Regular, 16 fl.oz	260	0	72
Sugar Free, 16 fl.oz	20	0	2
NOS, High Performance Energy,			
Grape, 16 fl.oz can	210	0	54
Av. other flavors, 16 fl.oz	200	0	55
Zero, 16 fl.oz	0	0	0
Nutrament *(Nestle),* 12 fl.oz	360	10	52
Nutrilite *(Amway):*			
BodyKey Meal Replacement Shakes:			
Powder, av. all flavors, 1.2 oz scoop	110	3	8
Ready To Drink, av. all flav., 11 fl.oz	140	3	15

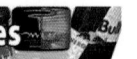
Energy/Protein Drinks (Cont)

	C	F	Cb
Optifast: *(Nestle):*			
800: Shake Mix, 1 pkg	160	3.5	18
Ready To Drink Shakes, 8 fl.oz	160	3.5	18
HP Shake Mix, 1 pkg	200	6	10
Optimum Nutrition:			
Gold Standard:			
100% Whey, av. all flavors, 1 oz scp	120	1	4
Gainer, av. all flav., 7.9 oz scoop	770	10	113
Hydro Whey, average. 1.4 oz scoop	140	1	3
Oats & Whey, average, 1.9 oz scoop	205	1.5	23
Optisource *(Nestle),*			
Very High Prot. Drink, Strawb., 8 fl.oz	200	6	12
OrGain: *Per*			
Nutr. Prot. Shake, Choc Fudge, 14 fl.oz	150	4	11
Prot. Shake, Iced Cafe Mocha, 11 fl.oz	255	7	32
Powerade,			
ION4, av. all flavors, 20 fl.oz bottle	150	0	35
PowerBar: Protein Shakes, 14 fl.oz	160	3	5
Perfect Energy Blends, av., 1 pouch	80	0	21
Power Gel, average, 1.5 oz pkg	110	0	27
Simple Fruits, av. all flav., 1 pouch	100	0	25
Premier Protein *(Premier Nutrition):*			
Powder, Choc./Vanilla, average, 1.65 oz	180	3.5	8
Shakes, average, 11 fl.oz bottle	160	3	5
Propel, Purified Water, 12 fl.oz	0	0	0
Protein2O, av. all flavors, 16.9 fl oz	60	0	2
Pure Protein: *Per 11 fl.oz Bottle or Can*			
23 Gram Shakes, average	115	0.5	8
35 Gram Shakes: Banana	150	1	1
Average other flavors	165	1.5	2
Powder, av., 1 scoop, 1.16 oz	130	2	6
Radioactive:			
Regular: 10.5 oz	150	0	37
16 oz	220	0	56
Sugar Free, all sizes	0	0	0
Red Bull:			
Energy Drink: Average, 8.4 fl.oz	110	0	28
12 fl.oz can	160	0	40
Sugar-Free, 8.4 fl.oz	10	0	3
Zero Calories, 8.4 fl.oz	0	0	0
Revival:			
Soy Mix, unsweetened:			
Plain, 2 scoops, 0.95 oz	105	1	4
Average all flavors, 2 scoops	115	2.5	5
Rhino's, Energy Drink, all flav., 100ml	50	0	11
Rip It, Energy Fuel, Citrus X, 16 fl.oz	200	0	52
Rockstar: *Per 16 fl.oz Can*			
Energy Drink: Punched, av.	270	0	62
Sugar Free	20	0	0
Rumble, Supershake, 12 fl.oz	250	8	28
Rush: *Per 8.4 fl.oz*			
Energy Drink: Regular	120	0	32
with Maca, 8 fl.oz	130	0	30

	C	F	Cb
Skratch Labs:			
Hydration Drink Mix: *16 fl. oz Prepared*			
Anytime Mix, all flav., 1 scoop, 0.46 oz	50	0	12
Hyper, Mango, 0.9 oz	70	0	16
Rescue, Lemons & Limes, 0.76 oz	70	0	17
Sport Mix, average, 1 scoop, 0.78 oz	80	0	20
Sport Recovery Mix, all flav., 1.76 oz	200	3.5	35
Slim-Fast:			
Original, Protein Shakes, av., 11 fl.oz	185	6	24
Advanced Nutrition:			
Meal Replacement Shakes, av., 11 fl.oz	180	8	6
Smoothies, Powder, av., 1 scoop, 0.9 oz	105	3.5	8
SoBe: *Per 20 fl.oz Can/Bottle*			
Citrus Energy Fruit Drink	250	0	64
Lifewater: Strawberry Kiwi	100	0	26
Coconut Water	80	0	21
O-Cal, all flavors	0	0	9
Note: Carb figure inlude 7-10g sugar alcohol			
Solixir, Energy Drink, av. all, 12 fl.oz	55	0	13
Special K,			
Protein Shakes, av. all flav.	185	5	23
Spiru-Tein:			
Energy Meal Shake Powder:			
Chai Latte, 1.2 oz scoop	130	0	16
Choc. Chip Cookie Dough, 1.2 oz	130	1.5	14
Gold: Strawberry, 1.3 oz scoop	130	0	20
Average other flavors, 1.2 oz	100	0	21
PureTrition, av., 1.3 oz scoop	115	0.5	10
Sport, average, 2.25 oz scoop	260	9	26
Whey, Cookies & Cream, 1.2 oz scp	125	2	15
Starbucks: Refreshers, av., 12 fl.oz	65	0	19
Doubleshot Energy ~ *See page 37*			
Steaz: Energy, all flav., 12 fl.oz	135	0	35
Zero Calorie, Berry, 12 fl.oz	0	0	0
The Sports Club/LA:			
Beachbody Whey Prot. Powder,			
Chocolate; Vanilla, av., 1 scoop, 1 oz	110	2	4.5
Twin Lab, MVP Fuel, all flav., 1 sc., 0.5 oz	25	0	6
Vega, Protein Shake, 11 fl.oz	170	5	14
Vemma: Bod-e Burn, 8 fl.oz can	110	0	12
Energy Drinks, 8.3 fl.oz can	80	0	21
Vemma, 8.3 fl.oz can	50	0	14
Venom: Mojave Rattler, 16 fl.oz	50	0	8
Av. other varieties, 16 fl.oz	235	0	57
Vital Whey, 100% Whey, 0.7 oz	85	1	2
Weider: 100% Whey, av., 1.4 oz sc.	155	3	11
Creatine ATP, ½ cup, 1.7 oz	210	0	37
Dynamic Wt Gainer, av., 4.5 oz	460	2	96
Mega Mass 2000, av., 3.5 oz	400	7	61
Pro Carb, Ult. Mass Gainer,			
6 scoops, average, 7 oz	770	6	161
XS *(Quixtar),* Energy Drink, 8.4 oz	10	0	0
Zola Acai: Original Juice, 8 fl.oz	125	2	25
Pomegranate, Blueberry, 8 fl.oz	120	2	25

Quick Guide — C F Cb

Orange Juice
Average ~ Fresh

	C	F	Cb
½ Cup, 4 fl.oz	55	0	13
Small Glass, 6 fl.oz	85	0	19
Regular Cup 8 fl.oz	110	0.5	26
Regular Glass, 12 fl.oz	160	0.5	39
10 fl.oz Bottle	140	0.5	32
11.5 fl.oz Can	160	0.5	37
16 fl.oz Bottle	225	1	52
20 fl.oz Bottle	280	1	64

Juices ~ Generic

Average All Brands:

	C	F	Cb
Aloe Vera Juice, unsweetened, 2 oz	10	0	0
Apple Juice: 8 fl.oz	120	0	29
10 fl.oz Bottle	145	0.5	36
16 fl.oz	235	0.5	58
Cactus Water, 1 Cup, 8 oz	25	0	6
Carrot Juice: Fresh, 6 fl.oz	35	0	8
Sweetened, 6 fl.oz	75	0	17
Coconut Water, 8 fl.oz	50	0.5	9
Cranberry Juice, Cocktail/Blend	140	0	34
Fruit Blends, average all, 8 fl.oz	110	0	27
Fruit Nectars, average all, 8 fl.oz	140	0	36
Grape Juice, 8 fl.oz	155	0	38
Grapefruit Juice, 8 fl.oz	95	0	22
Lemon/Lime Juice: 1 Tbsp	5	0	1
1 cup, 8 fl.oz	50	0.5	16
Concentrate, 1 tsp	0	0	0
Noni Juice:			
Tahitian, 2 Tbsp, 1 fl.oz	15	0	3
Tahiti Traders, 1 fl.oz	20	0	5
Papaya/Peach Nectar, av., 8 fl.oz	140	0	36
Passion Fruit Juice, Fresh:			
Purple, 1 cup, 8 fl.oz	125	0	34
Yellow, 1 cup, 8 fl.oz	80	1.5	14
Pear Nectar, 8 fl.oz	150	0	40
Pineapple Juice, 8 fl.oz	130	0	32
Pomegranate Juice, 8 fl.oz	160	0	40
Prune Juice, 8 fl.oz	180	0	45
Strawberry/Raspberry Juice, 8 fl.oz	100	0	23
Tangerine Juice, 8 fl.oz	105	0.5	25
Tomato Juice, 8 fl.oz	40	0	10
Vegetable Juice, 8 fl.oz	45	0	11
Wheat Grass Juice:			
1 fl.oz 'Shot'	10	0	1.5
2 fl.oz 'Shot'	20	0	3

Quick Guide — C F Cb

Fruit Smoothies (Jamba Juice; Smoothie King)
Average All Brands

	C	F	Cb
Fruit Only: 8 fl.oz	115	0.5	29
12 fl.oz	175	1	43
16 fl.oz	230	1	58
24 fl.oz	350	1	78
Fruit + Non-Fat Milk/Soy:			
12 fl.oz	135	0	29
16 fl.oz	155	0	37
24 fl.oz	265	1	59
Fruit + Non-Fat Frozen Yogurt/Sherbet:			
12 fl.oz	200	0.5	47
16 fl.oz	265	1	63
24 fl.oz	395	1.5	95

Juice ~ Brands

Per 8 fl.oz Unless Indicated

Apple & Eve:
100% Juice, No Sugar Added:

	C	F	Cb
Cherries & Berries; Cranb. Raspb., av.	120	0	29
Cranberry Apple	130	0	33
Cranberry Pomegranate	140	0	34
Fruitables, av. all flav., 6.75 fl.oz	60	0	14
Organic Quenchers, all flav., 6.75 fl.oz	40	0	10
Bolthouse Farms: Per 8 fl.oz			
Juice: 100% Carrot	70	0	15
100% Pomegranate	150	0	38
Acai + 10 Superblend	120	0	31
Mango Ginger + Carrot	110	0.5	27
Orange + Carrot	100	0	22
Fruit Smoothies: Amazing Mango	130	0	31
Berry Boost	120	0	27
Blue Goodness	170	1.5	41
C-Boost	110	0	27
Green Goodness	130	0	30
Strawberry Banana	130	0	32
Bright & Early (Minute Maid),			
Orange Flavored Drink, 8 fl.oz	110	0	30
Cactus Cooler, Orange Pineapple Blast,			
12 fl oz can	150	0	40
Campbell's:			
Tomato Juice: 5.5 fl.oz can	30	0	7
8 fl.oz	50	0	10

Juice Brands (Cont)   **C** **F** **Cb**

Per 8 fl.oz Unless Indicated

	C	F	Cb
Califia Farms: *Per 8 fl.oz Unless Indicated*			
Agua Fresca:			
Strawberry Basil	80	0	20
Watermelon Ginger Lime	60	0	14
Ginger Limeade	90	0	21
Meyer Lemonade	80	0	21
Orange Juice, 10. 5 fl.oz	140	0.5	32
Tangerine	100	0	24
Capri Sun: *Per 6 fl.oz*			
100% Juice, average,	85	0	21
Juice Drinks,			
(25% Less Sugar), all flavors	50	0	14
Roarin' Waters, all flav., 6 fl.oz	30	0	8
Clamato: *Per 8 fl.oz*			
Original Tomato Cocktail	60	0	12
Picante	60	0	13
Coco Joy, Coconut Water, 8.4 fl.oz	30	0	7
Coco Libre, Coconut Water, 11 fl.oz pkg	60	0	14
CocoZia, Coconut Water:			
100% Organic, 11.1 fl.oz pkg	70	0	16
Original, 8 fl.oz	40	0	10
Chocolate, 8 fl.oz	60	0.5	13
Dole: *Per 8 fl.oz*			
100% Pure, Chilled or Frozen, av.	120	0	28
Blended Juices, average all flavors	120	0	30
Florida's Natural: *Per 8 fl.oz*			
Apple Juice	120	0	29
Cranberry Ruby Red Cocktail	130	0	32
Orange, No Pulp	110	0	26
100% Blends: Orange Mango	110	0	27
Orange Pineapple	130	0	31
Orange Strawberry	110	0	26
Ruby Red Grapefruit, Original	90	0	22
Goya: *Per 12 fl.oz Can*			
Nectar: Guava; Tamarind	240	0	59
Mango	230	0	56
Papaya; Peach, average	220	0	55
Average other varieties	220	0	55

Per 8 fl.oz Unless Indicated

	C	F	Cb
Great Value *(Walmart):*			
100% Juice: *Per 8 fl.oz*			
Apple	110	0	28
Cranberry Pomegranate	140	0	35
Grape	160	0	40
Orange, all varieties	110	0	26
White Grape	150	0	38
Hansen's:			
Juice Box: *Per 6.75 fl.oz Box*			
Awesome Apple; Loud Lemonade, av.	90	0	23
Burstin Berry; Totally Tropical	100	0	24
Strawberry Banana	110	0	27
Junior Juice,			
100% Juice, av. of flavors, 4.23 oz box	60	0	16
Natural, (64 fl.oz Bottles): *Per 8 fl.oz*			
Apple	120	0	28
Apple Strawberry	110	0	27
Cranberry Apple	110	0	27
Cranberry Grape	140	0	35
Grape	120	0	33
White Grape	140	0	36
Hawaii's Own, Frozen Concentrate, 10% Juice, average all flavors, 8 fl.oz prepared	105	0	27
Hi-C Juice Drinks: *Per 6.75 fl.oz Box*			
Flashin' Fruit Punch	90	0	25
Orange Lavaburst	90	0	25
Poppin' Lemonade	100	0	27
Hood: *Per 8 fl.oz*			
Apple	120	0	31
Lemonade	110	0	29
Orange	120	0	30
Jamba Juice ~ *See Fast-Foods Section*			
Juicy Juice *(Nestle):*			
Average all flavors:			
4.23 fl.oz box	60	0	15
6.75 fl.oz box	100	0	24
Kerns:			
Nectars: *Per 11.5 fl.oz Can*			
Guava; Strawberry	210	0	53
Pear; Strawb. Banana, av.	220	0	53
Pineapple Coconut	280	8	53
L & A: *Per 8 fl.oz*			
All Cherry	180	0	45
All Cranberry	60	0	14
Papaya Delight	130	0	32
Pineapple Coconut	140	3	28

Juice Brands (Cont)

Per 8 fl.oz Unless Indicated

	C	F	Cb
Lakewood Organic: *Per 8 fl.oz*			
Blends: Acai Amazon Berry	130	1.5	29
Blueberry Blend	120	0	31
Cranberry Lemonade	100	0	24
Lemonade	100	0	25
Pineapple Coconut	190	8	29
Pomegranate Lemonade	100	0	26
Super Kale	100	0	24
Super Tomato	70	0	15
Super Veggie	60	0	13
Pure: Apple	120	0	30
Beet	100	0	23
Blueberry	110	0	26
Carrot	90	0	21
Cranberry	80	0	19
Noni	5	0	1
Orange	120	0	28
Pineapple	130	0	31
Pink Grapefruit	100	0	24
Prune	180	0	42
Langers: *Per 8 fl.oz*			
100% Juice: Apple Cider	120	0	28
Apple Juice	120	0	28
Red/White Grape Juice	160	0	40
Juice Cocktails (27% Juice):			
Blueberry Cranberry	135	0	34
Cranberry	140	0	35
Cranberry Grape	165	0	41
Cranberry Raspberry	140	0	35
20% Juice, all flavors	120	0	30
Martinellli's: *Per 8 fl.oz*			
Juice, 100% Apple, all varieties	140	0	35
Sparkling: Apple Cider	140	0	35
Apple-Cranberry	110	0	27
Apple Grape	120	0	31
Apple-Mango/Pomegranate	140	0	34
Apple-Pear/Marionberry, av.	125	0	31
Minute Maid:			
15.2 fl.oz Bottles: *Per Bottle*			
Apple Juice	210	0	52
Cranb. Apple Raspberry	230	0	61
Cranberry Grape	270	0	74
Pineapple Orange	220	0	55

Per 8 fl.oz Unless Indicated

	C	F	Cb
Minute Maid (Cont):			
Orange Juice,			
Pure, No Pulp, 8 fl.oz	110	0	26
Coolers, average all flavors, 6.75 fl.oz	100	0	26
Kid's Juice Boxes, 100% Juice,			
Apple White Grape, 6.75 fl.oz	90	0	22
Light Juices: Orange, 8 fl.oz	50	0	13
With Tea; Light Lemonade, 8 fl.oz	15	0	3
Soft Frozen Concentrate,			
Limeade, 3 fl.oz tube	70	0	19
Mott's:			
100% Juice:			
Original Apple, 8 fl.oz	120	0	29
Apple White Grape, 6.75 fl.oz	130	0	31
Fruit Punch, 4.23 fl.oz	60	0	15
Light, Apple, 8 fl.oz	50	0	12
Juice Drink:			
Fruit Punch Rush, 8 fl.oz	60	0	16
Strawberry Boom, 8 fl.oz	60	0	15
Wild Grape Surge, 8 fl.oz	60	0	16
Medleys:			
Apple, 8 fl.oz	110	0	25
Grape, 8 fl.oz	140	0	33
Mott's For Tots (47-54% Juice):			
40% Less Sugar:			
Apple Wh. Grape; Fruit Punch, 8 fl.oz	70	0	17
Average other flavors, 8 fl.oz	60	0	16
Naked Juice: *Per 15.2 fl.oz*			
100% Juice, No Sugar Added:			
O-J	210	0	51
Orange Mango	250	0	59
Pomegranate Blueberry	290	0	68
100% Juice Smoothie, No Sugar Added:			
Berry Blast; Strawb. Banana	250	0	55
Mighty Mango	290	0	68
Boosted: Acai Machine	300	6	59
Blue Machine	170	0	40
Green Machine	270	0	63
Power-C Machine	230	0	55
Red Machine	320	9	59
Coconut Water: Pure, 16.9 fl.oz	80	0	21
Kale Coconut, 16.9 fl.oz	120	0	30
Pineapple Coconut, 8 fl.oz	50	0	13

Juice Brands (Cont)

	C	F	Cb

Per 8 fl.oz Unless Indicated

Nantucket Nectars:

100% Juice: *Per 16 fl.oz*

	C	F	Cb
Peach Orange	270	0	64
Pineapple Orange Banana	290	0	69
Pomegranate Cherry	230	0	57
Premium Orange Juice	220	0	51
Pressed Apple	240	0	59
Juice Cocktail, Cranberry	240	0	59

Juice Drinks: *Per 16 fl.oz*

	C	F	Cb
Orange Mango	220	0	59
Pineapple Orange Guava	210	0	52
Pomegranate Pear	230	0	57
Red Plum	220	0	53
Watermelon Strawberry	220	0	55
Lemonade, Squeezed	180	0	47

Newman's Own: *Per 8 fl.oz*

	C	F	Cb
Lemonade, Regular; Pink	110	0	27
Limeade	140	0	34

Fruit Juice Cocktail:

	C	F	Cb
Gorilla Grape	110	0	29
Orange Mango Tango	130	0	33

Northland: *Per 8 fl.oz*

100% Juice:

	C	F	Cb
Blueberry Blackberry Acaí	110	0	25
Cranb. Blackberry/Raspberry, av.	110	0	25
Cranberry Cherry	140	0	35
Cranberry Grape	100	0	25
Cranberry Mango	120	0	29
Superfruits, Raspb. Pomegr. Goji	130	0	32

Ocean Spray: *Per 8 fl.oz*

Juice Cocktails:

	C	F	Cb
Blueberry; Cranberry	110	0	28

100% Juice Blends:

	C	F	Cb
Citrus Tangerine Orange	110	0	28
Cranberry Concord Grape	130	0	33
Cranberry Mango	120	0	30
Cranberry Raspberry	120	0	30

Juice Drinks:

	C	F	Cb
Cran-Apple	120	0	31
Cran-Grape	120	0	31
Cran-Tangerine	110	0	28
Diet Juice Drinks, all flavors	5	0	2
Light Juice Drinks, av. all flavors	50	0	13
Sparkling, av. all flavors, 8.4 fl.oz	85	0	22
Wave, average all flavors, 8 fl.oz	80	0	20

Per 8 fl.oz Unless Indicated

	C	F	Cb

Odwalla:

100% Juice: *Per 15.2 fl.oz Bottle*

	C	F	Cb
Berry Greens	160	0	39
Groovin' Greens	150	0	37
Orange	210	0	47

Smoothies: *Per 15.2 fl.oz Bottle*

	C	F	Cb
Citrus C Monster	240	0	58
Mango Tango	260	0	65
Mo' Beta	250	0	59
Original Superfood	240	0	58
Red Rhapsody	210	0	52
Strawberry C Monster	240	0	58

Orange Julius:

Originals: *Per Medium*

	C	F	Cb
Mango P'apple, 22.2 oz	450	0	114
Orange, 18.2 oz	270	0	68
Pina Colada, 21.6 oz	470	7	99
Strawberry Banana, 20.9 oz	530	8	114

Smoothies ~ *See Fast-Foods Section*

	C	F	Cb
Orangina, 10 fl.oz bottle	130	0	32

Pom Wonderful,

100% Juice (8 fl.oz Bottle),

	C	F	Cb
Pom Blueberry/Cherry/Pomegranate	150	0	37

R.W. Knudsen: *Per 8 fl.oz*

Organic, 100% Juice: Apple

	C	F	Cb
Apple	110	0	28
Concord Grape	150	0	39
Cranberry Blueberry	120	0	31

Natural, 100% Juice:

	C	F	Cb
Mango Peach	120	0	30
Papaya Nectar	130	0	32
Razzleberry	110	0	28
Rio Red Grapefruit	140	0	34

Just Juice:

	C	F	Cb
Just Blueberry	100	0	24
Just Black Cherry	150	0	36
Just Black Currant	110	0	25
Simply Nutritious: Mega C	120	0	30
Average other flavors	125	0	31
Sparkling: Blueberry; Cranberry, av.	110	0	28
Cherry; Pomegranate	130	0	32
Organic Pear	120	0	31

Juice Brands (Cont)   C   F   Cb

Per 8 fl.oz Unless Indicated

R.W. Knudsen (Cont):

	C	F	Cb
Sensible Sippers: *Per 4.23 fl oz*			
Organic Apple; Fruit Punch	30	0	7
Organic Berry	35	0	9
Very Veggie, Original, 8 fl.oz	60	0	12
RealLemon – RealLime:			
Lemon/Lime Juice (from concentrate):			
1 teaspoon	0	0	0
2Tbsp, 1 fl.oz	10	0	2.5
Santa Cruz: *Per 8 fl.oz*			
Organic, 100% Juice:			
Apple; Red Tart Cherry	120	0	30
Concord/White Grape	160	0	39
Orange Mango	120	0	29
Pear Nectar	130	0	33
Carbonated Beverages,			
Lemonade, 10.5 fl.oz can	130	0	32
Lemonade: Regular; Peach; Mango	90	0	22
Cherry	100	0	26
Raspberry; Strawberry, average	90	0	24
Simply Orange Juice Company:			
Lemonade; Limeade, average	120	0	31
Mixed Berry; Fruit Punch; Tropical	100	0	26
Orange Juice,			
with or without pulp	110	0	26
Snap•E•Tom,			
Tomato & Chili Cocktail,			
11.5 fl.oz can	70	0	15
Snapple: *Per 16 fl.oz Bottle*			
Juice Drink Blends:			
Go Bananas; Rasp. Peach, av.	225	0	55
Grapeade; Lemonade; Orangeade	190	0	46
Fruit Punch	200	0	48
Diet, Cranberry Raspberry	20	0	5
Ssips, Juice Boxes,			
av. all flavors, 6 fl.oz box	80	0	21
Stonyfield Farm: *Per 10 fl.oz Bottle*			
Smoothies: Strawb.; Wild Berry	230	3	39
Peach	230	3	42
6 oz Bottle, Strawb. Banana	140	2	25

Per 8 fl.oz Unless Indicated   C   F   Cb

SunnyD:

	C	F	Cb
Original: *Per 64 fl.oz Ctn*			
Orange, all var., 8 fl.oz	50	0	15
Blends, 64 fl.oz Containers,			
average all flavors, 8 fl.oz	60	0	15
Baja Juice: *Per 12 fl.oz Bottles*			
Red Punch	170	0	43
Other flavors	190	0	46
Chillers: *Pe 16 fl.oz*			
Blue Raspberry	110	0.5	28
Grape	120	0	30
Sunsweet: *Per 8 fl.oz*			
Plum Smart: Original	160	0	36
Light	60	0	15
Prune Juice: Original	180	0	42
Light	100	0	26
Trader Joe's:			
All Natural Pasteurized, 32/64 fl.oz Bottle: *Per 8 fl.oz*			
100% Cranberry	70	0	16
Blueberry Pomegranate	140	0	34
Just Blueberry	100	0	24
Just Pomegranate	150	0	37
Mango PassionFruit	130	0	32
Omega Orange Carrot	110	0	26
Organic, 32/64 fl.oz Bottle: *Per 8 fl.oz*			
100% Pomegranate	140	0	35
Apple Juice	120	0	30
Concord Grape Juice	160	0	39
Cranberry	70	0	18
Grapefruit Sunset; Lemonade	120	0	30
Mango Nectar	130	0	32
Pink Lemonade	130	0	32
Strawberry Lemonade	120	0	29
White Grape Juice	160	0	40
Joe's Kids: *Per 6.75 oz Box*			
From Concentrate: Apple	90	0	23
Apple Grape	100	0	24
White Grape	120	0	30
10% Juice, Lemonade	90	0	22
Sparkling Juices, 25.4 fl.oz Botle			
Blueberry, 8 fl.oz	120	0	30
Cranberry, 8 fl.oz	140	0	35
Pomegranate, 8 fl.oz	130	0	31

Juice Brands (Cont)   **C**   **F**   **Cb**

Per 8 fl.oz Unless Indicated

	C	F	Cb
Tree Top:			
100% Juice Concentrates:			
64 fl.oz Bottle: *Per 8 fl.oz*			
Apple Berry/Grape, average	125	0	32
Apple Cranb.; Or. Passionfruit, av.	115	0	28
11.5 fl.oz Can: *Per Can*			
Apple Berry/Grape, av.	180	0	46
6.75 fl.oz Box, average	105	0	26
Smoothie, Ban. Strawb., 4.5 fl.oz	100	0	23
Tropicana:			
20% Juice, 15.2 fl.oz Bottle,			
Cranberry	270	0	66
Farmstand, 32 fl.oz bottle,			
average all flavors, 8 fl.oz	120	0	27
100% Juice Pure Premium:			
Grapefruit, 15.2 fl.oz	170	0	42
Ruby Red Grapefruit, 15.2 fl.oz	250	0	59
Strawberry Kiwi, 15.2 fl.oz	230	0	58
Trop50, 50% less sugar, 59 fl.oz bottle,			
average all flavors, 8 fl.oz	50	0	13
Trop Twisters, 20 fl.oz bottle:			
Or. Strawb. Banana Burst	330	0	80
Tropicana Twister , 20 fl.oz	340	0	85
Tropics, 59 fl.oz container,			
average all flavors, 8 fl.oz	125	0	30
Tru Nopal:			
Cactus Water: 1 Cup, 8 fl.oz	25	0	6
16.9 fl.oz carton	50	0	12
Turkey Hill: *Per 8 fl.oz*			
All Natural Lemonade: Classic	100	0	26
Blackberry	110	0	27
Regular Lemonade flavors	120	0	29
Fruit Punch	100	0	26
Orangeade	110	0	26
V8 Juices & Drinks *(Campbell's)*:			
Original/Spicy 100% Vegetable Juice:			
5.5 fl.oz can	35	0	7
8 fl.oz cup	50	0	10
11.5 fl.oz can	70	0	14
12 fl.oz bottle	75	0	15
Blends: Pineapple Passion, 8 fl.oz	70	0	17
Red Radiance, 8 fl.oz	70	0	17
Healthy Greens; Carrot Mango, 8 fl.oz	60	0	14
V-Fusion: Average all flavors	115	0	28
Light Varieties, av. all flavors	50	0	13
Veryfine:			
100%: Apple, 8 fl.oz	120	0	29
Apple Strawb., Krazy Kiwi, 11.5 fl.oz	170	0	43
Orange, 8 fl.oz	120	0	30

Per 8 fl.oz Unless Indicated

	C	F	Cb
Vita Coco:			
Coconut Water: 8 fl.oz	45	0	11
with Pineapple, 8 fl.oz	60	0	15
Chocolate, 11 fl.oz	90	3	16
Walnut Acres: *Per 8 fl.oz*			
Organic: Apple; Cranberry, av.	110	0	28
Apricot; Raspberry	130	0	32
Cherry	140	0	34
Incredible Vegetable	50	0	12
Mango Nectar	120	0	29
Welch's: *Per 8 fl.oz Unless Indicated*			
100% Juice: Concord Grape	140	0	36
Red Grape juice	160	0	41
White Grape	140	0	38
White Grape Cherry/Peach	140	0	34
Fruit Shots, all flavors, 5.5 fl.oz can	90	0	22
Frozen Concentrates,			
100% Juice, Grape; all var., 2 fl oz	140	0	39
Light Juice, 52 fl.oz Bottle			
Concord/White Grape, 8 fl.oz	45	0	12
Sparkling Juice Cocktail:			
Blueberry Grape, 8 fl.oz	150	0	38
Other flavors, 8 fl.oz	160	0	40
Zola:			
Acai: *Per 12 fl.oz Bottle*			
Original	185	3	38
with Blueberry/Pomegranate	180	3	38
Coconut Water, 17.5 oz Can:			
Original,	50	0	13
Chocolate, 8 fl.oz	50	0	12
Espresso, 8 fl.oz	60	0	13

CALORIEKING PORTION WATCH

ORANGE JUICE	C	Cb
8 fl.oz	110	26
16 fl.oz	220	52
24 fl.oz	330	78
32 fl.oz	440	104

Quick Guide C F Cb

Cow's Milk ~ Average All Brands
Whole (3.25% fat):

	C	F	Cb
2 Tbsp, 1 fl.oz	20	1	1.5
1 Cup, 8 fl.oz	150	8	12
1 Large Glass, 12 fl.oz	220	12	17
1 Pint, 16 fl.oz	295	16	22
1 Quart, 946 ml	590	32	44

Reduced-Fat (2% fat):

	C	F	Cb
2 Tbsp, 1 fl.oz	15	0.5	1.5
1 Cup, 8 fl.oz	120	5	12
1 Large Glass, 12 fl.oz	180	7.5	18
1 Pint, 16 fl.oz	245	10	23
1 Quart, 946 ml	490	20	46

Light/Low-Fat (1% fat):

	C	F	Cb
2 Tbsp, 1 fl.oz	13	0.3	1.5
1 Cup, 8 fl.oz	100	2.5	12
1 Large Glass, 12 fl.oz	150	4	18
1 Pint, 16 fl.oz	205	5	25
1 Quart, 946 ml	410	10	49

Fat Free/Skim (0% fat):

	C	F	Cb
2 Tbsp, 1 fl.oz	10	0	1.5
1 Cup, 8 fl.oz	90	0.5	13
1 Large Glass, 12 fl.oz	135	0.5	19
1 Pint, 16 fl.oz	180	1	26

Half & Half ~ *See Page 89*

SWITCH & SAVE

Switch from whole milk to either 2%, 1% or 0% milk and save significant calories.

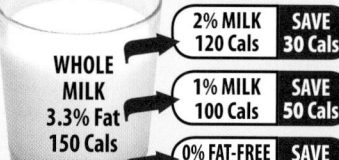

Per 8 oz Cup/Glass

WHOLE MILK 3.3% Fat 150 Cals

2% MILK 120 Cals	SAVE 30 Cals
1% MILK 100 Cals	SAVE 50 Cals
0% FAT-FREE 90 Cals	SAVE 60 Cals

Switching to low-fat or fat-free milk also greatly reduces saturated fat.

Other Milks C F Cb

Buttermilk: *Average All Brands*

	C	F	Cb
Reduced-Fat (2%), 1 cup, 8 fl.oz	120	5	10
Low-Fat (1%), 1 cup, 8 fl.oz	100	2.5	12

Lactose Free:

	C	F	Cb
Lactaid 100: Whole	160	8	13
2% Reduced-Fat	130	5	12
1% Low-Fat	110	2.5	13
Fat Free; Calcium Enriched	90	0	13
Smart Balance, FF + Omega-3s & Vit. E	100	0	14

Lower Calorie/Carb Dairy Drinks: *Per 8 fl.oz Cup*

Calorie Countdown (*Hood*):	C	F	Cb
2% Reduced-Fat: Plain	70	4.5	3
Chocolate	80	4.5	6
Fat-Free	35	0	4

Goat/Sheep Milk, Kefir

Goat's Milk (*Meyenberg*):

	C	F	Cb
Whole, 1 cup, 8 fl.oz	140	7	11
Low-Fat (1%), 8 fl.oz	100	2.5	11
Evaporated, reconst., 8 fl.oz	140	8	12

Kefir: *Per 8 fl.oz*

	C	F	Cb
Lifeway: Original, Plain	150	8	12
Greek, Plain, whole milk	210	14	12
Lowfat, average all flavors	140	1.5	20
Nancy's: Plain, low fat	140	3	17
Fruit flavors, average	205	2.5	38
Trader Joe's: Plain, 1%	110	2.5	8
Strawberry	160	2	21
Sheep's Milk, Whole, 1 cup	265	17	13

Canned & Dried Milk

	C	F	Cb
Condensed: Sweetened, 2 T., 1 fl.oz	130	3	22
Low Fat, 2 Tbsp	120	1.5	23
Fat-Free, 2 Tbsp	110	0	24
Evaporated: Whole, 2 Tbsp	40	3	3
Whole, ½ cup, 4 fl.oz	170	10	13
Carnation: Low Fat, 2 Tbsp, 1 oz	25	0.5	3
½ cup, 4 fl.oz	115	2.5	14
Fat-Free, 2 Tbsp, 1 oz	25	0	4
Dried: Whole, ¼ cup, 1 oz	160	9	12
Skim/Non-Fat, ⅓ cup	80	0	12
Made-up, 1 cup, 8 fl.oz	80	0	12
Buttermilk (sweet cream): 1 oz	110	2	14
Non-Fat, 1 Tbsp	25	0	3
Carnation, Malted, dry, 3 Tbsp, 0.7 oz	90	2	15
Horlick's, Malt Powder, dry, 1 oz	180	4	27

Soy/Non-Dairy Drinks ~ See Page 49

Quick Guide

C **F** **Cb**

Chocolate Milk:
Average All Brands:

	C	F	Cb
Whole Milk, (3.3%):			
8 fl.oz cup	220	8	29
1 Pint, 16 fl.oz	440	16	58
Reduced-Fat, (2%):			
8 fl.oz cup	190	5	30
1 Pint, 16 fl.oz	380	10	60
Low-Fat, (1%):			
8 fl.oz cup	160	3	26
1 Pint, 16 fl.oz	315	5	52

Flavored Milk ~ Brands

C **F** **Cb**

Ready-To-Drink: *Per 8 fl.oz Cup Unless Indicated*

	C	F	Cb
Albertson's, Choc Milk	180	2.5	29
Great Value *(Walmart)*,			
Low Fat Choc. Milk, 8 oz	140	2.5	21
Hood: Chocolate	220	8	30
Low-Fat (1%), Chocolate	160	2.5	28
Horizon Organic:			
Low-Fat:			
Chocolate with Omega 3	150	2.5	23
Vanilla with Omega 3	150	2.5	22
Kellogg's:			
To Go, Breakfast Shakes: *Per 10 fl.oz*			
Chocolate; Strawberry, av.	190	5	30
Mixes, average all flavors,			
1 packet	130	0.5	26
Kroger, Simple Truth,			
Choc Milk, Low-Fat, 1%	150	2.5	22
Land O Lakes: *Per 8 fl.oz*			
Grip 'n Go:			
Swiss Chocolate (2% red-fat)	190	5	26
Strawberry (whole milk)	190	8	22
Muscle Milk ~ *See Energy Protein Drinks*			
Nesquik: *Per 8 fl.oz*			
Low Fat, average all flavors	140	2.5	24
Chocolate: Fat Free, 8 fl.oz	95	0	24
No Sugar Added	100	2	13
Prairie Farms: *Per 8 fl.oz*			
Chocolate, 2% Reduced Fat	180	5	26
Strawberry, 1% Low Fat	160	2.5	28
Ralphs,			
Choc., Low-Fat, 8 fl.oz	210	2.5	36

Bottled Coffee Drinks ~ See Page 37

Flavored Milk ~ Brands (Cont)

Ready-To-Drink:
TruMoo:

	C	F	Cb
Chocolate/Strawberry:			
Whole, 8 fl.oz	220	8	29
1% Low-Fat: 8 fl.oz	140	2.5	20
14 fl.oz Bottle	250	5	35
Fat-free, 8 fl.oz	120	0	20
High Protein 1% (25g),			
average all flavors, 8 fl.oz	205	2.5	31
Yoo-Hoo: Chocolate,15.5 fl.oz bottle	230	2	51
Strawberry, 6.5 fl.oz	100	0.5	22

Bottled Coffee Drinks ~ *See Page 37*

Shakes

	C	F	Cb
Arby's: *Per Small Size*			
Jamocha, Ultimate Choc.,	440	12	75
Burger King: *Per Medium 16 oz*			
Hand Spun Shakes: Chocolate	760	21	131
Strawberry	640	15	113
Vanilla	580	15	98
Other flavors ~ *See Fast Food Section*			
Denny's: *Per 16 oz*			
Cake Batter	1090	52	147
Chocolate	870	43	111
Chocolate Peanut Butter	1080	66	111
Oreo	1050	56	125
Peanut Butter Banana	1030	65	99
Strawberry	760	34	110
Vanilla	800	43	97
Hardees, all flavors, av., 14 oz	710	33	87
McDonalds, McCafe Shakes:			
Chocolate/Strawberry, average:			
12 fl.oz cup	530	16	87
16 fl.oz cup	635	18	104
22 fl.oz cup	850	24	141
Other Restaurants ~ *See Fast-Foods Section*			

Smoothies

	C	F	Cb
Made Up Ready-To-Drink:			
8 fl. oz Milk/Soy + Fruit: *Per 12 fl.oz*			
Average all flavors:			
with Whole Milk	300	8	50
+ Ice Cream, 1 scoop	400	13	62
with Non-Fat Milk	240	0	50
Kroger/Ralph's Smoothies: *Per 8 fl.oz*			
Mixed Berry	210	2.5	40
Strawberry Banana	200	2.5	37
Freshens; Jamba Juice; TCBY ~ *See Fast-Foods*			

Nut, Rice & Cereal Drinks

Per 8 fl.oz Cup Unless Indicated

	C	F	Cb
Almond Breeze *(Blue Diamond):*			
Original: Regular	60	2.5	8
Reduced Sugar	30	2.5	1
Chocolate	100	2.5	19
Vanilla	80	2.5	14
Unsweetened: Original; Vanilla	30	2.5	1
Chocolate	40	3	2
Almond Dream:			
Almond Drink:			
Pumpkin Spice, ½ cup	50	1.5	9
Orig, Enriched Unswtn'd, 1 cup	130	11	4
Amazake, Oh So Original, Rice Shake	150	0	31
Better Than Milk:			
Rice Vegan Powder Mix,			
Orig.; Van., 2 Tbsp, 0.7 oz	70	0	17
Cacique, Horchata Rice Drink	230	5	46
Califia Farms: *Per 8 fl.oz Cup*			
Almond Milk: Original	60	4	6
Unsweetened	35	3	1
Vanilla	50	3	4
Toasted Coconut Almond	45	4	1
Don Jose: *Per 8 fl.oz Cup*			
Cereal Match	100	3	17
Horchata Rice Drink	140	4	25
Dream: *Per 8 fl.oz Cup*			
Boosted: Original Almond	120	7	6
Coconut	130	8	5
Enriched, unsweetened	70	2.5	1
Ultimate: Original Almond	150	11	9
Usweetened	130	11	4
Milkadamia: *Per 8 fl.oz Cup*			
Macadamia Nut Milk: Original	70	5	7
Original; Vanilla, unsweetened	50	5	1
Latte da	70	4.5	8
Pacific Foods: *Per 8 fl.oz Cup*			
Hazelnut: Original	110	3.5	18
Chocolate	130	5	19
Organic Almond:			
Original; Vanilla, av.	65	3	10
Chocolate, single serve container	100	3	19
Organic Oat, Original/Vanilla, av.	130	2.5	25
Rice Dream: *Per 8 fl.oz Cup*			
Organic Original Rice: Classic	120	2.5	23
Vanilla	130	2.5	26
Enriched: Unsweetened	70	2.5	11
Chocolate	160	3	34
Horchata, 8 fl.oz cup	160	2.5	32

Note: Rice/Oat/Nut drinks are very low in protein. Unless enriched with protein (and calcium), they are not suitable for infants as a substitute for milk or calcium-enriched soy drinks.

Nut & Rice Drinks (Cont)

Per 8 fl.oz Cup Unless Indicated

	C	F	Cb
Silk: *Per 8 fl.oz Cup*			
Almond: Original	60	2.5	8
Dark Chocolate	100	2.5	19
Unsweetened, Orig.; Vanilla	30	2.5	1
Cashew:			
Original	60	2.5	9
Unsweetened/ Vanilla	25	2	1
Chocolate	90	2	18
Trader Joe's: *Per 8 fl.oz Cup*			
Rice Drinks:			
Unsweetened:			
Original, Organic	120	2.5	23
Vanilla	130	2.5	26
WestSoy, Rice, Plain; Vanilla	110	2.5	20

Soy Milk ~ Ready-To-Drink

	C	F	Cb
365 Organic *(Whole Foods):* *Per 8 fl.oz Cup*			
Original, unsweetened	70	3.5	3
Chocolate	140	3.5	22
Vanilla	100	3.5	11
Light: Original	70	1.5	9
Vanilla	70	1.5	10
8th Continent: *Per 8 fl.oz Cup*			
Original	80	2.5	7
Complete Vanilla	80	2.5	8
Vanilla	100	2.5	11
Light: Original	50	2	2
Chocolate	90	1.5	12
Vanilla	60	2	5
Better Than Milk, Orig., 8 fl.oz cup	90	1.5	18
Edensoy: *Per 8 fl.oz Cup*			
Organic: Original	140	5	14
Unsweetened	120	6	5
Vanilla	150	3	24
Extra: Original	130	4	13
Vanilla	150	3	23
Great Value *(Walmart),*			
Vanilla Soy Milk, 8 fl.oz	100	3.5	10
Kikkoman ~ See Pearl *(next page)*			
Odwalla: *Per 15.2 fl.oz Bottle*			
Soy & Dairy Protein Shakes:			
Chocolate	410	8	53
Strawberry	320	7	37
Vanilla	380	7	46

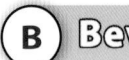 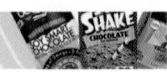
Soy Milk ~ Ready-To-Drink (Cont)

Per 8 fl.oz Unless Indicated

	C	F	Cb
Pacific: Per 8 fl.oz Cup			
Organic, Original, unsweetened	90	4	5
Select Soy: Original	70	2.5	9
Vanilla	80	2.5	11
Ultra: Original	140	5	12
Vanilla	140	5	14
Pearl (Kikkoman): Per 8 fl.oz Cup			
Chocolate	150	4.5	21
Coffee Flavor	150	4	24
Creamy Vanilla	110	3.5	11
Original	110	3.5	12
Unsweetened	80	2.5	6
Silk (Whitewave): Per 8 fl.oz Cup			
Original	110	4.5	9
Chocolate	120	3	21
Vanilla	100	3.5	12
Very Vanilla	130	3.5	18
Light: Original	60	2	5
Chocolate	90	1.5	16
Vanilla	70	2	7
Organic: Orig., unsweet'nd	80	4	4
Vanilla	100	3.5	10
Slim-Fast ~ *See Page 40*			
Soy Dream: Per 8 fl.oz Cup			
Enriched: Original	100	4	8
Vanilla	120	4	14
Organic: Original	130	4	16
Vanilla	140	4	18
Trader Joe's: Per 8 fl.oz Cup			
Soy Milk: Original	110	2	13
Chocolate	130	2.5	23
Vanilla	100	2	16
Organic: Original	130	3	17
Chocolate	120	3	17
Vanilla	130	3	19
WestSoy: Per 8 fl.oz Cup			
Organic Plus, (25% Less Sugar):			
Plain	110	4.5	11
Vanilla	110	4.5	11
Low-Fat: Plain	90	2	15
Vanilla	120	2	23
Non-Fat: Plain	70	0	10
Vanilla	80	0	12
Unsweetened: Plain	100	5	4
Vanilla	100	4.5	5

Soy Powder Mix

1 oz (¼ cup) mix makes 8 fl.oz Cup

	C	F	Cb
Soy Protein Isolate, dry, 1 oz	95	1	2
Better Than Milk:			
Original, 2 Tbsp	90	1.5	18
Vanilla, 2 Tbsp	90	1.5	18
Genisoy: Per Scoop			
Protein Shake Powder:			
Natural, 1 oz	100	0	0
Chocolate, 1.2 oz	120	0	17
Vanilla, 1.2 oz	130	0	18
Now:			
Soy Protein Isolate:			
Plain, ⅓ cup, 0.8 fl.oz	90	0.5	0.5
Natural:			
Chocolate, 1 level scoop, 1.6 oz	160	1.5	9
Vanilla, 1 level scoop, 1.6 oz	180	2.5	13
Revival: Per Packet			
Unsweetened Shakes: Plain	105	1	4
Chocolate	120	2.5	7
Strawberry Banana	115	2	4
Strawberry Smile	115	2	4
Vanilla Pleasure	120	2	6
Average other flavors	115	2	4
Whole Foods:			
Chocolate, with Spirulina, 1 oz	100	1	10
Vanilla, with Spirulina, 1 oz	100	0	11

Coconut Milk Drinks

	C	F	Cb
Silk: Per 8 fl.oz Cup			
Original	80	5	7
Unsweetened	45	4	0.5
Vanilla	90	5	10
Blends, Almond Coconut:			
Original	50	3	5
Unsweetned	35	3	0.5
So Delicious: Per 8 fl.oz cup			
Original	70	4.5	8
Chocolate	90	5	13
Vanilla	80	4.5	9
Unsweetened, Original	45	4.5	1
Trader Joes: Per 8 fl.oz cup			
Unsweetened	60	5	1
Vanilla	90	5	9
(Enriched with calcium + vitamins D & B12)			

Quick Guide 　C　F　Cb

Cola:

Drinks: *Average all Brands*

	C	F	Cb
8 fl.oz Cup/Can	100	0	26
12 fl.oz Can	150	0	39
16 fl.oz Bottle	200	0	52
20 fl.oz Bottle	250	0	65
24 fl.oz (Pepsi)	300	0	84
1-Liter Bottle (34 fl.oz)	400	0	100
2-Liter Bottle (68 fl.oz)	800	0	200

Other Soda Drinks: *Per 12 fl.oz, average all brands*

	C	F	Cb
Club Soda	0	0	0
Cream Soda	190	0	48
Ginger Ale	125	0	31
Lemonade, Regular/Pink	180	0	45
Orange	180	0	45
Root Beer	150	0	39
Tonic Water	125	0	32
Mineral Water: Plain	0	0	0
Sweetened/flavored	150	0	37
with Fruit Juice	120	0	30
Soda Water/Seltzer: Plain/Diet	0	0	0
Sweetened/flavored	155	0	39
with Fruit Juice	160	0	40

Fountain, Movie Theater & Take-Out

Average All Flavors

	C	F	Cb
Small Cup, 12 fl.oz: No Ice	160	0	40
with ⅓ Ice	120	0	30
Regular, 16 fl.oz: No Ice	215	0	53
with ⅓ Ice	160	0	40
Medium, 22 fl.oz: No Ice	295	0	73
with ⅓ Ice	220	0	55
Large, 32 fl.oz: No Ice	430	0	105
with ⅓ Ice	320	0	80

Note: ⅓ Cup of Ice = ¼ Cup Liquid

Soft Drink ~ Brands

Per 12 fl.oz Unless Indicated

	C	F	Cb
365 Organic *(Whole Foods)*,			
Spritzers, all flavors	110	0	28
A&W: Root Beer, 20 fl.oz	290	0	78
Ten, 20 fl.oz	10	0	3
Albertson's:			
Super Chill: Cola	160	0	43
Root Beer	180	0	48
Barq's, Root Beer	170	0	47
Big Red, Soda, 12 fl.oz	150	0	38
Blue Sky, Natural Soda, Cola	170	0	43

Soft Drink Brands (Cont)

Per 12 fl.oz Unless Indicated 　C　F　Cb

	C	F	Cb
Bubble Up, Lemon-Lime Soda,			
8 fl.oz	110	0	28
Cactus Cooler	150	0	40
Canada Dry:			
Club Soda; Diet Ginger Ale	0	0	0
Ginger Ale; Tonic Water, average	140	0	36
Cheerwine	150	0	42
Coca-Cola:			
Classic; Caffeine Free	140	0	39
Diet Coke, all varieties	0	0	0
Cherry Coke; Vanilla Coke	150	0	42
Crush:			
Grape; Orange	160	0	43
Peach; Pineapple, average	190	0	51
Strawberry	170	0	46
Dad's: Cream Soda	200	0	51
Root Beer	165	0	42
Diet Rite, Pure Zero	0	0	0
Dr Pepper: *Per 12 fl.oz Can*			
Regular	150	0	40
Cherry	160	0	43
Ten	10	0	3
Fanta: Orange	160	0	45
Other flavors	180	0	48
Fresca, all flavors	0	0	0
GuS, average all flavors	95	0	23
Hansen's: *Per 12 fl.oz*			
Natural Cane Sugar:			
Creamy Root Beer	170	0	45
Original Cola	160	0	41
Pomegranate	130	0	35
Diet, all flavors	0	0	0
Hawaiian Punch:			
Aloha Morning, 40% less sugar,			
Orange/Strawb./Mixed Berry Citrus	60	0	13
Average other flavors	60	0	14
Henry Weinhard's: Root Beer	170	0	43
Orange/Vanilla Cream, av.	180	0	44
Hires, Root Beer	170	0	45
IBC: Cream Soda; Black Cherry	175	0	44
Root Beer	160	0	40
Icee: Cola; Orange, 6 fl.oz	80	0	20
Lemon Lime	80	0	20
Raspberry Lemonade	80	0	21
Watermelon	80	0	20
Jarritos, all flavors, 8 fl.oz	110	0	28
Jelly Belly, all flavors	180	0	42
Jolt, Cola	150	0	41

Soft Drink Brands (Cont)

Per 12 fl.oz Unless Indicated

	C	F	Cb
Jones Soda:			
Regular, all flavors, 12 fl.oz	170	0	42
Stripped, all flavors, 12 fl.oz	30	0	8
Zilch, sugar free, 12 fl.oz	0	0	0
Kool Aid, Bursts, av., 6.75 fl.oz	35	0	9
Mello Yello, Regular	170	0	47
Mountain Dew: All flavors	170	0	46
Diet varieties	0	0	0
Dewshine	160	0	42
Black Label, 16 fl.oz	210	0	54
Mug, Root Beer	160	0	43
Natural Brew: Chai Cola	170	0	41
Draft Root Beer	170	0	43
Outrageous Ginger Ale	180	0	44
Vanilla Cream Soda	160	0	39
Nehi, Peach	190	0	51
Pepsi: *Per 12 fl.oz*			
Regular; Caffeine Free	150	0	41
Diet Pepsi; Jazz; Pepsi One	0	0	0
Pepsi Next	60	0	16
Pepsi True: 7.5 fl.oz can	60	0	17
12 fl.oz can	100	0	27
Perrier, Carbonated Water	0	0	0
Pibb, Xtra	155	0	39
RC Cola: Regular	160	0	43
Ten	10	0	3
Reed's, Ginger Brew,			
all varieties	145	0	38
7•UP: Lemon Lime; Cherry	140	0	39
Diet flavors	0	0	0
Ten, Lemon Lime	10	0	3
Safeway: *Per 8 fl.oz*			
Refreshe: Cola; Lem. Lime, av.	110	0	28
Grape	140	0	36
Mtn Breeze; Strawberry	120	0	30
Refreshe Ice, all flavors, 17 fl.oz	0	0	0
Santa Cruz, Lemonade, 12 fl.oz	130	0	32
Schweppes: Ginger Ale	120	0	33
Tonic Water	130	0	33
Shasta: Cream Soda	190	0	47
Cherry Cola	180	0	45
Club Soda; Diet, all flavors	0	0	0
Dr. Shasta	150	0	38
Ginger Ale	130	0	33
Tiki Punch; Pineapple; Orange	200	0	50
Average other flavors	170	0	41
Sierra Mist, Lemon Lime	120	0	30
Sprite: Regular, 12 fl.oz	140	0	38
Zero	0	0	0

Per 12 fl.oz Unless Indicated

	C	F	Cb
Squirt, Ruby Red	170	0	45
Stewarts: Root Beer	150	0	38
Grape; Orange 'n Cream	180	0	45
Sun Drop: Citrus Soda, 20 fl.oz	290	0	76
Diet Citrus Soda	10	0	1
Sunkist: Orange, with sugar, 20 fl.oz	170	0	44
Pineapple, 20 fl.oz	320	0	85
Surge, 16 fl.oz	230	0	62
TAB	0	0	0
Tampico: *Per 12 fl.oz*			
Punch: Blue Raspberry	90	0	21
Pineapple Coconut	105	0	26
Average other flavors	90	0	21
Soda, all flavors, 12 fl.oz	180	0	42
Thomas Kemper: *Per 12 fl.oz*			
Black Cherry	170	0	44
Ginger Ale; Vanilla Cream	150	0	36
Root Beer	160	0	41
Trader Joe's:			
Sparkling:			
French Berry Lemonade:			
1 cup, 8 fl.oz	130	0	31
1 bottle, 33.8 fl.oz	520	0	124
Lime Ade: 1 cup, 8 fl.oz	110	0	28
1 bottle, 33.8 fl.oz	440	0	108
Pink Lemonade: 1 cup, 8 fl.oz	130	0	31
1 Bottle, 33.8 fl.oz	520	0	124
Vernors, Ginger Soda, 20 fl.oz	240	0	65
Virgil's, Root Beer	160	0	42
Walgreens: *Per 20 fl.oz*			
Orchard Grape Soda	300	0	84
Cola; Zesty Lemon Lime, av.	225	0	65
Root Beer	225	0	75
Zevia, all flavors	0	0	4
(Contains between 4-7g Erythritol)			

Powdered Soft Drink Mixes

Per 8 fl.oz Prepared, Unless Indicated

	C	F	Cb
Country Time:			
Lemonade; Pink Lemonade	60	0	16
Strawberry Lemonade	80	0	19
Crystal Light *(Kraft):*			
Fruit Drinks, all flavors, 1/2 tsp	5	0	0
Pure Fitness, average all flavors, 1 pkt	15	0	4
Flavor Aid, 1/8 package	0	0	0
Kool-Aid, sweetened, 0.6 oz	60	0	16
Tang, Regular, 2 Tbsp, 1 oz	90	0	24

Quick Guide

C F Cb

Teas

	C	F	Cb
Regular: Bag, Loose or Instant			
Brewed, 1 cup, 8 fl.oz	2	0	0.5
(Add extra for sugar/milk)			
Herbal, av. all flav., 1 cup	2	0	0.5
Bubble Milk Tea, w/ Pearls, 8 fl.oz	175	0	41
Chai Tea Latte Mix, 1 oz	110	1	24
Kombucha Tea:			
Average all Brands:			
1 cup, 8 fl.oz	30	0	7

Iced Tea

Average All Brands

	C	F	Cb
Sweetened: 8 fl.oz cup	90	0	22
12 fl.oz glass/can	140	0	35
16 fl.oz bottle	180	0	45
20 fl.oz bottle	225	0	55
Unsweetened, 8 fl.oz	0	0	0

Iced Tea Mixes

Per 8 fl.oz Made-Up

	C	F	Cb
4C Iced Tea:			
Average all flavors, 0.67 oz	70	0	18
Totally Light, all flavors	0	0	0
Crystal Light, sugar free	5	0	0
Lipton:			
Sweetened: Lemon	70	0	17
Mango; Peach	80	0	19
Unsweetened	0	0	0
Diet, all varieties	5	0	1

Bottled & Canned Teas

	C	F	Cb
Arizona: *Per 8 fl.oz*			
Black: Cranberry	80	0	22
Sweet	90	0	23
with Ginseng	60	0	15
Green Tea, average all flavors	70	0	18
Bigelow: *Per 8 fl.oz*			
Green Tea, average all flavors	60	0	15
Half & Half Tea, Lemonade	70	0	16
Unsweetened Tea	0	0	0
Fuze, Iced Lemon	70	0	19
Gold Peak, Lemon, 12 fl.oz	120	0	30
Health-Ade, Kombucha Tea, 8 fl.oz	30	0	7
Honest Tea: *Per 16 fl.oz Bottle*			
Assam Black	35	0	9
Just Black/Green	0	0	0

Bottled & Canned Teas (Cont)

	C	F	Cb
Lipton:			
Iced Tea: *Per 20 fl.oz Unless Indicated*			
Citrus Green Tea, 8 fl.oz	70	0	19
Diet, all flavors	0	0	0
Half & Half	120	0	31
Lemon	120	0	32
Peach	120	0	30
Sparkling: Peach	70	0	18
Diet	0	0	0
Sweet Iced Tea, 12 fl.oz	130	0	35
White Tea, with Raspberry, 16.9 fl.oz	110	0	29
Nestea:			
Iced Tea, with Lemon:			
8 fl.oz	50	0	13
20 fl.oz bottle	125	0	33
Diet, Green/Lemon	0	0	0
POM:			
Antioxidant Super Tea: *Per 12 fl.oz*			
Pomegranate:			
Honey Green Tea	130	0	35
Lemonade Tea	140	0	35
Peach Passion White Tea	130	0	32
Sweet Tea	120	0	30
Snapple: *Per 16 fl.oz*			
Green Tea	120	0	31
Diet Green Tea	0	0	0
Lemon/ Raspberry Tea	150	0	37
Diet Lemon/Raspberry Tea	10	0	1
Straight Up Tea: *Per 18.5 fl.oz Bottle*			
Honey Green; Sorta Sweet	90	0	22
Rooibos	90	0	23
Sweet	180	0	45
SoBe, Elixir, Green Tea, 20 fl.oz	200	0	52
Ssips, Lemon Iced Tea, 6 fl.oz	70	0	17
Steaz, Iced Green Tea,			
lightly sweetened, av., 16 fl.oz	80	0	20
Tampico, Iced Tea,			
average all flavors, 12 fl.oz	135	0	35
Tazo, Org. Iced Black Tea, 13.8 fl oz	60	0	15
TeaZazz, all flavors, 12.8 fl.oz	70	0	20
Trader Joe's: *Per 8 fl.oz*			
Organic Tea & Lemonade	100	0	25
Pomegranate Green Tea	60	0	15
Turkey Hill: Iced Tea, 16 fl.oz	180	0	42
Peach Tea, 16 fl.oz	200	0	46
Green Tea, Mango, 16 fl.oz	180	0	42
365 Organic *(Whole Foods):*			
Unsweetened: Black Tea	0	0	0
Green Tea	0	0	0

Note: Most breads have similar calories on a weight basis. However, volume may vary.

For example, 1 oz of bread may equal 1 slice regular bread or 2 slices of a lighter bread. It is best to weigh bread used and calculate using: 1 oz bread = 70 calories, 14g carb.

Quick Guide C F Cb

Bread

White or Wheat: *Average Per Slice*

	C	F	Cb
Thin or Light, 0.75 oz	50	0.5	9
Sandwich slice, 1 oz	70	1	14
Thick or Large, 1.5 oz	105	1.5	18
Thick, 2 oz	140	2	23
Extra Thick, 3 oz	210	3	35
Whole Loaf: 16 oz	1120	15	185
24 oz Loaf	1680	24	280

Multi Grain/Whole Grain: *Per Slice*

Sandwich Slice, 1 oz	75	1.5	12
Thick Slice, 2 oz	150	2.5	25

Toast: *Based on same counts as White/Wheat as above*

1 Slice (1 oz fresh):

with 1 tsp butter/margarine	105	5	12
with 1 tsp "light" butter/marg.	90	3.5	12
with 2 tsp butter/margarine	140	9	12
with 2 tsp "light" butter/marg.	110	6	12

Breads

Per Slice Unless Indicated

	C	F	Cb
12-Grain, 1.5 oz	110	1.5	22
Bran style/Dark, 1 oz	70	1	14
Buttermilk, average, 1.5 oz	110	1	22
Challah, 0.75 oz	85	1.5	17
Chapati, 1 oz	110	3	18
Ciabatta, 2 oz	130	1	26
Cornbread, average, 3 oz	220	6	37
Cracked Wheat Sourdough, 1.5 oz	130	0.5	27
Croissants ~ *See Page 134*			
Crustless Bread, regular, slice, 0.75 oz	40	0.5	8.5
Crusts Only, regular slice, 0.25 oz	30	0	7
English Toasting, 2 oz	140	1.5	27
Flax & Grain, 1.5 oz	120	3	19
Foccacia: Plain, 2 oz serve	150	2.5	28
Cheese & Garlic; Pesto, 2 oz serve	160	6	21
Tomato & Olive, 2 oz serve	150	5	21

Breads (Cont) C F Cb

Per Slice Unless Indicated

	C	F	Cb
French Stick/Baguette, 1 oz	70	1	15
French Toast: Slices, 1.5 oz	140	2	26
Aunt Jemima, Sticks, av., 2 oz	110	2	18
Garlic Bread/Toast:			
Small slice + 1 tsp spread, 0.75 oz	80	5	7
Medium slice + 2 tsp spread, 1.5 oz	160	10	14
Thick slice + 3 tsp spread, 1.8 fl.oz	220	14	20
Pepperidge Farm, 1 slice, 1.4 oz	160	10	15
Hawaiian Sweet Bread, 1.5 oz	110	2	19
Hemp Bread, 1.2 oz	95	2	12
Italian Bread, 2 oz	140	1	28
Lower Carb, (higher protein/fiber), average all brands, 1 oz	60	1.5	9
MultiGrain, 1.5 oz	100	2	21
Naan Flatbread, 2 oz	160	3.5	29
Nut/Health Nut, 1.35 oz	90	1.5	18
Oatmeal/Oatbran Bread, 1.5 oz	90	0.5	19
Pita, average all types:			
Small (4" diam), 1 oz	90	0	18
Large (6½" diam), 2 oz	140	1.5	27
Extra Large (9" diam), 4 oz	300	1.5	60
Popovers, (1), without butter	130	2	18
Pumpernickel:			
Cocktail/Party size	30	0.5	6
Large slice, 1.35 oz	80	0	15
Raisin Bread, 1 oz	80	1	15
Rye: 1 thin slice, av., 1 oz	80	1	14
1 thick slice, 2 oz	150	2	25
Cocktail size, 0.4 oz	25	0.5	4
Sandwich Pockets, 2 oz	140	1.5	27
Sourdough: Regular, 1.5 oz	120	1	25
French Style, 1 oz	75	0	14
Spelt, 1.6 oz	130	1	26
Sprouted 7-Grain, 1.5 oz	110	0.5	18
Squaw, 1.1 oz	85	0.5	13
Tacos/Tortillas ~ *See Page 172*			
Turkish/Middle Eastern, 1 oz	80	1.5	16
Wheat-Free Breads: Spelt, 1.6 oz	130	1	26
Rice, with Fruit Juice, 1.5 oz	110	2	21
Healthseed Rye, 1.6 oz	90	1	20
Millet, 1.5 oz	100	1	20

Bread ~ Brands

C F Cb

Per Slice Unless Indicated

Ener-G, Gluten-Free Breads:

	C	F	Cb
Brown Rice Loaf,			
Regular, 1.3 oz	100	3	16
High Fiber Loaf, 1.4oz	90	4.5	16
Seattle Brown Loaf, 1.3 oz	90	3	15
Tapioca, regular, sliced, 1 oz	80	3	11

Ezekiel:

Sprouted: 7 Sprouted Grains, 1.2 oz	80	0.5	15
Sesame, 1.2 oz	80	0.5	14
Whole Grain, 1.3 oz	80	0.5	15

Francisco International:

Extra Sourdough Loaf,			
1 slice, 1.7 oz	130	1	24
French, 2 slices, 1.6 oz	120	1	22
Sourdough Sliced Bread, 2 sl., 1.4 oz	110	1	22

Oroweat:

3 Seed Oatnut, 1.34 oz	120	3	18
100% Whole Wheat, 1.34 oz	90	1	16
Dill Rye, 1.2 oz	80	0	16
Extra Grainy, 17 Grains & Seeds, 1.2 oz	110	2.5	18

Pepperidge Farm:

100% Whole Wheat	110	2	20
15 Grain	110	2	20
Family, White Sandwich	150	3	20
Italian, with Sesame Seeds	90	1.5	20
Light Style, av. all varieties	135	1	20

Frozen Breads:

Garlic Bread:			
Original	180	8	20
Five Cheese	200	10	20
Texas Toast, Cheddar	160	9	20
Roman Meal: Orig. Multigr., 2 slices	110	1.5	21
Honey Oat Bran, 1.5 oz	110	1.5	20
Sara Lee: Honey Wheat, 1 oz	70	0.5	13
100% Whole Wheat, 1 oz	60	1	12
Cracked Wheat, 1 oz	80	0.5	15
Schwan's, Frozen:			
Cheese Stuffed Breadsticks, 1.7 oz	130	5	15
French Baguette, 1/4 loaf, 1.7 oz	120	0	25
Trader Joe's: Gourmet White, 1.5 oz	120	3.5	19
Soft 10 Grain, 1.5 oz	90	1.5	16
Sprouted Rye, 1.2 oz	90	1	15

Biscuits, Bread Rolls & Buns

Biscuits: *Average, 2 1/2" diameter* C F Cb

	C	F	Cb
Plain/Butter Milk:			
Prepared from Recipe	210	10	27
Refrig. Dough, Baked	95	4	13
Brown 'n Serve, av., 1 oz	70	1	13
Refrigerated Dough:			
Pillsbury, Buttermilk Biscuit,			
(3), 2.25 oz	150	2	30

Buns:

Frankfurter/Hot Dog: 1.25 oz	110	1.5	21
1.5 oz	130	2	25
Hamburger: Regular, 1.5 oz	110	1.5	22
Large, 3 oz	210	3	40
Hoagie/Submarine, Plain, 2.3 oz	200	1	38

Rolls:

Ciabatta Roll, 3.5 oz	230	4	41
Crescent Roll, Original, 1 oz	100	6	11
Dinner:			
1 small, 1 oz	90	1.5	17
1 medium (3" diam),1.5 oz	110	1	23
French: 1 med, 1.3 oz	110	1.5	22
1 large, 3 oz	230	2.5	42
Kaiser:			
Small, 2 oz	200	2.5	35
Large, 3.5 oz	350	4	61
Plain, 6", average all, 2.5 oz	200	1	38
Sourdough, 1.3 oz	110	1	21
Wheat Rolls: Small, 1.2 oz	100	1	17
Medium, 1.8 fl.oz	130	1.5	23
Large, 3.5 oz	260	3	46

Breadsticks, Croutons

Breadsticks:

Salt Sticks, plain, 1 oz	110	1	20
Fresh baked (1), 2 oz	180	2.5	34
Stella D'oro: Original (1)	45	1	7
Sesame (1)	50	2	7
Croutons: Seasoned, 2 Tbsp, 0.3 oz	35	1.5	4
Pepp. Farm, Zesty Italian, 6 croutons	30	1	5

Bread Products

Bread Crumbs, dry:

Plain or seasoned: 1 oz	110	1.5	20
1 cup, 3.5 oz	385	5	70
Corn Flake Crumbs, 1 oz	120	0	29
Graham Cracker Crumbs *(Keebler),* 1 oz	110	2.5	20
Bread Dough, average:			
Frozen, 1 slice, 2 oz	140	2	26
Refrigerated: French, 1" sl.	60	1	13
Wheat; White, 1" slice	80	2	14
Coating Mixes, av., 2 Tbsp., 1 oz	100	0.5	20
Stuffing: Dry mix, average all,1 oz	110	1	10
Prepared, 1/2 cup, 4 oz	180	9	22

Quick Guide   **C** **F** **Cb**

Bagels
Average All Brands
Plain/Onion:

	C	F	Cb
1 mini/bagelette, 1 oz	65	0.5	13
1 small bagel, 2 oz	145	1	29
1 medium bagel, 3 oz	220	1.5	43
1 large bagel, 4 oz	290	2	57
Bagel Chips, 1 oz	130	4.5	19
Pizza Bagel Bites (Bagel Bites),			
average all varieties., 4 pieces, 3 oz	190	5.5	27
Bagel Crisps *(New York Style),*			
average all varieties, 6 crisps, 1 oz	130	5	17
Bagel Thins *(Thomas'),* 1, 1.5 oz	110	1	25

Bagel ~ Brands

Per Bagel

	C	F	Cb
Bubba's: Plain	220	1.5	45
Blueberry	150	0.5	32
Cinnamon Raisin	250	1.5	51
Costco Bakery: Plain	330	1.5	70
Cinnamon Raisin	340	1.5	73
Whole Grain	300	5	56
Lender's, Fresh, NY Style:			
Plain, 3.3 oz	240	2	46
Blueberry, 3.3 oz	240	2	46
Cinnamon, 3.3 oz	240	2	46
Whole Wheat, 3.3 oz	240	2	46
Panera Bread: Plain	290	1.5	58
Cinnamon & Raisin Swirl, 3.8 fl.oz	320	2	66
Everything, 4 oz	300	2	58
Whole Grain, 4.3 oz	330	2.5	67
Sara Lee: Mini, average, 1.3 oz	100	0.5	20
Plain, 3.4 oz	260	1	52
Blueberry, 3.4 oz	260	1	54
Cinnamon Raisin, 3.7 oz	260	0.5	54
Everything, 3.4 oz	270	3	50
Onion, 3.4 oz	260	1	53
Western, The Alternatives, av., 2 oz	120	0.5	29

Bagel Spreads

	C	F	Cb
Cream Cheese:			
Plain: 2 Tbsp, 1 oz	100	9	1
2 oz mini-tub	200	18	2
Reduced Fat: 2 Tbsp, 1 oz	60	5	2
2 oz mini-tub	120	10	4
Flavors: Lox, 1 oz	90	8	2
Honey Nut, 1 oz	80	7	4
Strawberry, 1 oz	90	7	5
Sundried Tomato, 1 oz	80	7	2
Vegetable, 1 oz	90	8	2

English Muffins   **C** **F** **Cb**

Average All Brands

	C	F	Cb
Plain/Whole Wheat: Regular, 2 oz	135	1.5	26
Heavier, 2.5 oz	155	2	31
Super Size, 3.2 oz	190	2	38
Raisin-Cinnamon, 2.2 oz	150	1	30

Note: Actual weight of packaged muffins can be 10-15% heavier than stated net weight.

Rice Cakes

	C	F	Cb
Regular size (1), average, 0.3 oz	35	0.5	7.5
Hain, Mini, White Cheddar (10), 1.2 oz	70	2.5	11
Lundberg: Brown Rice (1), 0.7 oz	60	0.5	14
Caramel Corn (1)	80	0.5	17
Cinnamon Toast (1), 0.8 oz	80	0	20
Quaker, Apple Cinn., 0.5 oz	50	0	11

Tortillas & Shells

Tortillas: *Per Tortilla*

	C	F	Cb
Corn Flour:			
White/Yellow: 6", 1 oz	55	1	11
7", 1.2 oz	75	1	14
Wheat Flour:			
6", 1.2 oz	100	3	16
8", 1.4 oz	130	4	20
10", 2.3 oz	200	6	31

Shells: *Per Shell, without Fillings*

	C	F	Cb
Corn Taco Shells:			
Mini, 3", 0.2 oz	25	1	3
Medium, 5", 0.5 oz	60	2.5	8
Large, 6½", 0.7 oz	100	4.5	13
Salad Shell, 10"	310	17	34
Tostada Shells, fried:			
White Corn, 5½" diam., 0.4 oz	55	2.5	8
Yellow Corn, 5½" diam., 0.5 oz	80	3.5	11
Sopes, 1 shell, 4" 2 oz	110	1.5	23
La Tortilla Factory:			
100 Calorie, Whole Wheat, 2 oz	100	1.5	24
Hand Made Style,			
White Corn & Wheat, 1.45 oz	90	1	15
Low Carb, Flour, 1 oz	45	1.5	10
Traditional, Flour,			
Soft Taco Size, 1.2 oz	130	3.5	18
Mission Foods:			
Corn, Yellow/White, Super Soft:			
Regular size, 2 Tortillas, 1.7 oz	100	1.5	20
Super size (1), 1.1 oz	70	1	13
Flour: Homestyle, 1 Tortilla, 2.2 oz	190	6	29
Super Soft, 1 Tortilla, 1.7 fl.oz	140	3.5	24

Quick Guide   **C** **F** **Cb**

Cooked Cereals

	C	F	Cb
Barley, pearled, cooked, 1 cup	195	0.5	44
Buckwheat Groats, roasted:			
Dry, 1/2 cup, 3 oz	285	2	61
Cooked, 1 cup, 6 oz	155	1	34
Bulgur: Dry, 1/2 cup, 2.5 oz	240	1	53
Cooked, 1 cup, 6.5 oz	150	0.5	34
Corn/Hominy Grits:			
Dry: Regular, 1/4 cup, 1.4 oz	140	0.5	32
Instant: 0.8 fl.oz packet	75	0	18
w/ Imitation Bacon Bits, 1 oz	100	0.5	22
Cooked, 3/4 cup, 6.5 oz	110	0.5	23
Cream of Rice, cooked, 3/4 cup, 6.5 oz	95	0	21
Cream of Wheat:			
Cooked: Regular, 3/4 cup, 6.5 oz	95	0.5	20
Instant, 3/4 cup, 6.5 oz	105	0.5	21
Quick, 3/4 cup, 6.5 oz	100	0.5	22
Farina, cooked, 3/4 cup, 6 oz	95	0.5	19
Millet, dry, 1/2 cup, 1.8 fl.oz	190	2	36
Oat Bran: Raw, 1/3 cup, 1 oz	70	2	19
Cooked, 1/2 cup, 3.8 fl.oz	45	1	13
Oatmeal:			
Dry: Regular, 1/3 cup, 1 oz	100	1.5	18
Instant: Regular, average, 1 oz	105	1.5	18
Flavored, average, 1.5 oz	165	2	34
Cooked: Regular, 3/4 cup, 6 oz	125	2.5	21
1 cup, 8 fl.oz	165	3.5	28
Whole Wheat, cooked, 3/4 cup, 6.5 oz	115	0.5	25

Brans, Wheat Germ, Add-Ons

	C	F	Cb
Bee Pollen Granules, 1 Tbsp, 0.3 oz	25	1	2
Bran:			
Oat Bran: Raw, 1 tbsp, 0.2 oz	20	0.5	3
1/3 cup, 1 oz	100	2	17
Rice Bran: Raw, 1 tbsp, 0.2 oz	15	1	2.5
1/4 cup, 1 oz	95	6	15
Fruit: Dried, average, 1 oz	70	0	18
Banana, 1/2 medium	55	0	14
Prunes in Syrup (5), 3 oz	90	0	23
Honey, 1 Tbsp, 0.75 oz	65	0	17
Lecithin Granules, 1 Tbsp, 0.4 oz	55	4	0.5
Nuts, Almonds (6), 0.3 oz	40	4	1.5
Psyllium Husks, 1 Tbsp, 0.2 oz	10	0	4
Wheat, unprocessed, 1 Tbsp	5	0	2
Wheat Germ: Raw, 1 Tbsp, 0.3 oz	25	0.5	4
1/4 cup, 1 oz	105	3	15

Hot/Cooked Cereals ~ Brands

Per Serving, Dry Mix only   **C** **F** **Cb**

	C	F	Cb
Albers,			
Quick Grits, 1/4 cup, 1.4 oz	140	0.5	31
B&G:			
Cream of Wheat Instant:			
Original, 1 oz	100	0	19
Cinn. Swirl; Maple Br. Sugar, 1.3 oz	130	0	29
Bobs Red Mill:			
Organic Kasha, 1/4 cup, 1.45 oz	160	1	33
Rolled Spelt Flakes, 1/2 cup, 1.4 oz	130	1.5	28
Whole Oat Groats, 1/4 cup, 1.6 oz	170	3	31
Dr. McDougall's: *Without Sugar*			
Mighty Omega Superfood, 2.6 oz	240	7	38
Milled Flax Oatmeal, 1.2 oz pkt	120	3	21
Superfood Chia Crunch, 1.3 oz pkt	140	3	24
Great Value *(Walmart):*			
Instant Oatmeal:			
Apple Cinnamon, 1.5 oz pkt	130	1.5	27
Maple & Brown Sugar, 1.5 oz pkt	160	2	33
McCann's:			
Instant Irish Oatmeal:			
Regular, 1 oz package	100	2	19
Apple & Cinn., 1.3 oz	130	1.5	27
Maple & Brown Sugar, 1.5 oz	160	2	32
Malt-O-Meal: Original; Choc., 1.2 oz	130	0.5	27
Maple Brown Sugar, 1/4 cup	170	0	37
Natures Path:			
Oatmeal: Flax Plus, 1 oz	110	1.5	23
Apple Cinnamon, 1.7 oz	210	2.5	40
Maple Nut, 1.7 oz	210	4	38
NutriSystem,			
Oatmeal, Apple Cinnamon, 1 pkt	130	1.5	26
Quaker:			
Instant Grits, av. all flavors, 1 oz	100	1	22
Quick Grits, Original, 1/4 cup, 1.3 oz	130	0.5	29
Instant Oatmeal:			
Maple & Brown Sugar,	160	2	32
Organic, Regular, 1 oz	100	2	19
Peaches & Cream, 1.3 oz	130	2	27
Old Fash'nd/Quick Oats, 1/2 c., 1.4 oz	150	3	27
Real Medleys:			
Apple, Pear, Pecan, 2.1 oz	250	8	41
Blueb. Hazelnut, 2.47 oz	270	7	49
Summer Berry, 2.47 oz	250	3	51
Super Grains: Ban. Walnut, 2.47 oz	280	8	49
Maple Pecan Raisin, 2.47 oz	270	7	49
Wegmans:			
Instant Oatmeal: Orig., 1.4 oz pkt	150	2.5	27
Maple & Spice, 1.4 oz pkt	150	2	28

B — Breakfast Cereals

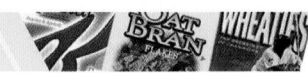

Quick Guide　　C　F　Cb

Cold Cereals
Average All Brands

	C	F	Cb
Bran Flakes, ³/₄ cup, 1 oz	95	0.5	24
Corn Flakes, 1 cup, 1 oz	100	0	22
Frosted Flakes, ³/₄ cup, 1 oz	110	0	27
Granola, 100% Nat., ¹/₂ cup, 1.7 oz	205	6	35
Oat Bran Cereal, ¹/₂ cup, 1.5 oz	145	3	25
Puffed Rice, 1 cup. 0.5 oz	55	0	13
Puffed Wheat, 1 cup, 0.5 oz	45	0	10
Raisin Bran, ¹/₂ cup, 1 oz	90	0.5	22
Rice Crisps, 1 cup, 1 oz	105	0.5	24
Shredded Wheat, 1 biscuit, 1 oz	85	0.5	20
Wheat Flakes, ³/₄ cup, 1 oz	105	1	24

Breakfast/Cereal Bars ~ *See Page 31*

Ready-To-Eat Cereal ~ Brands

Arrowhead Mills:

	C	F	Cb
Flakes: Amaranth, 1.2 oz	140	2	26
Kamut, 1 oz	120	1	25
Oat Bran, 1.2 oz	140	2.5	24
Spelt, 1 oz	120	1	24
Sprouted Wheat Berry & Quinoa, 1.5 oz	100	1	22
Puffed: Corn, 0.5 oz	60	1	12
Kamut, 0.5 oz	50	0	11
Millet, 0.5 oz	60	0.5	11
Rice, 0.5 oz	60	0	14
Wheat, 0.5 oz	60	0	12
Shredded Wheat:			
Bite Size:			
Regular, 1.7 oz	190	1	38
Sweetened, 1.8 fl.oz	200	1	42

Back to Nature: *Per ¹/₂ Cup*

	C	F	Cb
Granola: Apple Blueberry, 1.8 fl.oz	190	2.5	37
Chocolate Delight, 1.8 fl.oz	200	5	36
Classic, 1.8 fl.oz	200	2.5	38
Cranberry Pecan, 1.6 oz	180	5	34
Dark Chocolate Coconut, 1.76 oz	230	11	31
Sunflower & Pumpkin Seed, 1.8 fl.oz	210	7	31
Vanilla Almond Agave, 1.8 fl.oz	200	6	34
Granola Clusters:			
Peanut Butter, 1.8 oz	220	9	27
Av. other varieties, 1.8 oz	200	4.5	36

Barbara's Bakery:　　C　F　Cb
Classics, Organic & Sweetened:

	C	F	Cb
Brown Rice Crisps, 1.4 oz	150	1	33
Corn Flakes, 1.4 oz	150	0	35
Honest O's, Original, 1 oz	120	2	24
High Fiber Medley:			
Original, 2 oz	180	1.5	42
Cranberry, 2 oz	190	1.5	42
Morning Oat Crunch:			
Original, 2 oz	210	2	44
Cinnamon, 2 oz	230	3	43
Vanilla Almond, 2 oz	220	3	42
Puffins:			
Original; Cinnamon, 1 oz	90	1	24
Honey Rice, 1 oz	110	0.5	25
Multigrain; Pumpkin, 1 oz	110	0	25
PB/PB & Choc., av.,1 oz	115	1.5	24
Snackanimals, all varieties, 1 oz	110	0.5	26
Shredded Wheat, 2 biscuits, 1.4 oz	140	1	32
Spoonfuls, Multigrain, 1.1 oz	120	1.5	24
Squarefuls, Multigrain, 1.95 oz	200	1	47
Bear Naked, Granola:			
Fruit & Nut, 1 oz	140	6	20
Original Cinnamon, 1 oz	140	6	15
Triple Berry, 1 oz	120	2	23
Vanilla Almond, 1 oz	120	2.5	22
Bob's Red Mill,			
Muesli, Old Country, ¹/₄ cup, 1 oz	110	3	21
Cascadian Farm:			
Buzz Crunch, 2.1 oz	230	3	47
Cinnamon Crunch, 1 oz	110	2.5	22
Graham Crunch, 1 oz	110	2	23
Granola: Ancient Grains, 2 oz	240	6	41
French Vanilla Almond, 2 oz	250	7	42
Oats & Honey, 2.2 oz	260	7	46
Honey Nut O's, 1 oz	110	1	25
Multi Grain Squares,			
1 cup, 1.9 oz	210	1	44
Raisin Bran, 1.8 fl.oz	180	1	41
EnviroKidz: *Per 1 oz*			
Amazon Frosted Flakes, 1 oz	120	0	26
Gorilla Munch, 1 oz	120	1	26
Leapin' Lemurs, 1 oz	120	1.5	25
Panda Puffs, 1 oz	130	3.5	23
Erewhon:			
Corn Flakes, 1.2 oz	130	0	30
Crispy Brown Rice,			
Original/Cinn. av. 1 oz	110	0.5	24
Harvest Medley, 1 oz	110	1	24
Honey Rice Twice, 1 oz	120	0	26
Simply Vanilla Granola, 2 oz	240	6	41

Ready-To-Eat Cereal (Cont)

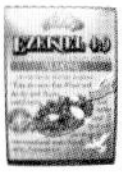

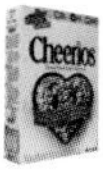

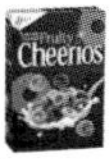

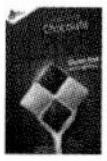

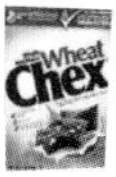

	C	**F**	**Cb**
Ezekiel 4.9:			
Sprouted Whole Grain Cereals:			
Original, ½ cup, 2 oz	190	1	40
Almond, ½ cup, 2 oz	200	3	38
Cinnamon Raisin, 2 oz	190	1	41
Golden Flax, ½ cup, 2 oz	180	2.5	37
General Mills:			
Cheerios: *Per ¾ Cup Unless Indicated*			
Original, 1 cup, 1 oz	100	2	20
Ancient Grains, ³/₄ c., 1 oz	110	2	22
Apple Cinn., ³/₄ cup, 1 oz	120	1.5	24
Chocolate, av., ³/₄ cup, 1 oz	100	1.5	21
Frosted, ³/₄ cup, 1 oz	100	1.5	22
Fruity, Nat Flav., ³/₄ c., 1 oz	100	1.5	21
Honey Nut, ³/₄ cup, 1 oz	110	1.5	22
Multi Grain, Regular, 1 c., 1oz	110	1.5	24
Protein: Cinn. Almond, 1¼ c., 2 oz	220	4.5	40
Oats & Honey, 1¼ cups, 2 oz	210	2.5	41
Chex: Choc., ³/₄ cup, 1 oz	130	2.5	26
Cinnamon, ¾ cup, 1 oz	120	2	25
Corn, 1 cup, 1 oz	120	0.5	26
Honey Nut, ³/₄ cup, 1 oz	120	0.5	28
Rice, 1 cup, 1 oz	100	0.5	23
Vanilla, ¾ cup, 1 oz	120	2	25
Wheat, ¾ cup, 1.7 oz	160	1	39
Cinn. Toast Crunch, ¾ cup, 1 oz	130	3	25
Fiber One: Original, ½ cup, 1 oz	60	1	25
Honey Clusters, 1 cup, 1.8 fl.oz	170	1.5	44
French Toast Crunch, ³/₄ cup, 1 oz	110	1	24
Kix: Original, 1¼ cups, 1 oz	110	1	25
Berry Berry; Honey,			
1¼ cups, 1.2 oz	120	1.5	28
Lucky Charms,			
Original; Chocolate, ³/₄ cup, 1 oz	110	1.5	23
Monsters: Count Chocula, ³/₄ c., 1 oz	100	1.5	23
Other varieties, 1.2 oz	130	1.5	28
Total, Whole Grain,1 oz	110	0.5	25
Trix, 1 cup, 1.1 oz	130	1.5	27
Wheaties, 1 oz	100	0.5	23
Great Value *(Walmart)*:			
Apple Blasts, 1.2 oz	120	0	29
Cinnamon Crunch, ¾ cup	130	3	23
Cocoa Crunch, ¾ cup, 1 oz	120	1.5	26
Corn Flakes, 1 cup	110	0	26
Crunchy Raisin Bran, 1.87 oz	190	1	20

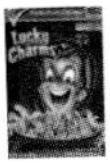

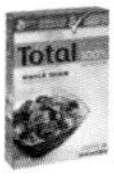

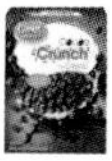

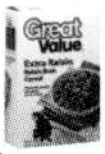

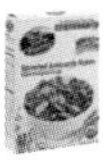

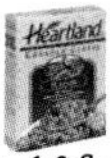

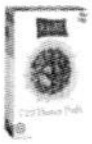

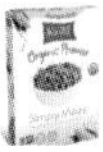

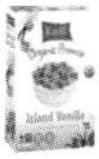

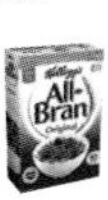

	C	**F**	**Cb**
Great Value Cont. *(Walmart)*:			
Extra Raisin Raisin Bran, 1 cup	200	1	43
Frosted Shredded Wheat, 1.9 oz	180	1	42
Fruit Spins, 1 cup	150	0	26
O's Oat, 1 oz	120	1	23
Sugar Frosted Flakes, 1 oz	120	0	28
Toasted Multi-Grain Spins, 1 cup	110	1.5	24
Health Valley:			
Crunch-Ems!, Rice, 1¼ cups, 1 oz	110	0	26
Organic Flakes:			
Oat Bran, 1 cup, 1.8 fl.oz	190	1.5	39
Sprouted Amaranth,			
1¼ cups, 2 oz	210	2	43
Heartland:			
Granola: Original, ½ cup, 2 oz	240	6	41
Fruit & Nut, ½ cup, 1.8 fl.oz	210	6	34
Harvest Spice, ½ cup, 1.8 fl.oz	210	5	37
Low-Fat var., ½ cup, 1.8 fl.oz	200	3	40
Oat Bran, ½ cup, 1.4 oz	160	3	23
Raisin, ½ cup, 2 oz	240	6	41
Kashi:			
7 Whole Grain: Flakes, 1 c., 1.8 fl.oz	170	0.5	41
Honey Puffs, 1½ cups, 1.4 oz	150	1	34
Nuggets, ½ cup, 2 oz	200	1.5	46
Whole Grain Puffs,			
1½ cups, 1.4 oz	150	1.5	32
GoLEAN: Original, 1¼ cups, 2 oz	180	2	40
Crunch: Original, ³/₄ cup, 2 oz	190	3	38
Chocolate, ³/₄ cup, 1.83 oz	220	7	32
Cinnamon Crisp, ³/₄ cup, 1.8 oz	180	4	32
Honey Almond Flax, ²/₃ cup, 2 oz	200	5	35
Heart to Heart:			
Oat Flakes & Blueb. Clusters, 1 c., 2 oz	200	2.5	42
Other varieties, ³/₄ cup, 1.2 oz	120	1.5	26
Organic Corn:			
Indigo Morning, 1.37 oz	140	1.5	32
Simply Maize, 1.37 oz	140	1.5	32
Organic Promise:			
Sprouted Grains, 1¼ cups, 2 oz	190	1	45
Sweet Potato Sunshine, 1 c., 1.8 fl.oz	180	1	43
Whole Wheat Biscuit,			
Island Vanilla, 27 biscuits	190	1	44
Kellogg's:			
All-Bran: Original, ½ cup, 1 oz	80	1	23
Bran Buds, ¹/₃ cup, 1 oz	80	1	24
Compl. Wheat Flakes, 1 oz	90	0.5	24
Apple Jacks, 1 cup, 1 oz	110	1	25
Cinnabon, 1 cup, 1 oz	120	2	25

continued next page...

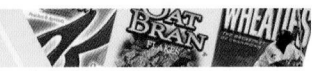

Ready-To-Eat Cereal (Cont)

Kellogg's (Cont):	C	F	Cb
Corn Flakes, Orig., 1 c., 1 oz	100	0	24
Cracklin' Oat Bran, ³/₄ cup, 1.8 fl.oz	200	7	34
Crispix, Original, 1 cup, 1 oz	110	0	25
Despicable Me 3 Minion, 1 c., 1.2 oz	120	1	27
Disney Princess, Strawb., 1.2 oz	120	1	27
Froot Loops: Orig., 1 c., 1 oz	110	1	25
Marshmallow, 1 c., 1 oz	110	1	26
Frosted Flakes: *Per 1 oz*			
Chocolate, ¾ cup	120	1	26
w/ Marshmallows, ¾ cup	120	1	26
Cinnamon, ¾ cup,	110	0	26
Original Flakes, ¾ cup	110	0	26
w/ Marshmallows, ¾ c.,	110	0	26
Honey Smacks, 1 oz	100	0.5	24
Krave, Double Choc., 1.1 oz	120	3.5	23
MarioKart, 1 pouch, 0.78 oz	70	0	17
Mini-Wheats, Frosted:			
Bite Size, Orig. (21), 1.8 oz	190	1	46
Little Bites: Orig., 1 c., 2 oz	200	1	47
Chocolate, 1 cup, 2 oz	200	2	46
Touch of Fruit In Middle, Raspberry (24), 2 oz	190	1	45
Mini Wheats, unfrosted:			
Bite Size (30), 1.8 oz	190	1	46
Little Bites, 1 cup, 2 oz	200	1	47
Mueslix, ²/₃ cup, 2 oz	200	3	41
Raisin Bran: Reg., 1 c., 2 oz	190	1	46
Crunch, 1 cup, 2 oz	190	1	45
Rice Krispies: Orig., 1.2 oz	130	0	29
Frosted, ³/₄ cup, 1 oz	120	0	27
Treats, ³/₄ cup, 1 oz	120	1	26
Smart Start, Orig. Antioxidants, 1 cup, 1.8 fl.oz	190	1	43
Special K:			
Apple Cinn. Crunch, 1.1 oz	120	1.5	27
Chocolate Almond, 1 oz	110	1.5	23
Cinn. Brown Sugar Crunch, 1.1 oz	110	1	22
Nourish, C'nut Cranb. Alm., 1.8 oz	200	4	40
Oats & Honey, ²/₃ cup, 1 oz	100	0.5	25
Protein, average, ³/₄ cup, 1.1 oz	115	1	21
Red Berries, 1 cup, 1.1 oz	110	0	27
Vanilla Almond, 1.1 oz	110	1.5	25
Super Mario, 1 cup, 1.2 oz	120	1	27
Kind: *Per ½ Cup, 1.8 oz*			
Clusters: Banana Nut; Raspb. Chia	190	3	36
Cinnamon Oat, with Flax	190	5	34
Dark Chocolate	190	4.5	30
Maple Quinoa, with Chia	200	4.5	34
Peanut Butter Whole Grain	210	6	28

Malt-O-Meal:	C	F	Cb
Apple Zings, 1 cup, 1.2 oz	130	1	29
Cocoa Dyno-Bites, ³/₄ c.	120	1	26
Coco Roos, ³/₄ cup, 1 oz	120	1.5	26
Frosted Flakes, ³/₄ cup, 1 oz	120	0	28
Frosted Mini Spooners,			
Blueberry, 1 cup, 1.95 oz	190	1	45
Golden Puffs, ³/₄ cup, 1 oz	100	0	24
Honey Nut Scooters, 1 cup, 1 oz	120	1.5	24
Raisin Bran, 1 cup, 2 oz	200	1	47
Nature's Path:			
Flax Plus: Flakes, 1 oz	110	1.5	23
Mesa Sunrise Flakes, 1 oz	120	1	24
Multibran Flakes, 1 oz	110	1.5	23
Pumpkin Raisin Crunch, 1.95 oz	210	4.5	40
Heritage Flakes, 1 oz	120	1	24
Honey'd Corn Flakes, ³/₄ cup, 1 oz	120	1	25
Kamut Puffs, 1 cup, 0.5 oz	50	0	11
Love Crunch, Dble Choc Chunk, 1 oz	135	4.5	21
Multigrain Oatbran Flakes, ³/₄ cup, 1 oz	110	1	24
Optimum Power, Blueb. Cinnamon Flax, 1 oz	120	1.5	25
Qi'a, Superfod, Original, 1 oz	140	7	13
New England Natural Bakers:			
Organic Granola:			
Berry Coconut, unsweeetened, ½ cup, 1.5 oz	250	12	31
Blueberry Harvest, ²/₃ cup, 2 oz	260	10	35
Cranberry Almond, ²/₃ cup, 2 oz	240	9	36
Pumpkin Spice, ½ cup, 2 oz	240	7	40
NutriSystem,			
Granola Cereal, 1 pkg	150	3	28
Peace:			
Clusters & Flakes:			
Blueberry Pomegranate, 2 oz	240	6	41
Blueberry Walnut, 1 oz	220	3	43
Coconut Chia Almond, 2 oz	220	3.5	42
Maple Pecan, 2 oz	240	6	42
Vanilla Almond, 2 oz	240	6	42
Granola: Coconut Craze, 2 oz	270	12	37
French Vanilla, 2 oz	240	6	41
Maple Pecan, 2 oz	250	8	40
Purple Corn Flakes, 1 oz	90	1	23
Raisin Bran, 1 oz	170	0.5	42

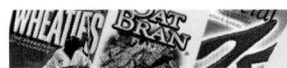

Ready-To-Eat Cereal ~ Brands (Cont)

Post:

	C	F	Cb
Alpha Bits, 1 cup, 1 oz	120	1.5	24
Bran Flakes, ³/₄ cup, 1 oz	100	0.5	24
CoCo Wheats, 1.1 oz	120	0	24
Good Mornings, 1 oz	120	1.5	25
Grape-Nuts: Original, 2 oz	210	1	47
Flakes, ³/₄ cup, 1 oz	110	1	24
Great Grains:			
Banana Nut Crunch, 1 cup, 2 oz	230	5	43
Cranb. Alm. Crunch, 1cup, 2 oz	210	3.5	41
Crunchy Pecan, ³/₄ cup, 2 oz	210	6	38
Honey Bunches of Oats:			
Chocolate, 1.2 oz	130	1.5	27
Honey Roasted, 1 oz	120	1.5	25
Pecan & Maple Brown Sugar	120	2.5	23
With Almonds, 1 oz	130	2.5	26
With Cinnamon, 1 oz	120	1.5	25
Honey-Comb, 1.1 oz	130	1	28
Malt O Meal ~ see Page 60			
Oreo O's, 2 cup, 1 oz	120	1.5	25
Pebbles, av. all varieties, ³/₄ cup, 1 oz	115	1	24
Raisin Bran, 1 cup, 2 oz	190	1	47
Shredded Wheat, Spoon Size:			
Original, 1.7 oz	170	1	40
Honey Nut, 2.1 oz	220	2	49
Waffle Crisp, 1 cup, 1 oz	120	1.5	25
Quaker:			
King Vitaman, 1¹/₂ cups, 1 oz	120	1	26
Life, all types, ³/₄ cup, 1 oz	120	1.5	25
Oatmeal Squares,			
all varieties, 2 oz	210	2.5	44
Quisps, 1 cup 1 oz	100	1.5	23
Simply Granola:			
Apple Cranberry Almond, 1.7 oz	200	5	37
Oats, Honey, & Almonds, 1.7 oz	200	6	35
Stop & Shop:			
Fiber Select, ¹/₂ cup, 1 oz	50	0.5	23
Granola,			
Oats & Honey, ¹/₂ c., 1.8 oz	230	9	31
Oats & O's, 1 cup, 1.1 oz	110	1.5	22
Raisin Bran, 1 cup, 2 oz	190	1	46
Shredded Wheat, Bite Size, 1 c., 1.5 oz	140	1	33
Sweet Home Farm:			
Blueberry, w/Flax, ³/₄ cup, 2 oz	250	8	40
Cinnamon, w/Raisins, ¹/₂ c., 1.8 oz	200	3	43
French Vanilla, w/Alm., ²/₃ c., 2 oz	250	8	40
Honey Nut, w/Alm., ¹/₂ c., 2 oz	260	10	37
Maple Pecan, w/Syrup, ¹/₂ c., 2 oz	250	8	40
Pumpkin Flax, ²/₃ cup, 2 oz	240	9	37

Trader Joe's:

	C	F	Cb
Bran Flakes, ³/₄ cup, 1 oz	100	0.5	24
Cinnamon Squares, 1 cup, 1.5 oz	170	3	31
Clusters: Raisin Bran, 1 cup, 2 oz	190	3	41
Super Nutty Toffee, ³/₄ cup, 2 oz	250	9	38
Vanilla Almond, ²/₃ cup, 2 oz	220	8	34
Av. other Flavors, 1 c., 2 oz	230	8	40
Cornflakes, 1 cup, 1 oz	110	0	26
Frosted Flakes, ³/₄ c., 1 oz	110	0	24
High Fiber Cereal: Reg., ²/₃ cup, 1 oz	80	0.5	23
Fruit & Nut, Multigrain, ²/₃ cup, 1 oz	90	1.5	25
Granola: Gluten Free, ³/₄ cup, 2 oz	60	12	35
Low Fat, av., ³/₄ cup, 2 oz	210	3	44
Org., Apple/Mango, av., ²/₃ cup, 2 oz	240	8	37
Joe's O's, 1 cup, 1 oz	110	2	20
Just The Clusters, av., ²/₃ cup, 2 oz	240	9	36
O's, av. all flavours, ³/₄ - 1 cup, 1 oz	120	2	24
Oatmeal (Instant): Per 1.4 oz Pkt			
Ancient Grains	160	6	24
Mango; Maple & Brown Sugar, av.	160	2	32
Unsweetened	160	3.5	27
Oatmeal Complete: Plain, 1.4 oz pkt	170	3	29
Maple Brown Sugar, 1.4 oz pkt	210	3	38
Raisin Bran: Regular, 1 cup, 1 oz	170	1	44
Clusters, 1 cup, 2 oz	190	3	41
w/ Pomegr. Blue. Flakes/Clusters, 1 c.	210	2	44
Shredded Wheat, 1 cup, 1.7 oz	180	1	38
Toasted Oatmeal Flakes, ³/₄ c., 1 oz	110	1	23
Udi's:			
Granola: Orig.; Cranb., ¹/₄ c., 1 oz	140	6	21
All Naturel; Vanilla, av., ¹/₄ cup, 1 oz	120	4	19
Uncle Sam:			
Original, Wheat Berry,			
³/₄ cup, 2 oz	210	6	37
Skinner's Raisin Bran, 1 cup, 2 oz	200	1	45
Weetabix, 2 bisc., 1.3 oz	130	1	29
Wegmans:			
Chocolaty Rice Crisps, 1 oz	120	1	26
Crunchy Raisin Bran, 1 cup, 1.8 oz	190	1	44
Granola, Vanilla & Almonds, 1 oz	140	4	22
Peanut Butter Corn Crunch, 1 oz	110	2.5	20
Shredded Wheat,			
Bite Size, 1 cup, 2 oz	200	1	44
Whole Foods 365:			
Corn Flakes, 1 cup, 1 oz	110	0	26
Frosted Flakes, 1 oz	110	0	27
Honey Flakes & Oat Clusters,			
³/₄ cup, 1 oz	120	1	25
Protein & Fiber Crunch, 1.8 oz	190	1	33
Raisin Bran, 1 cup, 2 oz	180	1	44
Wheat Squares:			
Bite Sized, 1.7 oz	180	1	38
Frosted, 1 cup, 1.9 oz	210	1	45

Ready-to-Eat   C   F   Cb

Per Piece/Slice

	C	F	Cb
Angel Food, Plain: without oil, 2 oz	145	0	33
with oil, 2 oz	145	1	27
with Cream Frosting	255	7	45
Almond Croissant, 5 oz	620	35	67
Apple Danish, 5 oz	450	18	67
Apple Pie ~ *See Pies/Tarts Page 134*			
Baklava, 1½″ square, 1.75 oz	200	10	27
Banana Cake, with Butter Cream, 2 oz	230	9	37
Banana Walnut Cake, 3 oz	270	11	40
Bear Claw, 4.5 oz	540	24	71
Black Forest, 3 oz	345	11	59
Brownie: Small, 2″ Square, 1 oz	130	8	14
Large, 3 oz	390	24	42
Bundt Cakes, average all types:			
3 oz slice	300	13	42
Mini-Bundt, 5 oz	500	22	70
Cannoli's: Mini, 1 oz	85	3	11
Regular, 2.5 oz	215	8	28
Carrot Cake: Plain, 3 oz	300	16	37
with Cream Cheese Frosting	400	22	48
Cheesecake:			
Small serving, 3 oz	240	13	26
Large serving, 5 oz	400	21	44
with Low-Fat Cheese/Fruit, 3 oz	170	4	28
Denny's, NY Style, 5oz	510	34	43
Chocolate Cake:			
with Chocolate Frosting, 4 oz	415	18	62
without Frosting, 1/12 of 9″, 3.5 oz	340	14	51
Chocolate Croissant, 4.25 oz	470	26	54
Chocolate Eclair, w/ custard, 3.5 oz	260	16	24
Chocolate Fudge Cake, 3 oz	270	12	40
Chocolate Meringue, 2.5 oz	320	13	48
Churros, 1 stick, 1.5 oz	165	8	21
Cinnamon Crumb Cake, 2.5 oz	260	9	40
Cinnamon Rolls: Small, 2 oz	220	8	34
Regular, 4 oz	440	16	68
Large, 6 oz	660	24	102
Brands ~ *See Page 67*			
Coffee Cake, 2 oz	180	6	30
Concha: Small, 2 oz	240	9	33
Large (5″ diameter), 5.5 oz	615	23	85
Cream Puff, custard filled, 4.6 oz	335	20	30
Cream Horn, 3 oz	210	5	36
Crumble Coffee Cake, 4.5 oz	500	25	65
Danish Pastries:			
Small, 2.5 oz	250	14	25
Large, 5 oz	500	28	50
Donuts ~ *See Page 66*			
Eclair, Chocolate, custard filled, 3.5 oz	260	16	24
Fig Bars, average	160	3	31

Ready-to-Eat (Cont)   C   F   Cb

Per Piece/Slice

	C	F	Cb
Fruit Cake, Dark/Light, 2 oz	185	5	34
Fudge Nut Brownie, 3.5 oz	380	18	54
Gingerbread, from mix, 3″ square	210	4	41
Honey Bun, 2.7 oz	310	15	39
Jelly Roll, 1/12 roll, 1.8 oz	150	2	32
Key Lime Pie, 4.3 oz	400	25	41
Kringles: Almond; Pecan, average	205	12	24
Blueberry: Cherry; Raspberry, av.	165	8	24
Lady Finger, 3 oz	310	4.5	59
Lemon Cake, 4 oz	440	24	49
Lemon Poppy Seed Creme, 1.6 oz	180	9	23
Marble Cake, 4 oz	430	23	50
Mississippi Mud Pie, 4 oz	480	22	67
Mud Cake, 4.5 oz	380	20	44
Muffins ~ *See Page 67*			
Palmier Cookie, large, 4.5 oz	490	25	62
Pineapple Upside Down Cake,			
2.5 oz	230	9	36
Peach Melba, 3.5 oz	300	8	52
Pecan Sticky Roll, 6.5 oz	690	22	91
Pecan Twirls, 1.3 oz	170	7	26
Pies & Tarts ~ *See Page 134*			
Pound Cakes: Iced Lemon, 3.5 oz	360	17	50
Marble, 3.75 oz	350	13	53
Raspberry Rugulah,			
1.2 oz	110	9	7
Scone, fruit, 2 oz	200	9	30
Sponge Cake: Plain, 2.5 oz	220	10	33
with Chocolate Frosting	290	12	45
with Cream & Strawberry Jam	390	12	69
Starbucks Cakes ~ *Page 244*			
Strawberry Cream Cake, 4.7 oz	400	27	33
Strudel Bites, 0.75 oz	60	2.5	9
Strudel, fruit, av., 4.5 oz	300	17	32
Swiss Rolls, 1 oz	135	6	19
Tiramisu, 4.5 oz	440	22	34
Turnovers, fruit, average, 3 oz	290	15	35

Cupcakes

Average all Varieties

	C	F	Cb
Regular:			
Cake only, 1.5 oz	140	5.5	20
Cake + Icing, 2.5 oz	260	13	34
Large, (Muffin Size):			
Cake only, 2.5 oz	235	9	34
Cake + Icing, 5 oz	520	27	67
Mini, (2-Bite):			
Cake only, 0.4 oz	40	1.5	5.5
Cake + Icing, 1 oz	110	5.5	13
Icing Only: Per 1 oz	115	7	13
Thick/Tall amount, 2.5 oz	290	17	32

Cakes ~ Brands	C	F	Cb
Albertson's Bakery:			
Ring Cakes: *Per 1/10 Cake*			
Angel Food	135	0	27
Cake Slices: *Per Slice Unless Indicated*			
Banana Nut Loaf	330	17	39
Butter Creme	110	6	20
Creme Cake (2), 3.2 oz	300	12	43
Cinnamon Streusel (2), 3.2 oz	350	18	43
Bimbo Bakery:			
Concha, Vanilla, 2 oz	260	6	35
Pound Cakes: *Per Slice*			
Panquecitos, 1.8 oz	170	4.5	29
Pecan, 2.3 oz	260	11	36
Raisin, 2.3 oz	240	9	38
Bon Appetit Bakery:			
Banana Bread, 4 oz	440	25	49
Cream Cheese Cake,			
4 oz slice	430	24	49
Danish: Apple (1), 5 oz	210	11	25
Bear Claw (1), 5 oz	240	13	27
Cheese & Berries (1), 5 oz	250	14	26
Vienna Cream (1), 5 oz	240	14	27
Slices: Cheesecake, 4 oz	430	24	49
Lemon Cake, 4 oz	430	24	49
Marble Cake, 4 oz	430	24	50
Walnut Brownie, 3.5 oz	380	18	54
Cheesecake Factory ~ *See Fast-Foods Section*			
Entenmann's: *Per Slice*			
Crumb Cake: Butter French, 1/8 cake	210	10	29
Cheese-Filled, 1/9 cake	200	10	25
NY Style, 1/9 cake	250	12	34
Danish: Cherry Cheese, 1/8 cake	180	6	28
Pecan Twist, 1/6 cake	260	16	27
Raspberry Twist, 1/8 oz	220	11	29
Dessert Cakes:			
Chocolate Fudge, 1/8 cake	240	10	37
Lemon, 1/8 cake	280	15	37
Marshmallow Devil's Food, 1/8 cake	260	13	36
Vanilla Bean Iced Cake, 1/6 cake	380	20	47
Loaf Cakes: Chocolate, 1/6 loaf	190	8	29
Cinnamon Crunch, 1/6 loaf	270	14	33
Glenny's:			
100 Calorie:			
Blondie, Choc. Chip, 1.5 oz	100	4	15
Brownies: Chocolate Chip, 1.5 oz	100	4	12
Peanut Butter, 1.5 oz	100	4	15
Muffins/Sweet Rolls ~ See Page 67			

Great American Cookies:	C	F	Cb
Cookie Cakes: *Per Slice*			
By the Slice, 4.5 oz	580	27	83
Heart Shaped, 3.5 oz	440	21	64
M&M, 4 oz	500	24	73
Great Value *(Walmart)*:			
Chocolate Cup Cake, (1), 2 oz	200	6	35
Snack Cakes: Fudge Swirl, (1), 1.3oz	165	8	23
Choc./Lemon Snack Cake, 1 oz	120	6	18
Swiss Roll Snack Cake (1), 1 oz	120	5	17
Hostess:			
Cup Cakes:			
100 Calorie Packs, av., 3 minicakes	100	2.5	21
8 Pack, Chocolate, 1 cake, 1.5 oz	160	6	26
Ding Dongs, (1)	165	9	22
Ho Hos, (1)	120	5	18
Twinkies:			
Original; Banana, av., (1)	140	5	24
Deep Fried: Original (1)	220	9	32
Chocolate (1)	220	8	36
Zingers, (2)	250	9	41
Donettes ~ Page 66			
Little Debbie:			
Boxed: Boston Creme Roll, (1)	270	12	40
Choc. Chip Cake, 2 oz	300	14	42
Choc. Cup Cake, Crm Filled (1), 1.9 oz	210	8	33
Cocoa Cremes, (1), 1.5 oz	170	8	24
Devil Cremes ,(1), 1.66 oz	200	9	29
Devil Squares, (2), 2.2 oz	260	11	38
Fancy Cakes, (2), 2.4 oz	310	15	43
Frosted Fudge Cake, (1), 1.5 oz	190	9	27
Fudge Brownie (1)	280	12	40
S'mores Cake Rolls, (1), 2.2 oz	260	11	40
Zebra Cake, (1), 2.6 oz	320	14	48
Ne-Mo's:			
Breads: Banana, 4 oz	460	23	57
Carrot, 4 oz	450	22	56
Cheese Coffee Cake, 4 oz	460	21	62
Wild Blueberry Bread, 4 oz	430	20	58
Brookie, (1), 1.5 oz	160	7	26
Bundt: Chocolate, 4 oz	380	14	62
Coconut Pineapple, 4 oz	410	18	60
Key Lime, 4 oz	440	18	67
Orange Dreamswirl	440	18	67
Cake Squares: Carrot, 3.6 oz	390	21	47
Banana; Chocolate, av, 3 oz	300	12	45
Crumble Cake: Blueberry (1), 4 oz	390	17	54
Cinnamon Streusel (1), 4 oz	420	18	59
Lemon Rasp. (1), 4 oz	400	19	55

Cakes ~ Brands (Cont)	**C**	**F**	**Cb**
Pepperidge Farm:			
3-Layer Cakes: *Per ⅛ Cake*			
Chocolate Fudge	240	13	30
Coconut 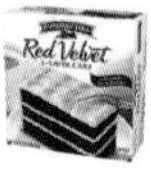	250	12	34
Creamy Red Velvet	240	13	30
Key Lime; Vanilla	240	12	34
Average other varieties	240	11	33
Turnovers (Frozen): 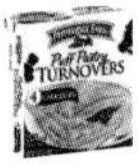			
Apple; Cherry (1)	260	13	31
Chocolate (1)	350	22	35
Peach; Raspberry (1)	270	13	34
Pop Tarts *(Kellogg's):* 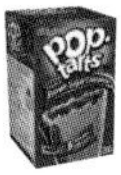			
Chocolate Chip	210	6	36
Fruit/Frosted/Unfrosted, av.	200	5	36
Wholegrain, Strawberry	180	2.5	38
Safeway Select,			
Molten Chocolate Lava Cake, 4.5 oz	440	26	50
Sara Lee:			
Banana Cake, ⅕ cake 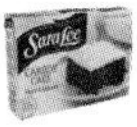	270	10	42
Carrot Cake, ⅙ cake	340	17	44
Cheesecakes:			
Classic: Cheesecake, ¼ cake	330	17	37
Cherry, ¼ cake	360	12	55
Strawberry, ¼ cake 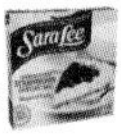	330	12	50
New York Style, ⅕ cake	480	29	48
French Style: Classic	410	26	38
Strawberry, ⅙ cake	310	18	35
NY Style: Original, ⅙ cake	510	30	52
Chocolate, ⅙ cake 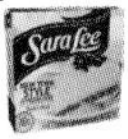	500	29	55
Pumpkin, ⅙ cake	480	30	46
Pound Cakes:			
All Butter, ⅙ cake	290	15	36
Blueberry, ¼ cake 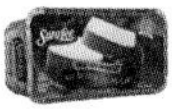	230	8	38
Lemon, ¼ cake	240	8	38
Slices: Original, 1.4 oz	150	5	24
Double Chocolate, 1.5 oz	150	5	24
Special K,			
Pastry Crisps, all varieties, (2), 1 oz	100	2	20
Tastykake:			
Choc Cupcakes:			
Chocolate Koffee Kake, 2.1 oz	220	7	36
Cream Filled, 2.1 oz 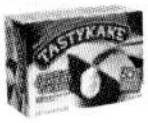	220	8	34
Banana Pudding, 2 oz	180	6	31

Tastykake (Cont):	**C**	**F**	**Cb**
Kandy Kake:			
Lemon Flavored, 2 oz 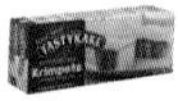	290	16	34
Peanut Butter, 1.4 oz	190	11	19
Krimpets, Spice Kake Cake, (2)	220	7	37
Mini Cupcakes, Koffee Kake (3)	180	8	25
Toaster Strudel *(Pillsbury): Per 2 oz*			
Boston Cream Pie 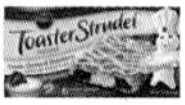	180	7	25
Cream Cheese,			
average all varieties	190	9	25
Fruit flavors, all var. 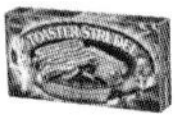	190	8	26
Trader Joe's:			
Bakery Fresh:			
Apricot Almond Tart, 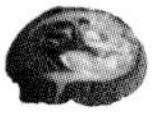			
4 oz slice	450	24	56
Cheesecake Brownie Bites (1)	110	7	9
Chocolate Ganache Cake, 3 oz slice	390	22	44
Flourless Chocolate Cake, 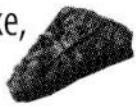			
1 slice, 2 oz	260	17	23
Lemon Cake, 3.3oz slice	350	19	43
Mini Carrot Cake, 5 oz	450	19	68
Whoopie Pie (1), 2.5 oz 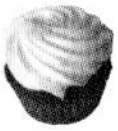	350	14	54
Bread Cake:			
Banana Bonanza, 2.6 oz slice	250	9	39
Pumpkin Nut, 2.6 oz slice	270	10	43
Walnut Streusel Coffee, 2 oz slice	180	8	25
Zucchini Carrot, 2 oz slice	200	7	32
Loaf Cake:			
Cranberry Pumpkin, 2 oz slice	140	2	30
Pumpkin Nut, 2.6 oz slice	270	10	43
Frozen:			
Apple Raspberry Turnover, 3.2 oz	280	14	34
Chocolate Dilemma Cheesecake:			
Plain, 3.5 oz	320	19	30
Choc. Chip; Triple Choc, av., 3.5 oz	345	20	35
Tuxedo, 3.5 oz	320	17	34
Choc Lava Cake, 4 oz 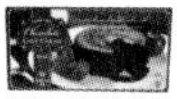	360	23	40
Karat Cake, 3 oz slice	320	19	37
N.Y. Style Cheesecake, 4.5 oz slice	400	28	32
Tiramisu Torte, 3.2 oz slice	230	12	24
Tarts 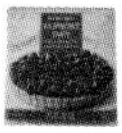			
Pear, 3.5 oz slice	250	9	39
Raspberry, 5 oz slice	290	10	51
Wild Blueberry, 3.5 oz slice	260	6	52

Cakes ~ Mixes	**C**	**F**	**Cb**

Prepared as Directed
Arrowhead Mills:
Brownie Mix:

	C	F	Cb
Regular, $^1/_{20}$ package, 1 oz	150	7	21
Gluten Free,			
Fudge Brownie, $^1/_{20}$ pkg., 1 oz	160	8	21
Cake Mix:			
Chocolate, organic, $^1/_{12}$ pkg., 1.75 oz	280	11	42
Vanilla, $^1/_{12}$ package, 1.7 oz	270	10	39

Betty Crocker: *Prepared as Directed*
Brownie Mix:

	C	F	Cb
Dark Choc. Fudge, $^1/_{20}$ pkg	160	6.5	24
Fudge, $^1/_{20}$ package	160	7	22
Low-Fat Fudge, $^1/_{18}$ pkg	140	2.5	28
Gluten Free, Chocolate, $^1/_{16}$ pkg	150	5	24
Premium:			
Chocolate Chunk, $^1/_{16}$ pkg	170	7	26
Original Supreme, $^1/_{16}$ package	190	8	27
P'nut Butter; Walnut, av., $^1/_{16}$ pkg	170	7	24
Triple Chunk, $^1/_{20}$ package	180	8	25
Ultimate Fudge, $^1/_{16}$ package	170	6.5	26

Gluten Free Cake Mix:

	C	F	Cb
Devils Food, $^1/_{10}$ Pkg	260	12	36
Yellow, $^1/_{10}$ Pkg	260	11	37

SuperMoiste Cake Mixes: *Per $^1/_{10}$ Package*

	C	F	Cb
Butter Recipe Yellow	240	9	36
Carrot	310	18	35
Cherry Chip	280	14	36
Devil's Food; French Vanilla	280	14	35
Lemon	280	14	36
Milk Chocolate	250	10	35
Triple Chocolate Fudge	280	14	34

If using No-Cholesterol Recipe, deduct 40 cals and 4g fat.

Dessert Bars: Reeses, 1 oz mix	180	12	20
Sunkist Lemon, 1 oz mix	140	4.5	24

Duncan Hines: *Prepared as Directed*
Brownie Mix:

	C	F	Cb
Chewy Fudge Brownie, $^1/_{20}$ pkg	150	7	22
Decadent, Caramel Turtle, $^1/_{15}$ pkg	170	7	25
Double Fudge, $^1/_{16}$ pkg	170	8	25

Cake Mix,

Classic, Dark Choc. Fudge, $^1/_{10}$ pkg	260	13	33

Decadent: *Per $^1/_{12}$ Pkg*

Classic Carrot	260	10	39
German Chocolate	290	14	37

Prepared as Directed
Duncan Hines (Cont):
Signature: *Per $^1/_{12}$ Pkg*

	C	F	Cb
Banana Supreme	270	12	36
French Vanilla; German Choc., av.	270	12	34
Red Velvet	250	12	33

Jell-O:
No Bake Cheesecake:

	C	F	Cb
Cherry, $^1/_8$ pkg, 2.2 oz	360	20	41
Real Cheesecake, $^1/_8$ pkg, 2.2 oz	350	16	49

Krusteaz:

Cinn. Swirl Crumb Cake, 2½x2" pce	210	5	39
Lemon; Key Lime Bar, 2" bar	140	3	26

Pillsbury:
Brownies, Premium Mix: *Dry Mix Only*

	C	F	Cb
Caramel Swirl, $^1/_{12}$ pkg, 1.2 oz	120	1	28
Cheesecake Swirl, $^1/_{15}$ pkg, 1 oz	110	1.5	25
Chocolate Extreme, $^1/_{15}$ pkg, 1 oz	120	2	24
Double Chocolate, $^1/_{16}$ pkg, 1 oz	100	0.5	24

Cakes:

	C	F	Cb
Funfetti: Bold Purple $^1/_6$ pkg, 1.4 oz	140	1.5	21
Neon Yellow, $^1/_6$ pkg, 1.4 oz	140	1.5	21
Moist Supreme: *Per $^1/_{10}$ Pkg, Dry Mix Only*			
Devils Food, 1.5 oz	150	2	34
White/Yellow, 1.5 oz	160	1.5	35

Cake Frostings			

Betty Crocker:
Rich & Creamy,

	C	F	Cb
average all flavors, 2 Tbsp, 1.2 oz	135	5	22
Whipped, av. all flavors.,2 T., 0.9 oz	100	4.5	15
Cool Whip, Original, 2 Tbsp, 0.3 oz	25	1.5	2

Duncan Hines:

Creamy Homestyle, av. all flav., 2T.	140	6	23
Whipped, av. all flavors, 3 Tbsp	150	7	21

Pillsbury: *Per 2 Tbsp*
Creamy Supreme:

	C	F	Cb
Choc Fudge; Milk Choc., 1.2 oz	130	6	21
Classic White; Vanilla, 1.2 oz	140	5	22
Fluffy, av. all flavors, 2 Tbsp, 0.8 oz	100	5	14
Funfetti, av. all flavors, 2 Tbsp,1.2 oz	140	5	23
Sugar Free, average, 2 Tbsp, 1.1 oz	100	6	16

Quick Guide   **C** **F** **Cb**

Donuts
Average All Brands

	C	F	Cb
Cake: Plain, 1.8 oz	205	12	23
Chocolate Iced, 2 oz	255	14	29
Sugared, 0.8 oz	205	10	29
Non-Cake, Glazed, 2 oz	225	11	29

Croissant-Donuts
(Includes Cronuts/Frissants)

Average all Brands

	C	F	Cb
Cream-filled, 3.5 oz	430	26	45
Custard-filled, 3.5 oz	360	19	45

Extra Listings ~ *See CalorieKing.com*
(Cronut is a trademark of Dominique Ansel Bakery, New York)

Donuts ~ Brands

Albertson's:
Donut Holes:

	C	F	Cb
Glazed Old Fashioned (4)	240	12	31
Powdered Sugar (4)	210	12	24
Gem Donuts: Plain Cake (3)	190	12	20
Cinnamon Sugar (3)	240	15	23
Glazed (1)	140	6	21

Bon Appetit:
Mini Donuts:

	C	F	Cb
Chocolate (4)	270	16	29
Crumb (4)	240	12	32
Powdered (4)	250	12	34

Dunkin' Donuts:

	C	F	Cb
Apple Crumb	320	15	42
Apple N' Spice	260	14	29
Barvarian Kreme	270	15	31
Blueberry Butternut	420	17	60
Blueberry Crumb Cake	380	18	50
Boston Kreme	300	16	37
Chocolate Frosted Cake	350	19	40
Chocolate Headlight	330	18	39
Choc. Peanut Butter Flav. Cream	360	19	44
Glazed Chocolate	340	19	38
Jelly Filled	270	14	32
Powdered	320	19	33
Vanilla Creme	330	20	35

Extra Listings ~ *See Fast Food Section*

Donuts ~ Brands (Cont)   **C** **F** **Cb**

Entenmann's:
8 Pack: *Per Donut*

	C	F	Cb
Plain	220	13	24
Crumb Topped	250	12	36
Glazed	260	13	34
Rich Frosted	290	19	30

Pop'ems:

	C	F	Cb
Pumpkin (4)	230	13	29
Rich Frosted (4)	320	23	28

Hostess:

	C	F	Cb
Mini Donettes: Crumb, 6-pack, 4 oz	430	18	63
Frosted, 6-pack, 3 oz	360	22	38
Powdered, 6-pack, 3 oz	340	17	43

Krispy Kreme:

	C	F	Cb
Apple Fritter, 3.5 oz	350	19	42
Chocolate: Iced Cake, 2.5 oz	280	13	37
Iced Custard Filled, 3 oz	300	15	37
Iced Glazed Cruller, 2.5 oz	260	10	40
Iced Glazed, 2.2	240	11	33
Iced Kreme Filled, 3 oz	350	19	41
Iced Glazed w/ Sprinkles, 2.3 oz	250	11	36
Cinnamon Twist, 1.9oz	210	11	26
Glazed Cruller, 1.9 oz	210	10	29

Glazed Doughnut Holes:

	C	F	Cb
Original (5)	220	11	25
Blueberry (4)	190	7	28
Cake (4)	190	8	28
Chocolate Cake (4)	180	7	27
Glazed Kreme Filled, 3 oz	340	19	40
Maple Iced Glazed, 2.2 oz	240	11	34
New York Cheesecake, 3.3 oz	310	17	35
Original Glazed, 1.7 oz	190	11	22
Powdered Cake, 2.3 oz	240	11	29
Traditional Cake, 2 oz	230	12	26

Little Debbie,

	C	F	Cb
Donut Sticks, 1.9 oz	270	16	29

Tastykake:

	C	F	Cb
Cinnamon, (3), 2 oz	230	11	31
Mini: Crunch, 3 oz pkg	330	13	50
Powdered Sugar, 2.5 oz pkg	300	14	41

Quick Guide   **C** **F** **Cb**

Muffins: Ready-To-Eat
Average All Brands

	C	F	Cb
Small, 1 oz	90	3.5	14
Medium, 2 oz	185	6.5	28
Large, 3 oz	275	10	42
Extra Large, 4 oz	365	13	57
Giant, 6 oz	550	20	84
Super Size, 8 oz	730	27	112

Muffins Ready-To-Eat ~ Brands

	C	F	Cb
Albertsons:			
Minis: Banana Nut (2)	200	12	20
Blueberry (2)	180	10	21
Honey Raisin Bran (2)	170	7	24
Entenmann's,			
Blueberry; Choc. Chip; Corn (1), av.	190	9	25
Garden Lites: Chocolate (1), 2 oz	120	4	21
Banana Choc. Chip (1), 2 oz	120	3	23
Blueberry Oat (1), 2 oz	120	2	25
Av. other flavors (1), 1 oz	70	2	13
Great Value *(Walmart):*			
Double Banana Filled,(1), 4 oz	360	16	52
Double Blueberry Filled, (1), 4 oz	430	16	65
Triple Chocolate Filled, (1), 4 oz	420	18	61
Little Debbie: Banana Nut (1), 1.9 oz	210	9	30
Blueberry (1), 1.9 oz	190	8	27
Chocolate Chip (1), 1.9 oz	210	9	28
My Favorite Muffin: *Per Large*			
Banana Nut	650	38	71
Blueberry	590	28	78
Boston Cream Pie	740	33	105
Chocolate Chip	790	39	100
Lemon Poppyseed	670	32	90
Otis Spunkmeyer:			
Banana, 2 oz	220	10	30
Blueberry, 2 oz	210	9	29
Choc. Chip Minis (3), 2.25 oz	270	14	32
Starbucks ~ *See Fast-Foods Section*			
Trader Joe's: *Per Muffin*			
Apple Cranberry, 4.8 oz	220	5	38
Banana Chocolate Chip, 4 oz	400	18	57
Carrot, 4 oz	320	11	52
Triple Berry, 4 oz	310	11	49
Vitalicious:			
VitaTops: Deep Choc./Choc Mint, 2 oz	100	1.5	26
Wild Blueberry, 2 oz	120	2	25
Protein, hoc. P'nut Butter, 2 oz	150	4	23
Sugar free, Velvety Choc., 2 oz	90	2	24
Weight Watchers:			
Blueb.; Double Choc, av., 2.5 oz	185	2.5	42

Muffin Mixes   **C** **F** **Cb**

Per Muffin, Prepared

	C	F	Cb
Betty Crocker: Banana Nut	170	8	22
Cinnamon Streusel	190	8	27
Wild Blueberry	160	6.5	24
Pouch Mix, with Milk:			
Banana Nut	130	4	24
Blueberry	130	3	23
Chocolate Chip	130	3	23
Krusteaz:			
Choc Chunk	260	12	33
Lemon Poppyseed	170	4	31
Oat Bran	180	4.5	32
Trader Joe's, Triple Berry	150	2	28

Sweet Rolls & Buns

Note: It is best to weigh for accuracy as actual weight can be 10-50% higher than label weight·

Per Sweet Roll or Bun Unless Indicated

	C	F	Cb
Bimbo, Bimbolete, 2.2 oz	250	10	36
Bon Appetit,			
Cinnamon Roll, 2.5 oz	230	8	34
Cinnabon: Classic	880	37	127
Caramel Pecanbon	1080	51	146
Cloverhill Bakery,			
Jumbo Glazed Honey Bun, 4.75 oz	600	35	64
Entenmann's, Cinn. Swirl Bun, 3 oz	320	14	44
Little Debbie:			
Honey Bun: 2.3 oz	280	16	32
Individual: 3 oz Bun	360	20	41
4 oz Bun	480	26	56
with White Icing, 4 oz	490	25	60
Pecan Spinwheels: Single, 1 oz	100	3.5	17
2 Pack, 2.1 oz	210	7	32
O&H Danish: *Per 1.95 oz*			
Kringles: Apple	180	7	26
Almond; Turtle, average	215	10	30
Cinn. Roll; Cream Cheese, average	205	11	26
Wisconsin,	170	5.5	28
Pillsbury:			
Sweet Rolls, Refrigerated: *Per Roll Unless Indicated*			
Cinnamon, w/ Crm Cheese Icing	140	4.5	23
Cinn., Flaky w/ Butter Cream Icing	160	7	23
Twists, Flaky Cinnamon, with Icing	160	7	23
Grands, Refrigerated: *Per Roll*			
Cinnabon: Cinnamon Roll,			
with Cream Cheese Icing	300	7	54
Caramel Rolls, with Icing, 3.5 oz	300	8	53
Flaky Supreme Cinnamon Roll,			
with Icing, 3.5 oz	360	17	47
7-Eleven: Iced Honey Bun, 6 oz	820	58	68
Glazed Honey Bun, 5 oz	620	35	70
Sara Lee, Cinnamon Roll, 2.4 oz	260	12	33

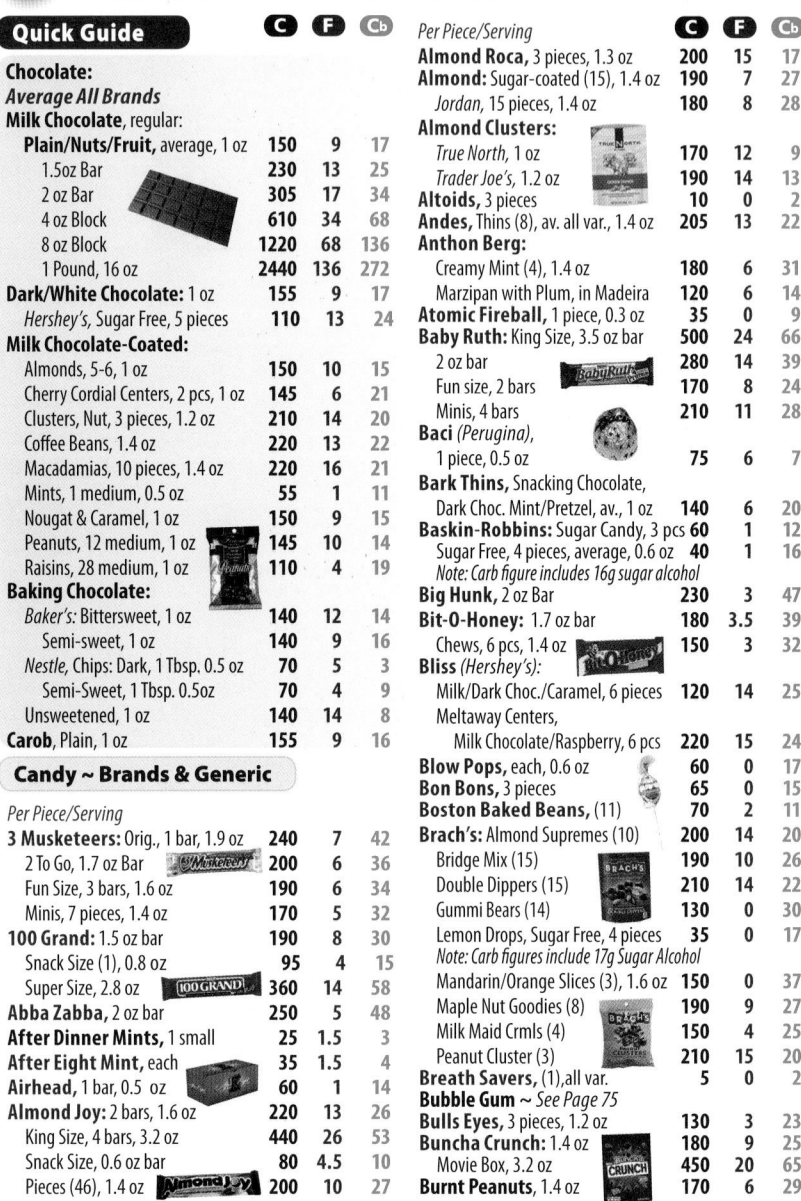

Quick Guide

C **F** **Cb**

Chocolate:
Average All Brands
Milk Chocolate, regular:

	C	F	Cb
Plain/Nuts/Fruit, average, 1 oz	150	9	17
1.5oz Bar	230	13	25
2 oz Bar	305	17	34
4 oz Block	610	34	68
8 oz Block	1220	68	136
1 Pound, 16 oz	2440	136	272
Dark/White Chocolate: 1 oz	155	9	17
Hershey's, Sugar Free, 5 pieces	110	13	24

Milk Chocolate-Coated:

	C	F	Cb
Almonds, 5-6, 1 oz	150	10	15
Cherry Cordial Centers, 2 pcs, 1 oz	145	6	21
Clusters, Nut, 3 pieces, 1.2 oz	210	14	20
Coffee Beans, 1.4 oz	220	13	22
Macadamias, 10 pieces, 1.4 oz	220	16	21
Mints, 1 medium, 0.5 oz	55	1	11
Nougat & Caramel, 1 oz	150	9	15
Peanuts, 12 medium, 1 oz	145	10	14
Raisins, 28 medium, 1 oz	110	4	19

Baking Chocolate:

	C	F	Cb
Baker's: Bittersweet, 1 oz	140	12	14
Semi-sweet, 1 oz	140	9	16
Nestle, Chips: Dark, 1 Tbsp. 0.5 oz	70	5	3
Semi-Sweet, 1 Tbsp. 0.5oz	70	4	8
Unsweetened, 1 oz	140	14	8
Carob, Plain, 1 oz	155	9	16

Candy ~ Brands & Generic

Per Piece/Serving

	C	F	Cb
3 Musketeers: Orig., 1 bar, 1.9 oz	240	7	42
2 To Go, 1.7 oz Bar	200	6	36
Fun Size, 3 bars, 1.6 oz	190	6	34
Minis, 7 pieces, 1.4 oz	170	5	32
100 Grand: 1.5 oz bar	190	8	30
Snack Size (1), 0.8 oz	95	4	15
Super Size, 2.8 oz	360	14	58
Abba Zabba, 2 oz bar	250	5	48
After Dinner Mints, 1 small	25	1.5	3
After Eight Mint, each	35	1.5	4
Airhead, 1 bar, 0.5 oz	60	1	14
Almond Joy: 2 bars, 1.6 oz	220	13	26
King Size, 4 bars, 3.2 oz	440	26	53
Snack Size, 0.6 oz bar	80	4.5	10
Pieces (46), 1.4 oz	200	10	27

Per Piece/Serving

C **F** **Cb**

	C	F	Cb
Almond Roca, 3 pieces, 1.3 oz	200	15	17
Almond: Sugar-coated (15), 1.4 oz	190	7	27
Jordan, 15 pieces, 1.4 oz	180	8	28
Almond Clusters:			
True North, 1 oz	170	12	9
Trader Joe's, 1.2 oz	190	14	13
Altoids, 3 pieces	10	0	2
Andes, Thins (8), av. all var., 1.4 oz	205	13	22
Anthon Berg:			
Creamy Mint (4), 1.4 oz	180	6	31
Marzipan with Plum, in Madeira	120	6	14
Atomic Fireball, 1 piece, 0.3 oz	35	0	9
Baby Ruth: King Size, 3.5 oz bar	500	24	66
2 oz bar	280	14	39
Fun size, 2 bars	170	8	24
Minis, 4 bars	210	11	28
Baci *(Perugina),* 1 piece, 0.5 oz	75	6	7
Bark Thins, Snacking Chocolate, Dark Choc. Mint/Pretzel, av., 1 oz	140	6	20
Baskin-Robbins: Sugar Candy, 3 pcs	60	1	12
Sugar Free, 4 pieces, average, 0.6 oz	40	1	16

Note: Carb figure includes 16g sugar alcohol

	C	F	Cb
Big Hunk, 2 oz Bar	230	3	47
Bit-O-Honey: 1.7 oz bar	180	3.5	39
Chews, 6 pcs, 1.4 oz	150	3	32
Bliss *(Hershey's):*			
Milk/Dark Choc./Caramel, 6 pieces	120	14	25
Meltaway Centers, Milk Chocolate/Raspberry, 6 pcs	220	15	24
Blow Pops, each, 0.6 oz	60	0	17
Bon Bons, 3 pieces	65	0	15
Boston Baked Beans, (11)	70	2	11
Brach's: Almond Supremes (10)	200	14	20
Bridge Mix (15)	190	10	26
Double Dippers (15)	210	14	22
Gummi Bears (14)	130	0	30
Lemon Drops, Sugar Free, 4 pieces	35	0	17

Note: Carb figures include 17g Sugar Alcohol

	C	F	Cb
Mandarin/Orange Slices (3), 1.6 oz	150	0	37
Maple Nut Goodies (8)	190	9	27
Milk Maid Crmls (4)	150	4	25
Peanut Cluster (3)	210	15	20
Breath Savers, (1),all var.	5	0	2
Bubble Gum ~ *See Page 75*			
Bulls Eyes, 3 pieces, 1.2 oz	130	3	23
Buncha Crunch: 1.4 oz	180	9	25
Movie Box, 3.2 oz	450	20	65
Burnt Peanuts, 1.4 oz	170	6	29

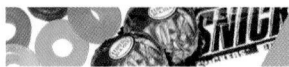

Candy ~ Brands & Generic (Cont)

Per Piece/Serving	C	F	Cb
Butterfinger: 2 oz bar	270	11	43
King Size (3 bars), 3.5 oz	480	18	75
Fun Size, (1), 0.8 oz	100	4	15
Giant, (Pieces in Choc.),			
¼ bar, 1 oz	150	8	21
Miniatures:			
1 piece, 0.4 oz	45	2	8
4 pieces, 1.4 oz	180	8	32
Crisp Bar: Original, 2 oz bar	270	11	43
King Size, 3 pieces, 2 oz	310	17	38
Minis, 2 bars, 1.4 oz	210	11	25
Snackerz:			
Single, 1.3 oz	170	8	23
Fun Size, 2 pcs, 1.2 oz	150	7	21
King Size, 10 pcs, 1.4 oz	190	8	25
Butter Mints, 7 pieces, 0.5 oz	50	0	12
Butterscotch: 3 pieces	60	0	15
Discs (Walgreens), 3 pieces, 0.6 oz	70	0	17
Cadbury: Caramello Bar, 1.6 oz	220	10	29
Caramel Egg, 1.2 oz	170	8	22
Dairy Milk Bar, 7 pcs, 1.4 oz	200	11	23
Mini Eggs (Candy), 12 pcs, 1.4 oz	190	8	28
Candy Apple, medium, 6.5 oz	280	0	60
Candy Cane, medium, 5", 0.5 oz	40	0	14
Candy Corn, 20 pieces, 1.4 oz	150	0	38
Candy Jar Mix (Jewel), 3 pcs, 0.6 oz	60	0	14
Candy Necklace (Smarties), (1), 0.8 oz	90	0.5	20
Caramels: Each, 0.4 oz	40	1	8
Chocolate, each, 0.3 oz	25	0.3	6
Creams (3), 1.3 oz	130	3	23
Caramel Popcorn, ⅔ cup	150	6	23
Cella's,			
Milk Choc. Cherries, 3 pieces, 1.5 oz	160	6	27
Certs, Breath Mints, 1 piece	5	0	2
Charleston Chew:			
Chocolate Bar (1), 1.4 oz	160	4.5	30
Mini Bars, 13 pieces	190	6	34
Charms: Blow Pop	60	0	17
Flat Pop, 0.5 oz	50	0	14
Chew-ets, Peanut Chews,			
Original (4), 1.6 oz	230	12	29
Chewz, 1 roll, 1 oz	120	1	28
Chick O Stick, 2 oz	240	9	42

Per Piece/Serving	C	F	Cb
Chunky Bar (Nestlé),			
King Size, 2.5 oz	340	19	44
Chupa Chups, 1 Pop	50	0	12
Cinn. Buttons (Walgreens), 3 pieces	60	0	16
Cinnamon Disks (Walmart), 3 pieces	70	0	18
Circus Peanuts (Spangler),			
6 pieces, 1.3 oz	165	0	41
CocoaVia, Orig., 0.8 oz	100	6	12
Coconut Stacks, (8)	320	16	46
Coffee Go, Candy, (4)	60	1	12
Conversation Hearts (Necco):			
Small (40), 1.4 oz	160	0	39
1 large	10	0	3
Cookie Dough Bites, 1.4 oz	200	10	27
Cote d'Or: Dark 86% Coca, 4 pcs	270	22	14
Dark, 70%, Orange, 3.5 oz	575	46	34
Dark, Raspberry, 3.5 oz	580	46	34
Milk, Intense, 3.5 oz	575	40	45
Cotton Candy, 1 oz	110	0	28
Cough Drops ~ See Page 75			
Cracker Jack, ½ cup, 1 oz	120	2	23
Creme Savers:			
3 pieces, 0.5 oz	60	1	11
Sugar-Free, 3 pieces	30	1	8
Crisped Rice, Choc Chip, 1 bar, 1 oz	115	4	20
Crows, 11 pieces, 1.4 oz	130	0	33
Crunch Bar ~ See Nestle			
Dots, 11 dots, 1.4 oz	130	0	33
Double Dip Stick, 1 stick	15	0.5	3
Dove:			
Milk Choc: Singles Bar, 1.4 oz	220	13	24
Large Tablet Bar, 9 pcs, 1.5 oz	230	13	25
Choc. Cov. Almonds, 13 pcs, 1.4 oz	220	15	19
Promises: Milk Choc., 1 pce, 0.3 oz	45	2.5	5
w/ Caramel, 1 piece, 0.3 oz	40	2	5
w/ Peanut Butter, 1 pce, 0.3 oz	45	3	4
Swirls, all var., 9 pieces 1.5 oz	230	14	25
Dark Choc: Singles Bar, 1.3 oz	220	13	24
Large Tablet Bar, 9 pcs, 1.5 oz	220	14	25
Choc. Cov. Almds, 13 pcs, 1.4 oz	210	15	19
Promises, Almond, 1 piece, 0.3 oz	40	3	4
Swirls, Raspberry, 9 pcs, 1.4 oz	220	14	24
Sugar Free, all flav., 5 pcs, 1.4 oz	195	15	21
Dum Dum Pops (Spangler), 1 pop	25	0	7
Drops (Hershey's):			
Cookies 'n' Creme, 14 pieces, 1.5 oz	210	11	26
Milk Chocolate, 15 pieces, 1.4 oz	200	12	25

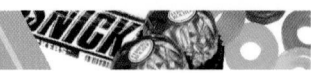

Candy ~ Brands & Generic (Cont)

Per Piece/Serving

	C	F	Cb
English Toffee, 1 piece, 0.4 oz	70	4	6
5th Avenue: 2 oz bar	260	12	38
King Size, 3.5 oz	440	20	64
Fannie May:			
Mint Meltaway (1)	230	15	24
Pixie (1), 1.5 oz	210	12	24
Trinidad (1), 1.5 oz	200	12	23
Fast Break (Reese's): 2 oz bar	260	12	35
3.5 oz bar	460	22	62
Ferrero Rocher: 1 piece	75	5	5
3 pieces, 1.3 oz	220	16	16
Rondnoir, 3 pieces, 1 oz	180	13	14
Fifty 50 Snack Bars:			
Milk Chocolate:			
5 pieces, 1 oz	135	11	14
Almond, 5 pieces, 1 oz	135	12	14
Crunch Bar, 7 pcs, 1 oz	140	12	16
Dark Chocolate, 5 pieces, 1 oz	120	11	15
Note: Carb figures include 9-12g Sugar Alcohol			
Fluffy Stuff *(Charms)*,			
Cotton Candy, 1.4 oz	150	0	40
Fondant: Choc-coated, 1.2 oz	125	3	27
Mint, 1 oz	105	0	25
Fran's: Gold Bar, Macadamia (1)	250	14	27
GoldBite, Almond (1)	120	7	13
Fruit Drops, (1), $\frac{1}{4}$ oz	20	0	4
Fruit Gems *(Sunkist)*, (4), 1.4 oz	130	0	33
Fruit Leathers, average, 0.5 oz	50	0.5	12
Fruit Pastilles *(Rowntree)*, 1 roll	185	0	45
Fruit Roll-Ups *(Betty Crocker/Sunkist)*,			
1 roll, 0.5 oz	50	1	12
Fruit Runts *(Walgreens)*,			
12 pieces	60	0	14
Fruit Flavored Shapes *(Betty Crocker)*,			
all varieties, 0.8 oz	80	0	19
Fudge:			
Chocolate; Mint, 1 oz	130	8	14
P'nut Butter & Choc., 1 oz	130	8	13
Brevin's: Cashew, 1 oz	195	9	28
Triple Decker, 1 oz	165	7	25
Ghirardelli:			
3 oz Bars: Dark Choc., 4 squares	220	17	23
Filled, P'nut Butter, 4 squares	250	17	22
Intense Dark Bars,			
Ev'ng Dream, 3 pcs	190	15	20
Squares:			
Dark Choc., (4), 1.5 oz	210	16	23
Milk & Caramel (3), 1.5 oz	220	12	27
Sea Salt Escape (4), 1.5 oz	210	15	24

Per Piece/Serving

	C	F	Cb
Godiva:			
Bars: Milk/Dark, av., 1.5 oz	230	14	26
Extra Dark: 75%, 1.5 oz	230	17	18
85%, 1.4 oz	260	21	14
Chocoiste: Dk Choc. Cherries (12)	190	7	30
Milk Chocolate Cashews (14)	230	15	19
Hearts: Dark Ganache (4)	200	12	23
Milk Praline (4)	220	13	23
Go Lightly:			
Assorted Toffee, 5 pieces, 1 oz	85	2	24
Fruit Chews, 5 pieces, 1 oz	95	2	26
Hard Candy, Assorted (4), 0.5 oz	45	0	15
Note: Carb figures include 15-25g sugar alcohol			
Goobers Peanuts, 1 package, 1.4 oz	200	13	21
Good & Plenty *(Hershey's)*, (33), 1.4 oz	140	0	35
GooGoo Clusters, 1 piece, 1.8 oz	240	12	30
Gum ~ *See Page 75*			
Gum Drops: 1 small, 0.1 oz	15	0	3
5 pieces, 0.5 oz	75	0	15
Gummi *(Shur Fine)*:			
Bears (15), 1.4 oz	130	0	29
Chewy Sweet Tarts (4)	160	0	36
Worms (9), 1.5 oz	140	0	31
Guylian:			
Bars: Dark Chocolate (3), 1 oz	150	12	11
Milk Choc. w/ Hazelnuts (3),1 oz	170	11	15
No Sugar Added Bars:			
Milk Chocolate, 3 squares	150	11	16
54% Cocoa, Dark Choc., 3 sqrs.	140	11	16
Seashells:			
Bar, 1.4 oz	210	13	21
Boxed, Originals (1), 0.4 oz	60	4	6
Truffles, (1), 0.4 oz	70	5.5	5
Heath: Original (1), 1.4 oz	210	13	24
King Size, 2.8 oz	410	22	49
Snack Size, 3 pieces, 1.5 oz	230	14	27
Hershey's:			
Cookie Layer Crunch, av., 1.4 oz	300	17	36
Cookies 'n' Creme, 1.55 oz Bar	230	12	26
Milk Chocolate:			
Bars: 1.55 oz	220	13	26
with Almonds, 1 bar, 1.4 oz	210	14	21
King Size, 1 Bar, 2.5 oz	370	22	44
Kisses, 9 pieces, av., 1.4 oz	200	12	25
Nuggets: 4 pieces, 1.4 oz	200	13	20
w/ Toffee & Alm., 4 pcs, 1.3 oz	200	13	21
Extra Dark Choc., 4 pcs, 1.4 oz	180	14	21
Simple Pleasures, 6 pcs, av.	180	8	29
Special Dark Choc., 1.5 oz bar	190	12	25
Sugar Free Choc., 5 pieces, 1.4 oz	160	13	24

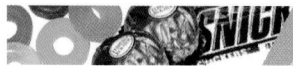

Candy ~ Brands & Generic (Cont)

Per Piece/Serving — **C F Cb**

Hershey's, (Cont):
Pot of Gold Chocolate Asstd:

Item	C	F	Cb
Carmel, 4 pieces, 1.4 oz	190	10	26
Av. other var., 4 pieces, 1.4 oz	210	12	24
Candy-Coated Eggs:			
Milk Chocolate: (8) 1.2 oz	170	8	27
w/ Almonds (8) 1.2 oz	200	12	18
Honeycomb: Plain, 1 oz	115	0	27
Choc-coated, 2 pieces	180	7	31
Hot Tamales, 20 pieces, 1.4 oz	150	0	36
Hugs ~ See Kisses			
Jawbreakers (Sathers), (15), 0.6 oz	60	0	16
Jells (Joyva), Raspb., 3 pieces, 1.6 oz	160	0	38
Jelly Beans, average all brands:			
Small Size (Jelly Belly): 1 bean	5	0	1
12 beans, 0.5 oz	50	0	13
Regular Size: 1 bean	10	0	2
10 beans, 1 oz	105	0	26
Large Size: 1 bean	15	0	3
10 beans, 1.5 oz	150	0	38
Sugar Free, average all brands, 25 beans, 1 oz	60	0	26

Note: Carb figure include 26g sugar alcohol

Item	C	F	Cb
Jelly Belly: 25 beans, 1 oz	105	0	26
3.5 oz package	360	0	90
Sugar Free, 25 beans, 1 oz	60	0	26

Note: Carb figure include 26g sugar alcohol

Item	C	F	Cb
Chocolate Dips:			
All flavors: 1 bean	4	0	1
10 beans	40	1	8
2.8 oz bag	300	8	62
Jelly Rings (Jewel), 5 pieces, 1.4 oz	110	0	26
Jolly Rancher:			
Bites: Soft, 15 pieces	150	1.5	32
Sours, 16 pieces	130	0	34
Crunch 'N Chew, 1 oz pkg	160	0.5	40
Filled Fruity Bites, 22 pieces	140	1	31
Gummies, 9 pieces	120	0	28
Hard Candy, 3 pieces	70	0	17
Jelly Beans/Sours, 1.4 oz	140	0	36
Lollipops (1), 0.55 oz	60	0	15
Jujubes, all varieties (52), 1.4 oz	110	0	28
Juju Bears, 5 pieces	130	0	34
Juju Mix (Sathers), 11 pieces, 1.5 oz	150	0	36
Jujyfruits, 16 pieces, 1.4 oz	120	0	32
Junior Caramels: 13 pieces, 1.5 oz	190	6	33
Mini, 2 boxes, 1 oz	130	4	23

Per Piece/Serving — **C F Cb**

Item	C	F	Cb
Junior Mints: 1.8 oz	220	4	45
16 pieces, 1.4 oz	170	3	35
Justin's, Peanut Butter Cups, Milk Choc, 2 cups, 1.4 oz pkg	200	14	18
Kinder Joy, 1 egg, 0.7 oz	110	6	12
Kisses (Hershey's):			
Milk Chocolate: (1), 0.16 oz	25	1.5	3
(9), 1.4 oz	200	12	25
with Almonds (9), 1.4 oz	200	13	22
Caramel Filled (9), 1.5 oz	190	9	27
Air Delights (11), 1.4 oz	200	12	24
Cookies 'n' Creme (9), 1.5 oz	220	12	26
Hugs (9), 1.4 oz	210	12	24
Special Dark, (9), 1.4 oz	180	12	25
Kit Kat (Nestle):			
Halloween:			
Miniatures, 1.34 oz bar	190	12	22
Snack Size: Triple Choc. 1.48 oz	200	11	27
White Choc., 1.48 oz	220	11	27
Milk Chocolate: 4 pce bar, 1.5 oz	210	11	28
Extra Crispy, 1.6 oz bar	220	12	29
King Size, 8 pcs, 3 oz bar	420	22	56
Minis, 5 pieces	210	11	28
Snack Size, 6 pcs, 1.5 oz	210	11	27
White Chocolate, 4 pcs, 1.5 oz	220	12	26
Lemon Drops (4), 0.6 oz	60	0	16
Walgreens, Sugar Free (3), 0.6 oz	50	0	17
Lemonhead, (26), 1.4 oz	140	0	36
Lance, Peanut Bar, 2.2 oz	340	19	29
Licorice:			
Average all varieties, 1 oz	100	0	25
Chews (Panda), (1)	10	0	3
Tid Bits (1)	10	0	2
Twists: Black/Red, av., 1 pc	35	0	8
Sugar Free, 1 piece	15	0	2.5
American Licorice Co.:			
Natural Vines: Black (9), 1.4 oz	140	1	33
Strawberry (9), 1.4 oz	150	1	34
Red Vines (4), 1.4 oz	140	0	34
Sip-n-Chew, 1 oz package	100	1	23
Snaps (31), 1.4 oz	140	0.5	33
Sour Punch (6), 1.4 oz	150	0.5	34
Super Ropes (1), 2 oz	200	0	46
Lifesavers: Large size, 1 candy	15	0	3
Regular: All flavors, 1 candy	10	0	3
1 Roll (14 candies), 1.2 oz	140	0	35
Creme Savers, 3 pcs, 0.5 oz	60	1	11
Pep-o-mint (3), 0.2 oz	20	0	5
Fruit Splosion (10), 1.4 oz	130	0	31
Sugar-Free, Pep-O-Mint (4), 0.5 oz	35	0	14

Note: Carb figure includes 14g sugar alcohol

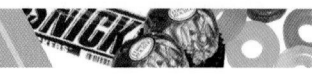

Candy ~ Brands & Generic (Cont)

Per Piece/Serving	C	F	Cb
Lik-m-aid (Nestle), Fun Dip, 1 package	50	0	13
Lindt: Lindor Truffles (1), average	75	6	5
Swiss Milk Chocolate Bars:			
70% Cocoa, 4 pieces	220	17	13
Classic, with Hazelnuts, 10 pieces	230	16	20
Raspberry filled, 7 pieces	200	10	25
Dark Choc. Truffles,			
with filling, 7 pieces	240	18	18
Lollipops: Mini, 0.3 oz	25	0	6
Small, 0.5 oz	50	0	12
Medium, 1 oz	100	0	25
Giant (4" diam), 7 oz	790	0	198
M & M's:			
Dark Chocolate: 1.5 oz package	210	10	29
Peanuts, 1.5 oz	220	12	25
Halloween:	210	10	29
Mini, Whitet Candy Corn Choc., 1.5 oz	220	11	29
White Pumpkin Pie Candy, 1.5 oz	210	11	29
Milk Chocolate: 28 piece, 1 oz	145	6.5	21
1.5 oz package	210	9	30
1.7 oz package	240	10	34
Almond Choc., 1.5 oz	220	12	25
Minis, 1 tube, 1 oz	150	7	21
Peanut: 28 pieces, 1 oz	155	8	17
1.75 oz pkg	250	13	30
Peanut Butter, 1.6 oz pkg	240	14	25
Premiums: Chocolate Trio, 1.5 oz	230	14	25
Mint Thrills, 1.5 oz	240	14	25
Pretzels, ½ pkg, 1.4 oz	180	6	29
Snack Mix, av. ⅓ cup, 1.5 oz	200	9	25
Mamba Sours, Fruit Chews,			
6 pieces, 1 oz	100	1	22
Marshmallow Egg, 1 egg, 1 oz	120	3	22
Mary Jane (Necco), 5 pieces, 1.4 oz	160	3.5	32
Marshmallows: Firm/Soft, 1 oz	90	0	23
Regular size, 4 pieces, 1 oz	100	0	24
Mini-Marshmallow, ⅔ cup, 1 oz	95	0	24
Joyva, Choc-coated Twists	95	2	10
Fluff, 2 Tbsp, 0.6 oz	60	0	15
Kraft: Creme, 0.5 oz	45	0	11
Funmallows, ⅔ cup, 1 oz	100	0	24
Jet-Puffed, 5 pieces, 1 oz	100	0	24
Mini, 1 oz	90	0	23
Marzipan, 2 Tbsp, 1.4 oz	160	4	29
Mauna Loa, Mountains, 4 pcs	230	17	21
Mexican Hats, (7), 1.4 oz	120	0	30
Mentos: Regular	10	0	3
Sugar Free	5	0	2
Mike & Ike:			
Original: 2.1 oz package	220	0	55
23 pieces, 1.4 oz	140	0	36
Milk Duds, 1 box, 1.8 oz	230	8	38

Per Piece/Serving	C	F	Cb
Milky Way (Mars):			
Bars: Single, 2 oz	240	9	37
Fun Size, 2 bars, 1.2 oz	160	6	24
To Go, 1.8 oz	230	9	36
Minis, 5 pieces, 1.5 oz	190	7	30
Midnight Bars: 1.8 oz	230	8	36
Minis, 5 pieces, 1.4 oz	190	7	30
Simply Caramel, 1.9 oz	250	11	37
Mints: Uncoated, 3 pieces	70	0	17
1 mint, medium	7	0	1
1 large mint	15	0	3
Mon Cheri (Ferrero), 4 pieces, 2 oz	260	18	20
Mounds: 1.75 oz bar	240	13	28
King Size, 4 pieces, 3.5 oz	480	26	56
Snack Size, 1 piece, 0.6 oz	80	4.5	10
Mr Goodbar: 1.8 oz bar	250	17	26
King Size, 2.6 oz bar	380	26	38
Munch Bar, 1.4 oz	220	15	18
Necco, Candy Wafers (40), 2 oz	220	0	56
Nestle: Original, 1.6 oz bar	220	11	30
Fun Size, 3 bars, 1.4 oz	180	9	26
Miniatures, 4 bars, 1.4 oz	200	10	27
Buncha Crunch, ⅓ cup, 1.2 oz	180	9	25
Crunch Crisp, 1.8 oz	240	13	32
Newman's Own:			
Milk Choc.: Caramel Cups (3)	160	8	21
Peanut Butter Cups (3)	180	12	17
Dark Choc.: Caramel Cups (3)	160	9	20
Peanut Butter Cups (3)	180	13	16
Nips, all varieties, 2 pieces, 0.5 oz	60	2	11
Nougat: 3 pieces, 1.5 oz	170	1	39
Chocolate Covered, 1 oz	125	4	22
Nuggets ~ See Hershey's			
Nutrageous Bar (Reese's), 1.8 oz	260	16	28
Oh Henry!: Fun Size, 0.9 oz	120	5	16
1.8 oz bar	230	11	33
Orange Slices:			
Jewel, 3 pieces, 1.5 oz	140	0	35
Walgreens, 4 pieces, 1.6 oz	160	0	39
Pastel Mints (Walgreens), 20 pieces	60	0	14
PayDay Bar: 1.8 oz bar	240	13	27
King Size, 3.5 oz bar	440	24	50
Snack Size, 0.7 oz	90	5	10
Avalanche, 1.8 oz bar	250	13	29
Peanut Bar (Planter's), 1.6 oz	240	14	21
Peanut Butter Cups ~ See Reese's; Newman's Own			
Peanut Brittle: 1 piece, 1.5 oz	190	5	32
Sugar Free (Russell Stover),			
4 pieces, 1.3 oz	140	10	24

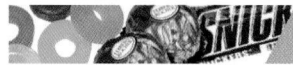 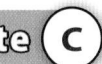

Candy ~ Brands & Generic (Cont)

Per Piece/Serving **C** **F** **Cb**

	C	F	Cb
Peanuts, choc-covered, 14 pieces	230	14	23
Pearson's, Mint Patties, (5), 1.3 oz	150	2.5	31
Peppermints: 7 small, 0.5 oz	60	0	15
Brach's, Star Brites (3)	60	0	16
Pez, 1 roll	35	0	9
Planters,			
Double Peanut Bar, 1.6 oz	240	14	21
Pop Rocks, 0.4 oz package	35	0	9
Pot of Gold *(Hershey's):*			
Assortment: Caramel, 4 pieces	190	10	25
Nut, 4 pieces	210	13	23
Pretzels: Choc-covered, Mini (6)	200	9	25
White Chocolate Bites (23), 1.4 oz	200	9	25
Pretzel Flipz *(Nestlé),* 8 pcs, 1 oz	130	5	20
Raisinets:			
Milk Choc: 1.58 oz pkg	190	8	32
Movie Pack, 3.5 oz	380	16	64
Dark Chocolate, 1/4 cup, 1.6 oz	180	8	32
Reese's:			
Clusters, 3 pieces, 1.5 oz	220	12	24
Crispy Crunchy Bar: 1.7 oz	260	18	22
2 pieces, 1.2 oz	170	10	19
King Size, 3 oz	480	32	40
Fast Break, 2 oz bar	260	12	35
Halloween: PB Pumpkins, 1.2 oz	180	10	18
Snack Size (2), 1.2 oz	180	10	19
P'nut Butter Chips, 0.5 oz	80	4	8
P'nut Butter Cups:			
Milk Choc: (2), 1.5 oz	210	13	24
Miniatures (5), 1.5 oz	220	13	26
Minis (11)	200	12	23
Big Cup (1), 1.4 oz	200	12	22
Sugar Free, Minis (5), 1.4 oz	180	13	27
Dark Chocolate (2), 1.5 oz	210	14	23
Pieces, Peanut Butter (51)	200	9	25
Sticks: 1.5 oz pkg	220	13	23
King Size, 3 oz pkg	440	26	46
Snack Size (1), 0.6 oz	90	5	9
Snacksters, 1 package, 0.8 oz	100	4	14
Whipps, 1.5 oz	230	9	37
Rice Krispies Treats *(Kellogg's),*			
1 bar, average all varieties, 0.8 oz	95	2.5	17
Riesen, Choc. Chew, 4 pcs, 1.3 oz	170	6	28
Rocky Road, Milk/Dark, 1.8 oz bar	240	11	34
Roca Thins, 3 pieces, av. all var.	210	14	24
Rolo: Regular, all var., 1.7 oz roll	220	10	33
Mini Chews, Caramel in milk choc. (11)	190	9	26
Root Beer Barrels, (3), 0.6 oz	60	0	17

Per Piece/Serving **C** **F** **Cb**

	C	F	Cb
Russell Stover Candy:			
Boxed Chocolates Choc. Coated:			
Assorted (2), 1.2 oz	150	7	22
Cherry Cordials (3), 0.4 oz	150	5	25
Dairy Crm Caramels (2), 1.2 oz	160	7	22
Elegant Collection (3), 1.6 oz	210	10	25
French Choc. Mints (4), 1.4 oz	220	13	22
Nut, Chewy & Crisp Centers (2)	160	8	21
Sugar Free:			
Ass'td Hard Candies (3), 1.6 oz	210	16	24
Bags: Caramel (3), 1.3 oz	180	8	25
Coconut (3), 1.5 oz	160	10	28
Mint Patty (3), 1.5 oz	180	12	26
Peanut Butter Cups (2), 1.2 oz	160	12	17
Pecan Delight (2), 1.2 oz	160	12	19
Note: Carbohydrate figures include sugar alcohol			
Salt Water Taffy *(Brach's),* (5)	170	2.5	36
Seashells *(Guylian),* (4), 1.6 oz	260	17	24
See's Candies:			
Almond Royal (5)	190	13	18
Butterscotch Chews (5)	210	12	27
Krispy's: Caffe Latte (5)	180	8	27
Mint (5)	170	8	27
Little Pops:			
Butterscotch (4), 0.5 oz	60	2	12
Av. other flavors (4)	55	3	10
Lollypops, average, 0.7 oz	90	3	17
Milk Molasses Chips (6), 1.4 oz	180	8	27
Milk Peppermints, 2 pieces, 1.3 oz	150	4	28
Peanut Brittle Bar, 1 oz	150	10	15
Peanut Butter Patties (2), 1.2 oz	170	10	16
Peppermint Twists (3)	60	0	15
Toffee-ettes, 3 pieces	270	21	18
Sugar Free:			
Dark Bar, 1.5 oz	180	16	24
Dark Walnut Clusters (4), 1.5 oz	230	21	17
Peanut Brittle, 1.5 oz	170	14	17
Note: Carbohydrate figures include 12-18 g sugar alcohol			
Skinny Cow:			
Dreamy Clusters, all var., 1 pouch	120	6	20
Heavenly Crips, all varieties, 1 bar	110	6	14
Skittles: Original, 2 oz	230	2.5	52
Sour, 1.8 oz	200	2	44
Tropical; Wild Berry, 2.2 oz	250	2.5	56
Fun Size, 1 bag, 0.5 oz	60	1	14
Tear & Share, 4 oz bag	420	4.5	93
Skor, Toffee Bar (1), 1.4 oz	200	12	25
Smarties: Candy Rolls (1), 0.3 oz	25	0	6
Giant, 1 roll, 1 oz	100	0	25

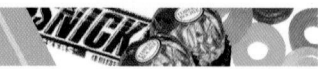

Candy ~ Brands & Generic (Cont)

Per Piece/Serving

	C	F	Cb
Snickers:			
Milk Chocolate: 1.9 oz bar	250	12	33
Fun Size, 2 bars, 1.2 oz	160	8	21
To Go Bar, 1.6 oz	220	10	29
Almond Bar, 1.8 oz	230	11	32
Protein Bar, 2 oz	200	7	18
P'nut Butter Squared, 2 bars, 1.8 oz	250	13	30
Miniatures: (4)	170	8	22
Sugar Free, 5 pcs	180	13	27
Dark Chocolate Bar, 1.8 oz	250	12	31
Sno Caps, ¹⁄₄ cup, 1.4 oz	180	8	30
Soft 'N Chewy, Butter Toffee, 1 piece	30	0.5	5
Sorbee, Crystal Light Hard Candy (4)	25	0	13
Note: Carb figure includes Isomalt which has fewer calories than sugar.			
Sour Patch: Kids, average, 2 oz	210	0	52
Extreme, 1.8 oz	190	0	47
Spearmint Leaves:			
Jewel, 5 pieces, 1.4 oz	140	0	35
Walgreens, 4 pieces, 1.6 oz	160	0	39
Spree Candies: Original, 15 pieces	50	0	13
Chewy, 8 pieces	60	0	13
Starburst:			
Candy Canes, 0.5 oz	70	0	18
Fruit Chews: Original (1)	20	0.5	4
8 pieces, 1.4 oz	160	3.5	33
Gummibursts, 9 pieces, 1.4 oz	130	0	31
Jellybeans, 1.5 oz	150	0	37
Starlight Mints, 3 pieces, 0.5 oz	60	0	15
Suckers *(Walgreens),* 1 piece, 0.4 oz	45	0	11
Sugar Babies, Original, 1.4 oz	160	1.5	37
Sugar Coated Peanuts, 1 oz	120	8	10
Sunbursts Sunflowers *(Kimmie):*			
ChocoRocks Milk, 3.5 oz	525	25	67
Habanero Corn, 3.5 oz	500	23	70
Sunburst Mix, milk, 3.5 oz	500	28	55
Swedish Fish, 7 pieces, 1.5 oz	150	0	38
SweeTARTS:			
Orig., 8 pieces, 0.5 oz	50	0	13
Mini Chewy, 23 pieces, 0.5 oz	50	0.5	12
Symphony *(Hershey's):*			
Milk Choc: 1.5 oz bar	220	14	23
Large Block: 5 pieces, 1.4 oz	200	12	22
w/ Alm. & Toffee, 5 pcs, 1.3 oz	200	13	21

Per Piece/Serving

	C	F	Cb
Taffy,			
Fruit Chews, 1 piece	20	0.5	4
Take 5 *(Hershey's):* Orig., 1.5oz	200	11	25
King Size, 2.3 oz	300	16	37
Snack Size, 2 pcs, 1 oz	150	8	19
3 Musketeers:			
Original, 1.9 oz	240	7	42
2 To Go, 1 bar, 1.6 oz	200	6	35
Fun Size, 3 bars, 1.6 oz	190	6	34
Minis, 7 pieces, 1.4 oz	170	5	32
Tang-a-Roos, 1 roll	25	0	6
Terry's: Chocolate Orange (5), 1.5 oz	230	12	27
Dark Chocolate Orange (5), 1.5 oz	240	13	28
Tic Tac, all flavors, 1 piece	2	0	0
Toblerone: 1.3 oz bar	190	10	22
1.8 oz bar	270	15	31
3.5 oz bar	540	30	63
5.3 oz Package, 5 pieces, 1.5 oz	230	13	27
Toffees, Regular, 1 oz	160	9	18
Tootsie Pops, (1), 0.6 oz	60	0	15
Tootsie Roll: 2.3 oz roll	245	2	55
Midgees, 1.4 oz	140	3	28
Truffles: Reg., 1 piece, 0.4 oz	60	4	6
Large *(Godiva),* 0.8 oz	110	6.5	12
Extra Large *(J. Schmidt),* 1.5 oz	220	13	24
Turtles: Original, 1 piece, 0.6 oz	85	5	10
Sugar Free, 1 piece, 0.4 oz	50	3.5	7
Twists, Licorice; Strawb., sugar free,			
7 pieces, 1.4 oz	90	0	25
Twix:			
Caramel: 2 cookies, 1.8 oz	250	12	34
Fun Size, 2 cookies, 1.7 oz	250	14	27
4 To Go, 1 cookie, 0.8 oz	110	5	15
6 To Go, 1 cookie, 0.5 oz	80	4	11
Minis, 3 pieces, 1 oz	150	7	20
Peanut Butter:			
Single, 2 cookies, 1.7 oz	250	14	27
4 to Go, 1 cookie, 0.8 oz	250	12	34
Twizzlers: Cherry Bites (17), 1.4 oz	140	0.5	32
Cherry Nibs, 29 pieces, 1.4 oz	140	1	32
Pull 'n' Peel, Cherry, 1 piece, 1.2 oz	110	0.5	26
Twists, Strawb., 1.3 oz	120	0.5	29
U-No Bar, 1.5 oz	250	17	22
Weight Watchers *(Whitman's):*			
Caramel Medallions (3)	160	9	24
Coconut (3)	150	9	23
English Toffee Squares (3)	150	9	21
Mint Patties (3)	150	9	23
Peanut Butter Cups (4)	180	8	31
Pecan Crowns (3)	160	10	24

Candy ~ Brands & Generic (Cont)

Per Piece/Serving **C F Cb**

Werther's:
	C	F	Cb
Hard Candy: Original (3), 0.5 oz	70	1.5	14
Sugar-Free Original (5)	40	1.5	15

Note: Carb figure includes 14g sugar alcohol

	C	F	Cb
Soft, Chocolate Caramel (4), 1.4 oz	190	8	28
Whatchamacallit: 1.5 oz Bar	230	12	28
King Size Bar, 2.5 oz	370	20	45

Whitman's, Boxed Chocolates:
	C	F	Cb
Sampler (4), 1.6 oz	220	12	27
12 oz Box, 3 pieces, 1.2 oz	170	9	21
Reserve, 7 oz Box, 2 pieces, 1.2 oz	160	9	21
Sugar Free, 10 oz Box, 3 pcs, 1.5 oz	190	13	25
Whoppers, av. all varieties, 18 pcs	190	7	31

Wonka:
	C	F	Cb
Bar (1), 2.5 oz	360	19	49
Exceptional Bars, average, 4 pieces	200	13	23
Gobstopper, 9 pieces, 0.5 oz	60	0	14
Laffy Taffy: Ropes, all var., 0.8 oz	80	1.5	18
Stretchy & Tangy, all var., 1.5 oz	150	3.5	29
Nerds, Giant, Chewy, 1.8 oz package	180	0	42

Yogurt Candy,
	C	F	Cb
Coated Raisins, 27 pieces, 1.4 oz	180	8	28
York: Mints, (3)	10	0	3
Peppermint Pattie, reg, 1.4 oz	140	2.5	31
Pieces (50)	170	8	28
Zagnut, 1.75 oz bar	220	9	35
Zero Bar: 1.8 oz bar	230	8	37
King Size, 3.5 oz	400	14	68

Gum

Per Piece **C F Cb**

	C	F	Cb
Bazooka	15	0	4
Beechies	6	0	2
Big League Chews	10	0	2
Bubble Yum: Original	25	0	6
Sugarless	10	0	3
Candilicious	30	0	2
Carefree, Sugarless/Regular	5	0	2
Chiclet	5	0	1
Dentyne	5	0	0.5
Double Bubble Ball	20	0	5
Estee, Bubble/Regular	5	0	2
Extra (Wrigley's), Sugar-Free	5	0	2
Freshen-Up	10	0	3
Hubba Bubba: Regular	25	0	6
Sugar-free, average	14	0	0.5
Ice Breakers	5	0	2
Jolt Gum	5	0	2
Super Bubble	15	0	4
Trident, Orig.; White	5	0	1
Wrigley's, all flavors	10	0	2

Carob Candy

C F Cb

Per Piece/Serving

	C	F	Cb
Carob, Plain/Natural, 1 oz	155	9	15
Carob Coated: Raisins, 1 oz	130	8	15
Almonds/Peanuts, 1 oz	150	10	14
Caramels, 1 oz	110	4	18
Dates, 1 oz	125	5	20
Malt Balls, 1 oz	135	8	15
Soybeans	145	9	16
Trail/Party Mix, 1 oz	150	9	15

Cough Drops

C F Cb

Per Drop/Piece

	C	F	Cb
Beech Nut, 1 drop	10	0	2
CVS, Honey Lemon Cough Drops	15	0	4
Diabetic Tussin	0	0	0
Halls, Defense Vitamin C: Regular	15	0	4
Sugar Free	5	0	3
Fruit Breezers	15	0	4
Menthol Drops: Regular	15	0	4
Sugar Free	5	0	4
Plus	20	0	5
Listerine *(Amer. Chicle)*, Lozenge	10	0	2
Luden's, Throat Drops: Reg., all var.	10	0	2
Sugar Free	0	0	0
Pine Bros, Cough Drops	10	0	2
Ricola, Cough Drops:			
Natural Herbs	10	0	3
Sugar-Free Lemon Mint	0	0	1
Rolaids, Sodium Free	5	0	1
Sathers, Peppermint Lozenges	15	0	3
Sucrets *(Beecham)*, Lozenges	10	0	2.5
Wintergreen, Lozenges	15	0	3

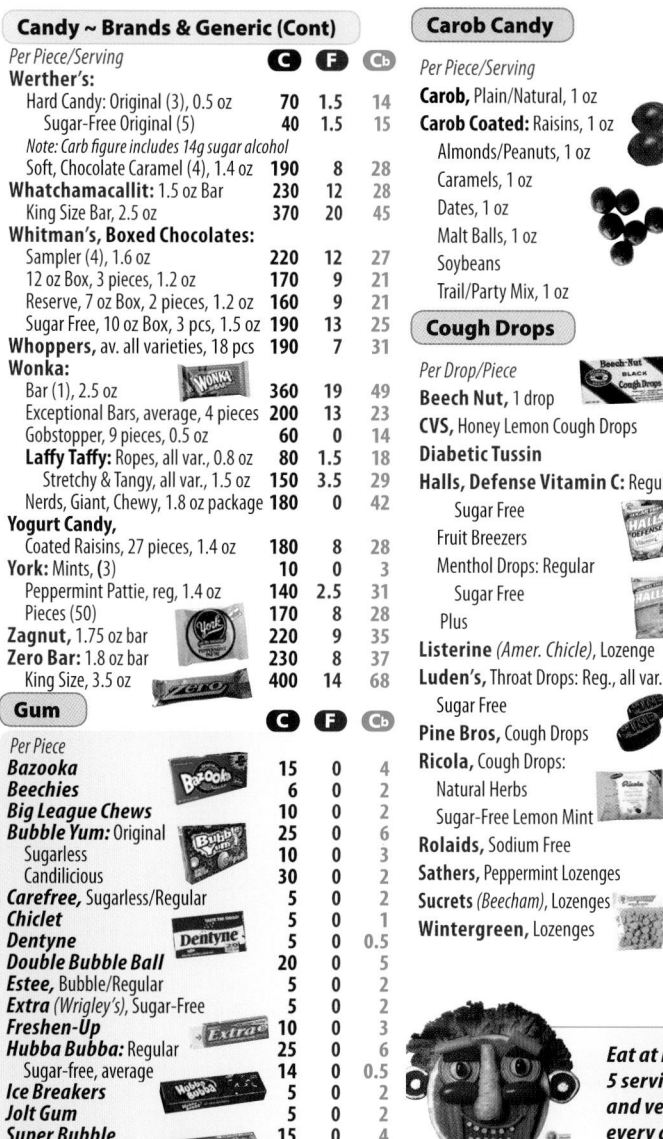

Eat at least 5 servings of fruit and vegetables every day . . . and Enjoy Better Health!

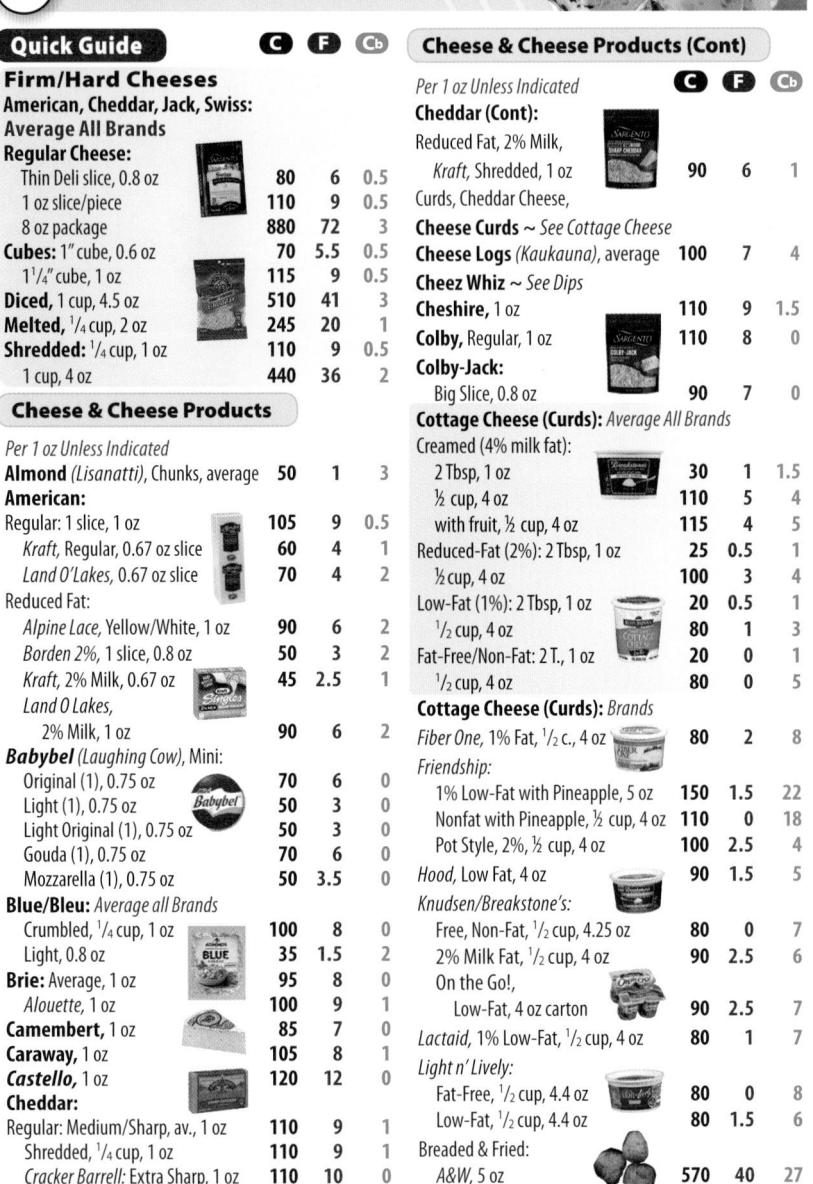

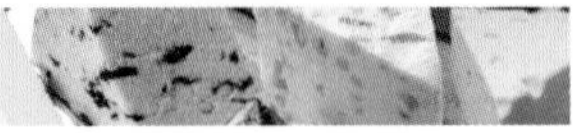

Quick Guide C F Cb

Firm/Hard Cheeses
American, Cheddar, Jack, Swiss:
Average All Brands
Regular Cheese:

	C	F	Cb
Thin Deli slice, 0.8 oz	80	6	0.5
1 oz slice/piece	110	9	0.5
8 oz package	880	72	3
Cubes: 1" cube, 0.6 oz	70	5.5	0.5
1¼" cube, 1 oz	115	9	0.5
Diced, 1 cup, 4.5 oz	510	41	3
Melted, ¼ cup, 2 oz	245	20	1
Shredded: ¼ cup, 1 oz	110	9	0.5
1 cup, 4 oz	440	36	2

Cheese & Cheese Products

Per 1 oz Unless Indicated

	C	F	Cb
Almond *(Lisanatti)*, Chunks, average	50	1	3
American:			
Regular: 1 slice, 1 oz	105	9	0.5
Kraft, Regular, 0.67 oz slice	60	4	1
Land O'Lakes, 0.67 oz slice	70	4	2
Reduced Fat:			
Alpine Lace, Yellow/White, 1 oz	90	6	2
Borden 2%, 1 slice, 0.8 oz	50	3	2
Kraft, 2% Milk, 0.67 oz	45	2.5	1
Land O Lakes,			
2% Milk, 1 oz	90	6	2
Babybel *(Laughing Cow)*, Mini:			
Original (1), 0.75 oz	70	6	0
Light (1), 0.75 oz	50	3	0
Light Original (1), 0.75 oz	50	3	0
Gouda (1), 0.75 oz	70	6	0
Mozzarella (1), 0.75 oz	50	3.5	0
Blue/Bleu: *Average all Brands*			
Crumbled, ¼ cup, 1 oz	100	8	0
Light, 0.8 oz	35	1.5	2
Brie: Average, 1 oz	95	8	0
Alouette, 1 oz	100	9	1
Camembert, 1 oz	85	7	0
Caraway, 1 oz	105	8	1
Castello, 1 oz	120	12	0
Cheddar:			
Regular: Medium/Sharp, av., 1 oz	110	9	1
Shredded, ¼ cup, 1 oz	110	9	1
Cracker Barrell: Extra Sharp, 1 oz	110	10	0
Vermont Sharp White, 1 oz	110	10	0

Cheese & Cheese Products (Cont)

Per 1 oz Unless Indicated C F Cb

	C	F	Cb
Cheddar (Cont):			
Reduced Fat, 2% Milk,			
Kraft, Shredded, 1 oz	90	6	1
Curds, Cheddar Cheese,			
Cheese Curds ~ *See Cottage Cheese*			
Cheese Logs *(Kaukauna)*, average	100	7	4
Cheez Whiz ~ *See Dips*			
Cheshire, 1 oz	110	9	1.5
Colby, Regular, 1 oz	110	8	0
Colby-Jack:			
Big Slice, 0.8 oz	90	7	0
Cottage Cheese (Curds): *Average All Brands*			
Creamed (4% milk fat):			
2 Tbsp, 1 oz	30	1	1.5
½ cup, 4 oz	110	5	4
with fruit, ½ cup, 4 oz	115	4	5
Reduced-Fat (2%): 2 Tbsp, 1 oz	25	0.5	1
½ cup, 4 oz	100	3	4
Low-Fat (1%): 2 Tbsp, 1 oz	20	0.5	1
½ cup, 4 oz	80	1	3
Fat-Free/Non-Fat: 2 T., 1 oz	20	0	1
½ cup, 4 oz	80	0	5
Cottage Cheese (Curds): *Brands*			
Fiber One, 1% Fat, ½ c., 4 oz	80	2	8
Friendship:			
1% Low-Fat with Pineapple, 5 oz	150	1.5	22
Nonfat with Pineapple, ½ cup, 4 oz	110	0	18
Pot Style, 2%, ½ cup, 4 oz	100	2.5	4
Hood, Low Fat, 4 oz	90	1.5	5
Knudsen/Breakstone's:			
Free, Non-Fat, ½ cup, 4.25 oz	80	0	7
2% Milk Fat, ½ cup, 4 oz	90	2.5	6
On the Go!,			
Low-Fat, 4 oz carton	90	2.5	7
Lactaid, 1% Low-Fat, ½ cup, 4 oz	80	1	7
Light n' Lively:			
Fat-Free, ½ cup, 4.4 oz	80	0	8
Low-Fat, ½ cup, 4.4 oz	80	1.5	6
Breaded & Fried:			
A&W, 5 oz	570	40	27
Culver's, Wisconsin, 5.3 oz	510	25	51

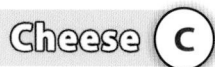

Cheese & Cheese Products (Cont)

Per 1 oz Unless Indicated	C	F	Cb
Cream Cheese: *Average All Brands*			
Regular/Soft:			
2 Tbsp, 1 oz	95	10	1
3 oz package	290	29	3.5
8 oz package	780	78	9
Light, Plain, 1 oz	60	4.5	2.5
Fat-Free, Plain, 1 oz	30	0	2
Better Than Cream Cheese (Tofutti),			
all varieties, 1 oz	85	5	9
Easy Cheese (Kraft),			
American, 2 Tbsp, 1.2 oz	80	6	1
Edam, 1 oz	100	8	0.5
Farmer, Low-Fat, 1 oz	40	2.5	0
Feta: Regular, 1 oz	75	6	1
Crumbled, ¹/₂ cup, 2.5 oz	190	15	3
Athenos, Reduced-Fat,			
1 oz	50	3	1
Fontina, 2 Tbsp, 1 oz	110	9	0.5
Galaxy, Cheese Substitute:			
Grated Parmesan Flavor, 2 tsp, 0.2 oz	15	0.5	0
Slices: Mozzarella, 1 slice, 0.6 oz	40	3	0.5
Cheddar, 1 slice, 0.67 oz	35	2	5
Goat's Milk Cheese:			
Chevre: Original, 2 Tbsp	75	6	0.5
Semi-Soft, 1 oz	100	8.5	1
Hard, 1 oz	130	10	0.5
Chavrie, Logs:			
Original, 2 Tbsp, 1 oz	80	7	1
Sundried Tomato & Garlic, 1 oz	80	6	2
Pyramid, Original, 1 oz	50	3.5	1
Gjetost, fresh, 1 oz	130	8	12
Myzithra, grated, 1 oz	80	4	2
Gorgonzola, 1 oz	100	8	0.5
Galbani, Dolcelatte, 1 oz	95	8	1
Gouda, 1 oz slice	100	8	0.5
Gruyere, 1 oz	115	9	1
Handi-Snacks *(Kraft):*			
Breadsticks 'n Cheez Single, 1 oz	110	4.5	14
Ritz Crackers 'n Cheez Dip, 1 oz	100	6	11
Havarti *(Land O'Lakes),* 0.7 oz	80	6	1
Jarlsberg: Average, 1 oz	100	8	0
Reduced Fat, shredded, 1 oz	70	3.5	0
Labneh, (Lebanese Cream Chse), 1.8 oz	70	4	4

Cheese & Cheese Products (Cont)

Per 1 oz Unless Indicated	C	F	Cb
Laughing Cow, Wedges:			
Creamy Asiago (1)	35	1.5	1
Swiss: Original Creamy (1)	50	4	1
Light Swiss (1)	35	1.5	1
Lifetime, Cholesterol Reducing,			
Low Fat, all varieties, 1 Slice, 1 oz	45	1.5	1
Limburger, 1 oz	95	8	0
Mascarpone, av., 1 oz	125	13	0.5
Mexican:			
Cacique: Asadero, sliced	70	5	1
Cotija	100	8	0
Enchilado; Manchego	90	7	0
Panela	80	7	0
Queso Fresco	80	6	0
Queso Quesadilla	90	7	0
Ranchero	80	6	0
Chi-Chi's, Salsa Con Quéso, Mild	45	3	4
El Mexicano: Asadero, Regular	90	7	0
Cotija, grated, 2 Tbsp	40	3	0
Kraft, Mexican Four Cheese; Taco,			
Shredded,	100	8	0
Sargento, 4 Cheese Mexican	110	9	2
Supremo, Quéso Chihuahua, 1 oz	100	8	0
Verole, Quéso Oaxaca, 1 oz	70	8	0
Monterey Jack:			
Regular, shredded, 1 oz	100	8	1
Land O Lakes, Co-Jack, 1 oz	110	9	1
Kraft, 1" cube, 1 oz	100	9	1
Mozzarella:			
Whole Milk: Average 1 oz	85	6.5	0.5
Land O'Lakes/Polly-O:			
Slice, average, 1 oz	80	6	1
String, 1 oz	90	6	1
Fat-Free,			
Kraft, Shredded, 1 oz	45	0	2
Reduced Fat,			
Kraft, 2% Milk Fat	70	5	0
Part Skim:			
Borden/Kraft, Shredded	80	5	2
Kraft, String	80	6	0
Polly-O, Shredded, 1 oz	80	5	0
Muenster:			
Regular, 1 oz	105	9	0.5
Low-Fat, 1 oz	85	5	1

Cheese & Cheese Products (Cont)

Per 1 oz Unless Indicated	**C**	**F**	**Cb**
Parmesan:			
Fresh/Block, Dry, 1 oz	110	7.5	1
Grated (Packaged): 2 tsp	20	1.5	0
1 oz	120	8	1
1/2 cup, 1.8 oz	215	14	2
Kraft, Reduced-Fat Topping, 1 Tbsp	20	1	2
Philadelphia:			
Cream Cheese: Original, 2 T. 1 oz	80	7	2
3 oz package	240	21	6
Flavored:			
Blueberry, 1.16 oz	80	4.5	7
Chive & Onion, 1.1 oz	80	7	2
Pinapple, 1 oz	70	4.5	5
Salmon, 1.1 oz	70	5	2
Strawberry, 1.1 oz	80	6	5
1/3 Less Fat: Plain, 2 T., 1 oz	70	5	3
Neufchatel, 2 T., 1 oz	70	6	1
Fat-Free, Plain, 1 oz	30	0	3
Cheesecake Filling, 3 oz	240	17	6
Milk/White Chocolate:			
2 Tbsp, 1.27 oz	110	6	12
Dark Chocolate, 2 T., 1.23 oz	100	5	12
Whipped:			
Original, 0.8 oz	50	4.5	2
Mixed Berry, 0.7 oz	50	3.5	5
Pizza Four Cheese, shredded, *Kraft/Sargento,* Regular, av., 1 oz	90	7	1
Port de Salut, 1 oz	100	8	0
Port Wine *(Kaukauna/WisPride):*			
10 oz Ball, 1 oz	100	6	4
10 oz Log, 2 Tbsp, 1 oz	100	7	4
11.3 oz Tub, 0.85 oz	80	6	3
Provolone: Regular, 1 oz	100	7.5	0.5
Alpine Lace, Reduced-Fat, 1 oz	80	6	1
Sargento, 1 slice, 0.67 oz	70	5	0
Pub *(President),* average all varieties	75	7	1
Quark: 40% fat	45	3	1
20% fat	30	1.5	1
Skim/Non-Fat	20	0	1.5
Rice Cheese Chunks *(Lisanatti),* average, 1 oz	60	3	2

Cheese & Cheese Products (Cont)

Per 1 oz Unless Indicated	**C**	**F**	**Cb**
Ricotta Cheese:			
Whole Milk: 1 oz	50	3.5	1
1/2 cup, 4.5 oz	215	16	4
Part Skim: 1 oz	40	2	1.5
1/2 cup, 4.5 oz	170	10	6
Light/Low-Fat: 1 oz	25	1	1.5
1/2 cup, 4.5 oz	125	5	6
Fat-Free, 1/2 cup, 4.5 oz	100	0	10
Baked Ricotta, 2 oz	130	9	3
Romano: Block/Loaf	110	8	1
Grated: 1 oz	120	9	1
1 Tbsp, 0.2 oz	20	1.5	0
Roquefort, 1 oz	105	9	0.5
Sheep's Milk, (Manchego), *Trader Joes/Wegman's,* 1 oz	120	10	1
Soy Cheese:			
Trader Joe's, Cheddar flavor, 0.7 oz	45	2	3
Soy Kaas: Cheddar, 1 oz	50	2	8
Monterey Jack, 1 oz	60	4	0
Soy Sation, Chunks, all varieties, 1 oz	60	3	2
Smoked Cheddar, average, 1 oz	110	10	0
Stilton, average, 1 oz	110	10	0
String:			
Regular, average all brands	80	6	0.5
Kraft, Twist-Ums & String-ums, Super Long, 1 stick, 1.1 oz	90	6	1
Light/Lite:			
Frigo, String (1), 0.85 oz	50	2.5	0.5
Polly-O, String, 2% Red-Fat, 1 oz	70	4.5	0
Sargento: 1 piece, 1 oz	80	6	1
Light, , 0.75 oz	50	2.5	1
Swiss: Regular, 1 oz	110	8	1.5
Alpine Lace, Reduced-Fat, 1 oz	90	6	1
Kraft Singles, 2% Milk, 0.75 oz	60	4.5	1
Tilsit, 1 oz	100	7.5	0.5
Tofutti, Better Than Cream Cheese, all flavors, 2 Tbsp	60	5	2
Tybo, 1 oz	100	7	0.5
Velveeta (Kraft):			
Original, 1 oz	80	5	3
Reduced Fat, 2% Milk, 1 oz	60	3	4
Mexican, 1 oz	60	4	3
Queso Blanco, Mild, 1 oz	70	4	3

Dips/Spreads | C | F | Cb

Per 2 Tbsp, 1 oz, Unless Indicated

Average All Brands

	C	F	Cb
Avocado/Guacamole	45	4	2
Baba Ghanoush (Eggplant/Sesame)	70	6	2
Cheese Fondue, $^1/_2$ cup, 4 oz	260	15	4
French Onion Dip	60	4.5	3
Hummus: 2 Tbsp	50	1	5
$^1/_2$ cup, 4.5 oz	220	4.5	23
Tzatziki (Cucumber/Yogurt)	30	2.5	2
Clearman's, Original Spread	150	16	0
De La Casa, 5 Layer Party Dip	45	2.5	4
Fritolay, French Onion Dip, 2 Tbsp	60	5	3

Fritos: *Per 2 Tbsp*

Dips:

	C	F	Cb
Bean; Hot Bean w/ Jalapeno	35	1	5
Jalapeno Cheddar Cheese	40	2.5	3
Mild Cheddar	40	3	3

Guiltless Gourmet,

	C	F	Cb
Black Bean/Spicy Black Bean Dip	40	0	7

Heluva Good Cheese,

	C	F	Cb
French Onion Dip, 2 Tbsp	50	4.5	2

Kaukauna *(Wisconsin)*:

Spreadable Cheddar,

	C	F	Cb
Sharp/Smokey Cheddar	80	6	3

Kemps: *Per 2 Tbsp*

Dips:

	C	F	Cb
French Onion	60	5	2
Ranch Style	60	5	2

Top The Tater,

	C	F	Cb
Taco Fiesta; Veggie Ranch, av.	60	5	3
Kroger, Dips, all varieties	60	5	2

Kraft: *Per 2 Tbsp*

Dips:

	C	F	Cb
Average all varieties	60	5	3
Cheez Whiz: Orig., 1.2 oz	90	7	4
Light	80	3.5	6

Salsa Con Queso ~ See Velveeeta

	C	F	Cb
Spreads: Olive & Pimento, 1.1 oz	80	6	3
Old English Sharp; Roka Blue, av	88	7	3

Marzetti: *Per 2 Tbsp*

Dips:

	C	F	Cb
Chocolate Fruit, 2 Tbsp	110	1	25
Old Fashioned Caramel, 1.25 oz	130	4	22
Veggie: Dill, Light, 1.1 oz	60	5	4
Ranch, 1 oz	110	12	2
Light Ranch, 1.1 oz	60	5	4

Dips/Spreads (Cont) | C | F | Cb

Per 2 Tbsp, 1 oz, Unless Indicated

Marie's:

	C	F	Cb
Dips: Buttermilk Ranch; Crmy Dill. av.	100	10	2
Guacamole	40	3	3

Naturally Fresh: *Per 2 Tbsp*

Dips:

	C	F	Cb
Chocolate, 1.3 oz	90	0	23
Crm Cheese Strawb., 1 oz	90	3	15
Caramel, 1 oz	100	4	16

Old Dutch:

Dips:

	C	F	Cb
French Onion, 1 oz	50	3	5
Mild Cheddar, 1 oz	40	3	2
Nacho Cheese, 1 oz	35	2.5	2

Old El Paso: *Per 2 Tbsp*

Dips:

	C	F	Cb
Cheese & Salsa, 1.2 oz	40	3	3
Thick N' Chunky Salsa	10	0	2

Price's: *Per 2 Tbsp*

Dips:

	C	F	Cb
Pimiento Cheese	90	7	4
Light Pimiento	50	3	3

Stop & Shop: *Per 2 Tbsp*

Dips:

	C	F	Cb
Veggie	100	10	3
Sour Cream French Onion	60	4.5	2

TGI Fridays,

	C	F	Cb
Spinach, Cheese & Artichoke Dip, 1 oz	30	2	2
Toby's, Original Tofu Spread, 2 Tbsp	80	8	2

Tostitos:

Dips:

	C	F	Cb
Chunky Salsa, 2 Tbsp	10	0	2
Creamy Spinach, 2 Tbsp	50	4	2
Salsa Con Queso, 2 Tbsp	40	2.5	5

Wise: *Per 2 Tbsp*

Dips:

	C	F	Cb
French Onion	60	5	3
Salsa con Queso	45	3	3

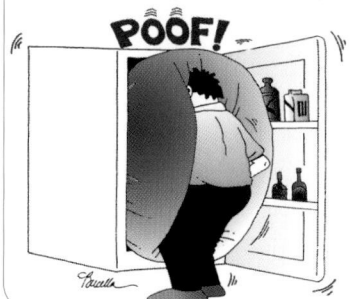

**New Diet Aid
- The Refrigerator Air Bag!**

POOF!

Condiments, Sauces | C | F | Cb

Average of Brands & Homemade

	C	F	Cb
Apple Sauce:			
Sweetened, $^1/_4$ cup, 2.5 oz	55	0	13
Unsweetened, $^1/_4$ cup, 2 oz	25	0	7
Barbecue Sauce:			
Regular, av. all flavors, 2 Tbsp, 1 oz	40	0	10
Bull's Eye, Original, 1 oz	60	0	14
Bearnaise Sauce, $^1/_4$ cup, 2.5 oz	190	19	5
Buffalo Wing Sce: Hon. Mustard, 1 T.	40	3	3
Average other varieties, 1 Tbsp	25	2	2
Cheese, h/made, $^1/_4$ cup, 2.5 oz	150	10	12
Chef-Mate, Hot Dog, $^1/_4$ cup	70	2.5	9
Chili Sauce *(Heinz),* 1 Tbsp	20	0	5
Cocktail Sauce: $^1/_4$ cup	110	0	15
Walden Farms, Fat-Free, 1 Tbsp	0	0	0
Cranberry Sauce, av. all varieties: 2 T.	45	0	11
$^1/_4$ cup, 2.5 oz	110	0	27
Demi Glaze Gold, 2 tsp	30	0.5	3
Honey Mustard *(French's),* 2 Tbsp	60	0.5	12
Horseradish: 1 tsp	2	0	0
Kraft, 1 tsp	15	1.5	1
Ketchup: Regular, 1 Tbsp	15	0	4
Heinz: Reduced Sugar, 1 Tbsp	5	0	1
Simply Heinz, 1 Tbsp	15	0	4
Mole:			
Dona Maria, av. all varieties., 2 T.	150	10	10
Rogelio Bueno, 2 Tbsp, 1 oz	160	11	12
Mushroom Sce, $^1/_2$ cup, 2 oz	50	2	5
Mustard, average, 1 tsp	5	0	0.5
Pesto Sauce, $^1/_4$ cup, 2 oz	270	28	2
Pizza Sauce, $^1/_4$ cup, 2 oz	30	0	6
Seafood Cocktail Sce, $^1/_4$ cup	60	0	15
Soy Sauce: Average all, 1 Tbsp	10	0	1
Kikkoman, Lite Soy, 1 Tbsp	10	0	1
Spaghetti Sce, $^1/_2$ cup, 4.5 oz	135	6	19
Steak Sauce:			
Kraft, A1, 1 Tbsp, 0.5 oz	15	0	3
Lea & Perrins, 1 Tbsp, 0.5 oz	20	0	5
Strawb. Puree Sauce, Unsweet., 2 T.	10	0	2
Sweet & Sour Sauce:			
Contadina, 1.2 oz	40	1	8
Kraft, 1 Tbsp	60	0	13
Tabasco Sauce, 1 tsp	2	0	0
Taco Sauce, average all, 2 Tbsp, 1 oz	10	0	1
Tartar Sauce: *(Heinz),* 2 Tbsp, 1 oz	120	11	4
Hellmann's, Regular, 2 Tbsp, 1 oz	80	7	4
McCormick, Fat-Free, 2 Tbsp, 1 oz	30	0	7
Teriyaki Sauce *(Kikkoman),* 1 T., 0.5 oz	15	0	2
Vinegar, White or Wine, 2 T.	4	0	1
White Sauce, $^1/_2$ cup, 5 oz	130	7	10
Worcestershire Sauce, 1 tsp	5	0	1

Pickles & Relish | C | F | Cb

Average All Brands

	C	F	Cb
Bread & Butter Pickles, 4 sl.,1 oz	25	0	6
Chutney, 2 Tbsp, 1.25 oz	50	0.5	11
Dill Pickles:			
Slices, 4 slices, 1 oz	4	0	1
1 large, ($3^3/_4$"x $1^1/_4$" diam.), 2.25 oz	12	0	3
Extra large (4"x $1^3/_4$" diam.), 5 oz	30	0	6
Halves: Small, 1 oz	3	0	0.5
Large, 2.5 oz	8	0	2
Gherkins, sweet, 1 medium, 1 oz	30	0	7
Green Chiles, chopped, 2 Tbsp	5	0	1
Horseradish, 1 Tbsp	10	0	2
Jalapenos, pickled (2), 2 oz	10	0.5	2
Jalapeno Relish, 1 Tbsp, 0.5 oz	5	0	1
Mustard, av. all brands, 1 tsp	5	0	0.5
Peppers, Hot/Mild (1), 1.5 oz	20	0	4
Pickled: Beets, $^1/_2$ cup, 4 oz	75	0	19
Cocktail Onion, 1 onion	2	0	0
Red Cabbage, $^1/_2$ cup, 3 oz	65	0	15
Pickles: Sweet, 2 Tbsp, 1 oz	35	0	8
Large (3"x $^3/_4$ diam.),1.25 oz	40	0	10
Pickle in a Pouch, 1 large	12	0	3
Relishes:			
Cranberry-Orange, 1 Tbsp	30	0	7
Hot Dog *(Heinz),* 1 T., 0.5 oz	17	0	3
S'wich Spread, 1 tsp	20	1	5
Sweet Pickle, 1 Tbsp, 0.5 oz	20	0	5
Sweet Cauliflower, 1 oz	35	0	8
Sugar Free Relish, 1 tsp	5	0	1
Sweet Gherkins (2), 1 oz	5	0	1
Sauerkraut,			
Drained, 1 cup, 5 oz	25	0	6

Salsa

Average all Types:

	C	F	Cb
Regular, w/out oil, 2 T., 1 oz	15	0	3.5
Made with oil, 2 Tbsp, 1 oz	40	3	8
La Victoria, 2 Tbsp, 1 oz	10	0	2
Old El Paso, 1 Tbsp, 1 oz	10	0	3
TGI Friday's, 1.2 oz	15	0	4

Quick Guide Ⓒ Ⓕ Ⓒb

Cookies:

Average All Brands: *Per Cookie*

	C	F	Cb
Biscotti: Small, 0.5 oz	70	3	10
Regular, 1 oz	140	6.5	18
Chocolate Chip:			
Small/Thin, 0.5 oz	70	3.5	9
Regular, 1 oz	140	7	18
Large (*Mrs Fields*), 3 oz	350	17	45
Extra Large, 4 oz	555	28	73
Oatmeal/Oatmeal Raisin:			
Small/Thin, 0.5 oz	65	2.5	10
Regular, 1 oz	130	5	20
Large (*Mrs Fields*), 2.5 oz	330	14	44
Extra Large, 4 oz	510	20	78
Peanut Butter:			
Small/Thin, 0.5 oz	70	3.5	9
Regular, 1 oz	135	7	17
Large (*Mrs Fields*), 2.5 oz	330	17	41
Extra Large, 4 oz	540	27	67
Low-Fat Cookies:			
Choc Chip (Low-Fat), (1), 0.5 oz	65	2	10
Oatmeal Raisin (Fat-Free), (1), 1 oz	95	0.5	22
Peanut Butter (Low-Fat), (1), 1 oz	105	5	15

Quick Guide

Crackers

Average All Brands: *Per Cracker Unless Indicated*

	C	F	Cb
Cheese Crackers:			
Plain: 1" square	5	0	0.5
Bag, single serving, 1 oz	140	7	16
Cheese/P'nut Butter filled	30	1.5	4
Crispbread, Rye	35	0	8
Grahams, 2½" square	30	0.5	5
Melba Toast, Plain, 1 piece	20	0	4
Matzo, Plain, 1 oz	110	0.5	23
Oyster/Soup, ½ cup	95	2	17
Rice: 1 crackers	70	1.5	11
Oriental Style, 1 oz	130	3.5	23
Saltines, 5 crackers	65	2	11
Snack-type, 1 round cracker	15	1	2
Soda Crackers (*Saltine*), 2	25	1	4.5
Water Cracker (*Carr's*), Original	15	0.5	2.5
Wheat:			
Wheat Thins	10	0.5	1.5
Cheese/Peanut Butter filled	35	2	4

Cookies & Crackers ~ Brands

Per Cookie/Cracker, Unless indicated Ⓒ Ⓕ Ⓒb

	C	F	Cb
Albertsons:			
Animal Crackers (6), 1 oz	130	3.5	22
Chocolate Chip:			
Original (3), 1 oz	150	7	20
Chewy (2), 1 oz	130	6	18
Chunky (1), 0.5 oz	80	3.5	10
Chocolate S'wich Cremes: (3) 1 oz	150	6	25
Double Filled (2), 1 oz	140	6	22
Fudge Graham (3), 1 oz	140	7	18
Fudge Wafer (3), 1 oz	140	8	18
Fudge Marshmallow Ring	120	5	19
Pinwheels, Chocolate Marshmallow	120	5	20
Vanilla Wafers (9), 1 oz	140	4	25
Graham: Cinnamon (2)	150	3	28
Honey (2), 1 oz	140	2	28
Annie's:			
Bunny Grahams:			
Honey, 1 oz	130	4	20
Other varieties, 1 oz	130	4.5	22
Gluten Free: Cocoa & Vanilla, 1 oz	120	3.5	22
SnickerDoodle, Cinn. Sugar, 1 oz	140	4.5	22
Crackers:			
Cheddar Bunnies:			
Regular, 1 oz Snack Pack	140	6	19
Extra Cheesy, 1 oz	150	7	18
White Cheddar; Whole Wheat, 1 oz	145	7	19
Arnott's:			
Tim Tams: Original; Chewy C'rml (2)	190	9	26
Classic Dark; Dark Mint (2)	190	10	25
Austin:			
Sandwich Crackers: *Per Package*			
Cheese: with Cheddar Cheese	190	10	23
with Peanut Butter	190	10	23
with PB & Jelly	190	9	25
Toasty			
Barbara's Bakery:			
Snackimals:			
Choc Chip; Vanilla, 1 oz	140	4.5	23
Oatmeal, 1 oz	130	4	20

Cookies & Crackers ~ Brands (Cont)

Per Cookie/Cracker, Unless Indicated **C** **F** **Cb**

BelVita *(Nabisco):*

Breakfast Biscuits:

	C	F	Cb
Crunchy, 1 pack (4 biscuits), average	**230**	8	36
Soft Baked, 1 biscuit, average	**190**	7	32
Bites, (46), av., 1.8 oz	**230**	8	37

Blue Diamond:

Nut Thins: Almond,(19),1 oz	**130**	2	24
Cheddar Cheese, 2 oz bag	**250**	7	41
Country Ranch (17); Pecan (16), 1 oz	**130**	3.5	23

Brent & Sam's:

Natural: *Per 2 Cookies*

Key Lime White Choc.	**120**	6	16
White Choc. Macadamia	**130**	7	14

Soft Baked: *Per 1 Cookie*

Choc. Chunk; Snickerdoodle	**130**	4.5	20
Oatmeal Raisin	**140**	6	20

Carr's:

Crackers: Orig.; Cracked Pepper (4)	**60**	1	10
Roasted Garlic & Herbs (4)	**50**	1	10
Rosemary (4)	**70**	2.5	11
Toasted Sesame (4)	**60**	1.5	10

Cheez•It ~ *See Sunshine, Page 87*

Chips Ahoy! ~ *See Nabisco, Page 85*

Country Choice:

Sandwich Cremes,

all varieties, 2 pieces	**130**	5	19

Snacking:

Ginger Snaps (5); Vanilla Wafers (7)	**140**	5	22
Iced Oatmeal (4)	**120**	4	21

Dr. Kracker:

Crispbread: Klassic 3 Seed (1)	**100**	4	15
Pumpkin Seed Cheddar (1)	**100**	4.5	13
Snackers, Pumpkin Seed Cheddar (8)	**125**	5	13

Erin Baker's:

Original Breakfast: *Per 3 oz*

Banana Walnut	**310**	8	55
Peanut Butter	**330**	11	50

Minis: *Per 1 oz Cookie*

Peanut Butter	**100**	3.5	16
Dble Chocolate; Oatmeal Raisin, av.	**100**	2.5	18

Famous Amos:

Bite Size: Choc. Chip,

4 Cookies, 1 oz	**140**	7	20
Choc. Chip & Pecans (4)	**150**	8	18

Per Cookie/Cracker, Unless Indicated **C** **F** **Cb**

Fig Newtons ~ *See Nabisco, Page 85*

Fifty50:

	C	F	Cb
Chocolate Chip (4)	**170**	9	22
Hearty Oatmeal (4)	**160**	7	24
Wafers, average all varieties, (4)	**150**	9	17

Gamesa:

Animalitos, 14 cookies, 1 oz	**110**	1	25
Arcoiris Marshmallow, 2 oz pkg, 6 cookies	**220**	5	38
Chocolatines Marshmallow, 2 cookies, 1 oz	**130**	5	18
Chokis, Chocolate Chip, 1.4 oz pkg	**190**	9	27

Emperador: Cream Cookie Sandwich

Lemon Creme, 1 pkg, 6 cookies	**270**	8	45
Av. other flavors, 1 pkg, 6 cookies	**360**	12	57
Fruitbars, average, 1 cookie, 1 oz	**110**	4.5	18
Giro, 3 cookies, 1 oz	**140**	6	20
Mamut, Choc Marshmallow, 1 cookie, 1 oz	**130**	5	19
Marias, 8 cookies, 1 oz	**120**	2	24
Sugar Wafers, (3), average, 1.2 oz	**160**	7	25

Girl Scouts Cookies:

Caramel DeLites/Samoas, (2), av.	**145**	8	18
Girl Scout S'Mores (2)	**180**	9	25
Peanut Butter S'wich, (3)	**170**	9	19
Shortbread (4)	**120**	4.5	19
Thin Mints (4)	**160**	7	22

Goldfish Crackers ~ *See Pepperidge Farm, Page 86*

Goya:

Lady Fingers , 1 oz	**130**	1	25
Maria, 5 cookies, 1 oz	**130**	3	24
Wafers, average all flavors, 4 wafers, 1 oz	**150**	7	20

Grandma's:

Homestyle: *Per Cookie*

Chocolate Brownie	**190**	8	27
Chocolate Chip	**200**	10	25
Minis, 1 pkg	**210**	8	31
Oatmeal Raisin	**180**	7	26
Peanut Butter	**190**	10	22

Sandwich Cremes:

Peanut Butter (5)	**200**	9	25
Vanilla (5)	**190**	9	27
Minis, 1 pkg	**240**	1	34

Cookies & Crackers ~ Brands (Cont)

Per Cookie/Cracker, Unless Indicated **C** **F** **Cb**

Great American Cookies:			
Chewy Choc. Supreme	200	9	29
Chewy Pecan Supreme	230	12	31
Double Fudge with Reese's	230	11	33
Original, w/ Reese's or M&M's	240	12	31
Peanut Butter w/ M&M's	250	14	29
White Chunk Macadamia	250	14	30
Double Doozies:			
Original, 5.3 oz	690	34	94
M&M Big Bite, 2.5 oz	340	17	46
Cookie Cakes:			
16", 3.5 oz	460	22	67
16" M&M, 4 oz	500	24	73
Heart Shaped, 3.5 oz	440	21	64

Great Value *(Walmart):*

Chocolate Chip Chippers:			
Chewy (2), 1 oz	150	6	21
Chunky (2), 1.3 oz	160	8	21
Classic (3), 1.64	170	8	22
Fig Bars, (1)	120	2	24
Fudge Marshmallow, (1)	130	5	20
Ginger Snaps, (4)	130	4	22
Pecan Shortbread, (2)	160	9	19
Twist & Shout, (3)	160	7	24
Crackers:			
Buttery, Whole Wheat (5)	70	3	9
Buttery Rounds, 0.5 oz	70	4	8
Buttery Smooth, 0.5 oz	70	2.5	11

Joseph's:

Sugar Free:			
Almond; Chocolate Chip (4)	95	5	13
Coconut (4)	95	4.5	14
Average other varieties (4)	95	4	15

Note: Carb figures include 6 grams Maltitol

Kashi: *Per Cookie*

Chocolate Almond Butter	130	5	19
Oatmeal:			
Dark Chocolate	130	5	20
Raisin Flax	120	4.5	20
Crackers:			
Original 7 Grain, (15)	120	3.5	20
Fire Roasted Veggie, (15)	120	3.5	20
Pita Crisps:			
7 Grain Sea Salt (11), 1 oz	120	3	23
Garlic Pesto (11), 1 oz	120	3	23

Per Cookie/Cracker, Unless Indicated **C** **F** **Cb**

Keebler:			
Animals:			
Crackers, Pouch, 1 oz	120	3.5	22
Frosted Cookies (8)	160	8	22
Chips Deluxe: Original (2)	160	8	19
Chocolate Lovers (2)	170	9	20
Coconut (2)	160	9	18
Deluxe Triple Choc (2)	150	8	20
Soft 'n Chewy (2)	140	6	21
Rainbow:			
Choc. Chip wih M&M's (2)	160	8	20
Choc. Chip Minis, with M&M's,			
5 cookies, 1 oz	140	7	19
Danish Wedding, (5)	160	8	22
E.L. Fudge: Original (2)	170	7	25
Chocolate (2)	170	7	26
Double Stuffed (2)	180	9	24
Vanilla (2)	180	7	26
Fudge Shoppe:			
Coconut Dreams (2)	140	8	17
Deluxe Grahams (3)	140	7	18
Fudge Sticks:			
Original (3)	150	8	20
Fudge Stripes:			
Birthday (2)	140	6	19
Original (2)	140	6	19
Mini, Original, 2 oz pkg	280	13	38
Grasshopper (4)	150	7	20
Gripz, Chips Deluxe, 0.9 oz pouch	120	5	18
Oatmeal: With Raisins (2)	130	6	19
Country Style (2)	130	6	19
Pitter Patter, P'nt Butter Creme (2)	140	6	19
Sandies Shortbread Cookies:			
Cashew (2)	170	9	19
Classic (2)	160	9	19
Pecan (2)	170	10	18
Toffee (2)	160	9	20
Simply Made Cookies:			
Butter (2)	140	7	18
Chocolate Chip (2)	140	7	17
Chocolate S'wich (2)	140	6	20
PB Chocolate Chip (2)	140	8	15
Soft Batch, Chocolate Chip (2)	150	7	21
Vienna Fingers:			
Creme Filled (2)	150	6	23
Reduced Fat (2)	140	4.5	24
Wafers, Vanilla (8)	140	5	23

continued next page...

C ⬦ Cookies ◇ Crackers

Cookies & Crackers ~ Brands (Cont)

Per Cookie/Cracker, Unless Indicated **C** **F** **Cb**

Keebler (Cont):
Crackers:

	C	F	Cb
Club: Original (4)	70	3	9
Reduced Fat (5)	70	2	12
Grahams: Original (8)	130	3.5	22
Honey (8)	140	4.5	24
Town House: Original (5)	80	5	9
Reduced Fat (6)	60	1.5	12
Flatbread Crisps, all flavors (8)	70	2	11
Pita: Mediterranean Herb (6)	70	2.5	12
Parmesan Cheese Basil (6)	70	2.5	11

Kroger:
	C	F	Cb
Chip Mates: Orig. (3), 1.5 oz	150	7	22
Chunky (2), 1 oz	120	6	17
Peanut Butter (2), 1 oz	120	7	15
White Chip (2), 1 oz	120	6	16
Chocolate Sandwich:			
Original (3), 1.2 oz	150	6	24
Double Filled (2), 1 oz	140	6	22
Olde Southern Pecan Shortbread (2)	150	9	16
Vanilla Wafers (7)	130	3.5	23
Crackers:			
Grahams, Orig.; Honey, (4)	120	3	20
Saltines, Original (5), 0.5oz	60	1.5	10

Lance: *Per Pack of 6 Cookies/Crackers*

	C	F	Cb
Choc-O-Lunch/Van-O-Lunch, av.	220	8	34
Crackers:			
Captain's Wafers:			
Grilled Cheese	190	9	25
PB & Honey	200	9	23
Cracker Sandwiches:			
Malt, with Peanut Butter Filling	180	8	20
Nekot, Peanut Butter	240	11	33
Nip Chee, Cheddar Cheese	200	9	24
Toastchee, Peanut Butter	220	11	25
Toasty, Peanut Butter	190	9	21
Wholegrain, Cheddar Cheese	200	10	26

Little Debbie:
	C	F	Cb
Crml Apple Oatmeal Pies (1), 1.23 oz	140	4.5	24
Chocolate Chip Cream Pie (1), 3 oz	380	16	58

Little Debbie (Cont):
	C	F	Cb
Cookies & Cream (1)	160	7.5	22
Happy Campers, Strawberry (1)	140	4	25
Marshmallow Puffs (1)	160	5	25
Oatmeal Creme Pie (1)	170	7	26
Star Crunch(1)	150	6	22

Lu:
	C	F	Cb
Petit Ecolier Dark Chocolate(2)	130	6	17
Petit Ecolier, Milk Chocolate (2)	130	6	17
Pim's, Orange(2), 0.9 oz	100	3	17

Manischewitz:
Crackers:

	C	F	Cb
Tam Tams: Original (10)	110	4	16
Everything; Garlic (10)	140	5	19

Mary's Gone Crackers:
	C	F	Cb
Chocolate Chip Cookies, (2)	130	6	19
Crackers:			
All Flavors, (13)	140	5	21
Super Seed, Classic (12)	160	8	9

Miss Meringue:
Meringue Classiques:

	C	F	Cb
Cappuccino (4), 1 oz	110	0	26
Mint Choc. Chip (4), 1 oz	120	1.5	25
Triple Chocolate (4), 1 oz	120	1.5	25
Vanilla Rainbow/Van. (4), 1 oz	110	0	27
Meringue Minis, Low Fat:			
Mini: Chocolate Chip (12), 1 oz	130	1.5	27
Mint Chocolate Chip (12), 1 oz	120	1.5	26
Meringue Minis, Fat Free:			
Peppermint Crush (9), 1 oz	110	0	25
Rainbw Vanilla; Vanilla (13), 1 oz	110	0	27
Meringue Petites: Cafe au Lait (7)	100	0	25
Toasted Coconut (6)	120	2.5	23

Mother's:
	C	F	Cb
Circus Animal, (7), 1 oz	150	7	20
Chocolate Chips, (4)	150	7	20
Coconut Cocadas, (4), 1 oz	140	7	17
Double Fudge, (2), 1.3 oz	190	8	27
English Tea, (2), 1.4 oz	190	8	28
Iced Oatmeal, (4), 1.2 oz	150	6	23
Taffy, (2), 1.3 oz	190	9	28

Mrs Fields Cookies ~ *See Page 219*

Cookies & Crackers ~ Brands (Cont)

Per Cookie/Cracker, Unless Indicated **C** **F** **Cb**

Nabisco Cookies:

	C	F	Cb
Chips Ahoy!, Chocolate Chip:			
Original:			
3 cookies, 1.2 oz	160	8	22
Single Serve, 2 oz	280	14	38
Reduced Fat (2), 1.2 oz	150	6	24
Mini Choc. Chips:			
Big Bag, 5 cookies, 1oz	150	7	19
Go Pak, 14 cookies, 1 oz	150	7	20
Snak Sak, 5 cookies, 1.1 oz	160	7	21
Chewy: Regular (2), 1.1 oz	140	6	21
Brownie Filled (1), 0.65 oz	80	3.5	12
Chunky: Choc. Chunk (2), 1.2 oz	160	8	20
White Fudge Chocolate (1)	80	4	11
Hot Cocoa (2), 1.1 oz	150	7	22
Oreo Creme, (2), 1.1 oz	150	7	21
Peanut Butter, (1), 0.7 oz	90	4	13
Lorna Doone:			
100 Calorie Pack,			
Shortbread Cookie Crisps (6), 0.7 oz	100	3	16
Shorbreads: 1 oz cookie	140	7	20
1.5 oz cookie	210	10	28
Mallomars (1), 1 oz	120	5	18
Newtons:			
100% Whole Grain:			
Blueberry (2), 1 oz	100	1.5	22
Fig (2), 1 oz	110	0	22
Strawberry 92), 1 o	100	2	21
Original Fig: 2 cookies, 1.1 oz	110	2	22
Fat-Free, 2 cookies, 1 oz	90	0	23
Nilla Wafers:			
8 wafers, 1 oz	140	6	21
Reduced-Fat (8), 1 oz	120	1.5	24
Vanilla, 1 oz pkg	120	3	22
Nutter Butter:			
Peanut Butter Sandwich:			
16 oz package, 2 cookies, 1 oz	140	6	19
4.8 oz package, 2 cookies, 0.9 oz	120	5	16
1.9 oz package	270	11	39
Bites, 1 package, 1.73 oz	240	10	34
Wafer, 5 patties, 1.2 oz	160	9	19
Oreo Berry, (2) 1 oz	140	6	20
Oreo Cool Mint, (2), 1 oz	140	7	21
Oreo Chocolate/Golden: *Average All fillings*			
100 Calorie Pack, Thin Crisps (6)	100	2	19
Original: 1 cookie	55	2.5	8
3 cookies, 1.2 oz	165	7	25

Per Cookie/Cracker, Unless Indicated **C** **F** **Cb**

Nabisco (Cont):

Oreo, Choc./Golden (Cont): *Average All Fillings*

	C	F	Cb
Original Continued:			
Reduced Fat (3), 1.2 oz	150	5	27
Mini Bite: Bite Size (9), 1 oz	130	6	21
15 oz Pack	200	8	30
Go-Paks, average, 3.5 oz	490	22	70
Chewy, 1.2 oz	150	7	21
Double Stuf:			
2 cookies, 1 oz	145	7	21
Single Serve, 1.5 oz	210	10	30
Fudge Cremes: 1 cookie	60	3	8
3 cookies	190	9	24
Thins, all flavors, 1 oz	140	6	21
Triple Double Chocolate (1), 0.75 oz	100	5	15
Oreo Peanut Butter Creme, (2) 1 oz	140	6	20
Teddy Grahams:			
Single Serve: Honey (24), 1 oz	120	4	21
Cinnamon (24), 1 oz	120	4	21
Nabisco Crackers:			
Barnum's Animals:			
8 crackers, 1 oz Pack	120	3.5	22
Snack Saks, 1.2 oz Pack	140	4	24
Cheese Nips:			
Cheddar: 29 pieces, 1 oz	150	6	19
Mini, Despicable Me, 1 oz Pack	130	4	19
Honey Maid:			
Grahams (8) average all varieties,	130	3	24
Honey, low fat (8), 1.24 oz	140	2	29
Premium:			
Original: 5 crackers, 0.5 oz	70	1.5	12
Minis (17), 0.5 oz	70	2	11
Unsalted Tops(5), 0.5 oz	70	1.5	13
Rounds: Original (6), 0.5 oz	60	1.5	12
Wholegrain (6), 0.5 oz	60	1.5	11
Soup & Oyster (22), 0.5 oz	60	1.5	11
Teddy Graham Crackers, 1 oz pkt	120	4	21
Triscuit: Original (6), 1 oz	120	3.5	20
Reduced Fat (6), 1 oz	110	2.5	21
Brown Rice & Wheat (6),			
average all varieties	130	3	22
Thin Crisps, Original (7)	130	4.5	21
Wheat Thins: *Per 9 oz Box*			
Original (16), 1.1 oz	140	5	22
Reduced Fat (16), 1 oz	130	3	22
Av. other flav. (14), 1.1 oz	140	5	21
Multigrain (14), 1.1 oz	130	4	22
Popped, av. all flavors, 24 pcs	125	3	23

C Cookies ◆ Crackers

Per Cookie/Cracker, Unless Indicated	C	F	Cb
Nana's: *Per Cookie*			
Choc. Chip; Oatmeal Raisin, av.	410	17	59
Coconut Chip; Peanut Butter, av.	370	18	50
Double Chocolate	420	20	58
Gluten Free: Choc. Crunch	360	12	62
Ginger	360	10	64
Lemon	360	14	60
Cookie Bars, average	150	6	23
Bites, P'Nut Butter (1), 1 oz	130	6	17
Newman's Own Organics:			
Alphabet: Chocolate (10)	110	3	21
Other varieties (10)	120	3	21
Double Choc Chip, (5)	150	8	22
Fig Newman's:			
Fat-Free (2)	100	0	24
Low Fat & Wheat/Dairy-Free (2)	110	1.5	23
Strawberry (2)	110	1.5	22
Newman-O's: Original (2)	130	5	20
Choc.; Hint O Mint Creme, (2), av.	130	5	20
Peanut Butter (2)	120	5	18
Oatmeal Chocolate Chip, (2)	140	6	23
Orange Chocolate Chip, (2)	160	7	22
Nonni's:			
Biscotti:			
Original, 1 piece, 0.8 oz	90	3	14
Av. other varieties, 1 piece, 0.8 oz	110	4	17
THINAddictives: Cranb. Alm., 1 oz	130	4.5	20
Chocolate varieties, average, 1 oz	140	5	21
Pistachio/Mango Coconut Alm., 1 oz	145	6	18
Oreo Cookies ~ *See Nabisco, Page 85*			
Payaso:			
Animalitos, 19 pieces	120	1.5	23
Marias, (8)	120	2.5	22
Orejitas Finas, (4)	100	5	13
Pepperidge Farm:			
Cookies:			
Chunk: *Per Cookie*			
Chesapeake, Dark Chocolate Pecan	140	8	20
Lexington, Milk Chocolate,			
Toffee Almond	130	7	16
Monauk, Milk Chocolate	140	6	22
Nantucket, Dble Dark Chocolate	140	7	19
Sausalito, Milk Choc. Macadamia	130	7	17
Tahoe,			
White Chocolate Macadamia	130	7	17

Per Cookie/Cracker, Unless Indicated	C	F	Cb
Pepperidge Farm (Cont):			
Brown Butter Rum, (3)	130	6	20
Brussels (3)	150	7	20
Lemon (4)	160	8	21
Geneva (3)	160	9	19
Milano: Crunchy Almond Slices (3)	150	8	17
Dark Chocolate (2)	180	9	22
Double Milk Chocolate (2)	130	7	17
Dulce De Leche (2)	130	7	16
Pirouettes, (2), av. all var.	120	5	19
Tahiti, Coconut (2)	170	10	17
Crackers:			
Cracker Trio, (3)	60	2	9
Golden Butter, (4)	70	2.5	11
Harvest Wheat, (2)	50	2	7
Goldfish Crackers:			
Cheddar: ½cup, 1.1 oz	140	5	20
Carton, small, 2 oz	280	10	40
Lunch Pack, 0.9 oz pouch	120	4.5	17
Flavor Blasted, av., (56)	140	4	20
Grahams, av., (35)	140	5	22
Parmesan, (60)	140	5	20
Pizza, (55)	140	5	20
Pretzel, (43)	130	2.5	24
Wholegrain Cheddar, (55)	140	5	19
Ritz:			
Originals: Original (5)	80	4.5	10
Roasted Veg. (5)	80	3.5	10
Whole Wheat (5)	70	2.5	10
Bits, Peanut Butter (12)	150	8	18
Crisp & Thins, all varieties (21)	130	4.5	21
Toasted Chips:			
Original (13)	130	4	20
Cheddar (12)	30	6	19
Sour Cream & Onion (12)	130	6	19
Safeway Select:			
Homestyle, Oatmeal Raisin, 1 oz	130	6	18
Indulgent: Double Choc Chunk, 1 oz	130	7	18
Milk Chocolate Macadamia Nut, 1 oz	140	8	17
Gourmet Sandwich Cremes:			
Maple Creme (2)	170	7	25
Raspberry Swirl (2)	130	5	20
Strawberry Swirl (2)	130	6	19
Sedano's:			
Cinnamon, (5)	160	6	24
Maria, (5)	120	3	22
Shar Gluten Free ~ *See CalorieKing.com*			

Cookies & Crackers ~ Brands (Cont)

Per Cookie/Cracker, Unless Indicated **C** **F** **Cb**

	C	F	Cb
Special K: *Per 1 oz Serving*			
Crackers, all varieties (14)	130	4.5	21
Cracker Chips, 0.9 oz pouch	100	3.5	18
Stella D'Oro:			
Breakfast Treats (1), av. all var.	90	2.5	15
Margherite: Chocolate (2)	130	6	19
Vanilla (2)	120	4	20
Roman Egg Biscuits, 1 oz	130	4.5	19
Swiss Fudge (3)	180	9	22
Toast & Sponge:			
Almond Toast (2)	100	1.5	20
Anisette Sponge (3)	90	1	18
Streit's:			
Flavored Wafers:			
Chocolate (3)	160	9	19
Vanilla (3)	170	11	18
Sunshine:			
Cheez-It:			
Crackers: Original, 1 oz	150	8	17
Grab & Go, 2 oz pouch	290	15	32
White Cheddar, 1 oz	140	7	17
Whole Grain, 0.75 oz pouch	100	3.5	14
Big, 1 oz	150	8	17
Snack Mix: Classic, 1 oz	140	5	20
Double Cheese, 0.9 oz	120	5	17
Trader Joe's:			
100 Calorie Packs, average	100	2.5	18
Almond Windmill (2)	140	6	18
Charmingly Chewy Choc Chip (2)	130	5	20
Cherry Granola (2)	110	4	18
Chocolate Chip: Small (4)	140	7	18
Large, singles, 1.7 oz	280	14	35
Deep Dish: 1/10 cookie, 1.6 oz	200	9	28
1/4 Cookie, 4 oz	500	23	70
Vegan (1)	130	6	18
Caramel Cashew (3)	140	7	16
Crispy Crunchy Choc. Chip (12)	150	9	19
Crispy Oatmeal Choc. Chip (12)	150	7	19
Dark Choc Chunks with almonds (3)	140	7	17
Dunkers: Chocolate Chip (2)	160	7	21
Choc. Coated Choc. Chip (2)	190	9	25

Per Cookie/Cracker, Unless Indicated **C** **F** **Cb**

Trader Joe's (Cont):

	C	F	Cb
Ginger Snaps, Gluten Free (5)	140	6	21
Highbrow Chocolate (2)	140	7	17
Joe Joe's Sandwich Cremes, Chocolate/Vanilla (2)	130	6	19
Macarons A La Parisienne (2)	90	3	10
Meringues, Vanilla (4)	110	0	27
Oatmeal Raisin, 1.8 oz	270	12	35
Pecan Southern Style (4)	150	9	15
Thins: Meyer Lemon (9)	130	4.5	22
Toasted Coconut (8)	130	4.5	22
Triple Choc Chunk, 1 oz	140	7	20
Ultimate Vanilla Wafers (5)	120	6	15
Way More Chocolate Chip (3)	160	11	14
Crackers:			
Multigrain (14)	150	6	22
Savory Thin Edamame (38)	120	2	21
Water (4)	60	1	12
Triscuits ~ *See Page 85*			
Voortman: *Per Cookie Unless Indicated*			
Almond Delight	120	6	16
Chocolate Chip	90	4	13
Coconut	100	5	9
Coconut Dark Chocolate	90	5	10
Fudge Striped Almonette	110	6	13
Iced Almonettes	100	4.5	11
Oatmeal Choc Chip	90	4	12
Sugar Free: Choc Chip	90	4.5	14
Fudge Striped Shortbread	130	8	17
Oatmeal	90	4.5	14
Wafers (3), average all flavors	140	8	18
Whole Foods (365 Organic):			
Chocolate Chip (2)	150	7	21
Classic Fig Bars (2)	140	2.5	27
Lemon Wafers (7)	110	3	19
Oatmeal (2)	130	4.5	20
Sandwich Cremes; Sugar, (2), average	130	5	20

Cookie ~ Mixes

As Packaged

	C	F	Cb
Betty Crocker:			
Cookie Mix: *Per 3 Tbsp Mix*			
Double Chocolate Chunk	110	2.5	21
Reeses PB & Choc. Chunk	130	5	20
Snickerdoodle	110	1.5	24
Walnut Chocolate Chip	120	3.5	20
Limited Edition,			
Snowball, 2 Tbsp Mix, 1 cookie	100	3	18

C Cookies ~ Refrigerated ◊ Crispbread

Thaw, Bake & Serve **C** **F** **Cb**

Per Cookie/Cracker Unless Indicated

Pillsbury Cookies:

Refrigerated Cookie Dough: *Per Cookie*

Chocolate Chip Cookie, 1 oz	130	6	17
P'nut Butter, 1.1 oz	130	6	19
Sugar, 1 oz	160	7	23

Ready To Bake:

Choc. Chunk?Chip Cookies, 1.34 oz	170	7	24
Choc. Chunk & Chip Cookies,	170	7	24
Sugar Cookies, 1 oz	120	5	18
Melts: Caramel Brownie (1)	140	5	22
S'mores Sensation (1)	150	6	23
Sugar Shapes, (2), av. all var.,1 oz	120	6	15

Refrigerated Sweet Buns/Rolls~ *See Page 67*

Toll House (Nestle):

Refrigerated Doughs: *Per Cookie*

Bars: Chocolate Chip	90	4	11
P'B Chocolate Chip	80	4.5	10
Sugar Bar	80	3.5	11
Walnut Chocolate Chip	90	4.5	11
Blueberry Lemon (1)	80	3	4
Peanut Butter (1)	130	7	15
Pecan Turtle Delight (1)	160	7	24
Triple Chip (1)	90	4.5	4

Ultimates Refrigerated Dough: *Per Cookie*

Chocolate Chip Lovers	180	9	23
Chocolate Pecan Deluxe	190	10	22
Choc. P'nut Butter Deluxe	180	9	23
Dark Chocolate Delight	160	8	21
Pecan Turtle Delight	160	7	23

Crispbreads **C** **F** **Cb**

Per Crispbread Unless Indicated

Finn Crisp:

Classic: Caraway	20	0	4
High Fibre	40	0.5	7
Sourdough	20	0.5	4
Traditional	40	0.5	7
Round: Multigrain	50	0	7.5
Original	45	0.5	8
New York Flatbread Crisps, Sesame, 0.4 oz	50	1.5	8
Ry-Krisp: Natural (2)	50	0	11
Seasoned (2)	50	0	11
Sesame (2)	50	0	9

Ryvita:

Crackerbreads, Original; Ched. Chse	20	0	4
Crispbreads, Original; Dark	35	0	6.5

WASA:

Crisp'n Light Thins:

Fiber (2), 0.7 oz	60	1	14
Hearty (1), 0.5 oz	50	0	12
Light Rye (2), 0.5 oz	60	0	15
Whole Grain (1), 0.5 oz	40	0	10

Matzos

Manischewitz:

Matzos: Egg & Onion, 1 oz	80	0.5	17
Thin Salted/Tea, average, 0.9 oz	95	0	20
Whole Wheat, 1 oz	110	1	21
Yolk Free, 1.2 oz	100	0	20

Crackers:

Tam Tam Snack:: Original (10), 1 oz	110	4	16
Everything; Onion (10), 1 oz	140	5	19
Rye (10), 1 oz	110	4	16

Streit's:

Lightly Salted, (1)	110	0.5	23
Unsalted Matzos, (1)	100	0	23

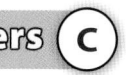

Quick Guide C F Cb

Cream
Average All Brands
Half & Half Cream:

	C	F	Cb
1 Tbsp, 0.5 oz	20	1.5	0.5
2 Tbsp, 1 oz	40	3	1
1/4 cup, 2 oz	80	6	2
Light: Coffee/table (20% fat): 1 Tbsp	30	3	0.5
2 Tbsp, 1 oz	60	6	0.5

Sour Cream:

Regular: 1 Tbsp, 0.5 oz	25	2.5	1
1 cup, 8 oz	445	45	7
Low-Fat/Light: 1 Tbsp, 0.5 oz	20	1.5	1
2 Tbsp, 1 oz	40	3	2
Fat-Free: Av., 2 Tbsp, 1 oz	20	0	3
Knudsen, 2 Tbsp, 1 oz	30	0	2
Kroger, 2 Tbsp, 1 oz	20	0	3

Sour Cream Substitute:

Albertson's, 2 Tbsp, 1 oz	60	5	2
Tofutti, Sour Supreme, 2 Tbsp, 1 oz	85	5	9

Whipping Cream:
Heavy, (37% fat):

1 Tbsp fluid/2 Tbsp whipped	50	5.5	0.5
1/2 cup whipped	105	11	1
1 cup whipped	410	44	3.5

Light, (30% fat):

1 Tbsp fluid/2 Tbsp whipped	45	4.5	0.5
1/2 cup fluid/1 cup whipped	350	37	3.5

Coconut Cream/Milk

Coconut Cream, (Canned):

Plain/unsweetened: 2 Tbsp, 1 oz	75	6.5	3
1/2 cup, 4 oz	285	26	12

Sweetened:

Coco Lopez: 1 oz	130	5	21
1/2 cup, 4 oz	520	20	84

Coconut Milk: (Canned):

Thai Kitchen: Lite, 1/3 cup, 2 fl.oz	50	4.5	1
Premium/Organic, 2 fl.oz	115	10	4
Unsweetened, 1/3 cup	140	14	3
Coconut Water, (Center), 1 cup	45	0.5	9

Whipped Toppings

Average All Brands

Cream (Pressurized): 2 Tbsp	20	1.5	1
1/4 cup	40	3.5	2
Cream Topping, Lite, 2 Tbsp	20	1	3

Whipped Toppings (Cont)

Kraft:

	C	F	Cb
Cool Whip: Regular, Original, 1/3 oz	25	1.5	2
Extra Creamy, 2 Tbsp	25	2	2
Lite, Sugar Free, 1/4 oz	20	1	3
Free, 2 Tbsp, 0.3 oz	20	0	3
Seasons Delight, Fr. Vanilla, 0.3 oz	25	1.5	2
Dream Whip Mix, 1/16 envolope	10	0	1

Reddi-wip:

Original, 2 Tbsp, 0.3 oz	15	1	1
Extra Creamy, 2 Tbsp, 0.3 oz	15	1	1
Fat-Free, 2 Tbsp, 0.3 oz	5	0	1
Chocolate, 2 Tbsp, 0.3 oz	15	1	1

Creamers (Non-Dairy)

Powder:
Coffee-Mate/Cremora/N-Rich:

Original: 1 tsp	10	0.5	1
Lite, 1 tsp	10	0	2
Flavors: Av., 0.4 oz	60	3	9
Fat-Free, average, 4 tsp	50	0	11
Sugar Free, Chocolate, 0.2 oz	30	0.5	2

Liquid/Refrigerated:
Per Tablespoon

Baileys, Coffee Creamer, all flavors, 1 Tbsp, 15ml	25	0.5	5
Califia Farms, all flavors, 1 Tbsp	15	0	4

Coffee-Mate: *Per Tbsp, 15 ml Unless Indicated*

Flavors: Average all flavors	35	1.5	5
Fat-Free, all flavors	25	0	5
Sugar free, all flavors	15	1	2
Shelf Stable, Ital. Swt Creme	35	1.5	5
Unflavored: Original	20	1	2
Fat-Free	10	0	1
2Go, all flavors, 5 ml	25	1.5	3
Natural Bliss, all flavors	35	1.5	5
Hood, Country Creamer, 1 Tbsp	20	1.5	2

International Delight: *Per Tbsp*
American/Classic/Coffee House:

Regular, all flavors	35	1.5	6
Fat-Free, all flavors	30	0	7
Sugar-Free, all flav.	20	2	1
Simply Pure, all flavors	30	1	5

Kroger: *Per Tbsp*

Coffee Creamers: Original	20	1	3
Caramel Vanilla; Hazelnut	35	1.5	6
Fat-free, Hazelnut	30	0	6
Silk: Almond, Vanilla	20	1	3
Soy: Original	20	1.5	2
Hazelnut	30	1.5	4

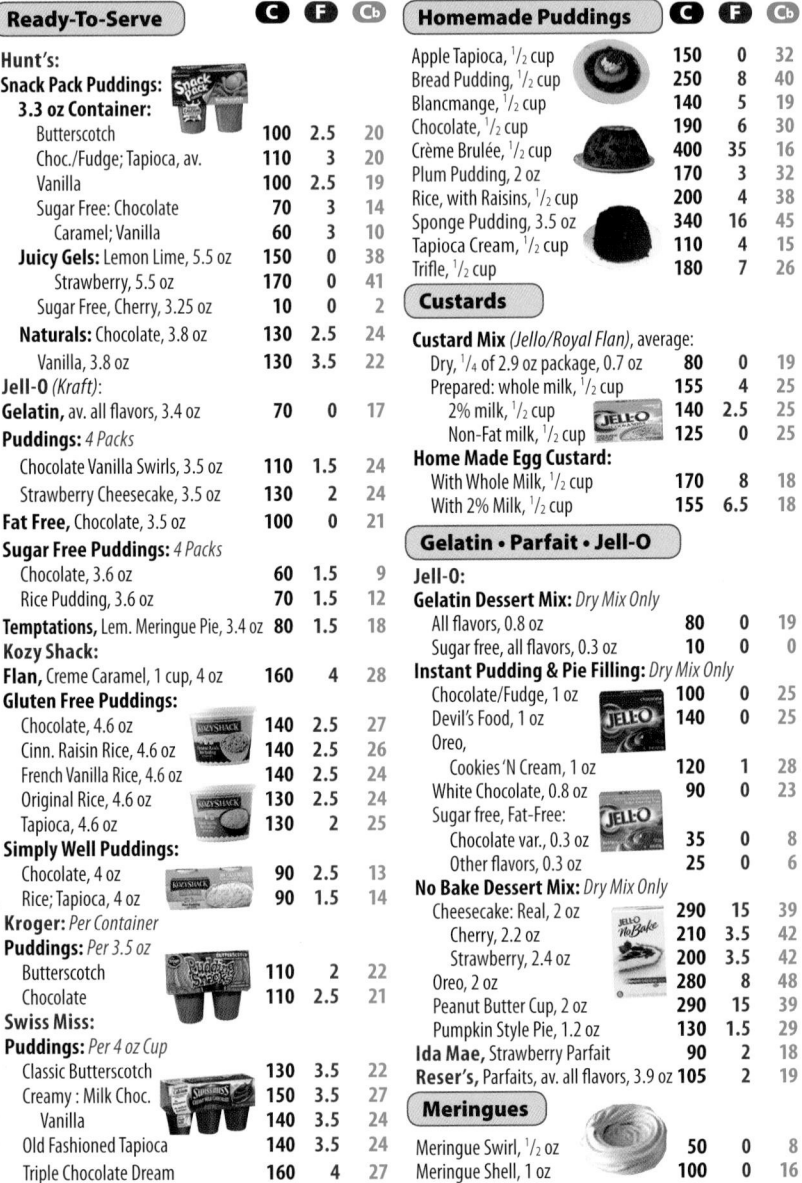

Ready-To-Serve | C | F | Cb

Hunt's:
Snack Pack Puddings:
3.3 oz Container:

	C	F	Cb
Butterscotch	100	2.5	20
Choc./Fudge; Tapioca, av.	110	3	20
Vanilla	100	2.5	19
Sugar Free: Chocolate	70	3	14
Caramel; Vanilla	60	3	10
Juicy Gels: Lemon Lime, 5.5 oz	150	0	38
Strawberry, 5.5 oz	170	0	41
Sugar Free, Cherry, 3.25 oz	10	0	2
Naturals: Chocolate, 3.8 oz	130	2.5	24
Vanilla, 3.8 oz	130	3.5	22

Jell-O *(Kraft):*

	C	F	Cb
Gelatin, av. all flavors, 3.4 oz	70	0	17

Puddings: *4 Packs*

	C	F	Cb
Chocolate Vanilla Swirls, 3.5 oz	110	1.5	24
Strawberry Cheesecake, 3.5 oz	130	2	24
Fat Free, Chocolate, 3.5 oz	100	0	21

Sugar Free Puddings: *4 Packs*

	C	F	Cb
Chocolate, 3.6 oz	60	1.5	9
Rice Pudding, 3.6 oz	70	1.5	12
Temptations, Lem. Meringue Pie, 3.4 oz	80	1.5	18

Kozy Shack:

	C	F	Cb
Flan, Creme Caramel, 1 cup, 4 oz	160	4	28

Gluten Free Puddings:

	C	F	Cb
Chocolate, 4.6 oz	140	2.5	27
Cinn. Raisin Rice, 4.6 oz	140	2.5	26
French Vanilla Rice, 4.6 oz	140	2.5	24
Original Rice, 4.6 oz	130	2.5	24
Tapioca, 4.6 oz	130	2	25

Simply Well Puddings:

	C	F	Cb
Chocolate, 4 oz	90	2.5	13
Rice; Tapioca, 4 oz	90	1.5	14

Kroger: *Per Container*
Puddings: *Per 3.5 oz*

	C	F	Cb
Butterscotch	110	2	22
Chocolate	110	2.5	21

Swiss Miss:
Puddings: *Per 4 oz Cup*

	C	F	Cb
Classic Butterscotch	130	3.5	22
Creamy : Milk Choc.	150	3.5	27
Vanilla	140	3.5	24
Old Fashioned Tapioca	140	3.5	24
Triple Chocolate Dream	160	4	27

Homemade Puddings | C | F | Cb

	C	F	Cb
Apple Tapioca, 1/2 cup	150	0	32
Bread Pudding, 1/2 cup	250	8	40
Blancmange, 1/2 cup	140	5	19
Chocolate, 1/2 cup	190	6	30
Crème Brûlée, 1/2 cup	400	35	16
Plum Pudding, 2 oz	170	3	32
Rice, with Raisins, 1/2 cup	200	4	38
Sponge Pudding, 3.5 oz	340	16	45
Tapioca Cream, 1/2 cup	110	4	15
Trifle, 1/2 cup	180	7	26

Custards

Custard Mix *(Jello/Royal Flan),* average:

	C	F	Cb
Dry, 1/4 of 2.9 oz package, 0.7 oz	80	0	19
Prepared: whole milk, 1/2 cup	155	4	25
2% milk, 1/2 cup	140	2.5	25
Non-Fat milk, 1/2 cup	125	0	25

Home Made Egg Custard:

	C	F	Cb
With Whole Milk, 1/2 cup	170	8	18
With 2% Milk, 1/2 cup	155	6.5	18

Gelatin • Parfait • Jell-O

Jell-O:
Gelatin Dessert Mix: *Dry Mix Only*

	C	F	Cb
All flavors, 0.8 oz	80	0	19
Sugar free, all flavors, 0.3 oz	10	0	0

Instant Pudding & Pie Filling: *Dry Mix Only*

	C	F	Cb
Chocolate/Fudge, 1 oz	100	0	25
Devil's Food, 1 oz	140	0	25
Oreo,			
Cookies 'N Cream, 1 oz	120	1	28
White Chocolate, 0.8 oz	90	0	23

Sugar free, Fat-Free:

	C	F	Cb
Chocolate var., 0.3 oz	35	0	8
Other flavors, 0.3 oz	25	0	6

No Bake Dessert Mix: *Dry Mix Only*

	C	F	Cb
Cheesecake: Real, 2 oz	290	15	39
Cherry, 2.2 oz	210	3.5	42
Strawberry, 2.4 oz	200	3.5	42
Oreo, 2 oz	280	8	48
Peanut Butter Cup, 2 oz	290	15	39
Pumpkin Style Pie, 1.2 oz	130	1.5	29
Ida Mae, Strawberry Parfait	90	2	18
Reser's, Parfaits, av. all flavors, 3.9 oz	105	2	19

Meringues

	C	F	Cb
Meringue Swirl, 1/2 oz	50	0	8
Meringue Shell, 1 oz	100	0	16

Chicken Eggs

C **F** **Cb**

Fresh Eggs: Raw:	C	F	Cb
Small	55	4	0
Medium	65	4	0
Large	70	5	0
Extra Large	80	5.5	0
Jumbo	90	6	0
Egg Yolk, 1 extra large	55	4.5	0
Egg White, 1 extra large	17	0	0
Dried Egg Powder:			
Whole Egg: 1/4 cup, 1 oz	170	12	0
1 Tbsp	30	2	0
Egg White, 1/4 cup, 1 oz	105	0	0
Egg Yolk, 1/4 cup, 1 oz	195	18	0

Egg Substitutes

1/4 Cup (Equivalent to 1 Egg) ~ Zero Cholesterol

	C	F	Cb
All Whites (Crystal Farms), 1.6 oz	25	0	0
Better 'n Eggs (Crystal Farms):			
Regular, 1/4 cup, 2 oz	30	0	1
Egg Beaters (ConAgra):			
100% Egg White 3 Tbsp	25	0	0
Original, 3 Tbsp, 1.6 oz	25	0	0.5
Southwestern Style, 3 Tbsp, 1.6 oz	20	0	0.5
Egg Replacer (Ener-g), 1.5 tsp	15	0	4
Egg Substitute (Albertson's), 1/4 cup	30	0	1
Naturegg (Burnbrae Farms),			
Simply Egg White, 1/4 cup, 2 oz	30	0	0
Vegan Egg Substitute:			
Aquafaba, 1/4 cup, 2 oz	10	0	2

Liquid from cooked/canned beans or chickpeas. Replaces eggs and egg whites in recipes.
Extra Info: www.aquafaba.com

Other Eggs

	C	F	Cb
Duck, 1 large, 2.5 oz	130	9.5	0
Goose, 1 large, 5 oz	280	19	0
Quail, 3 eggs, 1 oz	42	3	0
Turkey, 1 large, 3 oz	135	9.5	0
Turtle, 1 egg, 1.75 oz	75	5	0

Omega-3 Fat Enriched

	C	F	Cb
Egg·Land's Best, 1 large	60	4	0
Horizon Organic, 1 large	70	4.5	1

Note: Cholesterol content is the same as regular eggs.

Cooked Eggs

C **F** **Cb**

	C	F	Cb
Boiled Egg: *Same as Raw Egg*			
Hard-Cooked, Small, peeled	65	4	0
Fried Egg:			
With fat: 1 large egg	105	9	0.5
2 small eggs	175	13	1
No fat/nonstick pan, 1 large	75	5	0.5
Deviled Egg, 2 halves	145	13	0.5
Eggs Benedict, (2),			
on Toast or English Muffin	860	56	25
Eggs Florentine, (2),			
on Toast or English Muffin	890	59	25
Pickled Egg, 1 large	80	5.5	0
Poached Egg, 1 large	65	4	0
Quiche (Homemade):			
Egg & Bacon, 1 slice, 5.3 oz	580	43	27
Ham & Cheese, 1 slice, 5.3 oz	475	33	29
Scotch Egg, 1 egg	300	21	16
Scrambled Eggs:			
1 large egg:			
With 1 Tbsp milk + 1 tsp fat	120	9	1
With 1 Tbsp skim milk/no fat	85	5.5	1
2 large eggs:			
With 2 Tbsp milk + 2 tsp fat	260	20	2
With 2 Tbsp skim milk, w/o fat	180	11	2

Omelets

	C	F	Cb
1 Egg:			
Plain (with 1 tsp fat)	125	10	0.5
With: 1/2 oz cheese	175	15	0.5
1/2 oz cheese + 1/2 oz ham	200	16	0.5
2 Eggs:			
Plain (with 2 tsp fat)	250	20	1
With: 1 oz cheese	360	29	2
1 oz cheese +1 oz ham	410	32	2
3 Eggs:			
Plain (with 1 Tbsp fat)	360	29	1.5
With: 2 oz cheese	580	47	2.5
2 oz cheese+2 oz ham	680	53	2.5
Extras, Tomato/Onion/Veggies, 2 oz	20	0	4.5
Egg Substitute (EggBeaters):			
2 eggs (1/2 cup) + 1 tsp fat	100	4	2
3 eggs (3/4 cup) + 2 tsp fat	160	8	3
Extras: 1 oz Cheese	110	9	1
1 oz Ham	50	3	1

Egg Nog

Average all Brands,

	C	F	Cb
1/2 cup, 4 oz	170	9.5	17
Borden, Regular, 4 fl.oz	160	8	18
Hood, Golden, 1/2 cup, 4 fl.oz	180	9	22
Horizon, Light/Low-Fat,	130	3	23

Breakfast Sides   C   F   Cb

	C	F	Cb
Toast:			
Plain, 1 thick slice	85	1	13
With: 2 tsp butter/marg.	155	9	13
3 tsp/1 Tbsp fat	190	13	13
English Muffin:			
Plain, 2 oz	130	1	26
With 3 tsp fat	230	12	26
Bacon, 2 strips	70	5	0
Ham, lean, 2 oz	100	3	0
Hash Brown:			
1/2 cup, 3 oz	125	6.5	14
1 cup serving, 6 oz	250	13	28
Sausages, 2 oz link	180	16	1.5

Frozen Egg Breakfasts

	C	F	Cb
Jimmy Dean:			
Breakfast Sandwich: *Per Sandwich*			
Biscuit, Sausage, Egg & Cheese	410	29	26
Croissant, Egg, Red Peppers, Onions			
& Jack Cheese	290	16	27
Muffin, Meat Lovers	480	34	26
Omelets: *Per Omelet*			
Three Cheese	290	23	4
Ham & Cheese	250	19	4
MorningStar Farms,			
Breakfast Muffin Sandwich,			
Veggie Sausage, Egg & Chse	210	8	20
Pillsbury:			
Toaster Scrambles:			
Bacon	190	10	18
Bacon & Sausage	190	11	18
Ham	180	10	17
Red Baron:			
Biscuit Scrambles:			
Bacon (1), 5.85 oz	440	21	47
Sausage (1), 5.85 oz	430	20	47
Frozen Pancake/Waffles ~ *See Page 132*			
Toaster Pastries ~ *See Page 64*			

Frozen Egg Rolls

	C	F	Cb
Kahiki: *Each, without sauce*			
Chicken; Vegetable, av., 2.3 oz	150	3.5	26
Pork, 2.8 oz	190	5	31
Lotus Restaurant:			
Imperial, Chicken/Pork (1)	160	6.5	24
Vegetarian, (1)	120	5	20
Pagoda Express: *Each, with Sauce*			
Chicken	160	4	24
Pork	180	7	23
Pork & Shrimp	180	7	23
Vegetable	140	4	24

Fast-Foods/Restaurants   C   F   Cb

	C	F	Cb
Arby's,			
Bacon, Egg & Cheese Croissant	440	27	29
Au Bon Pain, 2 Egg on Plain Bagel	390	11	51
Bob Evans:			
Omelets, Low Calorie:			
Border Scramble	840	53	55
Western	740	43	52
Bojangles: Cheddar 'Bo'	510	31	42
Bacon, Egg & Cheese Biscuit	480	28	42
Bruegger's:			
Bagel: Egg & Cheese, 6.8 oz	450	14	62
Western, 9.2 oz	560	25	64
Burger King:			
Burrito, Egg-Normous	910	55	73
Croissan'wich:			
Bacon, Egg & Cheese	340	18	30
Ham, Egg & Cheese	330	16	31
King, with Double Sausage	700	51	31
Carl's Jr:			
Burrito: Bacon & Egg	570	35	32
Big Country	740	45	55
Loaded Breakfast	760	48	46
Steak & Egg	630	36	37
Chick-fil-A, Chicken, Egg & Cheese,			
on Sunflower Multigrain Bagel	480	18	51
Del Taco, Bacon Breakfast Burrito	640	36	38
Denny's: *With Hashbrowns, Without Bread*			
Omelette:			
Loaded Veggie	600	43	25
Ultimate	820	66	25
Dunkin Donuts:			
Bagel, Bacon, Egg & Cheese	520	18	67
Croissant, Saus., Egg & Cheese	700	50	41
Eat 'N Park:			
Omelette:			
Ham & Cheese	535	35	5
Meat Lovers	725	55	3
Hardee's:			
Biscuit: Loaded Omelet	490	28	40
Sausage & Egg	560	39	39
IHOP: 2 Eggs, Scrambled	220	17	2
Omelette, Spinach & Mushroom	890	70	20
Jack in the Box:			
Biscuit: Bacon, Egg & Cheese	410	25	26
Saus., Egg & Cheese	535	38	27
McDonald's:			
Biscuit, Bacon, Egg & Cheese, reg.	450	24	40
McMuffin, Egg	300	12	30
Whataburger, Breakfast Platter,			
with Bacon	740	52	36

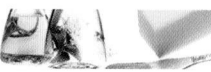

Quick Guide   **C** **F** **Cb**

Butter
Average All Brands

	C	F	Cb
Regular: 1 tsp, 0.2 oz	35	4	0
1 Tbsp, 0.5 oz	100	11	0
2 Tbsp, 1 oz	205	23	0
1 Stick, ½ cup, 4 oz	810	92	0
1 Pound, 2 cups, 16 oz	3255	368	0
Light: Regular, 40% Fat			
1 tsp, 0.2 oz	30	3	0
1 Tbsp, 0.5 oz	70	7.5	0
2 Tbsp, 1 oz	140	15	0
Whipped Butter: Regular			
1 tsp, 0.1 oz	20	2.5	0
1 Tbsp, 0.3 oz	65	7.5	0
1 Stick, 2.7 oz	545	62	0
Whipped Light Butter *(Land O Lakes):*			
1 tsp, 0.15 oz	15	1.5	0
1 Tbsp, 0.4 oz	45	5	0
2 Tbsp, 0.8 oz	90	10	0

Unsalted ~ *Same as Salted*

Flavored Butter/Spreads

Average All Brands

	C	F	Cb
Honey Butter, (60% Fat):			
1 Tbsp, 0.5 oz	90	8	4
Downey's, 2% Fat,			
1 Tbsp, 0.5 oz	60	1	11
Garlic Butter, (80% Fat):			
1 Tbsp, 0.5 oz	100	11	0
Sweet Cream Butter:			
Land O Lakes: Reguar, 1 Tbsp	100	11	0
Honey Butter Spread, 1 Tbsp	70	6	4

Butter & Butter Blends

Per 1 Tablespoon

	C	F	Cb
Challenge: Stick, 0.5 oz	100	11	0
Tub, Whipped, 0.3 oz	70	7	0
Brummel & Brown,			
Spread Made with Yogurt, 0.5oz	45	5	0
Land O'Lakes:			
Sticks, Original, 0.5oz	100	11	0
Tubs, Butter With Olive Oil, 0.5 oz	90	10	0

Ghee (Clarified Butter)   **C** **F** **Cb**

(Example ~ *Purity Farms*)
Note: Ghee is 100% fat compared to regular butter (80% fat + 20% water)

	C	F	Cb
1 tsp, 0.2 oz	45	5	0
1 Tbsp, 0.5 oz	120	14	0

Light & Reduced Fat Spreads

Per Tablespoon

	C	F	Cb
bestlife,			
Buttery Spread, 0.5 oz	60	6	0
Benecol: Regular, 0.5 oz	70	8	0
Light, 0.5 oz	50	5	0
Blue Bonnet:			
Stick, Light Spread, 0.5 oz	50	5	0.5
Tub, Orig. Soft Spread, 0.5 oz	60	6	0.5
Country Crock *(Shedd's):* Stick, 0.5 oz	80	8	0
Tubs: Original Spread, 0.5 oz	50	6	0
Light Spread, 0.5 oz	35	4	0
Churn Style, 0.5 oz	50	6	0
Fleischmann's:			
Orig., Soft Spread, 0.4 oz	60	7	0
Olive Oil Spread, 0.4 oz	60	7	1
Unsalted Spread, 0.4 oz	60	7	0
I Can't Believe It's Not Butter!:			
Tubs: Original Spread, 0.5 oz	60	6	0
Light, 0.5 oz	40	4	0
Olive Oil Spread, 1 Tbsp	60	6	0
Parkay:			
Original Spread, 0.4 oz	70	7	0.5
Spray, 5 sprays	0	0	0
Squeeze Bottle, 0.5 oz	70	8	0
Promise: Activ, Spread, 0.5 oz	45	5	0
Buttery Spread, 0.5 oz	80	8	0
Light Spread, 0.5 oz	45	5	0
Smart Balance:			
Tubs, Buttery Spread:			
Original, 0.4 oz	80	9	0
EVOO, 0.4 oz	60	7	0
Light EVOO, 0.4 oz	50	5	0
Light with Flaxseed Oil. 0.5 oz	50	5	0
Omega 3: Reg., 0.5 oz	80	9	0
Light, 0.5 oz	50	5	0

Butter Substitutes

	C	F	Cb
Butter Buds:			
Butter Flavored: Mix, 1 tsp	5	0	2
Sprinkles, 1 tsp	10	0	2
Earth Balance,			
Original, 1 Tbsp	100	11	0
Molly McButter, 1 tsp	5	0	1
Sunsweet, (Butter/Oil Replacement),			
Lighter Bake, 1 Tbsp, 0.7 oz	35	0	9

Updated Nutrition Data ~ www.CalorieKing.com
Persons with Diabetes ~ See Disclaimer (Page 22)

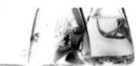
Animal Fats/Lards   C   F   Cb

Average All Types
Beef Tallow/Drippings, Lard (Pork),
Chicken, Duck, Goose, Turkey:

	C	F	Cb
1 Tbsp, 0.5 oz	115	13	0
2¼ Tbsp, 1 oz	255	28	0
1 cup, 7.3 oz	1850	205	0
½ pound, 8 oz	2040	227	0

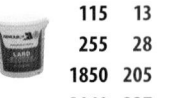

Ghee/Butter/ Oil ~ *See Page 93*

Vegetable Shortening

Average All Types

	C	F	Cb
1 Tbsp, 0.5 oz	115	13	0
2¼ Tbsp, 1 oz	250	28	0
1 cup, 7.3 oz	1810	205	0

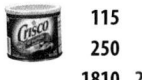

Vegetable Oils

Includes almond, avocado, canola, corn, coconut, flaxseed, grapeseed, linseed, mustard, olive, palm, peanut, rice bran, safflower, sesame, sunflower, soybean, wheat germ. Note: Oil is 100% fat.

	C	F	Cb
1 tsp, 0.2 oz	45	5	0
1 Tbsp, 0.5 oz	120	14	0
2 Tbsp, 1 oz	240	28	0
1 cup, 7.3 oz	1930	205	0

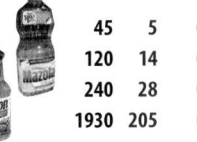

Fish Oils

Average All Types
(Includes Cod Liver, Herring,
Salmon, Sardines): 1 Tbsp, 0.5 oz   **125   14   0**

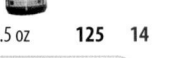

Cooking Sprays/Squeezes

Cooking Sprays: (PAM, Mazola, I Can't Believe It's Not Butter, Weight Watchers, Wesson):

	C	F	Cb
Pam: ¼ second spray	2	0	0
1-3 second spray	6	1	0
I Can't Believe It's Not Butter,			
Original Spray	0	0	0
Parkay, Buttery Spray	0	0	0

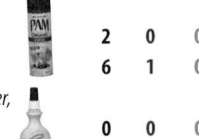

Olestra (Olean)   C   F   Cb

Olestra *(Olean)*   **0   0   0**
Note: Olean is Procter & Gamble's brand name for Olestra – a no-calorie cooking oil that gives snacks (like potato chips, tortilla chips and crackers) taste and texture without adding fat or calories.
Examples:
• *Frito-Lay,* Light Products
   (Lays, Ruffles, Tostitos, Doritos)
• *Pringles,* Fat-Free Potato Crisps

Quick Guide

Mayonnaise: C   F   Cb

Regular: *Per 1 Tbsp, 0.5 oz Unless Indicated*

	C	F	Cb
Average All Brands	90	10	0
Best Foods; Hellman's; Kraft:			
Original/Real	90	10	0
½ cup, 4 oz	720	80	0
Hain, Safflower Mayonnaise	100	11	0
Spectrum, Canola Mayo	100	11	0

Light/Reduced Fat: *Per 1 Tbsp, 0.5 oz*

	C	F	Cb
Best Foods/Hellman's	35	3.5	1
Kraft, Light/Olive Oil	35	3	1
Smart Balance, Omega	50	5	0
Spectrum, Light Canola Mayo,			
Eggless	35	3.5	0.5

Fat Free:

	C	F	Cb
Kraft: Original, 1 Tbsp	10	0	2
½ cup, 4 oz	80	0	16

Sugar Free:

	C	F	Cb
Dukes Mayo, 1 Tbsp	100	12	0

Mayonnaise Style Dressing:
Per 1 Tbsp, 0.5 oz

	C	F	Cb
Best Foods, Sandwich Spread	60	5	2
Kraft:			
Miracle Whip Dressing:			
Original	40	3.5	1
Light	20	1.5	1
Fat Free	15	0	3
Mayo:			
Chipotle	35	3	1
Horseradish-Dijon	35	3	1
Sandwich Shop, Hot & Spicy	100	11	0
Nasoya, Egg & Dairy Free:			
Nayonaise: Regular/Whipped	40	3.5	1
Light	20	1.5	1
Sir Kensington's, Egg/Dairy Free			
Fabanaise (Vegan Mayo)	90	10	0

Quick Guide

Fresh Fish

Low Oil: *Less than 2.5% fat*
White/Lightly-colored flesh. Examples:
Cod, Flounder, Haddock, Halibut, Mahi Mahi, Perch, Pike, Pollock, Snapper, Sole, Whiting.

	C	F	Cb
Raw, without bones, 4 oz	100	1	0
Steamed, broiled, baked, 4 oz	140	1.5	0
Fried: Lightly floured, 4 oz	210	8	3.5
Breaded, 4 oz	260	12	8
In Batter, 4 oz	320	16	27

Medium Oil: *2.5-5% fat*
Lightly-colored flesh. Examples:
Bluefin Tuna, Catfish, Kingfish, Orange Roughy, Salmon (Pink), Swordfish, Rainbow Trout, Yellowtail.

Raw, without bones, 4 oz	145	7	0
Baked/Broiled, 4 oz	195	8	0
Fried, 4 oz	230	11	8

High Oil: *Over 5% fat*
Darker-colored flesh. Examples:
Albacore Tuna, Mackerel, Salmon (Atlantic/Chinook/Sockeye), Sardines, Trout.

Raw, without bones, 4 oz	220	14	0
Baked/Broiled, 4 oz	275	17	0
Fried, 4 oz	340	23	12

Cooking Yields (Fin Fish):

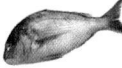

4 oz Raw wt. = 3.5 oz Cooked weight
4 oz Cooked wt. = 5 oz Raw weight

Calorie & Fat Variations:

The amount of fat/oil in fish varies with the species, season and locality. Within the same fish, fat/oil content is generally higher towards the head.

Fish & Shellfish

Edible Weights: (no bones/shell)

	C	F	Cb
Abalone: Raw, 3 oz	90	0.5	5
Fried, 3 oz	160	6	10
Ahi Tuna, grilled, 6 oz fillet (w/o fat)	235	2	0
Anchovy: Paste, 1 Tbsp, 0.5 oz	45	3	0
Canned in oil, drained, (5), 0.7 oz	40	2	0
Barracuda (Pacific), raw, 4 oz	130	3	0
Basa/Swai, raw, 4 oz fillet	70	2	0
Bass:			
Sea: Raw, 4.6 oz fillet	125	2.5	0
Baked, 3 oz	105	2	0
Striped: Raw, 1 fillet, 5.5 oz	150	3.5	0
Baked, 3 oz	105	3	0
Freshwater: Raw, 3 oz	95	3	0
Baked, 3 oz	125	4	0

Fish & Shellfish (Cont)

Edible Weights: (no bones/shell)

	C	F	Cb
Calamari/Squid:			
Raw, 4 oz	100	1.5	3.5
Baked, 1 cup	190	6.5	5.5
Fried, 3 oz	150	6	7
Catfish:			
Farmed: Raw, 1 fillet 5.6 oz	190	9.5	0
Baked, 1 fillet 5 oz	205	10	0
Wild: Raw, 1 fillet, 5.6 oz	150	4.5	0
Baked, 1 fillet, 5	150	4	0
Breaded, fried, 1 fillet, 3 oz	200	12	7
Caviar, black/red, 1 Tbsp, 16g	40	3	0.5
Clams: Raw (4 large/9 small), 3 oz	70	1	3
Breaded, fried (20 small), 6.6 oz	380	21	20
Canned, drained, 1/2 cup, 2.8 oz	115	1	0
Steamed (10 small), 3.3 oz	140	2	5
Cod:			
Atlantic: Raw, 4 oz	95	1	0
Baked, 3 oz	90	1	0
Canned, solids & liquid	90	0.5	0
Pacific: Raw, 4 oz	80	0.5	0
Baked, 3 oz	70	0.5	0
Crab:			
Alaska King, 1 leg, cooked, 4.7 oz	130	2	0
Blue: Raw, 1 crab, 6 oz	150	1	0
Steamed, 3 oz	70	0.5	0
Canned, drained, 6.5 oz can	105	0.5	0
Dungeness: Raw, 1 crab, 5.8 oz	140	1.5	0
Steamed, 4.45 oz	140	1.5	0
Crab Cakes *(Capt. D's)*, (1), 2.8 oz	250	16	16
Crayfish:			
Farmed: Raw, 3 oz	60	1	0
Steamed, 3 oz	75	1	0
Wild: Raw 3 oz	65	1	0
Steamed, 3 oz	70	1	0
Cuttlefish, raw, 3 oz	70	1	1
Dolphinfish ~ *See Mahi-Mahi*			
Eel: Raw, 3 oz	155	10	0
Baked, 3 oz	200	13	0
Fish & Chips *(Red Lobster),* battered, without condiments	700	33	61
Fish Sandwich *(Burger King),* without Tartar Sauce	340	9	49
Fish Oil, 1 Tbsp, 0.5 oz	125	14	0
Flounder/Sole:			
Raw, 4 oz	80	2	0
Baked, 3 oz	75	2	0
Frozen Fish ~ *See Pages 114-122*			

Fish & Shellfish (Cont) — C F Cb

Edible Weights: Without Bones or Shell

	C	F	Cb
Haddock: Raw, 4 oz	85	0.5	0
Baked, 3 oz	75	0.5	0
Smoked, 3 oz	100	1	0
Halibut:			
Atlantic: Raw, 4 oz	105	1.5	0
Baked, 1/2 fillet, 5.6 oz	175	2.5	0
Herring:			
Atlantic, raw, 4 oz	180	10	0
Canned: Plain, drained, 3 oz	130	8	0
In Tomato Sauce, 3.5 oz	140	8	2
Pickled, 2 pieces, 1 oz	75	5	3
Smoked, kippered, 4 oz	245	14	0
Jellyfish: Raw, 4 oz	30	0	0
Dried, Salted, 1 cup, 2 oz	20	1	0
Ling, raw, 4 oz	100	0.5	0
Lobster, Northern:			
1.5 lb Whole Lobster, edible portion:			
Raw, 6.3 oz	140	1.5	0
Boiled, 5 oz	140	1	0
Lobster Salads, average, 1/2 cup	220	13	5
Lobster Newberg, average, 3/4 cup	360	20	9
Lobster Thermidor, av., 1 serving	370	22	15
Lobster Tail (Rock),			
Red Lobster, grilled/roasted	230	6	2
Lox, Regular/Nova, 2 oz	65	2.5	0
Mackerel, Atlantic: Raw, 4 oz	230	16	0
Baked, 3 oz fillet	225	15	0
Pacific/Jack: Raw, 4 oz	180	9	0
Baked, 3 oz	170	9	0
Spanish: Raw, 4 oz	160	7	0
Baked, 3 oz	135	5.5	0
Mahi-Mahi/Dolphinfish:			
Raw, 4 oz	95	1	0
Baked, 4 oz	125	1	0
Monkfish: Raw, 4 oz	85	1.5	0
Baked, 3 oz	80	2	0
Mullet, Striped: Raw, 4 oz	135	4.5	0
Baked, 3 oz	130	4	0
Mussels:			
Raw: 4 oz (edible wt)	100	2.5	4
1 cup, 5.3 oz (edible weight)	130	3.5	5
Cooked, moist heat, 3 oz	150	4	6
Ocean Perch:			
Atlantic: Raw, 4 oz	90	2	0
Baked, 3 oz	80	1.5	0
Octopus:			
Common: Raw, 4 oz	95	1	3
Boiled, 3 oz	140	2	4
Orange Roughy:			
Raw, 4 oz	85	1	0
Baked, 3 oz	90	1	0

Fish & Shellfish (Cont) — C F Cb

Edible Weights: Without Bones or Shell

	C	F	Cb
Oysters, Common, Raw, 3 oz	70	2	4
Eastern:			
Farmed: Raw, 6 medium, 3 oz	50	1.5	5
Cooked, dry heat, 6 med., 2 oz	45	1.5	5
Wild: Raw, 6 medium, 3 oz	45	1.5	3
Cooked, dry heat, 6 med., 2 oz	45	1.5	3
Breaded & Fried, 6 med., 3 oz	175	11	10
Pacific: Raw, 1 medium, 1.8 oz	40	1	3
Steamed, 1 medium, 0.8 oz	40	1	3
Perch ~ *See Ocean Perch*			
Pike: Northern: Raw, 4 oz	100	1	0
Baked, 3 oz	95	1	0
Walleye: Raw, 4 oz	105	1.5	0
Baked, 3 oz	100	1.5	0
Pollock, Atlantic: Raw, 4 oz	105	1	0
Baked, 3 oz	100	1	0
Pompano, Florida, raw, 4 oz	185	11	0
Red Snapper ~ *See Snapper*			
Roe, raw, 2 Tbsp, 1 oz	40	2	0.5
Sablefish: Raw, 4 oz	220	17	0
Smoked, 3 oz	220	17	0
Salmon:			
Atlantic, Farmed: Raw, 4 oz	235	15	0
Baked, 3 oz	175	10	0
Steaks: Raw, 7 oz	410	27	0
Baked, 6 oz	365	22	0
Atlantic, Wild: Raw, 4 oz	160	7	0
Baked, 3 oz	155	7	0
Steaks: Raw, 7 oz	280	13	0
Baked, 6 oz	310	14	0
Chinook: Raw, 4 oz	205	12	0
Baked, 3 oz	195	11	0
Smoked, 3 oz	100	3.5	0
King: Raw, 3.5 oz	185	12	0
Kippered, 3.5 oz piece	265	16	0
Smoked & canned, 3.5 oz	150	6	0
Coho:			
Farmed: Raw, 4 oz	180	8.5	0
Baked, 3 oz	150	7	0
Wild: Raw, 4 oz	165	6.5	0
Steamed, 3 oz	155	6.5	0
Pink/Chum: Raw, 4 oz	145	5	0
Baked, 3.5 oz	155	5.5	0
Canned: Drained solids, 11 oz	435	16	0
Without skin & bones, 8.5 oz	330	10	0
Sockeye: Raw, 4 oz	160	6.5	0
Baked, 3 oz	145	5.5	0
Canned, Drained solids, 3 oz	140	6.5	0
Smoked, 3.5 oz	205	7.5	0
Salmon Cake (1), 3 oz	240	15	6

Fish & Shellfish (Cont) | C | F | Cb

	C	F	Cb
Sardines: *Canned, Average all Brands*			
Drained of Oil:			
¼ cup drained, 2.2 oz	130	9	0
3.75 oz can, drained, 3.3 oz	190	11	0
1 large/2 medium, ⅗", 0.8 oz	50	3	0
in Tomato Sauce, 3.8 oz	150	8	3
Sashimi ~ *See Japanese Foods, Page 171*			
Scallops: Raw, 6 lge/15 small, 3 oz	65	0.5	3
Breaded, Fried (6), 5 oz	385	20	39
Steamed, 3 oz	95	0.5	0
Sea Bass ~ *See Bass*			
Seafood Salad, Deli Style,			
½ cup, 3.5 oz	250	21	11
Shark: Raw, 4 oz	145	5	0
Baked, 4 oz	185	7	0
Batter-dipped, fried, 4 oz	260	16	7
Shrimp:			
Raw: Small/Medium (4), 0.8 oz	15	0	0
Large (4), 1 oz	20	0	0
Breaded & Fried, 4.8 oz	395	24	27
Steamed, in shell, 3 oz	100	1.5	0
Canned, 1 can, 4.5 oz	130	2	0
Snapper: Raw, 4 oz	115	1.5	0
Baked: 3 oz	110	1.5	0
6 oz fillet	220	3	0
Sole: Raw, 4 oz	80	2	0
Baked, 3 oz	75	2	0
Squid ~ *see Calamari*			
Surimi, (Imitation Crab), 4 oz	110	0.5	17
Swai/Basa, raw, 4 oz	70	2	0
Swordfish: Raw, 4 oz	165	7.5	0
Medium Steak, 6 oz	250	11	0
Baked: Small Steak, 4 oz	205	7	0
Medium Steak, 6 oz	290	13	0
Tilapia: Raw, 4 oz	110	2	0
Baked: 3 oz	110	2.5	0
Trout, Rainbow:			
Farmed: Raw, 4 oz	160	7	0
Baked, 3 oz	145	6.5	0
Wild: Raw, 4 oz	135	4	0
Baked, 3 oz	130	5	0
Tuna:			
Raw: Bluefin, 4 oz	165	5.5	0
Skipjack, Yellowfin, av., 4 oz	120	1	0
Baked: Bluefin, 3 oz	155	5.5	0
Skipjack, Yellowfin, av., 3 oz	110	1	0
Canned: *in Water, drained*			
Chunk Light: 2 oz	50	1	0
3 oz can	75	1.5	1
5 oz can	125	2.5	1.5

Tuna (Cont): *in Water, drained (Cont)* | C | F | Cb

	C	F	Cb
Solid White: 2 oz	60	0.5	0
5 oz can	150	1.5	0
7 oz can	210	2	0
in Oil, drained:			
Chunk Light: 2 oz can	80	4	0
5 oz can	200	10	0
Solid White: 2 oz can	90	4	0
6 oz can	270	12	0
Whitefish: Raw, 4 oz	150	6.5	0
Baked, 3 oz	145	6.5	1
Smoked, 3 oz	90	1	0
Whiting: Raw, 4 oz	100	1.5	0
Baked, 3 oz	100	1.5	0
Yellowtail: Raw, 4 oz	165	6	0
Grilled, 3 oz	160	6	0

Other Canned/Packaged Fish

	C	F	Cb
Bumble Bee: *Skinless, Boneless*			
Mackerel, in oil, drained, 1.9 oz	160	15	0
Pink Salmon, in oil, drained, 2 oz	60	1.5	0
Red Salmon, in oil, drained, 2.2 oz	100	5	0
Sardines, in oil, drained, 3 oz	210	15	0
Tuna Ready-To-Eat Kits: *with Crackers:*			
Sensations, Tuna Medley:			
Tom. & Basil, 3 oz can & 3oz Crackers	150	2.5	16
Thai Chili, 3 oz can & 3oz Crackers	180	2.5	23
Tuna, Snack on the Run!: *with Crackers Kit*			
Tuna Salad, 2.9 oz can, w/- Crackers	300	23	18
Tuna, Fat Free w/ Wheat Crackers,			
2.9 oz can	130	2.5	20
Tuna, White Albacore:			
Pouch, in water, 2 oz	70	1.5	0
Solid, in oil, drained, 2 oz	80	2.5	0
Chicken of the Sea:			
Pink Salmon: Skinless/boneless: 3 oz	80	2	0
Traditional, 14.75 oz can, 2.1 oz serve	90	5	0
Sardines, in oil, smoked, 3.75 oz can	150	10	0
Tuna: Lunch Solutions,			
Tuna Salad Cup & Crackers, 3.4 oz	80	0.5	7
To-Go-Cups, Tuna Salad, 2.8 oz	80	0.5	7
Starkist:			
Pouch: *Per 2.6 oz Pouch*			
Albacore White Tuna in water	80	1.5	0
Chunk, Light, Tuna in water	70	0.5	0
Lunch-To-Go Kit, Chunk Light Tuna			
with Light Mayo & Crackers, 4 oz	230	9	20
Tuna Creations: *Per 2.6 oz*			
Bold Hot Buffalo Style	70	1	0
Bold Thai Chili Style	90	1	7

Flours & Grains

	C	F	Cb
Amaranth Flour, ½ cup, 3.5 oz	365	6.5	65
Arrowroot Flour, ½ cup, 2.3 oz	230	0	56
Barley: Grain, regular, ½ cup, 2.6 oz	255	1	55
Pearled, raw, 3.5 oz	350	1	78
Buckwheat: Grain, ½ cup, 3 oz	290	3	61
Flour, whole-groat, ½ cup, 2 oz	200	2	42
Groats: Roasted, dry, ½ cup, 3 oz	285	2	62
Roasted, cooked, 3.5 oz	80	0.5	17
Bulgur: Dry, ½ cup, 2.5 oz	240	1	53
Cooked, ½ cup, 3.2 oz	75	0.5	17
Carob Flour, ½ cup, 1.8 oz	115	0.5	46
Corn Kernels, cooked, av., ½ cup	80	0.5	18
Corn Bran, ½ cup, 1.3 oz	85	0.5	33
Corn Flour/Masa, ½ cup, 2 oz	215	2.5	43
Corn Grits:			
Dry, ½ cup, 2.8oz	290	1	62
Cooked, ½ cup, 4.3 oz	70	0.5	15
Corn Germ, toasted, ½ cup, 4 oz	100	1.5	22
Cornmeal, average all varieties:			
3 Tbsp, 1 oz	105	0.5	22
½ cup, 2.5 oz	255	1	54
Mixes, same as above	230	1	48
Cornstarch: 1 Tbsp, 0.3 oz	30	0	8
½ cup, 2.3oz	245	0	58
Couscous: Dry, 1 oz	110	0	22
Cooked, 1 cup, 5.5 oz	175	0.5	37
Farina: Dry, ½ cup, 3 oz	325	0.5	69
Cooked, ½ cup, 4 oz	55	0	12
Flaxseed: Whole, 1 T., 0.3 oz	45	3.5	2
Ground, 2 Tbsp, 0.3 oz	60	4.5	4
Garbanzo, (Chick Pea), ½ cup, 1.6 oz	180	3	27
Gluten Free Flour, 3 Tbsp	100	0	24
Matzo Meal, ½ cup, 2.2 oz	230	0.5	48
Millet: Raw, ½ cup, 3.5 oz	380	4	73
Cooked, ½ cup, 3 oz	105	1	21
Oat Bran: Raw, ⅓ cup, 1 oz	75	2	21
Cooked, ½ cup, 3.8 oz	45	1	13
Oats, Rolled/Oatmeal:			
Dry/Groats, ½ cup, 1.5 oz	160	3	28
Cooked, ½ cup, 4.2 oz	75	1	13
Polenta ~ *See Cornmeal*			
Potato Flour, ½ cup, 2.8 oz	285	0.5	66
Psyllium Husks, 1 Tbsp, 0.2 oz	10	0	4
Quinoa: Dry, ½ cup, 3 oz	320	5	59
Cooked, ½ cup, 3.8 oz	130	2	24
Rice Bran, ½ cup, 2 oz	180	12	28
Rice Flour, ½ cup, 2.8 oz	290	1	63

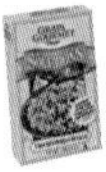

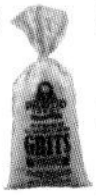

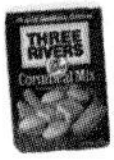

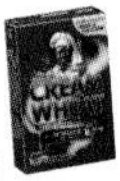

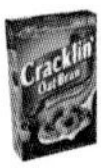

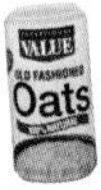

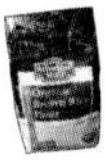

Flours & Grains (Cont)

	C	F	Cb
Rice Polish, ½ cup, 3.5 oz	360	0.5	80
Rye Flour:			
Dark, ½ cup, 2.3 oz	210	2	44
Light, ½ cup, 1.8 oz	190	1	41
Medium, ½ cup, 1.8 oz	180	1	40
Rye Grain: ½ cup, 3 oz	280	2	59
Flakes, ¼ cup, 1 oz	100	0.5	21
Semolina Flour, ½ cup, 3 oz	300	1	61
Sorghum, ½ cup, 3.4 oz	325	3	72
Soy Flour:			
Defatted, 1 cup, 3.5 oz	330	1	38
Low-Fat, 1 cup, 3 oz	325	6	33
Full-Fat, 1 cup, 3 oz	365	17	29
Soy Meal, defatted, 1 cup, 4.3 oz	415	3	49
Spelt Flour, ½ cup, 2 oz	190	1	41
Tapioca Pearl:			
Dry, ½ cup, 2.7 oz	270	0	67
3 Tbsp, 1 oz	100	0	25
Teff Seed Flour, 2 oz	215	2	42
Tortilla Flour Mix,			
½ cup, 2 oz	220	6	37
Triticale:			
½ cup, 3.4 oz	325	2	70
Flour, wholegrain, ½ cup, 2.3 oz	220	1	48
Wheat Bran, unprocessed, ½ cup, 1 oz	65	1	19
Wheat Flakes, ½ cup, 1.5 oz	160	1	35
Wheat Germ:			
Raw, ¼ cup, 1 oz	105	3	15
Toasted, ¼ cup, 1 oz	110	3	14
Wheat Flour:			
White, All Purpose/Self-Rising:			
1 level Tbsp, 0.3 oz	30	0	6
½ cup, 2.2 oz	230	0.5	48
1 cup, 4.4 oz	455	1.5	95
Whole Wheat, 1 cup, 4.2 oz	405	2	87

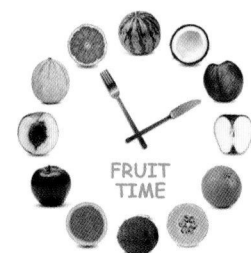

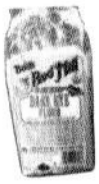

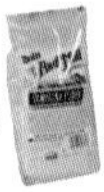

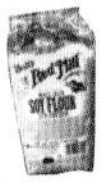

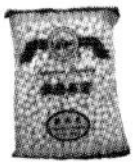

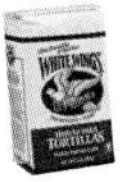

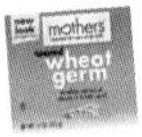

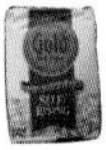

FRUIT TIME

Fruit ~ Fresh

Weights As Purchased

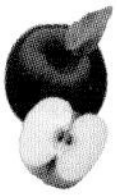

	C	F	Cb
Apples, all varieties, average:			
Whole, with skin:			
1 small, 4 oz	55	0	14
1 medium, 5.5 oz	75	0	19
1 large, 8 oz	110	0	28
1 extra large, 11 oz	145	0	36
Flesh only, no skin or core: 1 oz	15	0	3.5
Slices, 1 cup, 4 oz	55	0	14
Candy/Caramel Apple, 1 med., 6.5 oz	245	4	54
Chiquita, Apple Bites, 14 slices, 5 oz	80	0	20
Apricots: 1 small, 1.5oz	20	0	4
1 medium, 2 oz	25	0	6
1 large, 3 oz	40	0	10
1 extra large, 4 oz	50	0	12
Asian Pear, (Nashi Fruit), 1 med., 7 oz	85	0	21
Avocado:			
Fuerte (Florida) variety:			
¼ medium, 2.7 oz pulp	90	7.5	6
½ medium, 5.4 oz pulp	180	15	12
Mashed, 2 Tbsp, 1 oz	35	3	2
Hass variety (Californian/Mexican):			
Cubes, ½ cup, 2.5 oz	120	11	6
Mashed: 2 Tbsp, 1 oz	50	4	2
¼ cup, 2 oz	95	8	5
Pulp: ¼ medium, 1.5 oz	70	6.5	3
½ medium, 3 oz	140	13	7
1 medium (8.5 oz whole), 6 oz	280	26	14
Salad slices (3), 1 oz	50	4	2

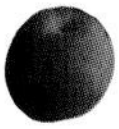

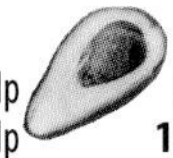

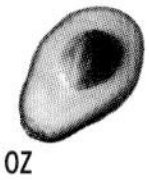

Note: The fat of avocados is heart-healthy. Avocados are very low in carbs ~ most is fiber. This benefits blood sugar and cholesterol levels. Use in place of butter and other high-fat spreads.

	C	F	Cb
Banana:			
Weight with skin:			
1 baby, 3 oz	50	0	12
1 small (5"), 4 oz	65	0	16
1 medium (7"), 5 oz	80	0	20
1 large (8"), 8 oz	120	0	30
1 extra large (9"), 9 oz	135	0	34
Flesh only, weight without skin:			
Mashed, ½ cup, 4 oz	100	0	25
Slices, ½ cup, 2.5 oz	65	0	16
Green Bananas, weight with skin:			
1 medium (7"), 5 oz	75	0	18
1 large (8"), 7 oz	110	0	27
Blackberries, 1 cup, 5 oz	60	0.5	14
Blueberries: ¼ cup, 1 oz	15	0	4
1 cup or ½ pint container, 5 oz	80	0	20
1 pint container, 10 oz	160	0	40

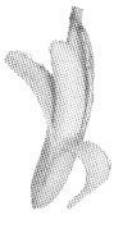

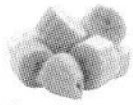

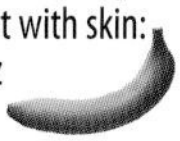

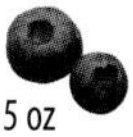

Weights As Purchased

	C	F	Cb
Boysenberries, 1 cup, 4.5 oz	60	4.5	14
Breadfruit, ½ cup, 4 oz	115	0	30
Cactus Fruit:			
1 small, 2 oz	15	0	4
1 medium, 5 oz	40	0	9
1 large, 7 oz	55	0	13
Pulp, no skin, 1 cup, 5.3 oz	60	0	14
Cantaloupe: Flesh, without skin, 1 oz	10	0	2
Pieces/Balls, 1 cup, 5.5 oz	55	0	13
Slices, ½ circle, without rind:			
1 thin (buffet), ⅛"), 0.5 oz	5	0	1
1 medium (¼"), 1 oz	10	0	2
1 thick (½"), 2 oz	20	0	5
Wedges, length cut, without skin:			
1 thin, 1/16 medium, 2 oz	20	0	5
1 thick, ⅛ medium, 4 oz	40	0	9
Whole, weight with seeds and skin:			
½ small, 20 oz	195	1	46
½ medium, 28 oz	270	1.5	65
½ large, 2.5 lb	370	2	90
Cape Gooseberries, 1 cup, 5 oz	70	1	15
Cherimoya: Pulp, ½ cup, 3 oz	60	0	14
1 Fruit (11 oz), 8 oz edible	170	1	40
Cherries, (Red/White), sweet, raw:			
6 medium or 4 large, 2 oz	30	0	7
1 cup, 4.5 oz	75	0	18
½ lb quantity	130	0	32
Sour, red, raw, 1 cup, 4 oz	50	0	12
Clementine, 1 medium, 2.6 oz	35	0	9
Coconut, raw:			
Young, sweet,			
Pieces: 1 piece (2" x 2"), 1.5 oz	35	2	4
½ cup, 3.5 oz	80	5	9
Mature, hard, 1 piece (2"x 2"), 1.5 oz	160	15	6
Crabapples, slices, ½ cup, 2 oz	40	0	11
Cranberries,			
fresh, ¼ cup, 1 oz	25	0	6.5
Custard Apple ~ *See Cherimoya*			
Dates: Medium (1), 0.3 oz	20	0	5
Large Medjool (1), 0.5 oz	40	0	10
Extra Large Medjool (1), 0.9 oz	65	0	16
Chopped, ½ cup, 3 oz	240	0	58
Dragon Fruit, (Pitahaya):			
1 medium, 4" long, 12 oz	60	0	12
1 large, 5"long, 16 oz	80	0	18
Durian, pulp, 4 oz	165	6	31
Elderberries, ½ cup, 2.5 oz	55	0.5	13

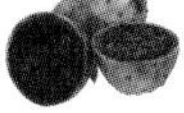

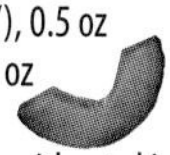

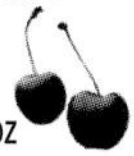

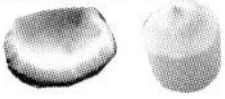

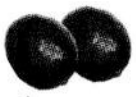

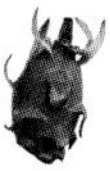

Weights As Purchased	C	F	Cb
Feijoa, (Pineapple Guava), 1 medium, 2 oz	30	0.5	5.5
Figs, green/black:			
1 medium, 2 oz	40	0	10
1 large, 3 oz	60	0	15
Gooseberries, raw, 1 cup, 5 oz	65	1	15
Grapefruit, all varieties, average:			
½ fruit, 10 oz (6 oz flesh)	55	0	13
1 cup sections w/ juice, 8 oz	75	0	18
Grapes: Average, 1 cup, 5.5 oz	105	0	28
1 small bunch, 4 oz	80	0	20
1 medium bunch, 7 oz	140	0	36
1 large bunch, 16 oz	315	0	82
Granadilla, pulp, ½ cup, 4 oz	110	0	27
Guanabana, pulp, ½ cup, 4 oz	75	0	19
Guava, 1 medium, 4 oz	80	1	16
Honeydew:			
1 slice, ¾" thick, 3 oz	30	0	7
1 wedge (⅛ of 7" diameter), 12 oz (with rind)	80	0	20
Cubes/Balls, 1 cup, 6 oz	60	0	14
½ small (4½ lb whole)	180	0.5	42
½ medium (6 lb whole)	230	1	56
Honey Murcots, 1 only, 5 oz	45	0	11
Jaboticaba, 1 cup, 5.5 oz	55	0	14
Jackfruit, flesh, ⅛, 4 oz	105	0	27
Kiwano, ½ medium, 5 oz	35	0	8
Kiwifruit:			
1 Medium, 2.7 oz	45	0	11
1 Large, 3.2 oz	55	0	13
Langsat, Duku, 1 medium, 2 oz	25	0	5
Lemons: 1 medium, 5oz	20	0	4
1 wedge, 1 oz	5	0	1
Limes, 1 medium, 2.4 oz	20	0	7
Loganberries, frozen, ½ cup, 2.5 oz	40	0	9
Longans, 5 fruit, 0.5oz	10	0	2.5
Loquats, 4 fruit, 2.3 oz	30	0	8
Lychees, 4 fruit, 2.3 oz	30	0	7
Mamey Apple, cubes, 1 cup, 6 oz	85	1	20
Mandarin Orange:			
1 small, 3 oz	35	0	9
1 medium, 4 oz	45	0	11
1 large, 6 oz	50	0	13
Mango:			
Slices, ½ cup, 3 oz	55	0	14
1 small mango, 7 oz	90	0.5	24
1 medium: 10 oz	130	0.5	34
Side cheek, 4 oz	60	0	14
1 large, 17 oz	220	1	58
1 extra large, 24 oz	310	1.5	82
Marionberries, 1 cup, 5 oz	75	1	15

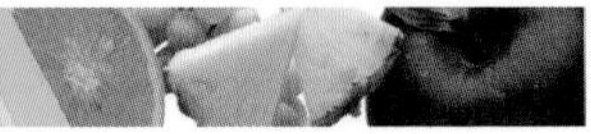

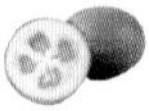

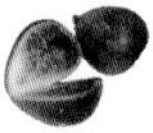

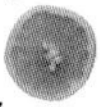

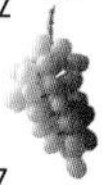

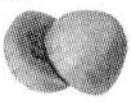

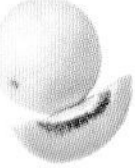

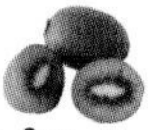

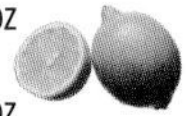

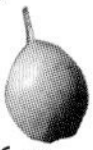

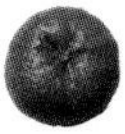

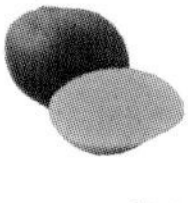

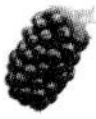

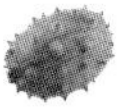

Weights As Purchased	C	F	Cb
Melons, all varieties, average, cubes/balls, 1 cup, 6 oz	60	0	14
Muloberries, 20 fruit, 1 oz	15	0	3
Nashi Fruit/Asian Pear, 1 med. 7 oz	85	0	21
Nectarines: 1 medium, 5oz	60	0	14
1 large, 7 oz	80	0	18
Oheloberries, ½ cup, 2.5 oz	20	0	5
Olives, Pickled: Green, 10 lge, 1.5 oz	60	6.5	1.5
Ripe, Greek Style, 10 medium, 1 oz	70	6	4
Ripe (Black) Californian:			
1 small/medium	5	0	0.2
1 large/extra large	6	0.5	0.5
1 jumbo	7	0.5	0.5
1 colossal	11	1	0.5
Oranges, all varieties, average, weights with skin:			
1 small, (2.5" diam.), 5 oz	45	0	11
1 medium (3") 7 oz	75	0	18
1 large, (3.5") 10 oz	105	0	25
1 extra large, (4"), 14 oz	130	0	30
Flesh/Pulp only, 1 cup, 6 oz	85	0	21
Peel, 1 Tbsp	0	0	0
California Navel (3"), 7 oz	70	0	17
California Valencia, 1 medium (2¾" diam.) 6 oz	60	0	14
Florida Orange, 1 med., 7 oz	70	0	17
Sunkist Navel, large, 14 oz	130	0	30
Papaya:			
1" pieces, 1 cup, 5 oz	60	0	15
1 medium, 16 oz	120	0	30
Green (unripe), ½ cup, 3.5 oz	20	0	5
Passionfruit:			
1 small, 1.5 oz	15	0	3
1 large, 2.7 oz	30	0	6
Pulp, ½ cup, 4 oz	110	0	27
Peaches: 1 baby/donut, 3 oz	30	0	7
1 small, 5 oz	50	0	12
1 medium, 6 oz	60	0	14
1 large, 7 oz	70	0	16
1 extra large, 9 oz	90	0	21
Pears, all varieties, average:			
1 mini, 2.5 oz	35	0	8
1 small, 5 oz	75	0	18
1 medium, 7 oz	100	0	25
1 large, 9 oz	130	0	33
1 extra large, 12 oz	170	0	42
Pepino, ½ medium, 4 oz	20	0	4
Persimmons: Native, 1 oz	35	0	9
Japanese (2½"d. x 2½"h), 7 oz	120	0	30
Maui, seedless, 1 medium, 5 oz	100	0	25

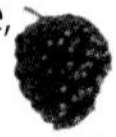

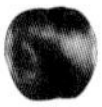

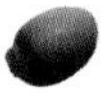

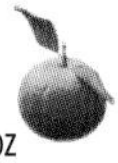

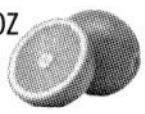

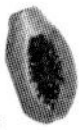

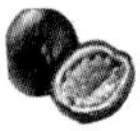

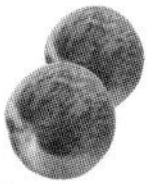

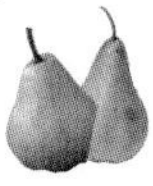

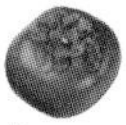

Weights As Purchased	**C**	**F**	**Cb**
Pineapple, average all varieties:			
Weights without skin: 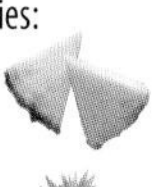			
1 thin slice (½"), 2 oz	30	0	7
1 thick slice (¾"), 3 oz	40	0	10
1 cup, chunks, 6 oz	80	0	20
Whole fruit, wt with skin: 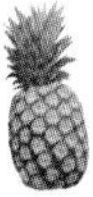			
Baby/Mini, 16 oz	150	0	39
Medium size, 3 lbs	450	1	118
Canned ~ See Page 102			
Pitanga, (Surinam-Cherry) (5), 1.2 oz	10	0	2
Plaintain:			
Fresh/Raw, weight with skin: 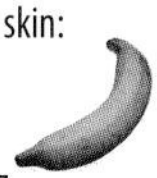			
1 medium, 10 oz	220	0	55
Slices, 1 cup, 5 oz	180	0	44
Cooked:			
Mashed, ½ cup, 3.5 oz	115	0	30
Slices, 1 cup, 5.5 oz	180	0	47
Fried in oil: 10 slices (¼"), 2 oz	160	6	26
1 cup, 4.2 oz	360	14	58
Plums, all varieties, average:			
1 mini/Damson, (1" diam), 0.5 oz	10	0	1.5
1 small (2"), 2.3 oz 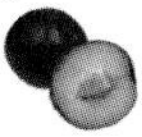	30	0	7
1 medium (2½"), 3.5 oz	45	0	10
1 large (3"), 5 oz	60	0	14
Plumcot, 1 medium, 6 oz	75	0	18
Pomegranate: 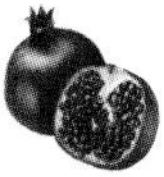			
1 small (3"), 5.5 oz	70	1	15
1 medium (3½"), 10 oz	125	2	27
1 large (4"), 16 oz	230	3	50
Seeds/Arils, ¼ cup, 2 oz	40	1	10
Pomelo, flesh, ½ cup, 3.5 oz	35	0	9
Prickly Pear ~ See Cactus Fruit			
Quince, 1 medium, 3.5 oz	55	0	14
Rambutan/Rambotang,			
Red/Yellow, 1 medium, 2 oz	15	0	4
Raspberries: ½ cup, 2 oz 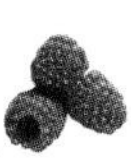	30	0	7
10 raspberries, 0.8 oz	10	0	2
1 cup, 4.3 oz	65	1	15
1 pint, 11 oz	160	2	37
Sapodilla: 1 medium, 6 oz	140	2	34
Pulp, 1 cup, 8.5 oz	200	2.5	45
Sapote: 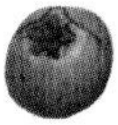			
Black: 1 medium, 4.5 oz	60	0	14
Pulp only, ½ cup, 4 oz	100	1	22
Mamey, piece, 1 cup, 6 oz	220	1	50
Satsuma Tangerine, 1 medium, 3 oz	45	0	11
Soursop, pulp, 1 cup, 8 oz	150	0.5	38
Starfruit, (Carambola): 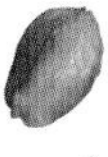			
1 medium, (3½" long), 3 oz	30	0	6
1 large (4½"), 4.5 oz	40	0	8
Strawberries: 1 cup, 5.5 oz 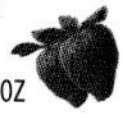	50	0.5	12
6 medium/3 large, 2 oz	20	0	4
1 pint container, heaping, 16 oz	130	1	32
Chocolate dipped, 1 large	45	2.5	6

Weights As Purchased	**C**	**F**	**Cb**
Sugar-Apple (Sweetsop), 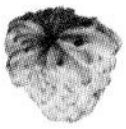			
pulp, ½ cup, 4 oz	120	0	28
Sugar Cane:			
Unpeeled, 1 baton (7" long), 4 oz	30	0	7
Peeled, 1 small stick (3"), 2 oz	35	0	8
Tamarillo, 1 medium, 3 oz 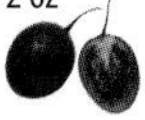	20	0	3
Tamarind: 1 fruit (3"x1")	5	0	1.5
Pulp, ½ cup, 2 oz 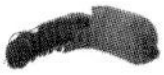	140	0.5	37
Tangelo: 1 small, 4 oz 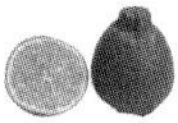	55	0	13
1 medium, 5 oz	70	0	17
1 large, 7 oz	95	0	23
Tangerine, 1 med., (2½" diam.), 4 oz	50	0	13
Tangor, 1 medium, 4 oz	35	0	7
Tomatillos: 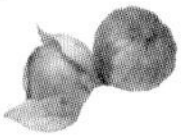			
3 medium, 3.5 oz	35	0.5	6
1 lb (16 oz) quantity	160	2	27
Tomatoes: 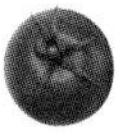			
1 small (2¼" diameter), 3 oz	15	0	3
1 medium (2¾"), 5 oz	25	0	5
Sliced: 2 thin slices, 1 oz	5	0	1
2 thick (⅜"), 2 oz 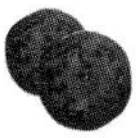	10	0	2
Wedge, ¼, 1.3 oz	6	0	1
1 large (3½"), 8 oz	40	0.5	9
1 extra large (4"), 12 oz	60	0.5	14
Cherry: 4 medium, 2 oz	10	0	2
1 cup, 5 oz 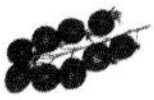	25	0	6
Grape, 5 medium, 2 oz	10	0	2
Yellow Tear Drop, 3 medium, 1 oz	5	0	2
Canned Tomatoes/Products ~ See Page 144			
Tree Tomato/Tamarillo, 3 oz	20	0	5
Ugli Fruit, Tangelo type, 5 oz 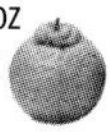	40	0	8
Watermelon:			
Flesh only, weights without skin:			
1 thin slice (½"), ¼ circle, 3 oz	25	0	6
1 thick slice (1"): ¼ circle, 6 oz	50	0	12
½ circle, 12 oz 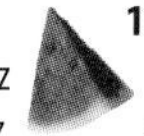	100	1	24
Buffet Slice, small, thin, 1 oz	8	0	2
Cubes or Balls, 1 cup, 5.5 oz	45	0	11
Round Seedless Melon, weight with skin:			
Medium size, 13 lb, (8" diam.):			
whole melon, 13 lb	1160	5	280
wedge, ⅛ whole, 26 oz	145	1	35
Mini size, 6 lb, (6.5" diam.): 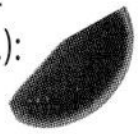			
whole melon, 6 lb	480	2.5	110
wedge, ⅛ whole, 12 oz	60	0	14

Dried Fruit

	C	F	Cb
Apples, 5 rings, 1 oz	80	0	19
Apricots, 8 halves, 1 oz	65	0	16
Banana Chips, ⅓ cup, 1 oz	180	9	16
Banana Flakes, 4 Tbsp, 1 oz	80	0	20
Cranberries *(Craisins)*:			
Original, ¼ cup	130	0	33
Reduced Sugar, ¼ cup	100	0	31
Chocolate Covered, ¼ cup, 2 oz	180	8	28
Dates ~ *See Dates in Fresh Fruit*			
Figs, 3 medium figs, 1 oz	90	0	23
Goji Berries, 3 Tbsp, 1 oz	100	0	21
Mango Slices, 5 pieces, 1.4 oz	25	0	6
Papaya Spears, 2 pieces, 1.4 oz	120	0	30
Peaches, 2 halves, 1 oz	60	0	15
Pears, 3 halves, 2 oz	140	0.5	34
Plums *(Sunsweet)*, (5), 1.4 oz	100	0	24
Prunes/Dried Plums:			
with pits, 3 medium, 1 oz	70	0	17
without pits, 4 medium, 1 oz	70	0	17
Cooked: with sugar, ½ cup, 5 oz	155	0	38
without sugar, ½ cup, 4.5 oz	135	0	33
Raisins: 2 Tbsp, 1 oz pack	85	0	20
½ cup, 2.8 oz	220	0.5	56
White Mulberries, 1 oz	90	0.5	22

Candied/Glazed Fruit

	C	F	Cb
Apricot, 1 medium, 1 oz	70	0	17
Cherry, Maraschino (1)	8	0	2
Citron/Fruit Peel, 1 oz	85	0	20
Ginger, 1 oz	90	0	21
Pineapple, 1 slice, 1.3 oz	120	0	29
Tamarind, dried, sweetened, 1 oz	70	0	17

Fruit Leather Rolls

	C	F	Cb
Betty Crocker: Fruit By The Foot,			
1 roll, 0.8 oz	80	0	17
Fruit Gushers, 1 oz	90	1	20
Fruit Roll-Ups, 1 roll	50	1	12
Stretch Island, Leathers, 1 pouch, 0.5 oz	45	0	12

Canned/Bottled Fruit

Solids & Liquids:
Per ½ Cup, 4½ oz Unless indicated

	C	F	Cb
Apricots/Peaches/Pears:			
in juice, light	60	0	15
in heavy syrup	105	0	28
in water/diet	35	0	8
Black/Blueberries:			
in heavy syrup	120	0	30
in light syrup	110	0	26

Canned/Bottled Fruit (Cont)

	C	F	Cb
Cherries, pitted:			
in heavy syrup	105	0	27
in light syrup	85	0	22
in water	55	0	15
Maraschino, 1 oz	50	0	12
Fruit Cocktail/Salad:			
in heavy syrup	95	0	25
in juice, light	60	0	16
in water/diet	35	0	10
Gooseberries, light syrup	90	0	24
Grapefruit, in light syrup	75	0	20
Lychees, ½ cup, 4.5 oz	105	0	26
Mixed Fruit: in fruit juices/light syrup	70	0	18
in heavy syrup	90	0	24
in water/diet	40	0	10
Pineapple, all varieties:			
in heavy syrup, 4.3 oz	110	0	28
in own juice, 4 oz	60	0	15
Prunes: with syrup, 3 oz	90	0	23
Stewed in water, ½ cup	135	0	35

Fruit Snack Cups

	C	F	Cb
Deli/Take-Out: Small, 6 oz	70	0	16
Large, 12 oz	140	0	32
Yogurt and Fruit Cup, 15 oz	380	4.5	75
Del Monte:			
Fruit & Veggie Fusions, all flav., 4 oz	70	0	17
Fruit Refreshers, average, 7 oz	95	0	24
Fruit Snack Cups in Gel, av., 4.5 oz	80	0	20
Light Fruit Cups, in Gel, av.,4.5 oz	50	0	12
Dole:			
Fruit Bowls In 100% Juice: *Per 4 oz Container*			
Diced Pears	90	0	22
Mixed Fruit	80	0	19
Fruit in Gel: *Per 4.3 oz Container*			
Mixed Fruit, in Black Cherry Gel	90	0	24
Average other fruits, in various Gels	95	0	24

Apple & Fruit Sauces

	C	F	Cb
Apple Sauce:			
Regular/sweetened, 2 Tbsp, 1 oz	20	0	6
4 oz package	90	0	22
Cranberry, Jellied, ¼ cup	110	0	25
Fruit Sauces & Purees:			
All fruit types, average: 2 Tbsp, 1 oz	25	0	6
½ cup, 4 oz	100	0	24
Mott's:			
Apple Sauce: Orig., sweeetened, 4 oz	90	0	24
Other Fruit Flavors, sweetened, 4 oz	90	0	23
Unsweetened Apple, 3.9 oz	50	0	13
Ocean Spray,			
Jellied Cranberry Sce, 3.5 oz	160	0	40

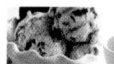
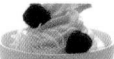

Ice Cream & Frozen Yogurt

Quick Guide

C F Cb

Ice Cream
Average all Flavors:
Regular (10% fat):
Examples: Dreyer's Grand, Hood, Friendly's

	C	F	Cb
½ cup, 4 fl.oz	140	7	16
1 cup, 8 fl.oz	280	14	32
1 pint, 16 fl.oz	560	28	64

Rich/Premium (16-17% fat):
Examples: Baskin Robbins, Ben & Jerry's, Haagen-Dazs

½ cup, 4 fl.oz	250	16	24
1 cup, 8 fl.oz	500	32	48
1 pint, 16 fl.oz	1000	64	96

Reduced-Fat/Light (5% fat):
Examples: Breyers ½ The Fat, Friendly's Light, Hood Light

½ cup, 4 fl.oz	140	5	21
1 cup, 8 fl.oz	280	10	42
1 pint, 16 fl.oz	560	20	84

Fat-Free:
Example: Breyers

½ cup, 4 fl.oz	90	0	21
1 cup, 8 fl.oz	180	0	42
1 pint, 16 fl.oz	360	0	84

Scoop Shops:
Average all Brands
Add extra for cone (see next column)

Kids, 3 fl.oz	125	8	12
Regular, 6 fl.oz	250	16	24
Large, 9 fl.oz	375	24	36

Soft Serve:
Average all Brands

Regular: ½ cup, 4 fl.oz	255	15	25
1 cup, 8 fl.oz	510	30	50
Light: ½ cup, 4 fl.oz	145	3	25
1 cup, 8 fl.oz	290	6	50

Quick Guide

Frozen Yogurt
Average all Brands

Hard: Low-Fat, ½ cup	110	3	19
Non-Fat, ½ cup	110	0	24
Soft: Low-Fat, ½ cup	120	4	17
Non-Fat, ½ cup	100	0	30

Brands ~ *See Ice Cream & Novelties Section*

Quick Guide

C F Cb

Gelato/Ices/Frozen Custard
Gelato: *Per ½ Cup*

	C	F	Cb
Milk base: Vanilla	160	6	25
Chocolate Hazelnut	230	15	21
Water base, ½ cup	100	0	26

Frozen Custard, Choc./Vanilla, av:

½ cup	210	11	23
Single Scoop, 5 oz wt	300	15	38
Double Scoop, 10 oz wt	600	30	76

Ice (Milk base): *Average all flavors*

Hard (4% fat),½ cup	100	3	15
Soft Serve (3% fat), ½ cup	110	2	19
Shaved Ice, average, 12 fl.oz	160	0	40
Sherbet, average, ½ cup	110	1.5	22
Sorbet, Fruit, fat free, ½ cup	70	0	19
Fruit Ice Pops	80	0	20

Sundaes

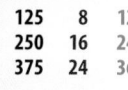

Baskin Robbins:

Classic: Banana Royale	680	33	90
Brownie	810	42	100
Classic Banana	970	39	146

Denny's,

Banana Split, 15 oz	760	30	116

Toppings ~ *See Page 195*
McDonald's:
Sundaes:

Hot Caramel, 6.4 oz	380	11	51
Hot Fudge, 6.3 oz	380	14	43
Toppings, Peanuts, 0.3 oz	50	4	2

Ice Cream Cones & Cups

Average all Brands

Wafer Cone/Cup, average	20	0	4
Sugar Cone, average	50	0	14

Waffle Cone:

Small	50	1	10
Large	90	0.5	19

Brands:

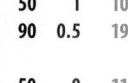

Comet, Sugar Cone	50	0	11
Keebler, Sugar Cone	50	0	10
Oreo, Chocolate Cone	50	1	10

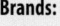

Ice Cream & Frozen Yogurt

Ice Cream ~ Brands   C   F   Cb

Amy's:

Non Dairy Frozen Dessert: *Per ½ Cup*

	C	F	Cb
Chocolate; Vanilla, average, 3.3 oz	175	12	15
Mint /Mocha Choc. Chip, av., 3.5 oz	230	16	20

Baskin-Robbins ~ *See Fast-Foods Section*

Ben & Jerry's:

Scoop Shop Ice Cream: *Hand Scooped, 3 oz Serving*

	C	F	Cb
Americone Dream	240	13	26
Bourbon Brown Butter	240	13	27
Butter Pecan	250	19	17
Choc. Chip Cookie Dough	230	13	26
Chocolate Fudge Brownie	220	11	26
Chunky Monkey	240	15	24
Coconut Seven Layer Bar	250	16	24
Coffee, Coffee, BuzzBuzzBuzz	260	17	23
Mint Chocolate Chunk	220	14	22
Strawberry Cheesecake	200	12	22
Sweet Cream & Cookies	210	12	23
Vanilla Toffee Bar Crunch	260	17	22

Ice Cream, 1 Pint Tubs: *Per ½ Cup*

	C	F	Cb
Banana Split	250	14	28
Cherry Garcia	260	15	27
Chubby Hubby	340	21	33
Everything But The; PB FudgeCore, av.	305	19	29
Milk & Cookies	280	17	28
Peanut Butter Cup	370	26	29
Salted Caramel Core	270	14	31
Red Velvet Cake	260	14	29
S'mores	310	16	36
Strawbery Cheesecake	260	15	28
Triple Caramel Chunk	270	15	32
Vanilla Caramel Fudge	290	16	33

Non Dairy: Chunky Monkey

	C	F	Cb
Chunky Monkey	260	14	31
Chocolate Fudge Brownie	200	11	23
Coffee Caramel Fudge	240	12	31
PB & Cookies	290	17	31

Fro Yo Frozen Yogurt: *Per ½ Cup*

	C	F	Cb
Cherry Garcia	170	3	32
Chocolate Fudge Brownie	180	2.5	35
Half Baked	180	3	35
Pfish Food, 3.6 oz	250	7	42

Greek: Peach Melba

	C	F	Cb
Peach Melba	130	4	12
Raspberry	140	5	21

Sorbet, all flavors | 80 | 0 | 20 |

Blue Bunny: C   F   Cb

Premium Ice Cream: *Pint Container*

	C	F	Cb
Banana Split, 2.65 oz	160	7	23
Bunny Tracks, 2.6 oz	190	11	22
Chocolate, 2.3 oz	130	7	17
Cocoa Bunny, 2.6 oz	170	8	22
Cookies 'n Cream, 2.3 oz	150	7	20

Sweet Freedom: *Per ½ Cup*

	C	F	Cb
Bunny Tracks, 2.5 oz	140	7	23
Butter Pecan, 2.53 oz	110	4.5	19
Double Strawberry, 2.53 oz	90	2.5	20

Note: Carbohydrate figures include 4-6 g sugar alcohols

Frozen Yogurt: *Per ½ Cup*

	C	F	Cb
Caramel Praline Crunch	130	4	21
Strawberry Banana	100	2	20
Vanilla Bean, 2.32 oz	100	2.5	18

Bars/Pops ~ *See Page 108*

Breyers:

Original Ice Cream: *Per ½ Cup*

	C	F	Cb
Butter Pecan, 2.2 oz	140	6	18
Cherry Van.; Cookies & Crm, av., 2.3 oz	130	4	22
Chocolate Truffle, 2.36 oz	170	9	21
Mint Chocolate Chip, 2.4 oz	150	8	17
Nat. Strawberry, 2.3 oz	110	5	14
Salted Caramel, 2.2 oz	130	3.5	23
Vanilla, Chocolate, 2.2 oz	130	7	16

Fat Free, av. all flavors | 90 | 0 | 21 |

Half The Fat: *Per ½ Cup*

	C	F	Cb
Cookies & Cream, 2.1 oz	120	4	20
Creamy Vanilla, 2 oz	100	3	17

No Added Sugar Dairy Dessert: *Per ½ Cup*

	C	F	Cb
Butter Pecan, 2 oz	100	5	13
Salted Cararmel Swirl, 2 oz	90	4	16
Vanilla Chocolate Strawberry, 2 oz	85	3.5	14

Note: Carbohydrate figures include 1-6g sugar alcohol and 0-2g fiber

Blasts!: *Per ½ Cup*

	C	F	Cb
Girl Scout Cookies, Thin Mint, 2.2 oz	140	4.5	23
Mrs Field's, 2.1 oz	140	5	23
Oreo, Cookies & Cream Mint, 2.1 oz	130	4.5	22
Waffle Cone, w/ Choc. Chips, 2.2oz	140	5	23

CarbSmart, average all flav., ¹/₂ cup | 115 | 6 | 14 |

Note: Carbohydrate figures include 5g sugar alcohol and 4g fiber

Bruster's:

	C	F	Cb
Ice Cream, Banana; Black Raspb., av., 5 oz	285	14	37

Fat Free, No Added Sugar:

	C	F	Cb
Coffee; Sea Salt Caramel, av., 5 oz	175	0	36
Fudge Ripple,; Mint with Fudge, 5 oz	200	0	43
Vanilla, Caramel Swirl, 5 oz	170	0	36

Frozen Yogurt: Chocolate, 5 oz

	C	F	Cb
Mint Chip; Peanut Butter, 5 oz	175	7	24

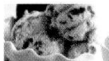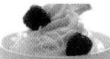
Ice Cream ~ Brands (Cont) Ⓒ Ⓕ ⓒⓑ

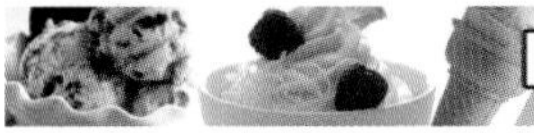

Carvel Ice Cream ~ *See Fast-Foods Section*
Coldstone Creamery ~ *See Fast-Foods Section*
Dairy Queen/Brazier ~ *See Fast-Foods Section*

Dannon:

Oikos Greek Frozen Yogurt: *Four Pack*

	C	F	Cb
Key Lime, 5.3 oz	150	4.5	16
Lemon Meringue, 5.3 oz	150	4.5	15
Average other flavors	150	5	15

YoCream Frozen Yogurt (Yogurt Shops): *Small 3 oz Cup*

	C	F	Cb
Premium, Peanut Butter	120	4	19
Custard, Vanilla	170	9	18
Low Fat: Chocolate Caramel Turtle	120	1.5	25
Dulce De Leche; Dutch Choc., av.	110	1.5	22
French Vanilla; Sweet Coconut, av.	110	1.5	21
Fudge Brownie Batter	110	0.5	24
No Sugar Added Nonfat:			
Cheesecake	80	0	18
Praline	90	0	18
Raspberry	80	0	17
Strawberry Banana	80	0	18

Note: Carbohydrate figure includes 0-5g sugar alcohol

Dippin' Dots:

Original Dots: *Per ½ Cup*

	C	F	Cb
Banana Split	160	8	20
Caramel Brownie Sundae	190	9	23
Cookies 'n Cream	200	11	22
Cotton Candy	160	8	18
Mint Chocolate	170	8	21
Strawberry	160	8	18
Vanilla	160	8	18

Dove:

Ice Cream: *Per ½ Cup*

	C	F	Cb
Mint/Vanilla Choc. Chunk	180	11	17
Unconditional Chocolate	200	12	23

Dreyer's/Edy's:

Classic Ice Cream: *Per ½ Cup*

	C	F	Cb
Chocolate; Vanilla, av.	140	7	16
Kit Kat	170	9	20
Mint Chocolate Chip	160	8	19
Mocha Almond Fudge	160	8	19
Rocky Road	160	8	20

Slow Churned, ½ The Fat: *Per ½ Cup*

	C	F	Cb
Butter Pecan	130	5	17
Chocolate	100	3.5	15
Coffee; Neapolitan	100	3	15
Neapolitan	120	4.5	17
Strawberry	100	3	16

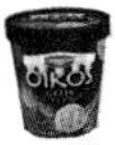

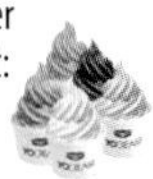

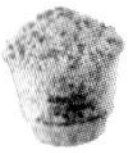

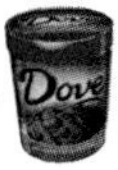

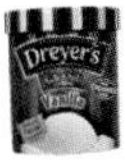

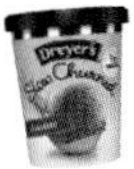

Friendly's: Ⓒ Ⓕ ⓒⓑ

Pure & Simple: *Per ½ Cup*

	C	F	Cb
Chocolate	160	10	15
Chocolate Fudge	160	9	18
Chocolate Peanut Butter	200	13	16

Rich & Creamy Ice Cream: *Per ½ Cup*

	C	F	Cb
Butter Crunch; Classic Chocolate, av.	150	7	18
Chocolate Almond Chip	160	9	17
Coffee	130	7	15
Strawberry; Vanilla, av.	140	7	16
Vienna Mocha Chunk	170	9	19

Light: *Per ½ Cup*

	C	F	Cb
Pistachio Almond	120	4.5	17
Vanilla	110	3.5	17

SundaeXtreme: *Per ½ Cup*

	C	F	Cb
Chocolate Fudge Brownie	150	5	25
Choc. Chip Cookie Dough	170	6	26
Chocolate P'nut Butter	190	9	22

Sherbet, Rasp Orange Lemon, ½ cup — 130 | 1.5 | 28

Yogurt Frozen,

Regular, average, ½ cup — 140 | 4.5 | 23

Gelati-da:

Gelato: *Per ½ Cup*

	C	F	Cb
Amaretto Chocolate	150	4.5	23
Choc Mint Milano	120	2.5	22
Coffee Fudge Latte	130	2	22
Limoncello; Vanilla Marsala, average	120	3	21
Red Raspberry	130	1.5	25

Great Value *(Walmart):*

Ice Cream: *Per ½ Cup*

	C	F	Cb
Chocolate Chip Cookie Dough	150	8	19
Coffee	130	7	15
Decadent Fudge Tracks	180	10	20
Homestyle Vanilla	140	7	17
Peanut Butter Cup	160	9	17

Sherbet, average all flavs — 110 | 0 | 26

Haagen-Dazs:

Tubs, Regular: *Per ½ Cup*

	C	F	Cb
Butter Pecan	300	22	20
Chocolate Peanut Butter	330	22	25
Dulce de Leche	270	16	28
White Chocolate Raspberry Truffle	280	16	31

Sorbet: *Per ½ Cup*

	C	F	Cb
Mango	150	0	38
Orchard Peach	140	0	34

Healthy Choice,

Greek Frozen Yogurt,

average all varieties, — 105 | 2 | 19

Bars ~*See Page 109*

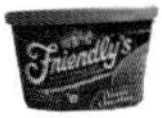

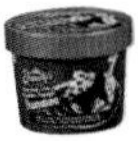

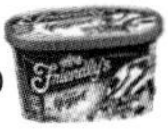

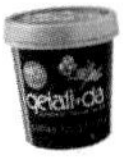

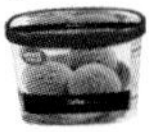

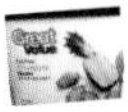

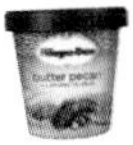

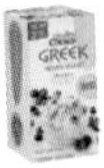

Ice Cream & Frozen Yogurt

Ice Cream ~ Brands (Cont)

	C	**F**	**Cb**
Hood:			
Classic: *Per ½ Cup*			
Chocolate	140	6	18
Classic Trio	140	7	17
Cookie Dough	170	8	21
Cookies 'N Cream	150	8	19
Creamy Coffee	140	7	16
Fudge Twister	140	6	20
Golden/Natural Vanilla; Patchwork	140	7	17
Maple Walnut	150	9	17
Churned, Light: *Per ½ Cup*			
Chocolate Chip	120	4.5	18
Coffee	100	3	16
Moosehead Lake Fudge	160	7	21
Under The Stars	160	8	18
Vanilla	110	3	16
Frozen Fat-Free Yogurt: *Per ½ Cup*			
Chocolate; Strawberry, av.	85	0	19
Mocha Fudge	100	0	22
Strawberry	80	0	19
New England Creamery ~ *www.CalorieKing.com*			
Jerseymaid *(Vons): Per ½ Cup*			
Ice Cream:			
Cookies & Cream	160	8	18
Choc Chip; Mint Choc Chip	150	9	16
Heavenly Hash	165	9	19
Mocha Almond Fudge; Chocolate	150	9	16
Neapolitan; Real Vanilla	140	8	15
Strawberry	130	6	17
Oberweis:			
Super Premium Ice Cream: *Per ½ Cup*			
Chocolate, 2.85 oz	480	31	43
Choc. Peanut Butter, 3 oz	280	19	21
Cookie Dough, 2.8	220	13	22
Espresso Caramel Chip, 3 oz	230	14	27
Mango Pomegranate, 2.9 oz	210	12	24
Vanilla, 2.75	210	14	18
Oikos *~ see Dannon*			
Pinkberry:			
Frozen Yogurt: *without Toppings*			
Original: Mini, 3.2 oz wt	90	0	19
Small, 4.9 oz wt	140	0	29
Medium, 8 oz wt	230	0	48
Large, 13 oz wt	370	0	78
Chocolate Hazelnut, 13 oz	560	15	96
Cookies & Cream, 13 oz	520	7.5	96
Mango, 13 oz	405	0	89

	C	**F**	**Cb**
Red Mango:			
Frozen Yogurt: *No Toppings included*			
Original: 3.3 oz wt	80	0	19
Small, 4.7 oz wt	120	0	27
Regular, 7.5 oz wt	190	0	43
Large, 11.4 oz wt	290	0	65
Blueberry: 3.3 oz wt	100	0	23
Small, 4.7 oz wt	150	0	33
Regular, 7.5 oz wt	230	0	53
Large, 11.4 oz wt	350	0	81
Dulce de Leche: 3.3 oz wt	80	0	18
Small, 4.7 oz wt	120	0	27
Regular, 7.5 oz wt	190	0	43
Large, 11.4 oz wt	290	0	65
Pomegranate: 3.3 oz wt	90	0	21
Small, 4.6 oz wt	130	0	30
Regular, 7.5 oz wt	210	0	48
Large, 11.4 oz wt	320	0	73
Rice Dream:			
Frozen Dessert: *Per ½ Cup*			
Cocoa Marble Fudge	170	6	31
Mint Carob Chip	180	7	28
Strawberry	170	6	30
Vanilla	160	6	26
Bars ~ *See Page 110*			
Skinny Cow:			
Bars/Sandwiches/Cones ~ *See Page 110*			
So Delicious: *Per ½ Cup*			
Almond Milk: Choc.; Mint Chip, av.	135	8	16
Mocha Almond Fudge	150	8	17
Vanilla	120	7	14
Cashew Milk: Cappuccino	150	7	21
Dark Choc. Truffle; Snickerdoodle, av.	185	9	24
Coconut Milk: Choc.; Coconut, av.	140	8	21
Choc. P'Nut Butter Swirl	200	14	22
Mocha Almond Fudge	160	8	23
No Sugar Added: Mint Chip	120	11	18
Vanilla Bean	100	8	18
Note: Carbohydrate Figure Includes 3g Sugar Alcohol			
Soy Milk: Chocolate Velvet	130	3.5	23
Cookie Dough	170	7	29
Creamy Van.; Neapolitan	120	3	24
Peanut Butter Zig Zag	210	11	28

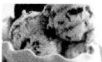 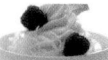
Ice Cream ~ Brands (Cont)

Soy Dream: 〇 〇 〇

Frozen Dessert: *Per ½ Cup*

	C	F	Cb
Butter Pecan	190	11	23
French Vanilla	170	9	21
Vanilla Fudge Swil	170	9	23

Stonyfield Farm:

Frozen Yogurt: *Per ½ Cup*

After Dark Chocolate	100	0	21
Creme Caramel	130	1.5	26
Gotta Have Vanilla	100	0	20

Stop & Shop:

Ice Cream: *Per ½ Cup*

Chocolate	150	8	18
Neapolitan; Vanilla, average	140	7.5	17
Vanilla Fudge Swirl	140	7	18
Light: Moose Tracks	130	5	18
Vanilla	100	3	17

Premium:

Cookies & Cream	170	9	21
Mint Chocolate Chip	160	9	18

Simply Enjoy:

Chocolate	210	12	22
Strawberry; Vanilla, average	225	13	25

Tasti D-Lite:

Soft Serve: *Per 3 oz Wt*

Banana	70	1	14
Blueberry Cheesecake	90	1.5	17
Brownie Batter Chocolate	90	2	16
Buttercrunch Mania	110	4	16
Coffee 'n Cream	80	1.5	16
Marshmallow Vanilla	90	1.5	17
Peanut Butter Fudge	90	3	15

Tofutti:

Premium Pints: *Per ½ Cup*

Better Pecan	250	15	27
Chocolate	210	13	20
Vanilla	210	13	21
Vanilla Almond Bark	240	15	24
Van. Fudge; Wild Berry Supreme, av.	190	9	25

TCBY ~ See Page 250

Turkey Hill: *Per ½ Cup*

All Natural:

Chocolate/Mint Chip	175	10	18
Salted Caramel	160	8	20

Turkey Hill (Cont): *Per ½ Cup* 〇 〇 〇

Light: Extreme Cookies 'n Cream

	C	F	Cb
Moose Tracks	140	6	20
Vanilla Bean	100	2	17

No Sugar Added:

Dutch Chocolate; Vanilla Bean, av.	70	0	20

Premium Ice Cream:

Black Cherry	130	6	18
Butter Pecan; Choco Mint Chip, av.	160	10	16
Chocolate Peanut Butter Cup	180	11	18
Cookies 'n Cream; Tin Roof Sundae	150	8	19
Rocky Road	170	8	23
Vanilla Bean	130	7	16

Stuff'd, average all flavors | 145 | 6 | 22 |

Frozen Yogurt: *Per ½ Cup*

Mint Cookies 'n Cream	110	1.5	22
Fat-Free: Chocolate Marshmallow	110	0	24
Other flavors	90	0	19

Sherbet, Fruit Rainbow | 120 | 1 | 26 |

Wawa:

Premium Ice Cream: *Per ½ Cup*

Butter Pecan; Mint Choc. Chip, av.	180	10	20
Chocolate; Vanilla Bean, average	160	8	20
Cookies & Cream	180	9	21
Strawberry Shortcake	160	7	22

Wegmans: *Per ½ Cup*

Regular: Chocolate | 130 | 7 | 15 |

French Van./ Vanilla, average	145	7	19

Light Extra Churned: Cookie Dough | 130 | 3 | 23 |

French Vanilla	120	3.5	19

Yoplait:

Go-Gurt!, average all flavors, 2.3 oz | 60 | 0.5 | 12 |

Frozen Yogurt: *Per ½ Cup*

Original Fruit flavors, average	115	2	21
Vanilla	110	2.5	19

Greek:

Fruit Flavors, average	130	2	21
Honey Caramel	140	2.5	22
Vanilla	100	2	18

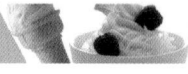
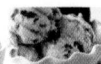

Ice Cream Bars & Pops ~ Brands

Per Bar/Serving Unless indicated   **C** **F** **Cb**

Ben & Jerry's:	C	F	Cb
Slices:			
Am. Dream; Choc Chip Cookie Dough, av.	285	18	30
Chocolate Fudge Brownie	250	16	27
Vanilla Peanut Butter Cup	300	22	24
Big Bear ~ See Klondike			
Blue Bunny:			
Single Bars: Big Alaska Bar, 3.3 oz	250	15	27
Chocolate Eclair, 2.8 oz	210	9	29
Cookies 'n Cream, 3 oz	240	11	33
Heath Bar, 3 oz	290	20	26
Hot Fudge Bar, 3.6 oz	360	24	33
Strawberry Shortcake, 2.8 oz	200	10	27
Turtle Bar, 3.5 oz	350	23	33
Tweety Bar, 2.8 oz	90	0	22
Snacks, Choc. Chip Cookie, 1.7 oz	150	8	19
Cones, 6 Pack:			
Caramel Lovers, 3.4 oz	310	16	38
Chocolate Lovers, 3.2 oz	270	12	36
Cookies 'n Cream, 3.2 oz	270	13	37
Big Dipper:			
Cookies 'n Cream, 3 oz	260	12	35
Chocolate Lovers, 3 oz	260	12	36
Big Swirls, Choc., Van., 3 oz	250	12	32
Ice Cream Sandwiches:			
Singles: Chips Galore, 3.4 oz	310	14	43
Cookies 'N Cream, 3 oz	240	10	37
8 Pack, Birthday Party, 2.6 oz	170	5	30
Big: Bopper, 5 oz	450	20	63
Double Strawberry, 3.9 oz	250	7	42
Mississippi Mud, 4 oz	280	8	47
Breyers:			
Carb Smart, 6 Pack:			
Fudge Bar, 1.7 oz	70	3	11
Vanilla Ice Cream Bar, 2 oz	150	11	13
Vanilla & Almond Ice Cream Bar, 2 oz	160	12	13

Note: Carbohydrate figure includes 4-5g sugar alcohol

Butterfinger *(Nestle)*,			
Loaded Ice Cream Bar	280	18	27

Per Bar/Serving Unless indicated   **C** **F** **Cb**

Cool Classics:	C	F	Cb
Arctic Blasters:			
Crispy Bar	160	11	15
Fudge Bar	100	1	21
Ice Cream Bar	150	10	13
Orange Cream	100	2.5	18
Strawberry Shortcake	150	8	20
Toffee Bar	160	11	14
Icepix: Grape; Cherry; Orange	35	0	8
Honeydew; Watermelon; Cantelope	35	0	9
Swirl Pops, Mango-Cherry	80	0	20
Creamsicles: *Per Bar*			
Box of 12, 100 Cal. Orange Crm Pops	100	1.5	19
Box of 18, Sugar-Free Cream Pops	30	0	6

Note: Sugar-Free carbohydrate figures include 5g Sucralose sweetener

Diana's Bananas:			
Banana Babies:			
Milk/Dark Chocolate (1)	130	6	18
Milk Choc. & Peanuts (1)	215	13	21
Banana Bites, (5), 2 oz	130	8	16
Dove:			
Single Bars: *Per 2.6 oz Bar*			
Milk Chocolate Vanilla:	250	16	24
And Almonds	250	17	21
Caramel Swirl & Cashews	250	16	23
Dark Chocolate Vanilla	250	17	24
Miniatures, Variety Pack,			
w/ Milk/Dark Choc., 5 pieces, av.	330	21	32
Sorbet Bars: Dark Chocolate Raspb.	150	8	19
Milk Chocolate Strawberry	150	7	20
Drumstick *(Nestlé)*:			
Classic Cones: Vanilla	290	15	34
Vanilla Caramel	300	15	38
Super Nugget: Van. Fudge	320	17	37
Strawberry	310	17	34
S'mores, Toasted Marshmallow	270	12	39
Strawberry, with Fudge	300	15	37
King Size: Triple Chocolate	350	14	51
Vanilla with Chocolate Layers	360	16	49
Lil' Drums: Choc. w/ Choc Swirls	130	6	16
Average other varieties	110	6	18
Simply Dipped: Mint	260	12	37
Vanilla	260	12	37

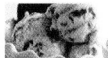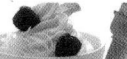

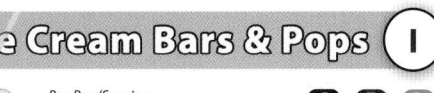

Ice Cream Bars/Pops ~ Brands (Cont)

Per Bar/Serving — **C** **F** **Cb**

Item	C	F	Cb
Edy's ~ *See Dreyer's*			
Eskimo Pie *(Nestle)*:			
Milk Chocolate, Vanilla	150	10	14
Dark Chocolate, No Sugar Added	150	10	13
Fat Boy:			
Sundae On A Stick:			
Nut Sundae	270	20	23
Toffee Crunch	280	20	26
Vanilla Dipped	260	19	22
Sandwiches: Chocolate, 3 oz	210	9	31
Cookies 'n Cream, 3 oz	220	8	34
Mint Chocolate Chip, 3 oz	220	9	33
Prem. Van.; Key Lime, 3 oz	210	8	31
Raspberry Cheesecake, 3 oz	210	7	35
Strawberry, 3 oz	210	7	35
Fresh & Easy, Vanilla Sundae Cone	260	15	29
Fudge Bar *(Nestle)*, Regular, 2.8 oz	110	2	21
Fudgesicle:			
100 Calorie: Fudge Bar	100	2	17
Low Fat Fudge Bar	60	1.5	12
No Sugar Added	80	1.5	19
Good Humor:			
Dessert Bars, Singles:			
Original Vanilla, 2.8 oz	240	14	27
Birthday Cake, 2.6 oz	200	10	25
Chocolate Eclair, 2.6 oz	190	9	27
Oreo 2.6 oz	210	11	26
Toasted Almond, 2.6 oz	200	11	24
Cones:			
Singles: Giant King Cone, Vanilla Chocolate, 5 oz	390	22	44
King Cone, Vanilla, 2.7 oz	230	14	25
4-Packs:			
Dessert Oreo Cone, 2.65 oz	200	9	29
King Cones, Vanilla, 3 oz	240	12	31
Sandwiches:			
Single, Giant, Neapolitan; Van., av.	220	5	40
4-Pack, Choc. Chip Cookie, 2.7 oz	250	10	40
Stickless: *4 or 6-Pack*			
Reese's PB Dessert Cup Bar: 2.4 oz	260	17	25
2.7 oz	280	19	22
Haagen-Dazs:			
Dark Chocolate Bar, Chocolate	280	20	22
Milk Chocolate Bars:			
Coffee & Almond Crunch	290	21	22
Vanilla & Almonds	290	21	21
Vanilla	270	19	22
Snack Size:			
Coffee & Almond Crunch	190	14	15
Vanilla & Almonds	195	15	13
Gelato, Vanilla Caramel Pizzelle	290	19	25

Per Bar/Serving — **C** **F** **Cb**

Item	C	F	Cb
Healthy Choice: Fudge Bar	80	0.5	15
Smoothie Bars:			
Mango Peach	70	0.5	14
Raspberry	80	0.5	15
Strawberry	70	0.5	13
Hershey's:			
Bars, Gluten Free: Banjo	170	11	17
Fudjo	120	0	24
Orange Blossom	80	2.5	13
Cones: Incredible	290	14	38
Moose Tracks	480	28	52
P-Nutty	260	15	30
Low fat, Cookies & Cream; Crazy, av.	120	1.5	25
Pops, all flavors	35	0	10
Sandwiches:			
99 Cent Vanilla Ice Cream	210	9	30
Giant:			
Andes Creme de Menthe	350	16	48
Neopolitan	320	14	43
Vanilla, 6 oz	300	12	43
Signature Bars: Chocolate Eclair	220	10	30
Cotton Candy	280	15	32
Strawb. Shortcake	240	11	32
Hood:			
Bars: Ice Cream Bar	130	7	14
Orange Cream	90	1.5	18
Hoodsie:			
Cups, Chocolate; Vanilla, 3 oz	100	5	12
Sundae Cups, 3 oz	120	5	19
Sandwich, av., 2.2 oz	175	6	29
Klondike:			
Bars:			
Single, Orig. Vanilla, 5.5 oz	300	17	34
4-Pack: Krunch, 3 oz	250	14	29
Mint Choc. Chip, 2.8 oz	230	14	26
Oreo Cookies & Cream, 2.6 oz	250	15	27
8-Count Snack Size: Orig., 1.4 oz	120	7	13
English Toffee, 1.3 oz	115	7	12
Choco Taco, Original, 4 oz	250	12	34
Kandy: Caramel & Peanuts, 3.5 oz	250	14	28
6 Pack: Cookies & Cream, 2.15 oz	200	10	24
Mint Fudge, 2.15 oz	190	11	23
Triple Chocolate, 2 oz	180	10	22
Sandwiches:			
Single: Mrs Fields, 3.9 oz	340	2	55
Oreo, 4.5 oz	220	7	37
4-Pack: Mrs Fields, 2.3 oz	210	8	34
Oreo, 2.4 oz	210	7	35
6-Pack, Vanilla, 2.7 oz	180	5	31

Ice Cream Bars & Pops — I

Updated Nutrition Data ~ www.CalorieKing.com
Persons with Diabetes ~ See Disclaimer (Page 22)

109

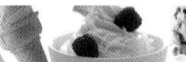

Ice Cream Bars/Pops ~ Brands (Cont)

Per Bar/Serving	C	F	Cb
Luigi's:			
Real Italian Ice:			
Cherry; Mango	100	0	26
Chocolate Fudge	150	0	36
Watermelon; Blue Raspberry	160	0	39
M&M's:			
Cone, Single, 2.6 oz	240	11	32
Cookie Ice Cream Sandwich, 2.9 oz	250	13	34
Magnum:			
Singles: Almond	270	18	25
Double Caramel	270	17	29
Minis, Classic	150	10	14
Multipacks: Dark Chocolate	240	16	23
Infinity Chocolate	270	18	25
White	240	15	24
Double: Choc. Hazelnut	280	19	26
Double Raspberry	260	16	28
Minute Maid, Juice Bars, 2.25 fl.oz	40	0	10
Nestlé:			
Bars: Crunch Bar	180	11	19
Orange & Cream	90	1.5	18
Strawberry Shortcake	210	9	31
Cones, Magical Minis	110	3.5	19
Dibs, Crunch, 4 oz container	340	24	30
Drumsticks ~ See Page 109			
Ice Pop, Wildberry & Zesty Lemon	90	0	22
Outshine Fruit Bars:			
Creamy Coconut	120	3	20
Peach	90	0	23
Other Fruit Flavors, av.	70	0	16
Sandwich, Vanilla	160	3.5	29
Toll House,			
Choc. Chip Cookie Sandwich	380	15	57
Popsicle:			
Firecracker, all flavors (1)	35	0	9
Hello Kitty; Scribbles (2)	60	0	14
Marvel Avengers Assemble (1)	40	0	10
SpongeBob Pop-Ups (1)	80	1	11
Slow Melts, Mighty Minis, 5 pieces	60	0	11
Reese's (Good Humor),			
P'nut Butter Ice Cream Cup, 2.4 oz	260	17	25
Skinny Cow: Per Item			
Bars: Fudge	110	1	22
Chocolate Truffle	100	2.5	19
Vanilla Almond Crunch	190	11	19
Candy Bars, av. all flavors	155	9	17
Cones, average all flavors	155	3	28
Sandwiches, all flavors	180	9	22
Snickers:			
Bars: Regular, 1.8 oz	180	11	18
Mini Bar, 1 piece, 0.9 oz	90	6	9
Cone, 2.9 oz	250	13	29
Ice Cream Brownie, 3.3 oz	300	13	41

Per Bar/Serving	C	F	Cb
Snow Cone (Wonder), av. all, 7 fl.oz	60	0	15
So Delicious (Turtle Mountain):			
Almond Based Minis:			
Bars, Mocha ALm. Fudge (1), 1.8 oz	150	10	14
Sandwich, Vanilla, 1.3 oz	90	3.5	13
Coconut Based Minis:			
Bars: Almond, 1.8 oz	180	13	17
Simply Strawberry, 2 oz	80	3.5	14
Soy Based Minis:			
Sandwiches, av. all varieties, 1.4 oz	90	2	18
Soy Dream: Almond Bar (1), 3 oz	140	16	24
Bites, Choc/Vanilla/Coconut, 15 pcs	140	16	22
Lil' Dreamers, Vanilla	100	4	15
Tampico, Freezer Pops, all var., 1.4 oz	30	0	7
Tofutti: Per Item			
Bars:			
Chocolate Fudge/Coffee Break Treats	30	0	6
Hooray Hooray Bar	120	8	8
Marry Me Bar	170	8	22
Totally Fudge Pops	95	1.5	19
Note: Carb figures include 0-7g sugar alcohols			
Cones, all flavors	220	13	24
Cuties, average all flavors	130	6	18
Turkey Hill:			
Bar, Vanilla Ice Cream, 3.3 oz	320	23	26
Sandwiches: Double Decker, 2.5 oz	190	7	30
Vanilla Bean, 2.5 oz	190	7	29
Sundae Cone, Van. Fudge	320	18	33
Twix, Ice Cream Bar, 3.3 oz	350	20	38
Wegmans:			
Bars: Fudge, low fat	100	1	20
Peanut Butter Sundae Crunch	200	11	22
Vanilla, Choc Coated, 2 oz	160	11	14
Sandwiches: Vanilla	160	5	26
Light Vanilla	150	3	29
Weight Watchers: Per Item			
Bars:			
Dulce de Leche, 1.83 oz	120	4.5	19
English Toffee Crunch (2), 2.4 oz	200	6	13
Giant, Chocolate Fudge Bar, 2.6 oz	90	1	21
Cones, Double Caramel Swirl, 1.45 oz	90	2	17
Sandwiches: Cherry Chseecake, snack	90	1	19
Round: Giant Vanilla	140	2	31
Mint	140	1.5	31
Yoplait ~ See Frozen Yogurt			
Yosicle, Swirlz, average all flavors, (1)	45	1	7

Canned & Packaged Meals ~ Brands

Amy's: *Per Serve*
Frozen:
Asian Meals:

	C	F	Cb
Stir-Fry Asian Noodle, 10 oz	300	7	50
Sweet & Sour Asian Noodle, 8 oz	250	3	46
Bowls: Asian Dumplings, 8.5 oz	400	13	5
Baked Ziti, 9.5 oz	370	13	53
Broccoli & Cheddar Bake, 9.5 oz	420	20	44
Paella, 8.5 oz	280	12	35
Pesto Penne w/ Brocc. & Tom., 9 oz	380	15	47
Pesto Tortellini, 9.5 oz	450	20	50
Burritos: Black Bean & Quinoa	220	5	36
Cheddar Cheese, Bean & Rice	260	8	37
Entrees: Cheese Enchilada, 4.5 oz	240	14	18
Cheese Lasagna, 10.3 oz	410	16	46
Macaroni & Cheese, 9 oz	400	16	47
Roasted Vegetable Tamale, 10.3 oz	280	7	45
Light & Lean: Bean & Cheese Burrito	280	5	49
Mattar Paneer	260	6	42
Spinach Lasagne	250	5	40
Pot Pies: Broccoli, 7.5 oz	460	24	50
Vegetable, 7.5 oz	430	20	54
Snacks: Cheese Pizza, 5-6 pieces	190	8	26
Cheese & Bean Nachos, 5-6 pcs	230	9	29
Swirls: Artichoke & Parmesan (2)	200	11	20
Cheddar Jalepeno (2)	210	9	25
Mushroom & Cheese; Pesto (2)	190	9	19
Veggie Burger Patties:			
All American	130	4	13
Black Bean	120	4	17
California	150	4.5	21
Wraps:			
Indian Samosa, 5 oz	250	9	35
Teriyaki, gluten free, 5.5 oz	250	6	38
Tofu Scramble B'fast, gluten free, 5.5 oz	300	13	35

Armour-Star:

	C	F	Cb
Beef Stew, 1 cup, 9 oz	230	11	21
Chili, with Beans, ½ of 15 oz can	280	11	26
Chili, No Beans, ½ of 14 oz can	330	23	15

Atkins: *Per 9 oz Tray/Bowl*
Frozen:

	C	F	Cb
Beef Merlot	300	21	9
Chicken & Broccoli Alfredo	290	18	9
Chili Con Carne	330	23	10
Crustless Chicken Pot Pie	300	19	8
Italian Style Pasta Bake	320	18	16
Meatloaf w/ Portobello Mshrm Gravy	330	21	11
Shrimp Scampi	290	19	19
Swedish Meatballs	390	22	24

Bagel Bites:

	C	F	Cb
Frozen:			
Cheese, Sausage & Pepperoni, 4 pcs	200	6	28
Supreme; Three Cheese, av., 4 pcs, 3 oz	195	5	31

B&M:
Baked Beans: *Per 16 oz Can, ½ cup, 4.6 oz*

	C	F	Cb
Original	170	2	31
Boston's Best	170	1.5	32
Maple Flavor	150	1	28
Vegetarian	160	1	25
Brown Bread, Raisin, ½ slice, 2 oz	130	0.5	29

Banquet:
Homestyle Bakes: *1 Cup, Prepared*

	C	F	Cb
Creamy Cheese Chicken Alfredo	330	15	37
Creamy Chicken & Biscuits	420	18	53
Frozen:			
Backyard BBQ & Mashed Potato, 8 oz	290	11	35
Chicken: Fingers, 6.5 oz	310	12	33
Fettuccine Chicken Alfredo, 8 oz	310	12	38
Fried Chicken, 10 oz	330	14	40
Parmesan, 8.5 oz	320	11	41
Strip Meal, 8.9 oz	440	19	45
Homestyle Patty, 10 oz	340	17	32
Lasagna, with Meat Sauce	250	9	31
Mac & Cheese, 8 oz	240	9	32
Meatloaf, 11.9 oz	330	11	43
Pepper Steak, 10 oz	320	13	39
Rigatoni & Italian Sausage, 8 oz	300	12	35
Salisbury Steak w/ Mshd Pot., 9.5 oz	350	14	44
Spaghetti & Chicken Nuggets, 7 oz	230	7	32
Spaghetti & Meatballs, 10 oz	320	14	34
Swedish Meaballs, 10.45 oz	370	17	39
Sweet & Sour Chicken, 8 oz	420	10	70
Turkey, 10 oz	280	11	29
Family:			
Gravy & Meat Loaf, 4 oz	120	6	9
Gravy, Salisbury Steak, Potatoes & Vegetables, 8 oz	180	8	21
Zesty Marinara Sce & M'balls, 5 oz	170	10	11

Breakfast Pies: *Per 7 oz*

	C	F	Cb
Deep Dish Cheesy Ham & Potato, 7 oz	440	25	46
Sausage & Gravy, 7 oz	450	33	44
Pot Pie: Chicken; Turkey, average	335	19	32
Chicken & Broccoli	330	18	31
Salisbury Steak Deep Dish, 7 oz	400	23	40

Barilla:

Microwaveables: *Per 9 oz Container*

	C	F	Cb
Marinara/Tomato & Basil Penne, av.	305	4	62
Sausage & Tomato Rotini	330	5	63

Betty Crocker:

Bowl Appetit:

	C	F	Cb
Herb Chkn Flav. Veggie Rice	250	3	51
Pasta Alfredo	350	9	55

Hamburger Helper: *Per 1 Cup, Prepared*

	C	F	Cb
Bacon Cheeseburger Macaroni	310	13	27
Beef Pasta	250	10	21
Ital. Four Cheese Lasagna	300	12	24
Philly Cheesesteak	310	13	25
Potato Stroganoff	280	12	27
Salisbury	270	10	24
Strogaoff	310	12	30
Three Cheese	340	14	30
Tomato Basil Penne	300	11	32

Potatoes: *Per Serving, Prepared*

	C	F	Cb
Casserole: Au Gratin, ½ cup	150	6	24
Cheddar & Bacon, ½ c.	150	6	24
Roasted Garlic, ½ cup	130	4	21
Scalloped, ⅔ cup	130	3	24
Sour Cream and Chives, ⅔ cup	130	3	24

Mashed Potatoes:

	C	F	Cb
Hearty Four Cheese, ⅔ cup	150	6.5	17
Homestyle Butter & Herb, ⅔ cup	150	7	17
Savory Roasted Garlic, ⅔ cup	160	9	18
Sweet Potato, ½ cup	200	9	27

Tuna Helper: *Per 1 Cup, Prepared*

	C	F	Cb
Cheesy Pasta	270	12	27
Average other varieties	265	10	30

Ultimate Chicken Helper: *1 Cup Prepared*

	C	F	Cb
Cheddar Broccoli	310	12	27
Creamy Parmesan Alfedo	340	13	30
Orange Chicken	310	9	36

Biggest Loser:

Refrigerated:

Simply Sensible: *Per ½ Package*

	C	F	Cb
Beef Pot Roast & Gravy	220	5	16
Beef ips & Gravy	200	3.5	21
Lasagna	200	5	28
Mediterranean-Style Chicken	250	6	36
Zing Chicken	230	1.5	38

Birds Eye:

Frozen:

Voila!: *Per 1 Cup Prepared Unless Indicated*

	C	F	Cb
Alfredo Chicken, 7.5 oz	240	7	27
Cheddar Chicken Potato, 8.6 oz	250	7	35
Chicken Florentine, 7.65 oz	220	5	28
Chkn & Pasta in Parmesan Sce, 9 oz	370	12	51
Fajita Chicken, 7.45 oz	170	2	26
Selects: Garlic Shrimp, 6.7 oz	230	7	31
Mongolian Style Beef, 7.7 oz	240	4.5	38
Sweet & Sour Chicken, 7.9 oz	230	1.5	42

Boca:

Frozen:

Burger:

	C	F	Cb
All American Flame Grilled, 2.5 oz	120	5	6
Cheeseburger, 2.5 oz	100	4.5	6
Grilled Vegetables, 2.5 oz	80	1	7
Original Vegan, 2.5 oz	70	0.5	6
Chik'n: Orig. Nuggets, 3 oz	180	7	17
Patties (1), 2.5 oz	160	6	15
Spicy Patties (1), 2.5 oz	160	6	15

Boston Market:

Frozen Dinners:

	C	F	Cb
Beef Steak & Pasta, 14 oz	470	14	52
Chicken Parmesan, 13 oz	500	13	70
Oven Roasted Chicken, 13 oz	280	7	31
Salisbury Steak, 14.5 oz	540	31	41
Swedish M'balls, 13 oz	660	30	67

Buitoni:

Refrigerated:

	C	F	Cb
Ravioli: Four Cheese, 3.7 oz	330	12	42
Spinach & Artichoke, 3.7 oz	290	8	42
Tortellini: Mixed Cheese, 3.7 oz	320	8	47
Tortelloni, Chkn & Proscuitto, 3.8 oz	330	9	46

Other Pasta Dishes ~ *See Page 133*

Bush's Best: *Per ½ Cup, 4.6 oz*

	C	F	Cb
Baked Beans: Original	140	1	29
Vegetarian	130	0	29
Average other varieties	150	1	32
Black Beans	100	0	18
Black Eyed Peas	80	0	15
Dark Red Kidney Beans	120	0	22
Garbanzo Beans	120	2	20
Grillin' Beans:			
Bourbon & Brown Sugar	170	0.5	35
Smokehouse Tradition	160	1	33
Southern Pit	170	0.5	35
Steakhouse	180	0.5	39
Pinto Beans, with Bacon	100	1	17
Refried Beans: Traditional	150	3	24
Fat Free	130	0	24

Campbell's:	C	F	Cb
Pork & Beans, 11 oz can,			
½ cup, 4.6 oz serving	130	0.5	27
Chunky Microwaveable Bowls:			
Firehouse; Roadhouse,			
Chunky Beef & Beans Chili, 1 cup	250	8	30
Spaghetti O's: *Per 1 Cup*			
Original, 8.9 oz	170	1	33
With Meatballs, 8.9 oz	230	7	31
With Sliced Franks, 8.9 oz	210	6	29
Chef Boyardee:			
Canned: *Per Cup*			
Beefaroni, 8.8 oz	240	9	30
Lasagna, 8.8 oz	230	8	31
Ravioli: *Per 1 Cup*			
Beef: Regular, 8.7 oz	220	7	33
Overstuffed, 9.2 oz	230	5	37
Cheese, 9 oz	210	2	40
Ital. Sausage, overstuffed, 9.2 oz	240	6	38
With Meaballs, 9 oz	290	12	33
Microwaveable: *Per 7.5 oz Cup*			
Beefaroni	220	8	28
Ravioli: Beef	200	7	28
Cheese	190	5	28
Mini Micro Beef	160	4	25
With Meatballs	250	10	32
Boxed Pizza Maker Kits: *Single Kits*			
Cheese, ¼ package, 4 oz	260	4.5	47
Pepperoni, ¼ package, 4 oz	280	8	42
Pizza Sauce, w/ Chse, ¼ c., 2 oz	35	1.5	4
Dennison's Chili: *Per Cup*			
Chili Con Carne:			
Original: with Beans	330	13	33
without Beans	260	14	17
Chunky, w/ Beans	330	13	33
Hot, with Beans	340	14	34
Vegetarian, 99% fat free	280	1.5	52
Devour ~ *See Heinz Page 114*			
Dinty Moore *(Hormel):*			
Big Bowl (Microwave): *Approx. ½ of 15 oz Bowl*			
Beef Stew, 8.3 oz	200	10	17
Chicken & Dumplings, 8.5 oz	210	6	29
Scalloped Potatoes & Ham, 8.7 oz	310	18	26
Dr. McDougall's: *Per 2 oz Package*			
Asian Noodles, Pad Thai	200	1.5	42
Pistachio Citrus Quinoa Salad	290	5	49
Sweet Potato Kale Salad	260	3.5	48

Eden Organics: *Per ½ Cup*	C	F	Cb
Brown Rice & Pinto Beans, 4.6 oz	120	1	24
Chili Black Beans & Quinoa, 4.4 oz	100	1	18
Curried Rice & Lentils, 4.6 oz	130	1	21
Mexican Rice & Black Beans, 4.6 oz	110	1	22
Farmhouse: *Per 1 Cup Prepared*			
Pasta: Fettuccine Alfredo	460	22	51
Wild Cheddar	380	14	51
Rice: Long Gr., & Wild Herbs & Butter	250	7	44
Mexican	230	5	42
Roasted Chicken Flavor	230	5	44
French's:			
French Crispy Fried Onions:			
Original; White Cheddar:			
2 Tbsp, 0.25 oz	45	3.5	3
¼ cup, 0.5 oz	90	7	6
1 cup, 2 oz	360	28	24
GardenBurger:			
Veggie Burger: *Per Burger*			
Original	110	3	16
Black Bean Chipotle	90	3	16
Portabella	100	2.5	16
Garden Lites:			
Entrees: *Per 7 oz Serving*			
Butternut Squash Souffle	180	2	33
Cheddar Broccoli Bake	210	6	29
Kale & Quinoa Souffle	200	6	23
Roasted Vegetable Souffle	170	3	28
Veggie Bites:			
Broccoli & Brown Rice (4)	130	5	16
Cornbread (4)	170	2.5	31
Italian (4)	130	5	16
Kale & Brown Rice (4)	130	5	17
Veggie Cakes: Kale & Quinoa (1)	90	5	10
Superblend (1)	100	6	10
Gorton's:			
Frozen:			
Battered Pollock Fillets,			
Crispy (2), 3.8 oz	230	13	24
Bites: Beer Batted Cod, 3 oz	220	14	16
Mac & Cheese Shrimp, 4 oz	260	11	32
Potato Crusted Cod, 3 oz	180	8	17
Breaded Pollock Fillets:			
Crunchy/Lemon Herb (2), av., 3.8 oz	230	11	24
Gourmet Cod: Parm. Crusted, 5.2 oz	330	17	31
Pub Style, Beer Battered, 5.2 oz	380	24	29
Grilled Fillets: *Per Fillet*			
Garlic/Lemon Butter Pollock, 3.5 oz	85	3	0
Signature Tilapia, 3.2 oz	80	2	2

continued nex page...

Gorton's (Cont):	C	F	Cb
Frozen:			
Shrimp:			
Cr. Butterfly Breadcrumbs, 3.5 oz	250	12	25
Popcorn (22), 3.5 oz	370	15	23
Simply Bake:			
Hadddock Garlic Herb Butter, 4.9 oz	130	2.5	7
Salmon, Rsted Garlic Butter, 4.4 oz	140	2.5	8
Tilapia, Signature Seasoning, 5.2 oz	130	3	6
Skillet Crisp, Lightly Battered,			
Tilapia, Garlic & Herb, 3.35 oz	180	8	15
Great Value *(Walmart):*			
Frozen:			
Breakfast Bowls: Bacon, 7 oz	430	27	19
Sausage, 7 oz	390	25	22
Sausage & Gravy, 7 oz	360	24	21
Steak & Egg, 7 oz	340	20	23
Meals: *Per 10 oz Pkg*			
Lean Chicken Parmesan & Spag.	320	7	45
Meatloaf & Mashed Potatoes	380	21	34
Rstd Turkey Breast w/ Mshd Potatoes	230	6	25
Salisbury Steak with Potatoes	330	18	25
Skillet Meal, Chsebgr Pasta, prep, 1 cup	320	12	27
Healthy Choice:			
Frozen:			
Cafe Steamers:			
Beef Teriyaki, 9.5 oz	280	5	42
Chicken & Noodles, 10 oz	260	7	31
Crustless Chicken Pot Pie, 9.6 oz	300	6	40
Four Chse Ravioli & Chkn Marinara, 10 oz	270	6	34
General Tso's Spicy Chicken, 10.3 oz	290	3.5	47
Portabella Spinach Parmesan, 9.8 oz	230	5	38
Spaghetti & Meatballs, 9.5 oz	280	7	35
Sweet & Sour Chicken, 10 oz	390	8	65
Sweet Sesame Chicken, 9.7 oz	300	6	43
Classics: Chicken Parmig., 11.6 oz	360	12	47
Lemon Pepper Fish, 10.7 oz	290	4	50
Simply Steamers: *Per Package*			
Beef & Broccoli, 10 oz	280	7	32
Chicken & Vegetable Stir Fry, 9.2 oz	190	4	15
Gr. Chicken & Broccoli Alfredo, 9.1 oz	190	5	8
Gr. Chicken Pesto & Veggies, 9.1 oz	200	5	11
Honey Balsamic Chicken, 9.87 oz	210	2.5	28
Meatball Marinara, 10 oz	280	6	36
Extra Product Listings ~ *www·CalorieKing·com*			

Heinz:	C	F	Cb
Beans, Original BBQ, ½ cup, 4.6 oz	190	0.5	39
Devour Frozen Meals: *Per Package*			
Bacon Topped Turkey w/ Garlic Sce	410	19	28
Buffalo Chicken Mac & Cheese	460	30	24
Cajun Syle Alfredo w/ Ssg & Chkn	410	19	34
Cheese Ravioli w/sundried Tom. Sce	490	19	59
Chicken Enchiladas Suiza	460	18	55
Italian Sausage Lasagna	470	23	41
Lasagna Alfredo w/Bacon & Ssg	570	37	33
Loaded Potato w/ Beef & Bacon	330	14	31
Pesto Ravioli w/Spicy Italian Ssg	670	37	55
Pulled Chicken Burrito Bowl	450	15	46
White Chedd. Mac & Cheese w/Bacon	710	41	54
Hormel:			
Chili with Beans: *Per Cup*			
Regular; Hot; Chunky, av. 8.7 oz	260	7	32
Turkey, 98% Fat-Free,8.7 oz	220	3	29
Vegetarian, 99% Fat Free, 8.7 oz	200	1.5	35
Chili No Beans: *Per Cup*			
Regular, 8.3 oz	260	14	19
Hot; Chunky, average, 8.3 oz	255	13	19
Turkey, 98% Fat-Free, 8.3 oz	190	3	16
Compleats, Comfort Classics:			
Beefy Mac & Cheese, 7.5 oz	230	4	37
Chicken & Noodles, 7.5 oz	180	6	20
Dumplings & Chicken, 7.5 oz	190	3.5	32
Noodles & Beef, 7.5 oz	170	2	28
Spaghetti & Meat Sauce, 7.5 oz	220	6	31
Compleats, Homesyle:			
Beef Pot Roast, 9 oz	200	6	20
Chicken Alfredo, 10 oz	350	18	30
Chkn Brst, Gravy & Msh'd Pot., 10 oz	220	4	28
Meatloaf, Gravy & Mashed Pot., 9 oz	300	14	28
Salisbury Steak, 9 oz	300	16	27
Swedish Mtballs, 9 oz	280	12	28
Refrigerated Meals: *Per Package*			
H'style Meat Loaf & Tom. Sce, 5 oz	220	9	14
Sliced Rst Turkey Brst & Gravy, 5 oz	110	2.5	3
Slow Simm. Beef Tips w/ Gravy, 4.3 oz	170	10	4
Side Dishes:			
Garlic Mashed Potatoes, 5 oz	170	10	17
HomeStyle Mashed Potatoes, 5 oz	170	10	18
Loaded Mashed Potatoes, 5 oz	200	12	18
Mashed Sweet Potatoes, 5 oz	170	6	27

Hot Pockets: **C** **F** **Cb**
Sandwiches: *Per Sandwich*

Crispy Buttery Crust:

	C	F	Cb
Cheddar Cheeseburger	290	10	41
Hickory Ham & Cheese	270	9	39
Steak & Cheddar	310	13	34

Crispy Crust:

	C	F	Cb
Five Cheese Pizza	340	16	38
Pepperoni Pizza	330	17	34

Croissant Crust:

	C	F	Cb
Applewood Bacon, Egg & Chse	320	14	37
Hickory Ham & Cheddar	300	13	37
Philly Steak & Cheese	310	14	37
Sausage, Egg & Cheese	320	15	35

Flaky Crust, Chicken Pot Pie | 230 | 8 | 31

Garlic Buttery Seasoned Crust

	C	F	Cb
Four Cheese Pizza	320	13	40
Four Meat & Four Chse	310	14	33
Meatballs & Mozzarella	310	13	38
Pepperoni & Sausage Pizza	320	14	38

Seasoned Crust: Beef Taco | 300 | 13 | 36
Philly Steak & Cheese | 300 | 11 | 40

Stuffed Pretzels:

	C	F	Cb
Cheesy Jalapeno	130	4	19
Chorizo Queso Fundido	140	5	19

Hungry Jack:
Casserole Potatoes: *Prepared*

	C	F	Cb
Cheddar & Bacon	160	7	20
Creamy Scalloped	170	7	24

Hashbrowns:

	C	F	Cb
Original, 1/3 cup prepared	100	4.5	14
Cheesy, 1/2 cup prepared	140	7	17

Mashed Potatoes, average,
Dry Mix only, 1/3 cup unprepared | 80 | 0 | 19

Hungry Man:
Dinners:

	C	F	Cb
Beer Battered Chicken	760	38	75
Boneless Fried Chicken	800	39	81
Country Fried Chicken	520	29	51
Home-Style Meatloaf	650	32	64
Mesquite Classic Fried Chicken	1050	72	60
Mexican Style Fiesta	570	18	90
Roasted Carved White Meat Turkey	420	11	60
Spicy Boneless Fried Chkn Patties	810	38	86
Salisbury Steak	590	33	52

Hungry Man (Cont): **C** **F** **Cb**
Selects: *Per Package*

	C	F	Cb
Boneless Fried Chicken & Waffles	800	28	110
Classic Fried Chicken	970	59	62

XXL Sandwiches: *Per Package*

	C	F	Cb
Angus Beef Charbroil	700	41	55
BBQ Pork Ribs	750	45	60
Buffalo Fried Chicken	660	27	70
Country Fried Pork	660	33	70

José Olé:
Breakfast Burritos:

	C	F	Cb
Egg & Bacon, 4 oz	260	10	30
Egg & Sausage, 4 oz	240	10	28

Burritos:

	C	F	Cb
Chicken Monterey (1)	270	7	39
Steak & Cheese (1)	310	11	40

Chimichangas:

	C	F	Cb
Chicken & Cheese (1), 5 oz	330	13	42
Steak & Cheese (1), 5 oz	310	11	40

Snacks:

	C	F	Cb
Mini: Chimichangas,			
Steak & Cheddar (3)	370	20	36
Nacho Bites, Chicken & Chse (3)	220	11	22
Quesadillas,			
Chicken & Cheese (3)	210	8	25
Tacos: Beef & Cheese (4)	220	11	23
Queso Chicken (5)	220	10	24

Taquitos: Chicken, Corn Tortillas, (3) | 200 | 8 | 26
Beef & Cheese, Flour Tortillas, (2) | 260 | 14 | 26

Kashi:
Entrees: *Per 10 oz Package*

	C	F	Cb
Amaranth Polenta Plantain	330	8	56
Black Bean Mango	310	8	55
Chimichurri Quinoa	240	7	41
Sweet Potato Quinoa	270	6	48

Kid Cuisine: *Per Meal*

	C	F	Cb
All Star Chicken Breast Nuggets	440	19	55
Beef Patty with Cheese & Bun	310	8	55
Cheese Pizza	450	14	62
Fish Sticks	340	11	46
Fun Shaped Chicken Breast Nuggets	430	19	51
Mac. & Cheese	440	11	70
Mini Corn Dogs	490	15	75
Pepperoni Pizza, Red. Fat	370	10	57
Popcorn Chicken	420	13	62
Spaghetti with Mini Meatballs	330	7	51

Knorr: *Sides, Dry Mix Only*	C	F	Cb
Cajun: Dirty Rice, 2.3 oz	230	2	48
Red Beans & Rice, 2.3 oz	230	2	47
Fiesta: Mexican Rice, 2.3 oz	230	1	48
Taco Rice, 2.2 oz	220	1	46
Italian, Creamy Pesto Pasta, 2.2 oz	220	2	44
Pasta:			
Alfredo; Parmesan, av.	245	4	42
Alfredo Broccoli, 2.2 oz	240	3.5	43
Butter & Herb, 2.2 oz	230	1.5	46
Cheesy Bacon Macaroni, 2 oz	220	1.5	43
Chicken Flavor, 2.2 oz	230	2	44
Rice: Beef Rice, 2.3 oz	230	1	49
Chedd. Brocc./Chkn Rice, av., 2.3 oz	240	2	49
Creamy Chkn Rice, 2.3 oz	240	1.5	49
Garlic Parm. Rice, 2.4 oz	250	2	50
Herb & Butter Rice, 2.3 oz	230	1	49
Mushroom Rice; Rice Pilaf, 2.3 oz	230	1	47
Kraft:			
Macaroni & Cheese:			
Original (7.25 oz Box):			
⅓ box, 2.5 oz (makes 1 cup)			
As Packaged	250	3	47
As Prepared, 1 cup	350	16	57
Deluxe: Original / 4 Cheese / Brocolli / Bacon, avg.			
¼ box, 3.5 oz (makes 1 cup)			
As Packaged	310	10	42
Microwave Bowls:			
Average all flavors, 1 bowl, 2 oz	220	4	41
Velveeta: *Per Container*			
Cheesy Bowls:			
Chicken Afredo	330	12	36
Chicken Chili Cheese Mac	310	10	33
Lasagna, with Meat Sauce	350	17	36
Ultimate Cheeseburger Mac	380	17	39
Cheesy Potatoes:			
Au Gratin, 2 oz dry	180	7	24
Bacon Scalloped, 2.1 oz dry	190	7	24
Southwest Diced, 1.9 oz dry	170	7	24
Shells & Cheese Microcups:			
Original; Queso Blanco, 2.4 oz dry	220	8	30
2% Milk, 2.4 oz dry	180	3	30

Kroger:	C	F	Cb
Kitchen Creation Skillet Dinners: *Per Cup, Prepared*			
Creamy Broccoli; Creamy Pasta	300	12	33
Double Cheeseburger	320	13	30
Lasagna	280	12	26
Frozen:			
Healthy Meals Made Simple: *Refrigerated, Per Cup*			
Braised Beef Pot Roast & Gravy	220	5	15
Lean Beef Tips & Gravy	210	4	20
Lem. Herb Chkn w/ Rice	170	1.5	23
Sweet & Spicy Chicken	270	1.5	48
Meals Made Simple:			
Beef Stir Fry, 1¾ cups	180	4	26
Chicken Florentine, 2¼ cups, 6.9 oz	320	18	22
Chicken Stir Fry, 1½ cups	180	2	25
Shrimp Fried Rice, 1¼ cups, 8 oz	240	0	44
Oven Ready:			
Breaded Calamari Rings (10), 3 oz	200	10	21
Coconut Shrimp (5),			
with 1 oz sweet Chili Sauce	350	20	34
La Choy:			
Family Meals, Canned: *Per 1 Cup*			
Beef Pepper Oriental, 8.9 oz	80	1	11
Beef Chow Mein, 8.7 oz	80	1	11
Chicken Chow Mein, 8.8 oz	100	3	10
Sweet & Sour Chicken, 8.9 oz	120	1	22
Lean Cuisine:			
Comfort: *Per Complete Meal*			
Baked Chicken	260	8	30
Cheddar Bacon Chicken	220	8	17
Chicken Carbonara	330	9	39
Chkn in Sweet BBQ Sce	290	9	30
Chicken Marsala	220	6	24
Chicken Parmesan	260	4	35
Glazed Chicken	240	3	34
Herb Roasted Chicken	160	3	18
Meatloaf w/ Mashed Potoes	240	7	25
Salisbury Steak with Mac & Cheese	280	8	28
Shrimp Alfredo	240	3	36
Steak Portabella	160	5	11
Craveables: *Per Package*			
Flatbread Melt, Chkn Ranch Club	370	9	52
Paninis: Chicken Club	350	9	45
Chicken, Spinach & Mushroom	350	9	45
Spinach, Artichoke & Chicken	320	9	44
Spring Rolls: Asian- Style Chkn (3)	170	7	19
Garlic Chicken (3)	180	8	21

Lean Cuisine (Cont):	C	F	Cb
Market Place: *Per Package*			
Apple Cranb. Chicken	280	4	48
Butternut Sq. Ravioli	260	4	46
Chicken Cashew Stir Fry	270	2	48
Chicken with Peanut Sauce	290	7	35
Creamy Basil Chicken w/ Tortellini	240	6	28
Fiesta Grilled Chicken	250	5	33
Garlic Sesame Noodles w/ Beef	300	6	46
Parmesan Crusted Fish	290	7	42
Pomegranate Chicken	180	3	20
Spicy Beef & Bean Enchil.	310	6	50
Spinach Artichoke Ravioli	280	7	41
Sweet & Spicy Korean-Style Beef	320	7	50
Sweet Sriracha Braised Beef	180	5	18
Pizzas ~ *See Page 136*			
Extra Product Listings ~ *www.CalorieKing.com*			
Lean Pockets:			
Sandwiches: *Per Single Pocket*			
Flaky Crust:			
Applewood Bacon, Egg & Cheese	260	8	36
Sausage, Egg & Cheese	280	8	41
Garlic & Herb Seasoned Crust:			
Mt'balls & Mozzarella	280	9	41
Pepperoni Pizza	280	8	42
Pretzel Bread:			
Chicken Japalpeno Cheese	260	7	36
Roasted Turkey, Bacon & Cheese	270	9	35
Uncured Ham & White Cheddar	270	7	39
Seasoned Crust:			
Philly Steak & Cheese	260	7	41
Lightlife (Meatless):			
Bowls: Chickpea Curry, 8 oz	310	7	50
Southwestern Quinoa & Black Bean	270	5	47
Gimme Lean Beef, 2 oz slice	60	0	7
Pasta: Veggie Sausage Ravioli, 8 oz	540	16	77
Wild Mushroom Ravioli, 8 oz	390	2	77
Smart Dogs: Veggie Hot Dog (1)	50	2	2
Jumbo Dog (1)	100	3.5	4
Smart Menue, Veggie Meatballs (3)	100	1.5	9
Smart Patties: Black Bean Burger	100	2.5	11
Garden Veggie Tempeh Burger (1)	100	3	10
Original, with Quinoa (1)	100	3	10
Smart Sausages: Chorizo	150	9	4
Harvest Apple	170	9	13
Italian	140	7	7
Tempeh: Fakin' Bacon, 4 slices	140	5	10
Three Grain, 3 oz	170	5	14

Lunchables: *Per Package*	C	F	Cb
Chicken Sliders	270	8	42
Lunch Combinations:			
Bologna Cracker Stackers, 2.43 oz	240	14	21
Cheese Pizza	220	10	27
Chicken Dunks	280	7	44
Pepperoni Flavored Sausage Pizza	220	10	25
Turkey & Cheddar Cracker Stackers	320	9	49
Lunchmakers *(Armour): Per Package*			
Bologna Cracker Crunchers	240	14	21
Cheese Pizza	220	10	27
Nachos	210	9	30
Pepperoni Flav Sausage Pizza	220	10	25
Turkey Cracker Crunchers	220	10	22
Marie Callender's:			
Beef: *Per Container*			
Beef & Broccoli	360	7	55
Meat Loaf & Gravy	380	13	45
Spaghetti w/ Meat Sce	540	18	75
Salisbury Steak	400	17	40
Slow Roasted Beef	260	9	32
Bowls: *Per Bowl*			
Creamy Vermont Mac & Cheese	570	22	71
Red Chili Grilled Chicken Burrito	360	10	44
Spicy Buffalo Style chicken Mac & Chse	540	25	53
Sweet & Savory Sesame Chicken	460	14	67
Chicken: *Per Container*			
Cheesy Chicken & Rice	430	14	54
Chicken Parmigiana	440	16	51
Cntry Fried Chkn & Grav	560	27	61
Sesame Chicken	500	17	69
Pasta: *Per Container*			
Fettuccini Alfredo & Garlic Bread	610	31	59
Fettuccini, Chicken & Broccoli	440	20	38
Grilled Chicken Alfredo Bake	460	19	45
Pot Pies: *Per 1 Cup, 7 oz*			
Beef	400	21	40
Broccoli & Cheddar	680	40	69
Cheesy Chicken & Bacon	510	32	41
Chicken	430	25	39
Chicken Corn Chowder	460	28	38
Creamy:			
Mushroom Chicken	430	25	39
Parmesan Chicken	430	26	36
Turkey	480	24	46
Family size: *Per 1 Cup*			
Beef, 7 oz	430	24	43
Chicken, 7 oz	370	21	35

Maruchan:	C	F	Cb
Bowls, all var., 3.3 oz	380	16	50
Ramen, Noodle Soup, average all, 3 oz pkg	380	16	52
Instant Lunch, average, 1 package	290	11	39
Yakisoba: Per 4 oz Pkg			
Chicken/Teriyaki Beef Flavor, av.	520	21	72
Sweet & Sour Chicken	560	22	78
Michael Angelo's:			
Organic: Chicken Parmigiana, 10 oz	310	6	47
Eggplant Parmigiana, 10 oz	240	12	22
Garden Vegetables w/ Penne Pasta	260	2	51
Lasagna with Meat Sauce, 10 oz	370	16	37
Signature: Chicken Alfredo, 11 oz	340	8	45
Florentine Lasagna, 11 oz	400	18	41
Shrimp Scampi, 10 oz	580	28	61
Minute Rice:			
Ready To Serve: Per 4.4 oz Container, Prepared			
Brown/Chicken Rice Mix, average	215	3	42
Fried/Yellow Rice Mix, average	220	2.5	44
Morningstar Farms (Meatless):			
Breakfast, Patties, all flavors (1)	70	3	3
Burgers:			
Grillers Original (1)	130	5	8
Medit. Chickpea (1)	120	4.5	13
Spicy Black Bean (1)	110	4.5	13
Chik Patties,			
Original (1)	170	7	20
Progressive Options:			
Indian Veggie Burger (1)	130	8	11
White Bean Chili Burger (1)	150	9	14
Veggie Classics: Buffalo Wings (5)	200	8	21
Chik'n Nuggets (4)	200	9	20
Corn Dogs (1)	150	2.5	26
Newman's Own:			
Complete Skillet Meal: Per ½ of 22-24 oz Package			
Chicken: General Paul's	400	16	47
Pad Thai	370	10	17
Teriyaki, w/ Low Mein Noodles	350	5	54
Nissin:			
Chow Mein: Per 4 oz Package			
Chicken Flavor	520	20	72
Spicy Chicken Flavor	560	28	66
Teriyaki Beef	480	20	66
With Shrimp	540	24	68
Parmigiana & Penne	490	25	47

Nissin (Cont):	C	F	Cb
Cup Noodles, all flavors, 1 cup	290	11	42
Very Veggie: Per ½ Pkg			
Spicy Chicken, 2.75 oz	340	11	53
Other var., 2.75 oz pkg	330	11	49
Raoh, ½ container, 1.9 oz	180	2	37
Souper Meals,			
av. all flavors, ½ pkg, 2.15 oz	280	13	38
Top Ramen, all flavors, 3 oz pkg	380	14	52
Old El Paso:			
Dinner Kits: Prepared with Chicken			
Chicken Soft Taco	330	13	30
Enchilada	400	14	27
Fajita	330	10	31
Pasta Roni: Per Cup, Prepared			
Angel Hair Pasta, with Herbs	270	9	38
Butter & Herb Italiano	300	12	42
Chicken & Broccoli	360	15	47
Chicken Flavor	300	12	39
Fettuccine Alfredo	440	24	48
Tomato Parmesan	270	9	39
White Cheddar & Broccoli	310	13	39
P.F. Chang's: Per ½ Package, 11 oz			
Entrees: Beef with Broccoli	310	11	23
General Chang's Chicken	370	12	48
Kung Pao Chicken	360	14	35
Mongolian Style Beef	310	9	39
Orange Chicken	440	14	57
Sesame Chicken	400	20	34
Shrimp Lo Mein	420	13	58
Sweet & Sour Chicken	340	9	51
Prego:			
Ready Meals: Per Pouch			
Creamy Three Cheese Alfedo Rotini	370	19	37
Creamy Tomato Penne	400	15	57
Marinara & Italian Sausage Rotini	350	9	55
Roasted Tomato &Vegetables Penne	300	4	55

Most packaged noodle soups are high in calories and fat.

Their promotion of 'O Grams Trans Fat' does not make them heart-healthy.

They are still high in saturated fat as well as salt/sodium.

Rice-A-Roni:	C	F	Cb
Classic Favorites: *Per Cup, Prepared*			
Beef; Herb & Butter; Rice Pilaf, av.	310	9	52
Cheddar Broccoli	350	16	47
Chicken & Garlic	250	8	41
Spanish Rice	260	7	45
Single Serve Cups:			
Cheddar Broccoli	230	4.5	41
Chicken Flavor	190	1	41
Creamy ereFour Cheese	240	6	43
Rosarita:			
Black Beans, 4.5 oz	110	0.5	19
Pinto Beans, 4.5 oz	120	0	22
Refried Beans:			
Traditional, 4.5 oz	120	2.5	18
No Fat, 4.5 oz	100	0	18
Safeway Select: *Per Tray*			
Frozen:			
Beef Salisbury Steak	400	25	23
Black Pepper Chicken	210	3.5	31
Chicken Cacciatore	290	10	34
Chicken Tikka Masala	260	5	36
Fettuccini Alfredo	480	15	75
H'style Baked Chicken	220	6	26
Lime Chili Chicken	260	3.5	43
Orange Chicken, Party Size, 6 oz	240	6	37
Penne Pasta, w/ Basil Cream Sauce	300	11	42
Pot Roast, w/ith Vegetables	200	6	22
S & W: *Per ½ Cup*			
Black Beans, 4.6 oz	120	0	22
Chili Beans, in Zesty Tom. Sauce, 4.6 oz	130	1.5	23
Kidney Beans, 4.6 oz	110	0	21
White Beans, 4.6 oz	100	0	19
Seapak ~ *See www.calorieking.com*			
Simply Asia:			
Noodle Bowls: *Per 8.5oz Bowl*			
Roasted Peanut	460	12	75
Sesame Teriyaki	390	3	82
Soy Ginger	420	6	84
Spicy Mongolian	430	6	86
Noodles & Sauce: *Per ⅓ Pkg*			
Sesame Teriyaki	300	3	60
Soy Ginger	320	4.5	60
Spicy Kung Pao	350	7	63
Quick Noodles: *Per 8.8 oz Tray*			
Honey Teriyaki	430	3.5	85
Pad Thai	460	3	93
Szechwan Garl. Chow Mein	460	7	83

Smart Ones *(Weight Watchers):*	C	F	Cb
Classic Favorites: *Per Meal*			
Angel Hair Marinara	180	2	34
Cheese Ravioli, in Mushroom Cream Sauce	230	5	35
Chicken Enchiladas Suiza	290	6	46
Lasagna Bake with Meat Sauce	250	5	39
Lasagna Florentine	310	9	45
Lemon Herb Chicken Piccata	210	2.5	32
Macaroni & Cheese	260	2	51
Pasta Primavera	200	2.5	35
Pasta w/ Ricotta & Spinach	290	5	44
Ravioli Florentine	210	3.5	37
Spagh. w/ Meat Sauce	280	3.5	50
Three Cheese Macaroni	300	6	48
Traditional Lasagna w/ Meat Sce	310	8	45
Tuna Noodle Casserole	250	3	44
Smart Anytime: *Per Meal*			
Brick Overn-Style Pepperoni Pizza	430	13	57
Chicken Quesadilla	170	6	17
Chicken Ranchero Mini Wrap	220	6	30
Chicken Slider	210	9	21
Spicy Chicken Slider	190	8	21
Smart Beginnings: *Per Meal*			
Breakfast Quesadilla	230	7	29
English Muffin S'wich, Egg White & Cheese	210	5	28
Three Cheese Omelet	200	7	20
Smart Creations: *Per Meal*			
Asian Style Beef & Broccili	160	4.5	16
Chicken Fettucini	300	4	45
Chicken Mesquite	250	3.5	33
Chicken Parmesan	280	5	37
Homestyle Turkey Breast, with Stuffing	280	6	36
Meatloaf	270	9	25
Teriyaki Chkn & Veggies	250	2.5	41
Stagg:			
Chili with Beans, 15 oz Can: *Per Cup*			
Chunkero, 8.7 oz	320	16	28
Classic, 8.7 oz	330	17	28
Dynamite Hot, 8.7 oz	330	17	29
Silverado, 8.7 oz	260	8	30
Vegetable Garden, 8.7 oz	210	1	41

Stouffer's:	C	F	Cb
Classics: *For One*			
Baked Chicken	240	8	17
Cheddar Potato Bake	270	17	21
Chicken a la King	360	12	44
Chicken Fett. Alfredo	570	27	55
Chicken Parmesan	410	14	47
Fettuccini Alfredo	630	35	63
Fish Filet with Mac & Cheese	400	19	35
Five Cheese Lasagna	330	14	33
Green Pepper Steak	240	4	32
Lasagna w/ Meat Sauce	350	11	38
Macaroni & Beef	410	16	45
Macaroni & Cheese, w/ Broccoli	480	20	52
Meat Lovers Lasagna	420	19	41
Roast Turkey	270	9	30
Spagh. w/ Meatballs	360	12	45
Stuffed Pepper	210	9	23
Tuna Noodle Casserole	450	20	45
White Meat Chicken Pot Pie	670	38	64
Creative Comforts: *For One*			
Chicken & Mushroom Marsala	300	7	40
Four Cheese Mac with Bacon	440	19	47
Honey Chipotle Chicken	430	19	42
Lasagna Italiano	290	12	30
Meatloaf w/ Swt Chipotle BBQ Sce	400	16	43
Mexican Style Lasagna	340	13	43
Rigatoni with Chicken & Pesto	400	15	44
Vegetable Lasagna	400	19	43
Fit Kitchen: *Per Package*			
Bourbon Steak	410	13	48
Moroccan Style Chicken	340	4	53
Pork Carnitas	380	12	45
Rotisserie Seasoned Turkey	330	10	37
Steak Fajitas	370	9	48
Teriyaki Chicken	325	9	46
Simply Crafted: *Family Size*			
Spicy Pomodoro Penne, 8.4 oz	260	6	41
White Cheddar Mac & Cheese, 7.94 oz	300	7	43
Urban Bistro: *For One*			
Aged Asiago Lasagna	350	12	40
Beer Glazed Meatballs	390	13	40
Smoked Gouda & Chorizo Mac	350	13	41
Spiced Chicken & Couscous	320	7	45

Swanson:	C	F	Cb
Dinners: *Per Package*			
Chicken Nuggets	590	25	71
Rib Style Boneless Pork	540	23	71
Salisbury Steak	450	22	44
Meat Pies: Beef	430	26	37
Chicken	370	20	37
Turkeuy	400	23	38
Skillets: *For Two*			
Alfredo Chicken	370	12	42
Beef Lo Mein	360	6	55
Chicken Parmesan	430	14	60
Garlic Chicken	420	15	51
Teriyaki Chicken	290	2.5	51
Tasty Bite:			
Mains: *Per ½ Package, 5 oz*			
Bengal Lentils	160	6	20
Bombay Lentils	130	3.5	19
Bombay Potatoes	140	4	22
Channa Masala	170	6	23
Coconut Vegetables	120	8	10
Jaipur Vegetables	150	10	12
Jodhpur Lentils	130	3.5	18
Madras Lentils	150	6	17
Punjab Eggplant	100	5	12
Thai Cashew Curry	140	9	12
TGI Friday's:			
Chicken Parmesan Sliders, 3 oz	260	13	27
Chkn Wings, Buffalo Style Sce, 4.2 oz	220	16	10
Cream Cheese Stuffed Jalap., 2.7 oz	220	11	20
Crispy Green Bean Fries & Sce, 3 oz	190	9	26
Dill Pickle Chips, w/ Horseradish Sce	200	11	22
Mozzarella Sticks (1), w/ Marinara Sauce	100	5	10
Thai Kitchen:			
Take-Out Meals: *Per ½ Package*			
Original Pad Thai	250	2	54
Thai Basil & Chili	250	3	50
Thai Peanut	270	5	51
Noodle Carts: *Per 9 oz Tray*			
Pad Thai	460	2	104
Thai Peanut	510	9	96
Rice Noodle Soup Bowls, average all varieties, 2.5 oz	240	2	50
Stir-Fry Rice Noodles: *Per ½ Package*			
Original Pad Thai	390	3.5	84
Thai Peanut	390	2	87

Tofurky: *Per Item*

	C	F	Cb
Chick'n:			
BBQ, 3.2 oz	200	5	14
Sesame Garlic, 3.2 oz	210	9	10
Tahai Basili, 3.2 oz	190	7	10
Tempeh: Original Soy Cake, 3 oz	170	4.5	12
Organic Five Grain, 3 oz	170	5	14
Sesame Garlic, 3 oz	130	3	14
Smoky Maple Bacon, 3 oz	130	1	17
Trader Joe's:			
Baked Beans, Organic, av., 1/2 cup	140	0	29
Black Beans:			
Regular, 1/2 cup	110	0	19
Cuban Style, 1/2 cup	100	0.5	19
Chicken Chili with Beans, 1 cup	290	9	32
Pasta, Shells & White Cheddar, 1 cup	280	6	47
Potatoes: Garlic Mashed, 1/2 cup	150	7	19
Cheddar Cheese Au Gratin, 1/2 cup	140	5	21
Turkey Chili w/ Beans, 1 cup	240	4.5	30
Frozen:			
Butter Chicken w/ Basmati Rice, 1 cup	270	8	33
Chicken Chow Mein, 1/3 pkg, 6.7 oz	210	2	35
Chicken Quesadilla (1), 6 oz	320	16	26
Citrus Glazed Chicken with Rice, 8 oz	270	5	40
Mac & Cheese: Regular, 1 cup, 7 oz	360	15	42
Reduced Guilt, 7 oz	270	6	40
Pies: Chicken Pot Pie, 1/2 pie, 8 oz	360	22	28
Shepherd's Pie, 1 cup, 8 oz	170	3	22
Shrimp Stir Fry, 6.4 oz	70	0.5	6
Spaghetti & Beef Meatballs,			
1 cup, 9 oz	380	13	48
Spicy Beef & Broccoli,			
1 3/4 cups	430	13	64
Thai Vegetable Kao Soi, 12.6 oz	430	20	55
Vegetable Pad Thai, 10.5 oz tray	520	21	74
Tyson:			
Any'tizers Snacks:			
Boneless Chicken Bites:			
Buffalo Style, 3 oz	180	9	12
Honey BBQ, 3 oz	210	9	20
Sriracha, 3 oz	200	11	12
Zesty Garlic Parmesan, 2.8 oz	170	9	12
Chicken Snackers:			
Buff. Ranch Style (1)	130	8	6
Chedd. Bacon Ranch (1)	140	9	7
Pepperoni Mozarella (1)	140	8	7
Chicken Twists: Original, 3 oz	250	12	23
Spicy, 3 oz	220	10	21
Homestyle Chicken Fries (7)	260	16	16
Popcorn Chicken, 3 oz	170	7	14

Tyson (Cont):

	C	F	Cb
Beef: Country Fried Steak, (1)	300	21	15
Steakhouse Seared,			
Seasoned Beef Steak Strips, 3 oz	120	3.5	1
Steak Fingers (2)	250	18	14
Breaded Chicken:			
Cheesy Chicken Nuggets 2.8 oz	220	13	14
Crispy Chicken Strips, 3 oz	190	8	18
Fun Nuggets, 2.75 oz	190	11	12
Southern Breast Tenderloins, 3 oz	180	9	12
Dinner Kits:			
Citrus Roasted Chicken, 6.4 oz	320	10	23
Crispy Adobe Chicken, 6.66 oz	430	20	34
Four Cheese Chkn & Broccoli Pasta	350	15	2
Lemon Parmesan Chicken, 10 oz	330	14	15
Roasted Ginger Chicken, 6.4 oz	320	11	21
Seasoned Steak & M'shrms, 10 oz	320	9	26
Grilled Chicken: Breast Fillets, 3.5 oz	110	2	2
Fajita Strips, 3 oz	110	4	1
Ital. Style Herb & Tomato Strips, 3 oz	120	2.5	3
Oven Rstd Diced Breast, 3 oz	100	2.5	1
Sweet Teriyaki Chicken Fillets, 3 oz	140	6	4
Uncle Ben's:			
Flavored Grains: *Dry Mix Only, as Directed*			
Average all flavors, 1 cup, cooked	200	0.5	42
Flav. Infusions, dry mix, av., 1.7 oz	155	0.5	34
Ready Rice: *Per 1 Cup, Heat & Serve*			
Brown Jasmin & Edamame	250	5	43
Brown Rice & Black Beans	210	3.5	37
Butter & Garlic Flav.	220	4	41
Cheddar & Broccoli Flav.	230	5	41
Creamy Four Cheese Flav.	220	5	40
Garden Vegetable	210	2.5	42
Jambalaya Flavored	200	2	40
Long Grain & Black Beans	220	4.5	40
Red Beans & Rice	210	2.5	41
Roasted Chicken Flavor	210	3	42
Teriyaki Style	220	3	42
Van Camp's:			
Baked Beans: Orig., 1/2 cup, 4.8 oz	150	0.5	30
Bacon Flavored, 1/2 cup, 4.8 oz	160	1	30
Beanee Weenee: Original, 7.75 oz	260	8	33
BBQ, 7.75oz	280	8	39
Smoked Hickory, 7.75 oz	320	8	48
Chilee, 7.75 oz	240	8	30

Van De Kamp's:	C	F	Cb
Appetizers:			
Crab Cakes, 3 oz	120	2	11
Crunchy Popcorn Fish, 4 oz	270	3	25
Fillets:			
Beer Battered/Crispy,3.8 oz	210	10	21
Crunchy, 1.8 oz	90	4	13
Fish Sticks,			
Crunchy, 3.6 oz	220	10	20
Fish For Tacos & Sandwiches:			
Fish Tenders, 3.6 oz	230	11	21
Sandwich: Original Recipe, 3 oz	190	10	18
Spicy Recipe, 3 oz	170	9	19
Flavor Crusted Fillets:			
Black Pepper & Salt Salmon, 4.5 oz	230	8	20
Garlic Herb Cod, 5 oz	260	10	26
Lemon Pepper Cod, 5 oz	280	10	26
Mediterranean Tilapia,, 5 oz	270	10	26
Parmesan & Rstd Garlic Tilapia, 5 oz	280	1	26
Whole Foods (365):			
Chickenless Nuggets,			
breaded (4), 2.8 oz	180	7	16
Meatless Meatballs (4), 2 oz	110	4	9
Meatless Burgers (1), 2.5 oz	120	4.5	7
Pasta Rings in Tomato Sauce, 1 cup	150	1	31
Vegetarian Chili, 1 cup	130	2	25
Worthington/Loma Linda:			
Big Franks: 1 link, 1.8 oz	110	6	3
Low-fat, 1 link, 1.1 oz	45	1.5	3
Chili, 1 cup, 8.10 oz	280	10	25
Choplets, Low Fat, 2 slices, 3.2 oz	90	1	4
Diced Chik, Low Fat, 2 oz	50	0	2
Fishless Tuna, 1.5 oz drained	60	1	5
FriChik, 2 pieces, 3.2 oz	140	8	3
Linketts (1), 1.3 oz	70	4	1
Little Links (2), 1.6 oz	90	5	3
Redi-Burger, Low Fat, 3 oz	120	2.5	7
Saucettes (1), 1.35 oz	90	6	1
Super Links (1), 1.1 oz	45	1.5	3
Tender Rounds w/ Gravy (6), 2.8 oz	120	4.5	6
Vegetarian Burger, 1/4 cup, 1.9 oz	70	1.5	3
Veja-Links (1), 1.1 oz	45	1.5	3

Yves Veggie Cuisine (Meatless):	C	F	Cb
Balls, Falafel (3)	150	7	17
Bites, Kale & Quinoa (4)	90	2.5	13
Breakfast, Veggie Patties (2)	80	2	5
Burgers: Gluten Free Veggie (1)	110	6	5
Kale & Root Vegetables (1)	110	6	5
The Good Veggie (1)	110	3.5	7
Deli Slices:	80	2.5	2
Bologna, 3 slices	60	1	2
Ham, 5 slices	80	1	5
Pepperoni, 10 slices	45	1	3
Salami, 5 slices	80	1	5
Turkey, 5 slices	80	1	4
Dogs: Good Dog (1)	45	1	2
Veggie (1)	50	0.5	2
Jumbo (1), 2.7 oz	110	2	4
Veggie Tofu (1)	50	1	2
Ground Rounds:			
Original, 1.9 oz	60	0.5	5
Garden Veggie Crumble, 1.95 oz	80	1.5	9
Taco Stuffers, 1.95 oz	80	3	6
Hot Dog:			
Good Dog (1), 2 oz	70	3.5	1
Hot Dog (1), 1.5 oz	50	0.5	2
Jumbo Hot Dog (1), 2.8 oz	110	3	5
Tofu Dog (1), 1.5 oz	45	1	2
Zatarain's:			
New Orleans Style: *Per Dry Mix Only*			
Black Beans & Rice, Original, 2.3 oz	230	1	47
Caribbean Rice Mix, 2.5 oz	250	2	52
Chicken Flavor Rice, 2 oz	210	0.5	45
Creamy Parmesan Rice Mix, 2.3 oz	240	4	45
Garlic & Herb & Rice Mix, 1.5 oz	130	0.5	29
Rice Pilaf, 2 oz	210	0.5	45
Smothered Chicken Rice Mix, 1.6 oz	160	0.5	34
Yellow Rice, 2 oz	200	0.5	43
Frozen Meals: *Per Meal*			
Blackened Chicken Alfredo, 10.5 oz	500	21	56
Dirty Rice with Beef & Pork, 10 oz	430	13	64
Jambalaya Flavored w/ Ssg, 12 oz	490	10	86
Red Beans & Rice w/ Sausage, 12 oz	540	17	79
Shrimp Scampi with Pasta, 10.5 oz	350	10	49

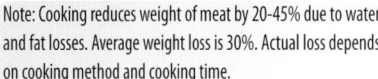

Note: Cooking reduces weight of meat by 20-45% due to water and fat losses. Average weight loss is 30%. Actual loss depends on cooking method and cooking time.

Examples:

4 oz raw weight = approx. 3 oz cooked weight

4 oz cooked weight = approx. 5½ oz raw weight

What 3 oz Cooked Meat Looks Like:

• Rectangular piece (4" x 2½" x ½" thick)

• Deck of cards (3½" x 2½" x ⅝" thick)

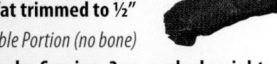

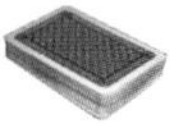

Quick Guide   **C** **F** **Cb**

Sirloin (Choice Grade):
External fat trimmed to ½"

Broiled, Edible Portion (no bone)

Small/Regular Serving, 3 oz, cooked weight:
(from 4-4½ oz raw)

Lean + external fat (⅛"), 3 oz	220	13	0
Lean + marbling, 3 oz	185	9	0
Lean only, 3 oz	160	6	0

(No external fat or marbling)

Medium Serving, 5 oz, cooked weight:
(from approximately 7 oz raw)

Lean + external fat (⅛"), 5 oz	365	22	0
Lean + marbling, 5 oz	310	15	0
Lean only, 5 oz	265	10	0

Large Serving, 8 oz, cooked weight:
(from approximately 11-12 oz raw)

Lean + external fat (½"), 8 oz	585	36	0
Lean + marbling, 8 oz	500	24	0
Lean only, 8 oz	425	15	0

Extra Large Serving, 12 oz, cooked weight:
(from approximately 16-17 oz raw)

Lean + external fat (⅛"), 12 oz	875	54	0
Lean + marbling, 12 oz	745	36	0
Lean only, 12 oz	640	22	0

Pan Fried:
Sirloin (Choice), medium serving,

Lean + external fat (⅛"), 5 oz	445	30	0

Other Steaks   **C** **F** **Cb**

Filet Mignon (Tenderloin):
1 Medium steak, 6 oz raw weight:
Broiled, with ¼" fat trim:

Lean + fat (¼"), 4 oz	360	27	0
Lean only, 3.5 oz	230	12	0

New York/Club Steak:
Top Loin/Short Loin:
1 steak, regular (9.25 oz raw, ¼" fat):
Broiled: Lean + fat (¼"), 6.3 oz

Broiled: Lean + fat (¼"), 6.3 oz	580	43	0
Lean + marbling, 5.5 oz	400	25	0
Lean only, 5.25 oz	360	20	0

Porterhouse Steak:
1 Medium, 6 oz raw weight, w/out bone, broiled:

Lean + fat (¼"), 4.3 oz	410	33	0
Lean only, 3.5 oz	210	11	0

1 Large, 12 oz raw weight, without bone, broiled:

Lean + fat (¼") 8.5 oz cooked	820	66	0
Lean only, 7 oz cooked	420	22	0

T̄-Bone Steak: *Broiled or Grilled*
Medium Size: *8 oz raw weight, without bone*
Approximately 6 oz cooked:

Lean + Fat (¼"), 5 oz	400	28	0
Lean only, 4 oz	265	12	0

Large Size: *12 oz raw weight*
Approximately 9 oz cooked:

Lean + fat (¼"), 7 oz, without bone	560	39	0
Lean only, 6 oz, without bone	400	18	0

Extra Large Size: *20 oz raw weight*
Approximately 16 oz cooked:

Lean + Fat (¼"), 12 oz, without bone	960	66	0
Lean Only, 10 oz, without bone	660	30	0

Also See Fast-Foods & Restaurants Section ~
Lone Star Steakhouse; Outback Steakhouse

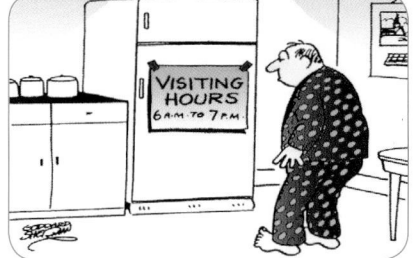

Beef – Individual Cuts   C   F   Cb

Average All Grades
Edible Weight, Without Bone

	C	F	Cb
Brisket, whole, braised:			
Lean + fat (¼" trim), 3 oz	330	27	0
Lean + marbling, 3 oz	250	17	0
Lean only, 3 oz	185	9	0
Chuck Blade, braised:			
Lean + fat (¼"), 3 oz	310	24	0
Lean + marbling, 3 oz	295	22	0
Lean only, 3 oz	245	13	0
Flank: Raw, 4 oz	175	8	0
Braised, 3 oz	225	14	0
Broiled, 3 oz	155	6	0
Round, bottom, braised:			
Lean + marbling, 3 oz	190	7.5	0
Lean only, 3 oz	185	6.5	0
Round, eye/tip, rstd:			
Lean + fat (¼"), 3 oz	205	11	0
Lean, w/ marbling, 3 oz	150	5	0
Round, top: *Per 3 oz, Cooked Weight*			
Braised, Lean + fat	210	10	0
Lean only	170	4	0
Broiled, Lean + fat	180	8	0
Lean only	160	5	0
Pan-fried, Lean + fat	235	13	0
Lean only	195	7	0

Beef Ribs

Back Ribs: *7" long, visible fat trimmed to ¼"*
10.3 oz raw w/ bone or 3.5 oz cooked, braised, w/o bone

	C	F	Cb
1 average rib	410	34	0
3 ribs	1230	102	0

Short Ribs: *2½" long, visible fat trimmed to ¼"*
6 oz raw with bone or 2.52 oz cooked, braised, w/o bone

	C	F	Cb
1 average rib	320	28	0
3 ribs	960	85	0

Ground Beef

Ground Beef, Raw: *Per 4 oz*

	C	F	Cb
70% lean (30% fat)	380	34	0
75% lean (25% fat)	335	29	0
80% lean (20% fat)	290	23	0
85% lean (15% fat)	245	17	0
90% lean (10% fat)	200	12	0
95% lean (5% fat)	155	6	0
Baked/Broiled: Regular (70%), 3 oz	230	16	0
Lean (80%), 3 oz	215	14	0
Extra lean (90%), 3 oz	185	10	0
Pan-Broiled:			
Regular (70%), 3 oz	230	15	0
Lean (80%), 3 oz	210	14	0
Extra lean (90%), 3 oz	195	10	0
Ground Beef Patties: *Average, 23% Fat*			
Raw, 4 oz	330	25	0
Broiled, 3 oz (from 4 oz raw)	250	19	0

Quick Guide   C   F   Cb

Roast Beef

Round (Eye/Tip, average): *Average All Cuts*
Small/Regular Serving: *3 oz*

	C	F	Cb
(2 thin slices/1 thick slice)			
Lean + fat (⅛" fat trim)	180	9	0
Lean only	145	4	0
Medium Serving: *5 oz*			
(3-4 thin slices)			
Lean + fat (⅛" fat trim)	300	15	0
Lean only	245	6.5	0
Large Serving, 8 oz: *3 thick slices*			
Lean + fat (⅛" fat trim)	480	24	0
Lean only	385	11	0

Roast Dinner Extras

	C	F	Cb
Gravy: Thin, 2 Tbsp	20	0.5	3.5
Thick, 2 Tbsp	50	2	0.5
1 Ladle/4 Tbsp	100	4	1
Veggies: Beans, green, ½ cup	20	0	5
Cauliflower with cheese sauce, 4 oz	135	9	15
Corn, kernels, ¼ cup	35	0	9
Carrots, ¼ cup	20	0	3
Peas, ¼ cup	35	0	6
Potato:			
Baked in jacket: Plain, 1 large	280	0	63
With sour cream, 2 Tbsp	270	5	64
With whipped butter, 1 Tbsp	350	8	63
Roasted with fat, 1 small	155	8	30
Sweet Potato/Yam, 1 medium	105	1	24
Yorkshire Pudding, 1 oz	90	3.5	11
Beef Kebab: *Cooked*			
Beef & Veggies, 2 oz	160	10	4
If very lean meat	100	4	4

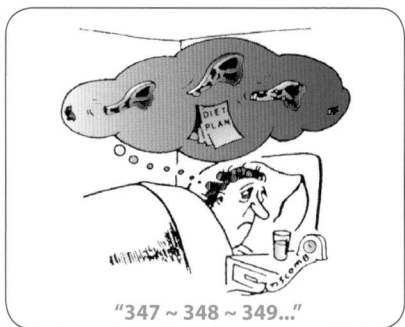

"347 ~ 348 ~ 349..."

Lamb

	C	F	Cb
Choice Grade:			
Leg (Whole), roasted:			
Lean + fat, 3 oz	220	14	0
Lean only, 3 oz	160	7	0
Leg (Sirloin Half), roasted:			
Lean + fat, 3 oz	250	18	0
Lean only, 3 oz	175	8	0
Leg (Shank Half), roasted:			
Lean + fat, 3 oz	190	11	0
Lean only, 3 oz	155	6	0
Loin Chop, broiled:			
1 chop (raw weight, 4.25 oz):			
Lean + fat (2.25 oz edible)	180	12	0
Lean only (1.6 oz edible)	85	3.5	0
Rib Chop, broiled:			
1 chop (raw wt., 3.5 oz):			
Lean + fat (2.5 oz edible)	255	21	0
Lean only (1.75 oz edible)	105	6	0
Shoulder (Arm/Blade):			
Braised: Lean + fat, 3 oz	295	21	0
Lean only, 3 oz	240	12	0
Broiled: Lean + fat, 3 oz	240	17	0
Lean only, 3 oz	170	8	0
Roasted: Similar to Broiled			
Cubed Lamb (Leg/Shoulder):			
For stew or kebab:			
Braised, lean only, 3 oz	190	8	0
Broiled, lean only, 3 oz	160	6	0

Veal

	C	F	Cb
Edible Weights:			
Leg (Top Round):			
Braised: Lean + fat, 3 oz	180	6	0
Lean only, 3 oz	175	5	0
Pan-fried, breaded:			
Lean + fat, 3 oz	195	8	9
Lean only, 3 oz	185	6	9
Pan-fried, not breaded:			
Lean + fat, 3 oz	180	7	0
Lean only, 3 oz	155	4	0
Roasted: Lean + fat, 3 oz	135	4	0
Lean only, 3 oz	130	3	0

Veal (Cont)

	C	F	Cb
Loin Chop: *1 chop, 7 oz raw weight*			
Braised: Lean + fat, 3 oz	240	15	0
Lean only, 3 oz	190	8	0
Roasted: Lean + fat, 3 oz	185	11	0
Lean only, 3 oz	150	6	0
Rib, roasted: *Lean + fat, 3 oz*	195	12	0
Lean only, 3 oz	150	7	0
Shoulder, Arm/Blade, roasted:			
Lean + fat, 3 oz	155	7	0
Lean only, 3 oz	140	5	0
Sirloin, roasted:			
Lean + fat, 3 oz	170	9	0
Lean only, 3 oz	145	6	0
Cubed for Stew, braised:			
Leg/Shoulder, lean only, 3 oz	160	4	0
(1 lb raw yields approximately 9.25 oz cooked)			

Pork

	C	F	Cb
Fresh Pork: *Cooked Weight, without bone:*			
4 oz raw weight = approx. 3 oz cooked weight			
BBQ, Pulled:			
2 oz	90	2.5	10
4 oz	180	5	20
8 oz	360	10	40
Blade Steak, broiled:			
Lean + fat, 3 oz	220	15	0
Lean only, 3 oz	190	11	0
Country Style Ribs, broiled/roasted:			
Lean + fat, 3 oz	280	22	0
Lean only, 3 oz	210	13	0
Spareribs, braised: *Lean & fat, 6 oz*			
(from 1 lb raw weight)	675	52	0
Leg (Ham), whole, roasted:			
Lean + fat, 3 oz	230	15	0
Lean only, 3 oz	180	8	0
Loin Chops, broiled: *Average*			
(From 1 chop: 5 oz raw weight with bone or 4 oz raw			
weight, without bone)			
Lean + fat, 3 oz	200	11	0
Lean only, 3 oz	165	7	0
Loin Roast, roasted:			
Lean + fat, 3 oz	210	13	0
Lean only, 3 oz	180	8	0
Rib Chops, (Boneless), broiled:			
Lean + fat, 3 oz	220	14	0
Lean only, 3 oz	185	9	0
Rib Roast:			
Lean + fat, 3 oz	215	13	0
Lean only, 3 oz	180	9	0

Pork (Cont)

	C	F	Cb
Sirloin Chop, broiled:			
Lean + fat, 3 oz	180	8	0
Lean only, 3 oz	165	6	0
Sirloin Roast, roasted:			
Lean + fat, 3 oz	175	8	0
Lean only, 3 oz	170	7	0
Tenderloin (Boneless), roasted:			
Lean + fat, 3 oz	125	4	0
Lean only, 3 oz	120	3	0
Ground Pork:			
Raw, average, 1/4 lb, 4 oz	300	24	0
Broiled, 3 oz	250	18	0
Pan-fried, drained, 3 oz	260	19	0

Bacon

	C	F	Cb
Raw: 1 med. slice, 0.75 oz	95	9	0
1 thick slice, 1.3 oz	175	17	0
(1 lb raw yields approximately 5 oz cooked)			
Broiled/Pan-Fried:			
1 medium slice, 0.3 oz	40	3	0
3 medium slices, 0.8	125	10	0
2 thin slices, 0.5 oz	75	6	0
1 thick slice, 0.9 oz	65	5	0
Canadian Bacon:			
Cooked: 1 slice, 1 oz	45	2	0.5
2 slices, 2 oz	90	4	1
Bacon Bits, 1 Tbsp, 0.3 oz	35	2	0
Breakfast Strips, Broiled, 1 sl., 0.4 oz	50	4	0

Ham

	C	F	Cb
Boneless Ham, cooked:			
Regular, (approximately 13% fat):			
Roasted, 3 oz	150	8	0
Extra Lean (5% fat),			
Roasted, 3 oz	125	5	0
Whole Ham, cooked:			
Lean + fat (as purchased)			
Roasted, 3 oz	210	15	0
Lean only, Roasted, 3 oz	135	5	0
Canned Ham: *Similar to boneless ham*			
Chopped, canned, 3 oz	200	16	0
Ham Patties, cooked, (1), 2.3 oz	220	20	1
Ham Steak, extra lean, 2 oz	70	2.5	0
Lunch Slices ~ *See Deli Meats, Page 128*			

Game & Other Meats

	C	F	Cb
Bison Steak,			
lean, 6 oz (raw)	205	4	0
Boar (wild), roasted, 3 oz	140	4	0
Buffalo Steak,			
New West Foods, 4 oz	70	3	0
Caribou, roasted, 3 oz	140	4	0
Deer/Venison, roasted 3 oz	135	3	0
Goat (Capretto):			
Raw, 3 oz	95	2	0
Roasted, 3 oz	120	2.5	0
Ostrich:			
Blackwing Ostrich Meats:			
Sausage Patties (2) 2 oz	60	0.5	0
Sport Jerky, 0.5 oz piece	25	0	0
New West Foods:			
Ground Ostrich, 4 oz	165	7	0
Ostrich Steak, 4 oz steak	130	2.5	0
Rabbit: Roasted, 3 oz	165	7	0
Stewed, 1 cup, diced, 5 oz	290	12	0

Variety & Organ Meats

	C	F	Cb
Brain (Lamb): Braised, 3 oz	125	9	0
Pan-fried, 3 oz	230	19	0
Chitterlings, pork, simmered, 3 oz	260	25	0
Ears, pork, simmered, 1 ear, 4 oz	185	12	0
Feet, Pork: Simmered, 3 oz	200	14	0
Cured, pickled, 3 oz	170	14	0
Hormel, 3 oz	80	6	0
Head Cheese (Pork Snouts/Ears/Vinegar/Spices),			
1 oz slice	50	4	0
Heart, Beef, braised, 3 oz	140	4	0
Jowl, pork, raw, 4 oz	750	80	0
Kidneys, braised, 3 oz	140	5	0
Liver (beef): Raw, 4 oz	150	4	4
Braised, 3 oz	140	4	3
Pan-fried, 3 oz	185	7	7
Pancreas, pork, braised, 3 oz	185	8	0
Pork Cracklins, 0.5 oz	80	6	0
Pork Hocks, 1 piece, 6 oz	340	23	0
Scrapple, pork, 2 oz	120	8	8
Spleen, pork, braised, 3 oz	130	3	0
Stomach, pork, raw, 4 oz	185	12	0
Sweetbreads:			
Beef,/Lamb, cooked, 3 oz	125	9	0
Tail, pork, simmered, 3 oz	340	31	0
Tongue: Raised Veal, 3 oz	170	9	0
Beef/Lamb/Pork, av., 3 oz	235	17	0
Tripe, beef, raw, 3 oz	85	3.5	0

Quick Guide   C F Cb

Franks & Weiners
Average All Brands
Regular (Pork Mix): *Per Frank*

	C	F	Cb
Regular, 1.5 oz	140	13	1
Bun Length/Jumbo, 2 oz	185	17	2
Extra Long, 2.75 oz	255	24	2
Small/Cocktail, each	30	3	0.5

Beef Franks: *Per Frank*

	C	F	Cb
Regular, 1.5 oz	140	13	2
Bun Length/Jumbo, 2 oz	175	17	2.5
$1/4$ lb Dog, 4 oz	375	33	5

Franks & Weiners

Ball Park: *Per 2 oz Frank Unless Indicated*
Angus Beef:

	C	F	Cb
Original; Bun Size, 2 oz	170	15	3
Lean, 1.8 oz	70	5	2
Beef: Original, Bun Size, 2 oz	190	16	4
Deli Style, Regular, 1.8 oz	150	12	2
Grillmaster, Hearty, 3 oz	250	21	3
Lean, 1.76 oz	80	5	2
Park's Finest, 2 oz	170	15	2
Foster Farms, Chicken; Turkey, 2 oz	140	12	1

Hebrew National: *Per Frank*
Beef:

	C	F	Cb
Regular, 1.7 oz	150	13	2
$1/4$ Pounder, 4 oz	350	31	4
Jumbo, 3 oz	260	23	3
97% Fat-Free, 1.6 oz	45	1	2
Bun Length Beef Frank, 2 oz	170	15	2

Jennie-O: *Per Frank*
Turkey Franks:

	C	F	Cb
1.2 oz	70	6	1
Jumbo, 2 oz	120	10	1
Turkey Bratwurst, 3.8 oz	170	10	2

Oscar Mayer: *Per Frank*
Angus Beef:

	C	F	Cb
Classic, 1.5 oz	130	12	1
Bun Length, 1.76 oz	170	15	2
Turkey, Classic, 1.6 oz	100	7	2

Shelton's: *Per Frank*

	C	F	Cb
Chicken, uncured, 1.2 oz	80	7	0
Turkey, Regular, 1.2 oz	60	4.5	1
Zacky Farms, Chkn; Turkey, av, 2 oz	115	10	4

Quick Guide   C F Cb

Fresh Sausages
Pork/Beef: *Average All Types*

	C	F	Cb
Small: Raw, 4" link, 1 oz	85	7.5	0
Broiled/Pan-fried	80	7	0
Medium: Raw, 2 oz	170	15	0
Broiled/Pan-fried	165	14	0
Large: Raw, 3 oz	255	22	0
Broiled/Pan-fried	245	21	0
Italian: Raw, 3.2 oz	315	28	1
Cooked, 2.4 oz	230	18	3
Chorizo: Beef Chorizo, 2.5 oz piece	250	23	5
Pork Chorizo, 2 oz piece	250	23	5

Note: Fat is lost in broiling/pan frying.
Cooked weight = approx. 60-70% raw weight

Smoked Sausages
Per Link:

	C	F	Cb
Butterball, Turkey, 2 oz	100	6	4
Eckrich:			
Original (1)	230	18	6
Cheddar (1), 2.36 oz	210	18	3
Hillshire Farm:			
Cheddarwurst, 2 oz	180	16	2
Chicken Hardwood, 2 oz	100	7	3
Polska Kielbasa, 2 oz	180	16	0

Johnsonville ~ *See CalorieKing.Com*

Breakfast Sausages/Patties

Butterball: *Fully Cooked*

	C	F	Cb
Turkey: B'fast Sausage Links (3), 2 oz	90	5	0
Patties (2), 2 oz	90	5.5	0

Jimmy Dean: *Fully Cooked*
Heat 'N Serve Sausage Links:

	C	F	Cb
Pork, Regular (3), 1.9 oz	210	19	2
Turkey (3), 2 oz	130	8	2

Heat 'N Serve Sausage Patties:

	C	F	Cb
Pork, Original (2), 1.8 oz	200	17	2
Turkey (2), 1.8 oz	120	8	1
Maple Pork Sausages,(3), 2.4 oz	260	22	3
Pork Patties, (2), 2.3 oz	270	24	2

Breakfast Sandwiches ~ *See Page 92*
Jones Dairy Farm:
Golden Brown Sausages: *Fully Cooked*

	C	F	Cb
Mild Pork Sausages (3), 2 oz	250	24	1
Maple Pork Sausages (3), 2 oz	240	22	2

Vegetarian Patties:
Boca ~ *See Page 117*
GardenBurger ~ *See Page 114*

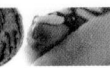

Bagel, Corn & Hot Dogs C F Cb

Hot Dogs, Ready-To-Go:
Includes Ketchup/Relish

	C	F	Cb
Regular, 1.5 oz frank, 1.5 oz bun	260	15	22
Bun Length, 2 oz frank, 1.5 oz bun	290	18	21
Jumbo Dog, 2 oz frank, 2 oz bun	360	20	36
$^1/_4$ lb Beef Dog, 2 oz bun	480	15	36
Mile Long Dog, 2.6 oz dog, 1.5 oz bun	360	24	23

Corn Dogs:
	C	F	Cb
Beef/Pork Frank, average, 2.6 oz	170	10	16

Foster Farms:
Corn Dogs:
	C	F	Cb
Chili Cheese (1), 2.7 oz	190	9	21
Honey Crunchy:			
Regular (1), 2.7 oz	190	9	18
Jumbo (1), 4 oz	280	14	27
Mini (4), 2.7 oz	220	13	19

State Fair: *Per Dog*
	C	F	Cb
Beef Corn Dog, 2.7 oz	230	11	26
Classic Corn Dog, Reg., 4 oz	330	11	34
Mini Classic (5), 3.3 oz	270	14	29

Bagel Dogs:
Hebrew National:
	C	F	Cb
Beef Bagel Dogs, 4 pieces, 2.75 oz	240	13	22
Schwanns, Bagel Dogs,			
with Cheese, 1 piece, 4.5 oz	370	16	40

Vienna Beef:
	C	F	Cb
Bagel Dog: 5.5 oz	410	19	44
6.5 oz	490	19	58
Mini (5), 4.6 oz	310	18	31

Hot Dog Toppings/Extras:
	C	F	Cb
American Cheese, 1 slice, 1 oz	110	9	1
Chili Con Carne, ¼ cup	50	2	5.5
Ketchup, 1 Tbsp	15	0	4
Mustard, 1 Tbsp	20	0	1
Onions, chopped, 1 Tbsp	5	0	1
Pickle Relish, 1 Tbsp	20	0	5
Sauerkraut, ½ cup	20	0	5

Deli/Lunch Meats & Sausage

	C	F	Cb
Beef Jerky/Meat Snacks,			
Berliner (pork/beef), 1 oz	65	5	1
Beerwurst (Beef):			
Small (2¾"diam), ¹⁄₁₆" slice	20	2	0
Large (4" diam), ⅛" slice	75	7	0.5
Beerwurst (Pork):			
Small (2.75"diameter), ¹⁄₁₆" slice	15	1	0
Large (4"diameter), ⅛" Slice	55	4	0.5
Blood Sausage, 1 oz	100	9	0.5

Deli/Lunch Meats & Sausages (Cont)

	C	F	Cb
Bologna:			
Beef Bologna: 1 slice, 1 oz	90	8	0
Light, 1 slice, 1 oz	60	4	2
Oscar Mayer: Regular, 1 oz	90	8	1
98% Fat Free, 1 oz	40	1.5	1
Light, 1 slice, 1 oz	60	4	1
Boar's Head, Ring, 2 oz	150	13	1
Pork Bologna: 1 Slice, 1 oz	65	6	1
Fat-Free, 1 slice, 1 oz	20	0	2
Turkey Bologna, average, 1 oz	60	5	0.5
Bratwurst: Average, 1 oz	80	7	1
Bob Evan's, Beer B'wurst, 2.2 oz link	170	14	0
Braunschweiger, (Pork/Liver/Sausage),			
Oscar Mayer, 2 oz slice	190	17	0
Chicken, average:			
1 thick or 2 thin slices, 1 oz	30	1	1
2 oz slice	60	2	2
Hillshire Farm,			
Rotiss. Seasoned Chicken Breast, 2 oz	50	0.5	2
Corned Beef, average, full fat, 1 oz	60	5	0.5
Ham, Sliced:			
Baked/Broiled, 1 oz slice	35	1	1
Oscar Mayer, Baked, Lean,			
3 slices, 2.3 oz	80	2.5	1
Honey/Brown Sugar, av., 1 oz	35	1	1
Prosciutto, average, 1 oz	70	5	0
Ham & Cheese Loaf, average, 1 oz	70	5	1
Italian Sausage, 2.6 oz	250	20	3
Kielbasa: Polish Sausage, 2 oz	65	5	1
Beef, 2 oz link	190	17	1
Knockwurst, av., 1 oz	90	8	0.5
Linguica *(Gaspar's),* 2 oz	130	9	1
Liverwurst, 1 oz	65	5	2
Liver Pate, fresh, average, 1 oz	90	8	1
Mortadella, 1 oz	105	9	0
Olive Loaf: Average, 1 oz	70	5	3
Oscar Mayer, 1 oz	80	6	1
Pancetta, *Boars Head, 1 slice*	50	4.5	0

Deli/Lunch Meats & Sausages (Cont)

	C	F	Cb
Pastrami (Beef):			
Boar's Head:			
1st cut Brisket, 2 oz	90	4	2
Cap-Off Top Round, 2 oz	80	3	1
Hillshire, Deli Select,			
Ultra Thin. 2 oz	60	1.5	0.5
Peppered Beef, 1 oz slice	40	2	1
Pepperoni, 5 slices, 1 oz	140	13	0
Pickle Loaf, average, 1 oz	70	5	5
Pickle & Pepper Loaf,			
Boars Head, 2 oz	150	13	2
Proscuitto/Proscuitti, av., 1 oz	70	5	1
Roast Beef, Lean, 1 oz	40	2	0
Salami: Beef, av., 1 oz	80	7	1
Oscar Mayer, Hard, 1 slice, 1.8 oz	100	8	0.5
Beer Salami, average, 1 oz	50	4	0.5
Oscar Mayer: Cotto, 1 slice, 1 oz	70	6	0.5
Beef Cotto, 1 slice, 1 oz	60	5	0.5
Dry, Hard, average, 4 slices, 1 oz	100	8	1
Genoa: Average, 1 oz	100	8	1
Stick, 1.8 oz	175	14	2
Bridgford, Italian, 1 oz	120	11	0
SPAM (Hormel): *Per 2 oz*			
Classic: 2 oz serving	180	16	1
7 oz can	630	56	3.5
12 oz can	1080	96	6
Spam Lite: 2 oz	110	8	1
12 oz can	660	48	6
Other Spam Products: *Per 2 oz*			
Hickory Smoked	180	16	1
Hot & Spicy	160	16	2
Oven Roasted Turkey	80	4.5	1
Spam Spresd	140	12	1
Spam with Bacon	180	16	1
Spam with Cheese	170	15	1
25% Less Sodium	180	16	1
Spam Singles: *Per 3 oz*			
Classic, 2.5 oz package	210	18	2
Lite, 2.5 oz package	130	9	2

Deli/Lunch Meats & Sausages (Cont)

	C	F	Cb
Summer Sausage:			
Armour, Beef, 2 oz	190	17	2
Hillshire Farm, 2 oz	190	16	1
Treet *(Armour),* Luncheon Loaf,			
Original, 2 oz	140	11	4
Turkey, average: 1 oz slice	30	1	0.5
0.8 oz slice	22	0.5	0.5
Turkey Breast:			
Butterball, Oven Roasted:			
1 slice 1 oz	30	0.5	1
Deli Inspirations,			
Extra Thin Slices, 4 slices, 2 oz	50	1	3
Hillshire, Deli Select,			
Oven Roasted, 6 slices, 2 oz	50	0.5	2
Turkey Ham, 1 slice, 1 oz	35	1.5	0.5
Turkey Loaf, 1 oz	30	1	0.5
Turkey Pastrami, 1 oz	35	1.5	1
Turkey Roll, 1 oz	40	2	0.5
Vegetarian Deli ~ See Page 118			

Meat Spreads

	C	F	Cb
Average All Brands:			
Chicken, white meat, 2.1 oz	140	11	2
Corned Beef, 2.1 oz	140	11	1
Ham, Deviled, 2.1 oz	180	15	1
Liverwurst	160	13	4
Roast Beef	130	10	2
Turkey	110	7	2
Underwood: *Per 2 oz*			
Chicken, White Meat	140	11	2
Deviled Ham	180	15	1
Liverwurst	160	13	4
Roast Beef	130	10	2

Paté

	C	F	Cb
Les Trois Petit Cochons: *Per 2 oz*			
Pate: de Campagne 2 oz	240	22	2
de Canard a l'Orange; Forestier, 2 oz	210	18	3
Paysan, 2 oz	150	12	2
Rustique, 2 oz	240	22	2
Venison, 2 oz	200	16	4
Wild Boar, 2 oz	180	15	4
Old Wisconsin Pate,			
Braunschweiger, 2 oz	210	18	3

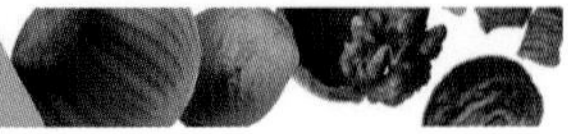

Nuts

Per 1 oz Unless Indicated	C	F	Cb
Acorns, raw 1 oz	110	7	12
Almonds: Dried/Dry Roasted:			
Whole: 12 medium size, 0.5 oz	85	7.5	3
23-25 medium size, 1 oz	170	15	6
½ cup, 2.5 oz	420	37	13
Ground, 1 cup, 3.4 oz	545	47	20
Sliced, ½ cup, 1.6 oz	260	22	10
Slivered, ½ cup, 2 oz	310	27	12
Chocolate Coated (5-6), 1 oz	150	10	15
Honey Roasted, 1 oz	170	14	8
Oil Roasted (*Blue Diamond*), 1 oz	170	16	5
Brazil Nuts, 8 medium, 1 oz	185	19	3.5
Cashews, dry or oil roasted:			
14 large/18 med./26 small: 1 oz	165	14	9
½ cup, 2.4 oz	375	31	20
Honey Roasted, 1 oz	165	13	10
Chestnuts:			
Average, dried, 1 oz	105	1	22
Raw/Fresh, 5-6 nuts, 1 oz	60	0	13
Canned, water chestnuts, sliced/whole/drained, 1 oz	30	0	7
Coconut, Fresh:			
1 piece, 2"x2"x ½ ", 1 oz	185	18	7
Shredded, fresh, ½ cup, 1.4 oz	140	13	6
Dried (Desiccated):			
Sweetened: Shredded, 1 oz	145	10	14
Grated, ½ cup, 1.3 oz	185	13	18
Unsweetened, 1 oz	185	18	7
Cream (canned), ½ cup, 5.2 oz	285	26	12
Milk (canned), unsweetened, ¼ cup, 2 fl.oz	100	10	3
Water (center liquid), ½ cup, 4.3 oz	25	0	4.5
Filberts or Hazelnuts:			
Shelled, 18-20 nuts	180	17	4.5
Chopped, ¼ cup, 1 oz	180	18	5
Ground, ¼ cup, 0.6 oz	120	12	3
Ginkgo Nuts, canned, 14 med., 1 oz	32	0.5	6.5
Hickory, 30 small nuts, 1 oz	200	18	5
Macadamia Nuts, Shelled:			
Raw or Dry Roasted, avg:			
12 small or 8 med., 1 oz	200	21	4
6-7 large, 1 oz	200	21	4
½ cup, 2.3 oz	480	51	10
Mixed Nuts: Raw, 18-22 nuts, 1 oz	170	15	7
Oil Roasted, all types	170	16	6
Sweet Roasts, 26 pieces, 1 oz	160	12	10
Planters, Dry Roasted/Honey	160	12	9
Nut Toppings, chopped, 1 Tbsp, 0.3 oz	40	4	1.5

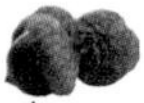
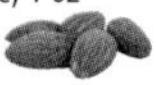
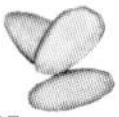
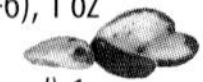
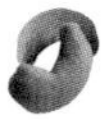

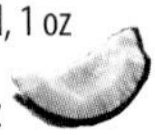
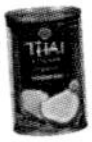

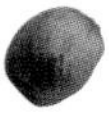
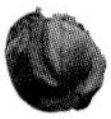
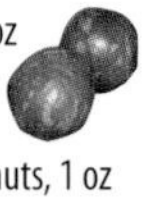
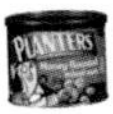

Per 1 oz Unless Indicated	C	F	Cb
Peanuts:			
Dry or oil roasted, average:			
Small handful, 0.5 oz	85	7	3
⅕ cup, 1 oz	165	14	6
½ cup, 2.5 oz	415	35	15
3 oz bag	500	42	18
7 oz bag	1160	98	42
Raw: Shelled, 1 oz	160	14	4.5
In shell, 1 oz	115	110	3
Planters:			
Cocktail, all varieties	170	14	5
Honey Roasted	160	13	7
Spanish Redskins	170	15	4
Sweet N' Crunchy	140	8	15
Japanese Style Peanuts, Coated in Crunchy Shell	150	8	13
Pecans, roasted:			
10 halves, 0.5 oz	95	10	2
20 Halves, 1 oz	195	20	4
1 cup, halves, 3.5 oz	680	71	14
Pilinuts, dried, 1 oz	215	24	1
Pine Nuts, dried, 1 Tbsp, 0.3 oz	70	7	1.5
Pistachios, raw:			
Shelled, 45 nuts, 1 oz	160	13	8
Unshelled, 2 oz	165	14	7
Lance, Roasted, 1.5 oz	120	9	6
Sesame Nut Mix, 1 oz	160	13	9
Soy Nuts: Dry Roasted	130	6	9
½ cup, 3 oz	390	18	28
Dr Soy, Chocolate coated, 1 oz pkg	140	7	13
Trail Mix *(Planters):*			
Daybreak, Berry Almond, 1.5 oz	180	7	27
Energy Mix, 1.5 oz	250	20	14
Fruit & Nut	140	9	14
Nut & Chocolate, 1.3oz	150	9	14
Nuts, Seeds & Raisins, 1 oz	160	11	11
Spicy Nuts & Cajun Sticks	150	11	10
Sweet & Nutty, 1 oz	150	9	13
Walnuts, average all types:			
7-10 halves, 0.5 oz	90	9	2
15-20 halves, 1 oz	175	17	3
Chopped, ½ cup, 2.2 oz	380	36	6
Ground, ¼ cup, 0.7 oz	130	13	3

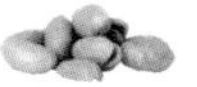
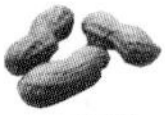
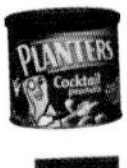

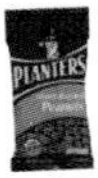

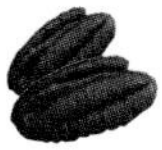
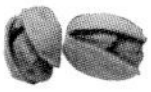
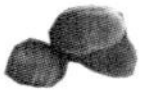
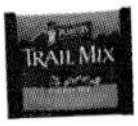

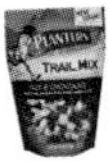

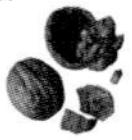

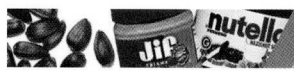

Quick Guide   C   F   Cb

	C	F	Cb
Peanut Butter: *Average All Brands*			
1 level tsp, 0.2 oz	35	3	1
1 level Tbsp, 0.6 oz	100	8.5	3.5
1 oz Quantity	165	14	6
½ cup, 5 oz	835	72	29

Peanut Butter ~ Brands

	C	F	Cb
Jif: Regular, all varieties, 2 Tbsp	190	16	8
Natural, average all varieties, 2 Tbsp	185	15	10
Reduced Fat, all varieties, 2 Tbsp	190	12	15
To Go: Crmy/Crunch, av.,1.5 oz cup	250	21	11
Chocolate Silk, 1.5 oz cup	250	18	18
Whipped: Creamy, 2 Tbsp	140	12	6
Chocolate flavored, 2 Tbsp	150	11	11
Laura Scudder's, Natural,			
Smooth; Nutty, average, 2 Tbsp	190	16	5
Peter Pan:			
Natural, Creamy/Crunchy, av., 2 T.	205	17	6
Creamy/Crunchy, Red.-Fat, 2 Tbsp	200	13	14
Plus Creamy, 2 Tbsp	210	17	7
Planters, Creamy/Crunchy, 2 Tbsp	180	15	8
Smucker's, Goober,			
Grape/Srawberry, 3 Tbsp. 2 oz	240	13	24
Skippy: Natural, Creamy/Chunky, 2 T.	190	16	6
Reduced Fat, all varieties, 2 Tbsp	180	12	15
PB Bites, average all, 15 pcs, 1 oz	160	10	14

Peanut Butter & Jelly Sandwich

	C	F	Cb
1 sandwich: *With 2 oz Bread*			
Thin Spread, 1 Tbsp Peanut Butter			
+ 1 Tbsp Jelly	310	10	48
Thick Spread, 2 Tbsp Peanut Butter			
+ 2 Tbsp Jelly	480	19	67

Nut & Chocolate Spread

	C	F	Cb
Nutella:			
1 Tbsp, 0.7 oz	110	6	11
2 Tbsp, 1.3 oz	200	11	22
Note: Nutella contains approx. 50% sugar & 13% hazelnuts			

Other Nut & Seed Butters

Per 1 Tbsp, 0.5 oz	C	F	Cb
Almond Butter	100	10	3.5
Cashew Butter	95	8	4.5
Hazelnut Butter; Pecan Butter	110	10	2
Pistachio Butter	90	6.5	4.5
Sesame Butter (Tahini)	90	8	3
Soy Nut Butter	75	5	4

Seeds   C   F   Cb

	C	F	Cb
Alfalfa Seeds,			
sprouted, ½ cup, 0.5 oz	5	0	1
Caraway/Fennel, 1 tsp	7	0.5	1
Chia Seeds: 1 Tbsp, 0.4 oz	45	3	4
3 Tbsp, 1 oz	140	8.5	12
Cottonseed Kernels,			
roasted, 1 Tbsp	50	3.5	2
Flax Seeds,			
3 Tbsp, 1 oz	140	9	9
Lotus Seeds,			
dried, ½ cup, 0.5 oz	55	0.5	10
Poppy Seeds, 1 tsp	15	1	1
Pumpkin/Pepita Seeds, whole:			
Roasted/Tamari: 1 oz	150	12	4
½ cup, 4 oz	590	48	15
Dried (hulled), ¼ cup, 1 oz	155	13	5
Safflower Kernels, dried, 1 oz	150	11	10
Sesame Seeds:			
Dried, 1 Tbsp, 0.3 oz	50	4.5	2
Roasted/Toasted, 1 oz	160	14	7.5
Sunflower Kernels/Seeds:			
Dried, ¼ cup w/out hulls, 0.3 oz	200	18	7
Dry Roasted: 1 Tbsp, 0.3 oz	45	4	2
¼ cup, 1 oz	165	14	7
Oil Roasted, ⅛ cup, 1 oz	170	14	6.5
Watermelon Seeds,			
dried, ¼ cup, 1 oz	150	13	4

*N*ut eaters are healthier and live longer, say scientists.

Nuts are a nutritious source of protein, vitamins, minerals, fiber, healthy fats, and antioxidants.

The fat and fiber of nuts can help reduce blood cholesterol. Their protein and fiber also promotes meal satiety (fullness) and reduces hunger levels – of benefit in weight control.

Eat nuts instead of high-sugar snacks, candy and soft drinks. Add chopped nuts to breakfast cereals.

Quick Guide | C | F | Cb

Pancakes:

Plain: *Average All Types*

	C	F	Cb
Small (3" diameter), 0.8 oz	50	2	6
Medium (4" diameter), 1.3 oz	85	3.5	11
Large (6" diameter), 2.5 oz	175	7.5	22

Add Extra for Syrups/Butter

	C	F	Cb
Pancake Syrup: Regular, 1 Tbsp	50	0	12
¼ cup, 4 Tbsp	185	0	49
Lite, 1 Tbsp	25	0	6.5
¼ cup, 4 Tbsp	100	0	27
Butter/Margarine:			
Regular, 1 Tbsp	100	11	0
Whipped, 1 Tbsp	65	7.5	0

Waffles:

	C	F	Cb
Homemade, 7" waffle, 2.5 oz	220	11	25
Frozen + Toasted, (4" diam.), 1 oz	105	3	16

Pancake Brands

Prepared as Directed

Aunt Jemima: *Prepared*

Mixes: *Makes 4" Pancakes*

	C	F	Cb
Original (4)	250	8	36
Original Complete (2)	160	1.5	32
Buttermilk (4)	160	3	27
Whole Wheat Blend (3)	200	6.5	30

Bisquick: *Prepared with Water*

Pancake/Waffle Mix: *Makes 3 Pancake*

	C	F	Cb
Complete, Buttermilk, 2 oz	200	3	40
Shake 'n Pour, Buttermilk, 2.2 oz	230	3.5	45

Hungry Jack:

Pancake & Waffle Mixes: *Makes 4" Pancake*

Complete Mixes: Just Add Water

	C	F	Cb
Chocolate Chip (3)	190	2.5	39
Extra Light & Fluffy (3)	180	1	38
Wheat Blends (3)	180	1.5	39

Easy Packs: *Dry Mix Only*

	C	F	Cb
Buttermilk, 1.9 oz	190	1	39
Chocolate Chip, 1.9 oz	190	2.5	39

Traditional: *Dry Mix Only*

	C	F	Cb
Original, 1.7 oz	160	1	34
Buttermilk, 1.7 oz	160	1	34
Extra Light & Fluffy, 1.6 oz	150	1	32

Northern Pines,

	C	F	Cb
Premium Mix (3), 4", 3.5 oz, prep'd	200	3.5	38

Frozen Breakfasts | C | F | Cb

Aunt Jemima:

	C	F	Cb
French Toast: Cinnamon, 2 slices	210	4	35
Homestyle, 2 slices	210	4	34
Sticks, Cinnamon (4)	260	10	39
Pancakes: Blueberry (3)	260	6	45
Buttermilk (3)	260	7	44
Homestyle (3)	240	6	41
Mini Pancakes (10)	280	8	45
Low-Fat (3)	200	3	39

Eggo *(Kellogg's):*

	C	F	Cb
French Toaster Sticks: Original (2)	220	6	35
Cinnamon (2)	220	6	38
Pancakes: Blueberry (3)	260	8	42
Choc. Chip (3)	270	9	42
Waffles: Buttermilk (2)	190	8	27
Strawberry (2)	180	6	29

Krusteaz:

	C	F	Cb
French Toast, Cinnamon Swirl, Regular Cut, 3 slices	320	7	53
Pancakes:			
Blueberry (3)	290	4	55
Buttermilk (3)	290	3.5	57

Pillsbury:

	C	F	Cb
Pancakes, Buttermilk; Homestlye, (3)	230	4	45

Frozen Waffles

	C	F	Cb
Aunt Jemima: Buttermilk (2)	190	5	29
Homestyle (2)	180	5	30

Eggo *(Kellogg's):*

	C	F	Cb
Blueberry (2)	180	6	29
Chocolatey Chip (2)	200	7	31
Strawberry (2)	180	6	29
Nutri-Grain:			
Blueberry (2)	180	6	30
Whole Wheat (2)	170	6	27
Kashi, all varieties (2)	150	5	26

Nature's Path:

	C	F	Cb
Ancient Grains (2)	180	6	30
Buckwheat Wildberry (2)	190	7	33
Chia Plus; Homestyle; Maple Syrup, (2)	210	7	34
Dark Chocolate Chip (2)	220	7	34
Flax Plus (2)	190	8	27
Van's: 8 Wh. Grains, Multigrain, 2.7 oz	150	5	25
Belgian, Homestyle (2)	250	10	37
Gluten Free, Apple Cinnamon (2)	200	6	35
Mini, Chocolate Chip (8), 2 oz	160	5	29

Spaghetti/Pasta — C F Cb

- Pasta includes all shapes and sizes; (e.g. spaghetti, fettuccini, elbows, shells, twists, sheets, cannelloni, linguini, tubes, ziti).
- All regular pasta products have the same cals/fat/carbs on a weight basis.
- 1 oz Dry = approximately 2.5 -3 oz cooked.

Dry Spaghetti/Pasta

	C	F	Cb
1 oz quantity	105	0.5	21
1lb box/pkg, 16 oz	1685	7	339
Elbows, 1 cup, 4 oz	380	2	80
Shells, small, 1 cup, 3.3 oz	330	1.5	69
Spirals, 1 cup, 3 oz	305	1.5	64

Cooked Spaghetti/Pasta

Plain, All Types (no added fat):

	C	F	Cb
Firm/Al Dente (8-10 minutes), 1 oz	42	0.5	8.5
Medium (11-13 minutes), 1 oz	37	0.5	7.5
Tender (14-20 minutes), 1 oz	32	0.5	7

Longer cooking increases water absorbed

	C	F	Cb
Spaghetti: ½ cup, 2.5 oz	90	0.5	18
Medium serving, 1 cup, 5 oz	225	1.5	44
Large serving, 2 cups, 10 oz	450	3	88
Extra large, 3 cups, 15 oz	675	5	132
Elbows/Spirals, 1 cup, 5 oz	220	1.5	43
Small Shells, 1 cup, 4 oz	180	1	36
Protein-fortified: Dry, 1 c., 3.4 oz	350	2	63
Cooked, 1 cup, 5 oz	230	0.5	45
Spinach/Vegetable: Dry, 1 cup, 3 oz	310	1	61
Cooked, 1 cup, 5 oz	180	0.5	38
Whole-wheat: Dry, 1 cup, 3.8 oz	365	1.5	79
Cooked, 1 cup, 5 oz	175	1	37

Fresh Pasta (Refrigerated)

Average All Brands:
Plain/Spinach/Tomato:

	C	F	Cb
As purchased, 4.5 oz	370	3	70
Cooked, 1 cup, 5 oz	185	1.5	35
Home-made, w/o egg, cooked, 1 c. 5 oz	175	1	35
Buitoni:			
Cut Pasta:			
Angel Hair, 3 oz	230	2	43
Fettuccine/Linguine, 3 oz	240	2	45
House Foods:			
Tofu Shirataki Noodles:			
Angel Hair/Fettuccini, Macaroni/Spaghetti, 4 oz	20	0.5	3
Nasoya,			
Shirataki Spaghetti, Pasta Zero, ⅔ cup, 4 oz	15	0	4

Buitoni: *Per 1 Cup Unless Indicated*

	C	F	Cb
Agnolotti, Mushroom, 3.8 oz	280	10	34
Ravioli, Four Cheese 3.7 oz	330	12	42
Tortellini: Mixed Cheese, 3.7 oz	320	8	47
Spinach Cheese, 3.7 oz	320	7	49
Tortelloni: Swt Italian Sausage, 4 oz	350	10	51
Cheese & Roasted Garlic, 3.7 oz	280	8	39

Other Varieties ~ *See Page 112*
Pasta Sauces ~ *See Page 144*

Macaroni & Cheese

Packaged (Kraft) ~ *See Page 116*
Restaurant: *Average*

	C	F	Cb
Side Serve, 6 oz	265	13	26
Medium serve, 1 cup, 9 oz	350	17	34
Large serve, 2 cups, 18 oz	700	34	68

Noodles

	C	F	Cb
Plain/Egg: Dry, 1 oz	110	1.5	20
1 cup, 1.4 oz	145	1.5	27
Cooked: 1 oz	40	0.5	7
½ cup, 2.8 oz	110	1.5	20
1 cup, 5.5 oz	220	3.5	40
Stir-Fried: 1 cup, 5.5 oz	270	9	40
2 cup serving, 11 oz	540	18	80
Low Carb Noodles,			
Quest Pasta, 4 oz	10	0	3

Note: Carbs are from glucomannan fiber

Yolk Free (Cooked):

	C	F	Cb
Manischewitz, Yolk Free, 2 oz	200	1	41
Chinese: Cellophane/Rice, dry, 1 oz	100	0	25
Chow Mein/hard, dry, 1 oz	150	9	16
Japanese: Soba: Dry, 1 oz	95	0.5	21
Cooked, 1 cup, 4 oz	115	0.5	24
Somen: Dry, 1 oz	100	0.5	21
Cooked, 1 cup, 6 oz	230	0.5	49
Japanese Style Pan Fried,			
Yaki-Soba (*Maruchan*), av., 5.6 oz	260	3	50

Ramen Noodles ~ *See Page 118*

	C	F	Cb
Rice Noodles: Dry, 3.5 oz	365	0.5	83
Cooked, 1 cup, 6.2 oz	190	0.5	44
Yakisoba, Stir Fry, 3.5 oz	430	6	52
House Foods, Tofu Shirataki, 4 oz	20	0.5	3
Chikara, Udon, average, 7.5 oz pkt	250	1	52

Simply Asia/Thai Kitchen ~ *See Pages 119 & 121*

Egg Roll/Won Ton Wrappers

	C	F	Cb
Egg/Spring Roll (1), 0.8 oz	65	0	15
Won Ton Wrapper (1), 0.3 oz	20	0	4

Quick Guide   C   F   Cb

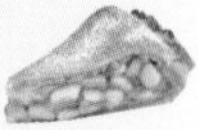

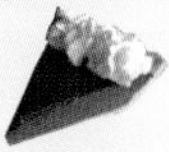

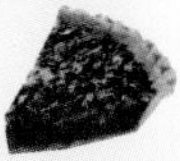

Fruit Pies: *Average All Brands, 9" Pie*
Apple; Blueberry; Cherry:

	C	F	Cb
Small Serving,			
⅛ pie, 4.8 oz	350	16	49
Medium Serving,			
⅙ pie, 6.5 oz	465	22	65
Large Serving			
¼ pie, 9.5 oz	700	33	98
Whole Pie (9"), 38 oz	2800	131	392

Other Pies: *Per Serving, ⅙ of 9" Pie*

	C	F	Cb
Chocolate Cream Pie	345	22	38
Custard: Egg Pie	220	12	22
Coconut Pie	330	18	35
Lemon Meringue Pie	305	10	53
Peach Pie	260	12	39
Pecan Pie	440	23	57
Pumpkin Pie	315	14	41
Shoo-Fly Pie	400	13	70

Dessert/Fruit Pies ~ Brands

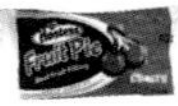

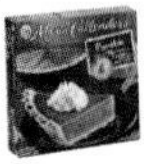

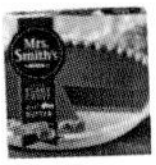

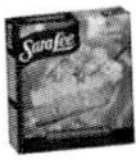

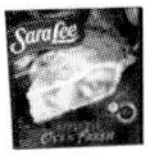

	C	F	Cb
Hostess:			
Cherry Pie, 4.5 oz	480	20	69
Lemon Pie, 4.5 oz	510	25	65
Marie Callender's:			
Banana Cream, 4.2 oz slice	310	18	35
Peach Cobbler, 4 oz slice	350	19	43
Pumpkin, 4.5 oz	340	14	49
Turtle, 4.7 oz	560	36	55
Mrs Smith's:			
Original Flaky Crust: *Per ⅛ Pie*			
Apple, 4.6 oz	340	17	45
Cherry, 4.4 oz	350	17	47
Peach, 4.6	340	19	41
Pumpkin, 4.6 oz	300	13	42
Very Berry, 4.4 oz	340	17	44
Sara Lee:			
Creme Pies:			
Chocolate, ⅕ pie, 3.9 oz	450	27	50
Coconut, ⅙ pie, 4.5 oz	370	20	44
Key Lime, ⅕ pie	410	17	60
Oven Fresh Pies: *⅛ pie, 4.27 oz Unless Indicated*			
Apple	320	16	41
Cherry	330	16	43
Dutch Apple	320	14	46
Pumpkin Pie, 4.4 oz	250	10	37
Southern Sweet Potato	270	9	41
Tastykake: Apple (1), 4 oz	270	11	40
Tasty-Klair (1), 4 oz	308	21	48

Croissants   C   F   Cb

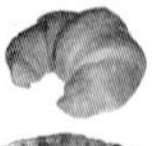

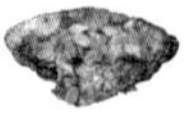

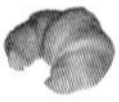

Average all Brands

	C	F	Cb
Plain/Butter/Cheese: Mini, 1 oz	115	6	13
Small, 1.5 oz	170	9	19
Medium, 2 oz	230	12	26
Large, 2.5 oz	290	15	32
Sweet Croissants:			
Almond Filled, 3 oz	330	18	39
Chocolate Filled, 3 oz	360	19	43
Dunkin' Donuts, Plain Croissant	340	18	37
Sara Lee:			
French Style: Original, 1.8 oz	185	9	21
Mini, 1 oz	230	11	26

Croissant Sandwiches ~ *See Page 165*

Pastry & Pie Crust

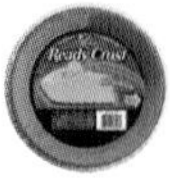

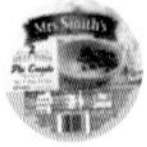

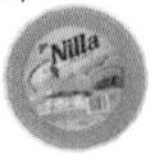

	C	F	Cb
Pie Crust, Baked, 9" diameter shell:			
1 Pie Shell, 6.5 oz	970	64	87
2-crust Pie, 9", 11.3 oz	1660	109	150
Filo Pastry: 4 sheets, 2.5 oz	210	2.5	40
Athens, Filo Dough, 5 sheets, 2 oz	170	1	36
Puff:			
Pepperidge Farm: ½ sheet	480	30	48
Bake & Fill Shell (1)	180	11	18
Arrowhead Mills,			
Graham Cracker Pie Crust, ⅛ of 9"	110	5	14
Keebler:			
Ready Crust: *Per ⅛ of 9" Crust*			
Chocolate	100	4.5	14
Graham: Regular	100	5	14
Reduced Fat	100	3.5	15
Shortbread Crust	100	5	14
Marie Callenders,			
Pie Crust, ⅛ pie, 1 oz	130	9	12
Mrs Smith's,			
Deep Dish, ⅛ pie, 1 oz	130	7	14
Nabisco:			
Honey Maid,			
Graham Cracker, ⅙ pie, 1 oz	150	5	14
Nilla, Pie Crust,			
⅙ of Pie, Crust, 1 oz	140	6	13
Pillsbury,			
Rolled, ⅛, 0.9 oz	100	6	12
Trader Joe's, Pie Crust, ⅛ pie, 1.2 oz	190	13	17

Pie Fillings ~ Canned

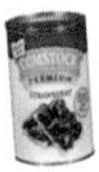

	C	F	Cb
Apple/Blueb./Cherry/Strawb., average:			
Sweetened: ⅓ cup, 3.2oz	90	0	22
1 cup, 9.5 oz	270	0	66
1 can, 21 oz	600	0	150
Light/Lite, ⅓ cup, 3.2 oz	60	0	15
Unsweetened, ⅓ cup, 3.2 oz	35	0	8
Lemon Crm/Creme, ⅓ cup, 3.2 oz	130	1.5	28

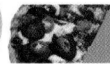

Pizzas ~ Ready to Eat C F Cb

Figures Based On Pizza Hut Unless Indicated

Cheese

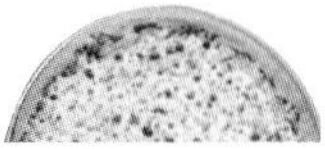

Medium Size (12"):
Hand Tossed Crust:

	C	F	Cb
⅛ Pizza (1 slice)	210	8	26
½ Pizza (4 slices)	840	32	104
Whole Pizza (8 slices)	1680	64	208
Original Pan: ⅛ Pizza (1 slice)	240	10	28
½ Pizza (4 slices)	960	40	112
Whole Pizza (8 slices)	1920	80	224

Thin 'N Crispy Crust:

⅛ Pizza (1 slice)	180	7	22
½ Pizza (4 slices)	720	28	88
Whole Pizza (8 slices)	1440	56	176

Ham & Pineapple

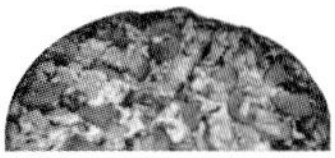

Figures Based On Domino's
Medium Size (12"):
Hand Tossed Crust:

⅛ Pizza (1 slice)	210	6	28
½ Pizza (4 slices)	840	24	112
Whole Pizza (8 slices)	1680	48	224
Handmade Pan: ⅛ Pizza (1 slice)	290	13	31
½ Pizza (4 slices)	1160	52	124
Whole Pizza (8 slices)	2320	104	248

Thin Crust:

⅛ Pizza (1 slice)	145	6.5	15
½ Pizza (4 slices)	580	26	60
Whole Pizza (8 slices)	1160	52	120

MeatZZA

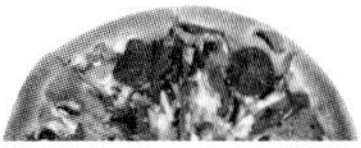

Medium Size (12"):
Hand Tossed Crust:

⅛ Pizza (1 slice)	270	12	27
½ Pizza (4 slices)	1080	48	108
Whole Pizza (8 slices)	2160	96	216
Handmade Pan: ⅛ Pizza (1 slice)	350	19	30
½ Pizza (4 slices)	1400	76	120
Whole Pizza (8 slices)	2800	152	240
Thin Crust: ⅛ Pizza (1 slice)	215	13	15
½ Pizza (4 slices)	860	52	60
Whole Pizza (8 slices)	1720	104	120

Pepperoni C F Cb

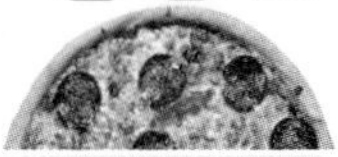

Medium Size (12"):
Hand Tossed Crust:

	C	F	Cb
⅛ Pizza (1 slice)	220	9	26
½ Pizza (4 slices)	880	36	104
Whole Pizza (8 slices)	1760	72	208
Handmade Pan: ⅛ Pizza (1 slice)	300	15	29
½ Pizza (4 slices)	1200	60	116
Whole Pizza (8 slices)	2400	120	232
Thin Crust: ⅛ Pizza (1 slice)	160	9	14
½ Pizza (4 slices)	640	36	56
Whole Pizza (8 slices)	1280	72	112

Large Pizzas

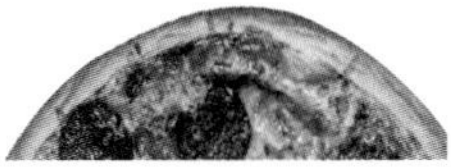

Large (14")
Hand Tossed Crust:

Cheese: ⅛ Pizza (1 slice)	290	10	36
½ Pizza (4 slices)	1160	40	144
MeatZZA: ⅛ Pizza (1 slice)	370	17	37
½ Pizza (4 slices)	1480	68	148
Pepperoni: ⅛ Pizza (1 slice)	300	12	35
½ Pizza (4 slices)	1200	48	140

Extra Large, Single Slice

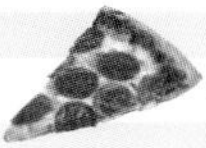

Figures Based On Sbarro

Cheese	430	15	51
Ham & Pineapple	490	16	60
Sausage	520	24	50
X-Treme Pepperoni	620	32	53

Individual Personal Pizzas

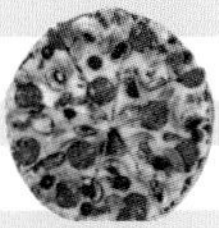

Pan (6"): Figures Based On Pizza Hut

Buffalo Chicken	640	24	72
Cheese	600	24	68
Pepperoni	640	28	68
Supreme	720	36	68
Veggie Lovers	560	20	72

Chicago-Style Deep Dish: Individual
Figures Based On Uno Pizzeria

Cheese & Tomato, 18.8 oz	1700	115	110
Chicago Classic, 25.8 oz	2220	157	112
Prima Pepperoni, 18.5 oz	1720	118	110
Sausage & Spinach Alfredo, 22.7 oz	1900	143	79

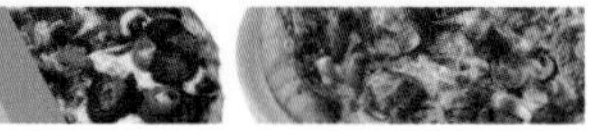

Frozen Pizzas	C	F	Cb
Amy's: *Per ⅓ Pizza*			
Cheese Pizza	290	12	33
Margherita	280	12	32
Mushroom & Olive	260	10	33
Pesto	310	12	39
Roasted Vegetable	280	9	42
California Pizza Kitchen:			
Crispy Flatbreads: *Per Piece*			
BBQ Recipe Chicken, 3.3 oz	200	6	24
Margherita, 3 oz	190	8	20
Sicilean Recipe, 4.3 oz	210	9	22
Crispy Thin Crust: *Per ⅓ Pizza*			
Margherita	320	16	31
Sicilian Recipe	360	18	30
Signature Pepperoni	350	19	29
White	320	17	30
Gluten-Free:			
BBQ Recipe Chicken, ½ pizza	330	11	43
Margherita, ⅓ pizza	220	9	27
Organic: Five Cheese & Tomato	270	10	33
Mushroom & Green Onion	240	8	33
Celeste: *Per Pizza*			
Pizza For One: Original	320	14	42
Deluxe	340	15	42
Four Cheese	330	15	38
Pepperoni	340	13	43
Sausage & Pepperoni	380	19	41
Zesty Four Cheese	350	16	43
Daiya *(Vegan):*			
Cheese Lovers, ⅓ pizza	390	17	54
Mushroom & Garlic, ⅓ pizza	390	14	58
Pepperoni Style, ⅓ pizza	470	21	64
Supreme, ¼ pizza	340	14	45
DiGiorno: *Per Slice, Unless Indicated*			
Cheese Stuffed Crust:			
Bacon Cheeseburger, ⅙ pizza, 4.5 oz	300	11	33
Five Cheese, ⅕ Pizza, 5.3 oz	370	15	41
Pepperoni, ⅕ pizza, 5.3 oz	380	16	41
Three Meat, ⅙ pizza 4.8 oz	300	12	31
Supreme, ⅙ pizza, 5 oz	350	16	35
...ic **Thin Crust**, Supreme, ...za, 5 oz	320	15	32

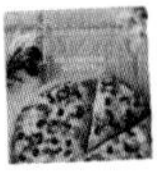

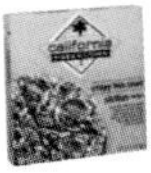

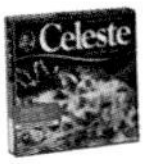

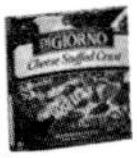

DiGiorno (Cont):	C	F	Cb
Garlic Bread: *Per ⅙ Pizza*			
Pepperoni, 5 oz	360	14	41
Supreme, 4.3 oz	280	12	32
Original Rising Crust: *Per ⅙ Pizza*			
Four Cheese, 4.7 oz	290	10	36
Italian Sausage, 5 oz	330	14	37
Spicy Chicken Supreme, 5.3 oz	290	8	37
Small Pizzas: *Per ½ Pizza*			
Cheese Stuffed Crust:			
Four Cheese, 4.2 oz	330	15	33
Pepperoni, 4.2 oz	330	16	33
Three Meat, 4.6 oz	360	18	34
Traditional Crust:			
Pepperoni, 4.6 oz	360	17	41
Three Meat, 4.7 oz	370	17	43
Freschetta:			
Brick Oven: *Per ⅕ Pizza Unless Indicated*			
5 Italian Cheese, ¼ Pizza, 5.2 oz	380	18	40
Chicken Club, ¼ Pizza, 5.5 oz	360	15	41
Pepp. & Italian Style Cheese, 4.6 oz	340	17	33
Roasted M'shrms & Spinach, 4.6 oz	270	10	34
Three Meat Medley, 4.6 oz	350	18	33
Zesty Italian Supreme, 4.6 oz	310	14	34
Naturally Rising: *Per ⅙ Pizza Unless Indicated*			
4 Cheese Medley, ⅕ Pizza, 5 oz	380	14	47
Canada Style Bacon P'apple, 4.5 oz	290	9	40
Classic Supreme, 5 oz	350	15	41
Old Fashioned Sausage, 4.7 oz	340	13	40
Signature Pepperoni, 4.5 oz	330	13	40
Jeno's: *Per Pizza*			
Crispy 'N Tasty:			
Cheese, 5 oz	310	14	38
Pepperoni, 5 oz	340	17	37
Kroger:			
3 Minute Microwave: *Per 8 oz Pizza*			
3-Meat	500	17	64
Cheese	490	16	66
Combination	520	20	64
Pepperoni	530	20	65
Supreme	490	18	63
French Bread, Pepperoni, 5 oz	380	17	42

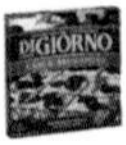

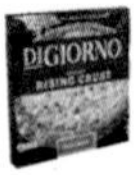

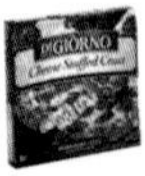

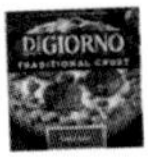

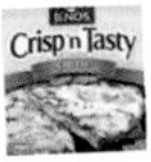

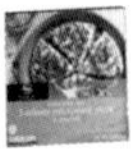

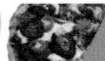

Frozen Pizzas (Cont)

C F Cb

Lean Cuisine:
	C	F	Cb
Craveables: Four Cheese, 6 oz	380	7	60
Pepperoni, 6 oz	410	9	61
Supreme, 6 oz	330	7	49
Deep Dish:			
Three Meat, 6 oz	420	9	62
Spinach & Mushroom, 6 oz	350	7	54
Thin Crust: BBQ Chicken, 6 oz	390	9	55
Margherita, 6 oz	320	4	55

Red Baron:
Brick Oven: *Per ¼ Pizza*
	C	F	Cb
Cheese Trio, 4.4 oz	320	14	36
Meat Trio, Pepperoni, 4.6 oz	340	16	36
Sausage Supreme, 4.7 oz	320	14	37

Classic Crust: *Per ¼ Pizza*
	C	F	Cb
4 Cheese, 5.2 oz	390	17	42
Sausage & Pepp., 5.3 oz	400	19	42
Supreme, 4.7 oz	320	15	34

Deep Dish Minis:
	C	F	Cb
Cheese, 4 pieces, 5.4 oz	390	14	50
Pepperoni, 4 pieces, 5.6 oz	430	20	50

Deep Dish Singles: *Per Pizza*
	C	F	Cb
Hawaiian Style, 5.3 oz	350	13	48
Meat-Trio, 5.6 oz	400	17	48
Sausage, 5.8 oz	420	19	48

Scrambles: Bacon, 5.85 oz | 440 | 21 | 47
	C	F	Cb
Sausage, 5.85 oz	430	20	47

Thin & Crispy Crust: *Per ⅓ Pizza*
	C	F	Cb
5 Cheese, 5 oz	360	16	40
Pepperoni, 5.3 oz	390	19	41
Supreme, 4.4 oz	300	15	31

Safeway Select:
Pizzeria Crust:
	C	F	Cb
Cheese Trio, ¼ pizza	340	15	34
Fajita Chkn Ole, ⅕ pizza	250	10	29
Pepperoni & Sausage, ⅕ pizza	320	17	30

Self Rising: *Per ⅙ Pizza*
	C	F	Cb
Four Cheese	300	9	41
Pepperoni	350	14	41
Sausage & Pepperoni	340	13	41

Smart Ones *(Weight Watchers):*
Classic Favorites, Thin Crust,
	C	F	Cb
Cheese Pizza, 6 oz	290	6	42

Smart Anytime, Brick Oven Style,
	C	F	Cb
Pepperoni Pizza, 6 oz	430	13	57

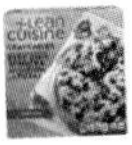

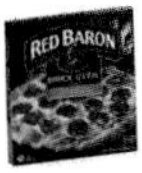

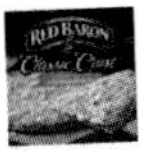

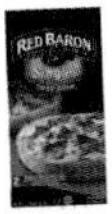

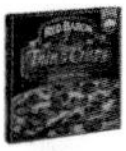

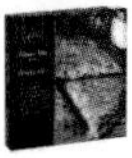

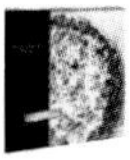

Stouffer's:
French Bread Pizzas:

C F Cb

Two Per Box:
	C	F	Cb
Deluxe (1)	430	21	44
Grilled Vegetable (1)	340	12	44
Sausage & Pepperoni (1)	460	24	43
Three Meat (1)	470	25	43

Nine Per Box:
	C	F	Cb
Cheese (1)	380	16	43
Pepperoni (1)	430	21	44

Tombstone:
Original: *Per ¼ Pizza*
	C	F	Cb
Canadian Style Bacon	310	11	35
Five Cheese	350	16	34
Pepperoni	360	18	35
Pepperoni & Sausage	350	16	35

Brick Oven Thin Crust:
	C	F	Cb
Cheese, ⅓ pizza	330	14	36
Pepperoni; Supreme, av., ¼ pizza	310	16	27

Garlic Bread Crust:
	C	F	Cb
Pepperoni, ⅙ pizza	340	15	39
Supreme, ⅙ pizza	330	13	40

Roadhouse:
	C	F	Cb
Bring on The Meat, ⅕ pizza	330	21	20
Double Down Deluxe, ⅕ pizza	310	18	21
Piled High Pepperoni, ⅕ pizza	330	21	20

Tony's:
Pizzeria Style Crust: *Per ¼ Pizza*
	C	F	Cb
Bacon Cheeseburger, 4.8 oz	360	16	39
Cheese, 4.8 oz	330	13	41
Meat Trio, 5 oz	360	16	41
Pepperoni, 4.7 oz	330	14	40
Sausage & Pepperoni, 4.87 oz	350	15	41
Supreme, 5.3 oz	350	15	42

Totino's:
Crisp Crust Party Pizza: *Per ½ Pizza*
	C	F	Cb
Canadian Bacon	320	14	37
Cheese	310	14	37
Combination	350	17	37
Hamburger	340	16	37
Pepperoni	350	18	37
Pepperoni Trio	350	18	37
Sausage	350	17	37
Triple Meat	340	16	37

Pizza Rolls:
	C	F	Cb
Pepperoni (6), 3 oz	220	9	29
Pepperoni Trio (6), 3 oz	230	10	29
Other var., (6), 3 oz	210	8	29

Trader Joe's:
	C	F	Cb
3 Cheese, ⅓ pizza	310	9	42
Parlanno, ¼ pizza	340	16	34
Pizza 4 Formaggi, ⅓ pizza	310	9	42
Spinach, ⅓ pizza	300	12	38

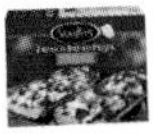

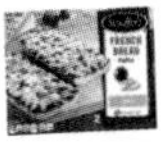

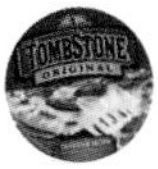

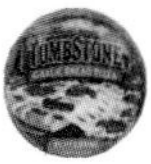

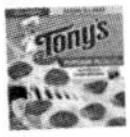

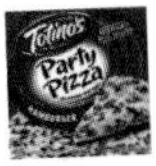

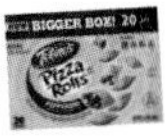

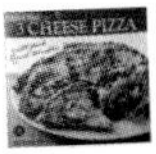

Quick Guide

	C	F	Cb

Chicken
From 3lb ready-to-cook chicken
Breast/Wing Quarter:

	C	F	Cb
Roasted: with skin	300	15	0
without skin	185	5	0
Fried, batter dipped	530	30	17

Leg Quarter:
Thigh & Drumstick:

	C	F	Cb
Roasted: with skin	270	16	0
without skin	185	8	0
Fried, batter dipped	435	25	15

KFC ~ *See Fast-Foods Section*

Per 4 oz Edible Portion

Average of Light Meat: *Per 4 oz without Bone*

	C	F	Cb
Roasted: with skin	250	12	0
without skin	175	4.5	0
Stewed: with skin	230	12	0
without skin	180	4.5	0
Fried: Batter-dipped, with skin, 4 oz	315	17	11
Flour-coated, with skin, 4 oz	280	14	2

Average of Dark Meat: *Per 4 oz without Bone*

	C	F	Cb
Roasted: with skin	290	18	0
without skin	235	11	0
Stewed: with skin	265	17	0
without skin	220	10	0
Fried: Batter-dipped, with skin, 4 oz	340	21	11
Flour-coated, with skin, 4 oz	325	19	5

Chicken Parts

Broilers or Fryers: *Edible Weights (no bone)*
Breast: *Per ½ Breast*

	C	F	Cb
Raw: with skin, 5 oz	250	14	0
without skin, 4.25 oz	140	3	0
Roasted: with skin, 3.5 oz	195	8	0
without skin, 3 oz	140	3	0
Stewed: with skin, 4 oz	200	8	0
without skin, 3.3 oz	145	3	0
Fried: Batter-dipped, w/ skin, 5 oz	365	19	13
Flour-coated, with skin, 3.5 oz	220	9	2

Drumstick: *Per Drumstick*

	C	F	Cb
Roasted: with skin, 2 oz	115	6	0
without skin, 1.5 oz	75	2.5	0
Stewed: with skin, 2 oz	115	6	0
without skin, 1.5 oz	80	3	0
Fried: Batter-dipped, w/ skin, 2.5 oz	195	11	6
Flour-coated, with skin, 1.8 oz	120	7	1

Chicken Parts (Cont)

	C	F	Cb

Broilers or Fryers (Cont): *Edible Weights (no bone)*
Thigh Portion:

	C	F	Cb
Raw: with skin, 3.3 oz			
(4¼ oz with bone)	200	14	0
without skin, 2.4 oz	80	3	0
Roasted: with skin, 2.3 oz	155	10	0
without skin, 2 oz	110	6	0
Stewed: with skin, 2.5 oz	160	10	0
without skin, 2 oz	105	5	0
Fried: Batter-dipped, with skin 3 oz	240	14	8
Flour-coated, with skin, 2.3 oz	165	9	2

Wing: *Per Wing, Bone In*
Raw Weight, 3.2 oz

	C	F	Cb
Raw: with skin	110	8	0
without skin	35	1	0
Roasted: with skin	100	7	0
without skin	45	2	0
Fried: Batter-dipped, with skin	160	11	5
Flour-coated, with skin	105	7	1
Stewed, with skin, 4 oz	100	7	0

Buffalo Wings ~ *See Fast-Foods Section*

	C	F	Cb
Neck: Simmered, with skin	95	7	0
without skin	30	2	0

Skin Only: *Skin from ½ Chicken*

	C	F	Cb
Raw skin, 3 oz	275	26	0
Roasted skin, 2 oz	255	23	0
Stewed skin, 2.5 oz	260	24	0
Fried, flour-coated, 2 oz	280	24	5
Fried, batter-dipped, 6.8 oz	750	55	44

Roasters: *Average of Light & Dark Meat*

	C	F	Cb
Roasted: with skin, 4 oz	250	15	0
without skin, 4 oz	190	8	0
Dark Meat, without skin	200	10	0
Light Meat, without skin	175	5	0

Stewing Chicken: *Per 4 oz, average of Light & Dark Meat*

	C	F	Cb
Stewed: with skin	325	22	0
without skin	270	14	0
Dark Meat, without skin	290	17	0
Light Meat, without skin	240	9	0

Capon Chicken:

	C	F	Cb
Roasted: with skin, 4 oz	260	13	0
½ Chicken, with skin, 22.5 oz	1460	74	0

Chicken Offal & Stuffing:

	C	F	Cb
Giblets: Simmered, 1 cup	230	7	0.5
Fried, flour-coated, 1 cup	400	20	6
Gizzard, simmered, 1 cup	210	4	0
Heart, simmered, 1 cup	270	12	0.2
Liver: Raw, 4 oz	130	5.5	0
Simmered, 1 cup	215	8.5	1
Liver Pate, fresh, 1 Tbsp, 0.5 oz	30	2	1
Stuffing, average, ½ cup	180	9	22

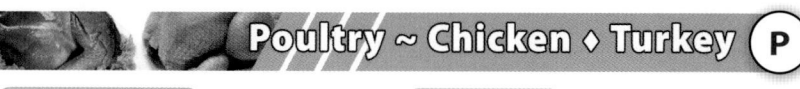

Chicken Products **C** **F** **Cb**

Bumble Bee:
Chicken In Water: *Per 2 oz Drained*

		C	F	Cb
Premium White		70	1.5	0
Premium Breast		70	1	1

Foster Farms:

	C	F	Cb
Chicken Breast Strips, grilled, 3 oz	100	2	1
Wings: Chipotle, 3 wings, 3 oz	190	13	4
Honey BBQ Glazed, 3 wings, 3 oz	190	11	7
Hot 'n' Spicy, 3 wings, 3 oz	190	14	1

Tyson:
Anytizers, Frozen:
Wings:

	C	F	Cb
Hot Wings, Buffalo Style (3)	190	13	1
Honey BBQ Seasoned (3)	190	12	8

Wyngz, Boneless:

	C	F	Cb
Buffalo Style, 3 pieces, 3 oz	150	7	8
Sweet Garlic Glazed, 3 pcs, 2.8 oz	130	5	10

Duck, Goose, Quail

Duck, Roasted:

	C	F	Cb
with skin, 3 oz	290	24	0
without skin, 3 oz	170	10	0
½ duck, with skin, 13.5 oz	1290	108	0
Goose: Roasted with skin, 3 oz	260	19	0
without skin, 3 oz	200	11	0
Pheasant, cooked, 3 oz	210	10	0
Quail, cooked, 1 whole, 6 oz	385	24	0

Turkey

Fryer-Roasters: *Per 3 oz Serving*
Roasted:

	C	F	Cb
Light Meat: with skin	140	4	0
without skin	120	1	0
Dark Meat: with skin	155	6	0
without skin	140	4	0

½ of Whole Turkey: (Approx. 3.3 lbs raw weight without neck and giblets; 1.8 lbs cooked weight)

	C	F	Cb
Roasted: with skin	1650	74	0
without skin	1125	31	0

Ground Turkey, raw: (4 oz raw wt. = 3 oz cooked wt.)

	C	F	Cb
85% lean, regular, 4 oz	170	10	0
93% lean: Average, 4 oz	160	8	0
Jennie-O, 4 oz	170	8	0
Trader Joe's, 4 oz	150	8	0
94% lean,			
Foster Farms, 4 oz	150	7	0
Breast, no skin, 4 oz	115	1	0
Patties: Small, 3 oz	130	7	0
Medium, 4 oz	170	10	0

Turkey Parts **C** **F** **Cb**

Roasted, Edible Weights, without bone:
Breast, (½), (from 17.3 oz raw weight with bone):

	C	F	Cb
with skin, 12 oz (no bone)	525	11	0
without skin, 10.8 oz	415	2	0
Back (½): with skin, 4.5 oz	265	13	0
without skin, 3.5 oz	165	6	0

Leg (Thigh & Drumstick):
(from 1 lb raw weight with bone)

	C	F	Cb
with skin, 8.5 oz (without bone)	410	13	0
without skin, 7.8 oz (w/out bone)	355	8.5	0

Wing: (From 7.3 oz raw weight)

	C	F	Cb
with skin, 3 oz (without bone)	185	9	0
without skin, 2 oz (w/out bone)	100	2	0
Neck: Simmered, 1 neck, 9 oz (with bone)	275	11	0
Giblets, simmered, 1 cup, 5 oz	240	7	3

Young Hens (Roasted)

Light Meat:

	C	F	Cb
with skin, 3 oz	175	8	0
without skin, 3 oz	135	3	0
Dark Meat: with skin, 3 oz	200	11	0
without skin, 3 oz	165	7	0

Young Toms ~ *Similar to Young Hens*

Turkey Products

Foster Farms,
  Meatballs, cooked,

	C	F	Cb
Homestyle (3)	160	9	3
Hormel, Canned Turkey Breast, in water, 2 oz	50	1	0

Jennie-O:

	C	F	Cb
Bacon, 1 slice, 0.5 oz	30	2.5	0
Bratwurst, lean, raw, 1 link, 3.85 oz	170	10	2
Burgers, raw, All Natural, White Meat, 5.3 oz	200	10	0
Meatballs, Fully Cooked: Italian, 3 oz	180	13	2
Home Style, 3 oz	180	13	3
Spam, Oven Roasted Turkey, 2 oz	80	4.5	1

Trader Joe's,

	C	F	Cb
Italian Turkey Meatloaf, 3 oz	140	8	5

Valley Fresh, 100% Natural, Canned White Turkey Breast,

	C	F	Cb
in water, 2 oz	50	1	0

White Rice   **C** **F** **Cb**

Raw:

	C	F	Cb
Glutinous, 1 cup, 6.5 oz	685	1	151
Long Grain, 1 cup, 6.5 oz	675	1	148
Short Grain, 1 cup, 7 oz	715	1	158
Wild Rice, 1 cup, 5.5 oz	570	2	120

Cooked Rice: *Boiled/Steamed*
Short/Medium Grain:

	C	F	Cb
½ cup, 3.3 oz	140	0	30
1 cup (½ Pint), 7.2 oz	265	0.5	59
2 cups (1 Pint), 13 oz	480	1	106
Long Grain: ½ cup, 2.8 oz	100	0	22
1 cup, 5.5 oz	205	0.5	44
Glutinous/Sticky, 1 cup, 6 oz	170	0.5	37
Parboiled, ½ cup, 3 oz	105	0.5	22

Precooked/Instant:

	C	F	Cb
Dry, ½ cup, 3.5 oz	380	1	82
Cooked, ½ cup, 3 oz	95	0.5	21
Wild Rice, Cooked, 1 cup, 5.8 oz	165	0.5	35

Brown Rice

Average of Short or Long Grain

	C	F	Cb
Raw/Dry: ½ cup, 3.3 oz	340	2.5	71
1 cup, 6.5 oz	685	5.5	143
Cooked: ½ cup, 3.5 oz	110	1	22
1 cup, 7 oz	220	2	46

Rice Dishes   **C** **F** **Cb**

	C	F	Cb
Chinese Fried Rice:			
½ cup, 2.5 oz	140	4.5	21
1 cup, (½ Pint), 5 oz	280	9	42
2 cups, (1 Pint), 10 oz	565	18	84
Mexican Style Rice:			
Taco Time, Seasoned, 4.6 oz	200	3	40
Rice-A-Roni ~ *See Page 119*			
Rice with Raisins/Pinenuts, 1 cup	400	11	60
Rice Pilaf: Restaurant, 1 cup	275	7.5	46
O'Charley's, side dish, 1 portion	160	4	27
Rice Pudding,			
Kozy Shack, Original, 1 pudding cup	130	2.5	24
Risotto, 1 cup	420	12	70
Saffron Rice, 4 oz	175	7	25
Spanish Rice: 1 cup, 5 oz	390	9	72
El Pollo Loco, Small, 4.5 oz	170	2.5	33
Sticky Rice, 1 cup, 5 oz	155	0.5	34
Sushi Rice: 1 Tbsp	25	0	5
1 cup, 5.2 oz	390	0	77
Other Packaged Rice Products:			
Uncle Ben's / Zatarain's ~ *See Page 121*			

CalorieKing.com Recipes

See the CalorieKing website for a *salubrious selection of healthy recipes* – all analyzed for calories, fat, protein, carbohydrate, fiber and sodium.

Choose from:
- *Starters/Appetizers*
- *Salads*
- *Entrees: Meat, Fish and Chicken*
- *Vegetarian*
- *Desserts*
- *Cakes, Cookies*
- *Drinks*

www.CalorieKing.com/recipes

HEALTHY RECIPE TIPS

- **Use non-fat milk** in place of whole or 2% milk
- **Use low-fat yogurt** in place of sour cream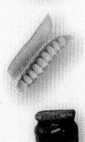
- **Skim fat** from surface of soups and casseroles after cooling
- **Add extra vegetables** to soups and hot entreés
- **Cakes/cookies/muffins:** Replace most or all the fat/oil with applesauce and/or prune puree (Example, *Sunsweet Lighter Bake*)
- **Drinks:** Replace sugar with no-calorie sweeteners such as *Equal, Stevia, Splenda* and *Sweet 'N Low*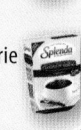

Deli Salads

	C	F	Cb
Average All Outlets			
Antipasto Salad, 1/2 cup	135	8	13
3-Bean Salad, 1/2 cup	90	4.5	12
Bulgur Salad, 1/2 cup	70	2	12
Caesar Salad, Classic, 1 cup	200	14	15
Side Salad, without Dressing	25	0	6
Carrot Raisin: with Dressing, 1/2 cup	135	12	6
without Dressing, 1/2 cup	20	0	5
Chef's Salad: Regular, w/o Dressing	620	37	8
with 2 oz Thousand Island Drssng	860	61	8
Chicken Salad, 1/2 cup/scoop, 4 oz	280	21	2
Coleslaw: Traditional, 1/2 cup	150	8	18
w/ Low Cal Dressing, 1/2 c.	50	2	8
Corn, Mexican, 1/2 cup	240	12	33
Cucumber: Non-Oil Dressing, 1/2 cup	60	0	14
with Oil Dressing, 1/2 cup	140	12	8
Eggplant Salad, 1/2 cup	75	5	7
Fettucini, with veges, 1/2 cup	135	6	16
Garden Salad, without Dressing, 1 cup	10	0	2
Greek Salad, 1 cup	105	8	7
Greek Vegetables, 1 cup	110	8	6
Lobster Salad, 1/2 cup, 4 oz	250	21	11
Macaroni Salad, 1/2 cup, 5 oz	360	26	26
Nicoise, 1 cup	450	32	18
Pasta Salad, 1/2 cup	200	11	19
Potato Salad: Dijon, 3 oz	120	7	13
with Mayonnaise, 1/2 cup, 4 oz	215	15	17
Lowfat, 1/2 cup	110	1.5	21
Rice Salad, 1/2 cup	150	10	13
Saffron Rice, 4 oz	175	7	25
Spinach Salad, 1 cup	180	13	13
Tabouli, 1/2 cup	125	7	13
Three Bean Salad, 1/2 cup	90	4.5	12
Tomato & Mozzarella, 1/2 cup	180	14	10
Tortellini, with Basil Pesto, 1/2 cup	150	9	15
Waldorf, with Mayo, 1/2 cup	110	7	12
Signature Salads: *Per 6 oz Serving*			
(Supplied to Deli's and Institutions)			
Antipasto Salad	510	50	4
Artichoke Salad, marinated	400	41	8
California Medley	120	7	15
Cheese Agnolotti	250	8	23
Chicken Salad	420	33	11
Crabmeat Flavored	450	38	20
Egg Salad	300	23	14
Fresh Button Mushroom	190	16	6

Signature Salads (Cont): *Per 6 oz*	C	F	Cb
Fresh Button Mushroom	190	16	6
Ham Salad	400	32	14
Prima Pasta Salad	360	30	18
Seafood Pasta Del Mar	170	10	21
Seafood, Crab & Shrimp	420	34	20
Shrimp Salad	360	32	8
Tuna Salad	450	36	14

~ Also See Fast-Foods & Restaurants Section

Fresh Salad Packs

Pre-Packaged (Supermarkets):	C	F	Cb
Dole:			
Kits: *Per 3.5 oz, with Dressing*			
Caesar: Original	150	12	8
Kale	210	15	11
Chopped:			
Chipotle & Cheddar	120	9	10
Sesame Asian	160	16	13
Southwest	120	9	9
Salad Blends: *Without Dressing*			
American; Mediterranean, 3 oz	15	0	3
Arugula; Baby Spinach, 3 oz	20	0	3
Fresh Express:			
Complete Salad Kits: *Per 3 1/2 oz, Prepared*			
Asian	120	5	17
Caesar: Classic	150	12	7
Lite	90	6	7
Supreme	160	14	6
Pear Gorganzola	130	6	17
Gourmet Cafe: *Per Package*			
Chopped Santa Fe	290	19	18
Tuscan	330	28	9
Ready Pac:			
Bistro Bowls: *Per Container, with Dressing*			
Apple Bleu Pecan, 4.5 oz	230	14	23
Caprese, 5 oz	210	17	12
Cranb. Walnut, 4.5 oz	210	9	26
Kale, Apple Veggie, 5.5 oz	240	13	31
Spinach Dijon, 4.76 oz	280	19	20
Turkey & Bacon Cobb, 7.3 oz	290	22	6

Salad Toppings

	C	F	Cb
Bac'n Pieces,			
McCormick, 1Tbsp, 0.3 oz	30	1	2
Bacon Bits *(Hormel)*, 1Tbsp	25	1.5	0
Bac-Os, Bits *(Betty Crocker)*, 1 Tbsp	30	1	2
Chow Mein Noodles,			
dry, 1/2 cup	120	7	13
Croutons, 2 Tbsp, 0.3 oz	40	1	7
Salad Toppins,			
McCormick, 4 tsp	35	1.5	3
Sunflower Seeds, 1 Tbsp, 0.3 oz	45	4	1.5
Toasted Sliced Almonds, 2 T., 0.5 oz	85	7	3

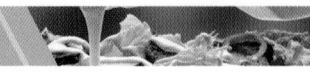

S — Salad Dressings

Quick Guide

C **F** **Cb**

Salad Dressings

Average All Brands: *Per 2 Tbsp, Approx 1 fl.oz*

	C	F	Cb
Balsamic Vinaigrette:			
Regular	90	9	3
Light, 2 Tbsp	45	4	2
Fat Free, 2 Tbsp	25	0	6
Blue Cheese: Regular, 2 Tbsp	145	15	1.5
Regular, ¼ cup, 2 oz	280	30	3
Light, 2 Tbsp	30	1	4
Caesar: Regular, 2 Tbsp	165	17	1
Regular, ¼ cup, 2 oz	310	34	2
Light, 2 Tbsp	35	1.5	5.5
Coleslaw: Regular, 2 Tbsp	125	11	8
Regular, ¼ cup, 2 oz	245	21	15
Light, 2 Tbsp	110	7	14
French: Regular	145	14	5
Regular, ¼ cup, 2 oz	260	25	9
Light, 2 Tbsp	65	4	9
Fat/Oil-Free, 2 Tbsp	40	0	10
Italian: Regular, 2 Tbsp	85	8.5	3
Regular, ¼ cup, 2 oz	165	16	6
Light, 2 Tbsp	55	5.5	2
Fat/Oil-Free, 2 Tbas	15	0	2.5
Ranch: Regular, 2 Tbsp	145	16	2
Regular, ¼ cup, 2 oz	290	30	4
Light, 2 Tbsp	60	4	6.5
Fat-Free, 2 Tbsp	35	0.5	8
Thousand Island: Reg., 2 T.	115	11	4.5
Regular, ¼ cup, 2 oz	210	20	9
Light, 2 Tbsp	60	3.5	7
Fat-Free, 2 Tbsp	40	0.5	10

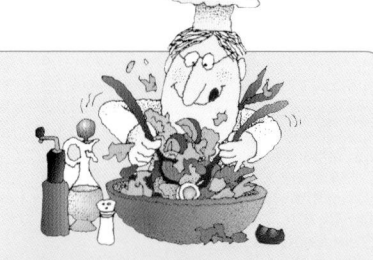

Enjoy a healthy salad but don't drown it in high-fat salad dressings.

Use 'light' dressings to halve the fat and calories.

Brands ~ Salad Dressings

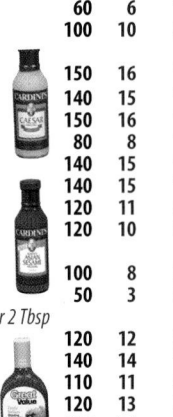

	C	F	Cb
Annie's Naturals: *Per 2 Tbsp*			
Organic: Goddess Dressing	120	12	2
Green Garlic	80	8	2
Papaya Poppy Seed	90	8	5
Thousand Island	90	8	5
Vinaigrettes:			
Red Wine & Olive Oil	140	14	1
Sesame Ginger	90	8	4
Shitake & Sesame	120	13	1
Bernstein's: *Per 2 Tbsp*			
Creamy Caesar	120	13	1
Herb Garden French	130	12	6
Italian	110	12	1
Restaurant Recipe Italian	120	12	1
Fat-Free, Cheese & Garlic Italian	10	0	2
Light Fantastic: Cheese Fantastico	30	1.5	3
Roasted Garlic Balsamic	45	3.5	3
Best Foods: *Per 1 Tbsp Unless Indicated*			
Dijonnaise, 1 tsp	5	0	0
Mayonnaise: Real	100	11	0
Light	35	3.5	1
Low-Fat	15	1	2
Canola	40	4	1
Olive Oil	60	6	1
Mayonesa, Lemon-Lime	100	10	0
Cardini's: *Per 2 Tbsp*			
Aged Parmesan Ranch	150	16	1
Caesar: Original	140	15	1
Garlic Lemon	150	16	1
Light Caesar	80	8	1
Red Jalapeno	140	15	1
Three Cheese	140	15	1
Honey Mustard	120	11	6
Roasted Asian Sesame	120	10	6
Vinaigrette, Balsamic:			
Regular	100	8	5
Lite	50	3	5
Great Value *(Walmart):* Per 2 Tbsp			
Caesar	120	12	2
Ranch: Bacon	140	14	1
Buttermilk	110	11	2
Chipotle	120	13	2
Classic	130	14	1
Zesty Italian	60	4.5	3
Hampton Creek *(Vegan):* Per 1 Tbsp			
Just Mayo:			
Original	90	10	0
Chipotle	60	6	1
Garlic	100	10	0
Sriracha	90	10	1

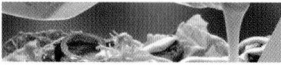

Brands ~ Salad Dressings (Cont)

Hidden Valley: *Per 2 Tbsp*

	C	F	Cb
Greek: Creamy Caesar; Cucumber Dill	60	5	3
Lemon Garlic	60	5	4
Ranch	60	5	3
Ranch: Bacon	140	14	1
Buffalo	110	1	2
Fiesta Salsa, Light	60	5	3
Ranch	60	5	3
Southwest Chipotle	100	10	2
Simply Ranch: Chili Lime	120	12	2
Classic Ranch	110	12	2
Cucumber Basil	110	12	2

Kraft: *Per 2 Tbsp*

Regular Dressings:

	C	F	Cb
Asian Toasted Sesame	80	6	2
Blue Cheese	120	12	1
Buttermilk Ranch	100	12	1
Catalina Classic	90	6	3
Classic Caesar	110	11	3
Creamy Balsamic	90	8	1
Creamy Italian	80	7	1
Cucumber Ranch	110	11	1
Honey Mustard	90	6	3
Zesty Catalina	90	6	3
Zesty Italian	60	4.5	1
Fat Free: French Style	45	0	4
Italian	15	0	1
Thousand Island	50	0	4
Lite: Catalina	60	1	4
House Italian	35	1	2
Raspberry Vinaigrette	30	1	2
Zesty Italian	25	1	1

Seven Seas:

	C	F	Cb
Green Goddess	100	8	2
Viva Italian Anything	50	4.5	1

Marie's: *Per 2 Tbsp*

Classics:

	C	F	Cb
Chunky Blue Cheese	160	17	1
Coleslaw	140	13	7
Creamy Caesar	120	13	1
Creamy Italian Garlic	180	19	1
Creamy Ranch	180	19	1
Super Blue Cheese	160	17	1
Thousand Island	150	15	3
Ranch: Buttermilk	150	16	1
Parmesan	170	19	1
Vinaigrette: Blue Cheese	120	11	4
Garlic Parmesan	110	11	2
Mango Chardonnay	120	11	6
Mediterranean	110	12	2
Rst'd Tomato w/ Parmesan & Basil	130	13	2

Marzetti's: *Per 2 Tbsp*

	C	F	Cb
Creamy: Aged Parm. Ranch	140	14	2
Asiago Peppercorn	130	14	2
Chunky Blue Cheese	150	15	1
Cilantro Avocado	110	12	1
Classic Ranch	160	17	1
Creamy Caesar	120	12	2
Fat Free Sweet & Sour	45	0	12
Potato Salad	160	15	6
Light: Chunky Blue Cheese	90	7	4
Classic Ranch	80	8	2
Honey French	80	3.5	12
Original Slaw	90	7	7
Poppyseed	90	5	9
Supreme Caesar	70	7	2
Simply Dressed: Avocado Ranch	120	13	1
Blue Cheese	130	14	1
Caesar	120	12	1
Cucumber Ranch	80	8	2
Thousand Island	130	12	5
Vinaigrette: Balsamic	90	9	4
Champagne	80	8	2
Pomegranate	60	4.5	6

Newman's Own: *Per 2 Tbsp*

	C	F	Cb
Regular: Creamy Balsamic	100	8	7
Creamy Caesar	150	16	1
Family Recipe Italian	130	13	1
Honey Dijon Mustard	140	13	6
Roasted Garlic	50	4	3
Light: Balsamic Vinaigrette	45	4	2
Caesar	70	6	3
Italian	60	6	1

Wish-Bone: *Per 2 Tbsp*

	C	F	Cb
Creamy: Caesar	180	18	1
Deluxe French	120	11	5
Italian	110	10	4
Ranch	130	13	2
Russian	110	6	14
Thousand Island	130	12	5
Light: Blue Cheese	70	6	2
Creamy Caesar	70	6	2
Honey Dijon	70	5	6
Italian	35	2.5	3
Parmesan Peppercorn Ranch	60	5	2
Ranch	70	5	4
Thousand Island	60	5	4
Fat-Free:			
Chunky Blue Cheese	30	0	7
Ranch	30	0	6
Oil & Vinegar:			
Balsamic Vinaigrette	60	5	3
House Italian	110	10	3
Red Wine Vinaigrette	70	5	6
Robusto Italian	80	7	4

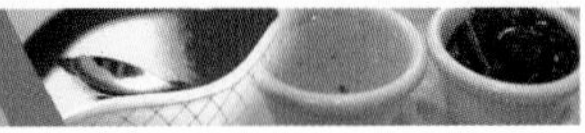

Gravy

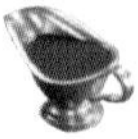
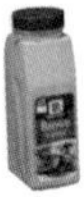

Gravy	C	F	Cb
Homemade Gravy, average:			
Thin, little fat, 2 Tbsp, 1 oz	20	1	3
Thick: 2 Tbsp, 1.3 oz	50	2	9
¼ cup, 2.5 oz	100	4	18
McCormick:			
Brown, 1 Tbsp	25	0.5	3
Turkey, 1 Tbsp	20	0.5	4

Gravy-In-Jars

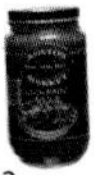
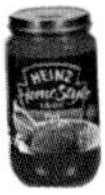

Gravy-In-Jars	C	F	Cb
Boston Market, Classic Beef, ¼ cup, 2 oz	30	1	4
Campbell's, Beef/Chicken/Turkey, ¼ cup, 2 oz	25	1	3
Heinz: *Per ¼ Cup, 2 oz*			
Homestyle: Bistro Au Jus	20	0.5	2
Classic Chicken	30	2	3
Pork; Rich Mushroom	20	0.5	3
Roasted Turkey	25	1	3
Savory Beef	30	1	4
Safeway, all varieties, ¼ cup, 2 oz	20	0.5	4

Tomato Products

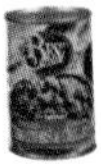
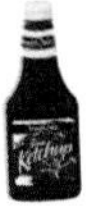
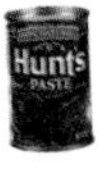
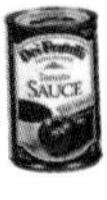
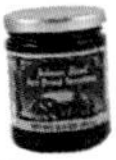

Tomato Products	C	F	Cb
Whole/Chopped/Crushed/Diced:			
Regular: 1 cup, 8.5 oz	50	0	10
In Aspic, ½ cup	50	0	12
with Green Chili, 1 c., 8.5 oz	60	0	16
Stewed, ½ cup, 1.7 oz	40	1.5	7
Wedges in Tomato Juice, 1 cup	70	0.5	18
Salsa, average, 2 Tbsp, 1 oz	25	0	6
Tomato Ketchup:			
Regular: 1 Tbsp, 0.5 oz	15	0	4
Single Serve, 1 packet	10	0	3
Heinz, Simply Heinz 1 Tbsp, 0.5 oz	15	0	4
Tomato Paste:			
Regular: 2 Tbsp, 1 oz	25	0	6
¾ cup, 6 oz	140	1	32
Tomato Puree, ½ cup, 4.5 oz	50	0	10
Tomato Sauce:			
Regular, ½ cup, 4.4 oz	50	0	11
Spanish Style, ½ cup, 4.3 oz	40	0	9
with Mushr., ½ cup, 4.3 oz	45	0	10
with Onions, ½ cup, 4.3 oz	50	0	12
Tomato Seasoning, 3 tsp	20	0	4
Sundried Tomatoes:			
Natural, 5-6 pieces, 0.4 oz	20	0	5
In Oil, drained, 6 pieces, 0.5 oz	40	2.5	4

Sauces ~ Brands

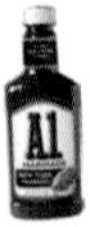
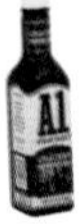
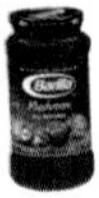
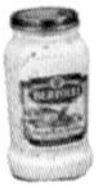
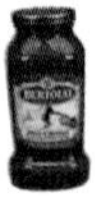
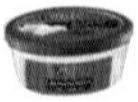
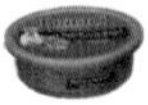
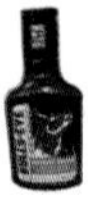
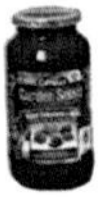

Sauces ~ Brands	C	F	Cb
A-1:			
Marinades: *Per Tbsp, ½ oz*			
Chicago Steakhouse	20	1	1
Classic	15	0	1
New Orleans Cajun	25	0	2
New York Steakhouse	20	0	2
Steak Sauce: Original	15	0	1
Bold & Spicy	20	0	1
Cracked Peppercorn	15	0	1
Sweet Hickory	25	0	2
Thick & Hearty	25	0	2
Barilla:			
Pasta Sauces: *Per ½ Cup, Unless Indicated*			
Chunky Traditional	60	1	13
Creamy Alfredo	70	6	4
Garlic Alfredo	60	5	4
Marinara	70	1	14
Meat Sauce; Mushroom	60	1	13
Sun-Dried Tomato Pesto, ¼ cup	130	10	7
Traditional Basil Pesto, ¼ cup	200	19	5
Bertolli:			
Alfredo Sauces: *Per ¼ Cup*			
Creamy Basil	100	10	2
Four Cheese Rosa	110	10	5
Garlic Romano w/ Parmesan	100	10	2
Traditional: *Per ½ Cup*			
Five Cheese	90	3.5	14
Portobello Mushroom	70	2.5	9
Vodka	150	9	11
Buitoni:			
Pasta Sauces:			
Alfredo: Regular, ¼ cup	150	14	3
Light, ¼ cup	90	6	4
Marinara, ½ cup	70	3	9
Pesto: with Basil, ¼ cup	290	27	5
Reduced Fat, ¼ cup	230	18	8
Bull's-Eye: *Per 2 Tbsp*			
BBQ Sauce: Original	50	0	4
Hickory Smoke	60	0	5
Regional, average all varieties	50	0	4
Catelli: *Per ½ Cup*			
Pasta, Garden Select Six Vegetable:			
Country Mushroom	70	1.5	11
Diced Tomato & Basil	70	1	12
Meat Sauce	80	2.5	11
Pizza Sauce, all varieties	60	1.5	11

Sauces ~ Brands (Cont)	C	F	Cb
Cento:			
Arrabbiata, ½ cup	60	3.5	6
Italiano, ¼ cup	25	0	6
Marinara, ¼ cup	60	3.5	6
Porcini Mushroom Sauce, ½ cup	80	4	7
Puttanesca, ½ cup	70	4.5	6
Vodka, ½ cup	100	5	8
Classico:			
Alfredo: *Per ¼ Cup*			
Creamy	60	4.5	3
Roasted Garlic	60	4	4
Family Favorites: *Per ½ Cup*			
Meat	60	1	10
Parmesan & Romano	70	2	10
Traditional	80	2.5	13
Riserva: Arrabbiata, 4.4 oz	60	1	11
Eggplant & Artichoke, 4.4 oz	60	1.5	10
Puttanesca			
Tomato Cream Sauces: *Per ½ Cup*			
Creamy Tomato & Rsd Garlic	35	1.5	5
Four Cheese Tomato	40	2	5
Spicy Tomato & Parmesan	40	2	5
Contadina:			
Pizza Sauce: *Per 2.2 oz*			
Flavored with Pepperoni	35	1	6
Original; Four Cheese	30	0.5	6
Tomato Sauce, average	20	0.5	4
Crosse & Blackwell:			
Meat: Ham Glaze, 1 Tbsp	25	0	7
Mint Meat Sauce, 1 tsp	5	0	2
Seafood:			
Cocktail, ¼ cup, 2.5 oz	90	0	21
Shrimp Sauce, ¼ cup, 2.5 oz	90	0	21
Dave's Gourmet:			
Pasta Sauce: *Per ½ cup*			
Butternut Squash	100	4	17
Creamy Parmesan Romano	120	8	8
Hearty Marinara	70	3.5	9
Red Heirloom	45	1.5	7
Rstd Garlic & Sweet Basil	70	4.5	8
Spicy Heirloom Marinara	45	1.5	7
Wild Mushroom	80	3	11
Del Monte:			
Pasta Sauces: *Per ½ cup*			
Four Cheese; Traditional, av.	60	1	12
Mushroom	60	1	11
Average other varieties	60	1	13
Sloppy Joe Sauce: *Per ¼ cup*			
Hickory	60	0	14
Original	60	0	13

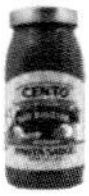

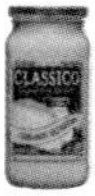

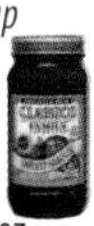

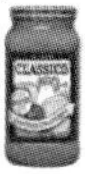

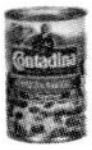

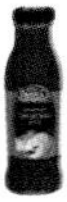

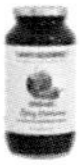

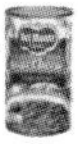

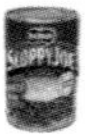

	C	F	Cb
Emeril's:			
Alfredo, Four Cheese Sauce, ¼ cup	60	5	4
Pasta Sauces: *Per ½ Cup*			
Homestyle Marinara	90	3	14
Kicked Up Tomato	80	3.5	11
Roasted Gaaahlic	80	3.5	12
Roasted Red Pepper	70	3.5	9
Vodka Sauce	110	7	12
Francesco Rinaldi:			
Alfredo, all flavors, ¼ cup	90	8	2
Cheese,			
Three Cheese, ½ cup	70	1	15
Garden, all var., ½ cup	60	1	12
Meat: Meat Flavored, ½ cup	70	2.5	13
Sicilian Family, Sausage, ½ cup	70	2.5	11
Pizza, ¼ cup	20	0	4
Tomato, Marinara, ½ cup	60	1	12
French's,			
Worcestershire Sauce, 1 tsp	0	0	1
Heinz: *Per 1 Tbsp*			
57 Steak Sauce	20	0	4
Chili Sauce	20	0	5
Cocktail Sauce, Original,			
¼ cup, 2.2 oz	70	0	18
Horseradish Sauce	75	6	3
Tomato Ketchup: Regular	20	0	5
Reduced Sugar	5	0	1
Worcestershire Sauce	5	0	1
House of Tsang:			
Bangkok Peanut Sce, 1.16 oz	70	5	9
Classic Sauce, 0.6 oz	25	0.5	5
Ginger Sriracha Sauce, 1.23 oz	15	0	4
General Tsao, 0.67 oz	45	0.5	10
Green Thai Curry Sauce, 1.1 oz	60	4	6
Korean Teriyaki Sauce, 0.67 oz	35	1	6
Oyster Flavored Sauce, 0.63 oz	30	0	7
Saigon Sizzle Sauce 0.63 oz	45	1	8
Sweet & Sour Sauce, 0.63 oz	35	0	8
Hunt's:			
BBQ Sauce, Original, 2 Tbsp	60	0	16
Hickory & Brown Sugar BBQ Sce, 2 Tbsp	50	0	13
Manwich, Sloppy Joe Sauce,			
Original, ¼ cup, 2.3 oz	35	0	8
Pasta Sauce: *Per ½ Cup*			
Four Cheese	60	1	10
Garlic & Herb	40	1	8
Meat Flavor	60	1	10
Mushroom	50	0.5	10
Traditional	60	1	11

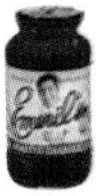

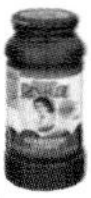

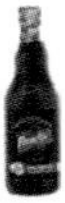

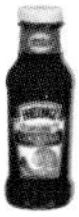

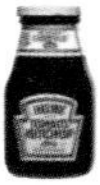

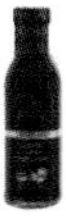

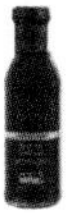

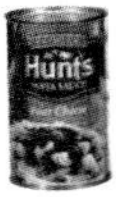

Brands (Cont)

	C	F	Cb
Kikkoman: *Per Tablespoon*			
Marinade: Gourmet Teriyaki	30	0	7
Honey & Mustard	30	0	6
Roasted Garlic & Herbs	20	0	4
Toasted Sesame	40	0.5	8
Asian Authentics: *Per Tbsp, Unless Indicated*			
Katsu	20	0	5
Kotteri Mirin	50	0	12
Plum Sauce, 2 Tbsp	90	1	21
Sukiyaki	20	0	4
Tempura	5	0	1
Unagi Sushi Sauce	40	0	10
Wasabi Sauce, 1 tsp	15	1	1
Knorr:			
Classic Sauce: *Per Whole Package*			
Bernaise, dry mix only	100	0	20
Hollandaise, dry mix only	100	0	20
Kraft:			
Barbecue Sauce, 2 Tbsp	60	0	5
Coleslaw 1.2 oz	80	4.5	3
Horseradish, 1 oz	100	9	1
Sandwich Spread, 1 Tbsp	30	2	1
Tartar, 1 Tbsp	60	5	1
Las Palmas: *Per ¼ Cup*			
Green Enchilada Sauce, all varieties, 2 oz	25	1.5	3
Red Chili Sauce,	15	0.5	3
La Victoria,			
Red/Green Enchilada Sauce, av., 2 oz	15	0.5	3
Lawry's:			
30 Minute Marinade: *Per Tbsp*			
Caribbean Jerk	30	0	7
Herb & Garlic; Lemon Pepper	10	0	2
Mesquite, w/ Lime Juice	10	0	2
Sesame Ginger, w/ Mandarin	30	0	7
Steak & Chop, w/ Garl. Pepp.	5	0	0.5
Packet Seasonings: *Dry*			
Fajitas; Taco, average, 2 tsp	15	0	3
Other varieties, average, 2 tsp	20	0	4
Lea & Perrins:			
Steak Sauce, Bold, 1 Tbsp	20	0	5
Worcestershire Sauce: Original 1 tsp, 5 ml	5	0	1
Reduced Sodium	5	0	1

	C	F	Cb
McCormicks:			
Seafood Sauces: *Per 2 Tbsp*			
Asian	50	1.5	7
Cajun Style	15	0	3
Lemon Butter Dill	100	9	4
Lemon Herb	140	15	0.5
Mediterranean; Santa Fe Style	20	0	4
Scampi	160	17	2
Mrs. Dash			
Marinades: *Per 1 Tbsp*			
Garlic Herb	15	0	3
Lemon Pepper	10	0	2
Lime Garlic	15	0	3
Sweet Teriyaki	35	0	9
Newman's Own: *Per ½ Cup*			
Pasta Sauce: Five Cheese	80	2.5	11
Marinara; Sockarooni	70	1	12
Roasted Garlic	60	1.5	11
Tomato & Basil Bombolina	70	2	11
Vodka	140	9	11
O Organics *(Von's): Per ½ Cup*			
Marinara; Roasted Garlic, av.	60	1.5	9
Mushroom; Tomato Basil	50	1.5	8
Old El Paso:			
Enchilada Sauce:			
Green, ¼ cup, 2.15 oz	25	1.5	4
Red, ¼ cup, 2.1 oz	20	0	4
Taco Sauce, all varieties, 1 Tbsp	5	0	1
Pace: *Per 2 Tbsp*			
Picante Sauce	10	0	2
Salsa: Thick & Chunky, av.	10	0	3
Fire, Chipotle & Jalapeno	10	0	2
Restaurant Style, Peach Mango	10	0	3
Prego: *Per ½ Cup, Unless Indicated*			
Alfredo, average all varieties, ¼ cup	70	6	3
Classic Italian:			
Fresh Mushroom; Traditional	70	1.5	12
Marinara	90	5	8
Tomato Basil Garlic	70	2.5	11
Farmers Market: Classic Marinara	90	5	9
Four Cheese; Roasted Garlic, av.	80	3.5	9
Garden Vegetable	60	2	8
Mushroom; Trad. Basil, average	70	2.5	9
Pizza Sauce, Pizzeria Style, ¼ cup	35	1	6
Pemium Pasta: Creamy Vodka	140	7	15
Italian, with Bacon & Provolone	100	3	15
Pesto Marinara	90	3	13
Spicy Sausage	110	4	15
Premier Japan,			
Hoisin; Teriyaki, 1 Tbsp	15	0	3

Brands (Cont)

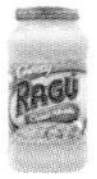

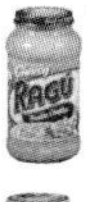

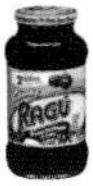

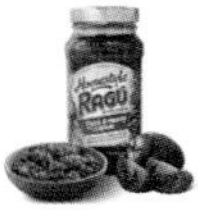

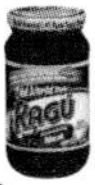

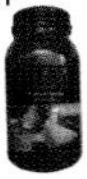

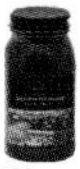

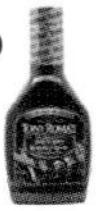

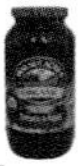

	C	F	Cb
Ragu:			
Cheesy: *Per ¼ Cup*			
Classic Alfredo	90	8	2
Creamy Tomato	90	8	4
Double Cheddar	100	9	2
Four Cheese	80	8	2
Light Parmesan Alfredo	60	4	2
Roasted Garlic Parmesan	100	9	3
Six Cheese	90	2.5	14
Chunky: *Per ½ Cup*			
Roasted Garlic	90	2.5	14
Average other varieties	90	2.5	14
Homestyle, Thick & Hearty: *Per ½ Cup*			
Four Cheese	90	2	14
Meat	90	2.5	15
Mushroom	90	2.5	16
Roasted Garlic	90	2.5	15
Rstd Peppers & Garlic	70	1	14
Tomato & Basil	90	2.5	15
Traditional	100	2.5	16
Old World Style: *Per ½ Cup*			
Flavored with Meat	80	2.5	10
Marinara	80	2.5	11
Traditional	80	2	13
Pizza: Homemade Style, ¼ cup	30	1	5
Quick Sauce, Traditional, ¼ cup	45	1.5	6
Safeway Select:			
Salsa, all varieties, average, 2 Tbsp	15	0	3
Select Sauces: *Per ½ Cup*			
Arrabbiata	110	8	10
Artichoke Pesto	60	2	9
Four Cheese	80	3.5	11
Marinara	60	2	10
Spicy Red Bell Pepper	50	1	9
Sundried Tomato & Olive	60	1.5	11
Tomato Alfredo; Vodka	130	10	9
Taco Bell, Creamy Jalapeno Sauce,			
1 Tablespoon, 0.5 oz	70	7	1
Tony Roma's:			
Bold & Spicy BBQ Sauce, 2 Tbsp	50	0	12
Carolina Honeys BBQ Sauce,			
2 Tablespoons	70	0	18
Trader Joe's:			
BBQ Sauce,			
Kansas City Style, 2 Tbsp	60	0	15
Tomato Basil Marinara, ½ cup	80	4.5	10
Walnut Acres,			
Organic Pasta Sauces,			
average all var., ½ cup, 4.5 oz	60	1	11

Seasonings & Flavorings

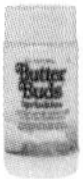

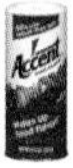

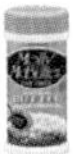

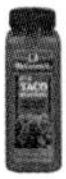

	C	F	Cb
Auromatic Bitters *(Angostua)*, 1 tsp	15	0	4
Bacon Bits, average, 1 Tbsp	35	2	2
Bacon Chips *(Durkee)*, 1 Tbsp	30	1	2
Bac-Os *(Betty Crocker)*,			
1Tbsp	30	1.5	2
Blends *(Mrs Dash)*, 1 tsp	0	0	0
Butter Buds, 1 tsp	5	0	2
Flavor Enhancer *(Accent)*, 1 tsp	0	0	0
Flavor Sprinkles *(Molly McButter)*,			
Natural/Cheese, 1 tsp	5	0	1
Garlic Bread Sprinkle, 1 tsp	8	0.5	1
Garlic Salt, 1 tsp	2	0	0
Italian Seasoning, 1 tsp	4	0	1
Lemon Pepper Seasoning,			
1 tsp	7	0	1
Meat Tenderizer, av., 1 tsp	7	0	1
Salad Crunchies *(McCormick)*,			
1 tsp	10	0.5	2
Salt, Reg., Sea Salt, Lite Salt	0	0	0
Seasoning *(Old Bay)*, ¼ tsp	0	0	0
Seasoning Mix *(Vegit)*, ¼ tsp	0	0	0
Seasoning Mixes, av., ¼ pkg	70	1	9
Taco Seasoning, av., ¼ pkg	30	0.5	4
Bragg's, Liquid Aminos	0	0	0
Old El Paso: Chili Season. Mix, 1 Tbsp	8	0.5	1.5
Cheesy Taco Seasoning Mix, 1 Tbsp	10	0.5	2
Taco/Burrito Seasoning Mix, 2 tsp	15	0	4
Fajita Seasoning Mix, 1 tsp	5	0	1.5

Spices & Herbs

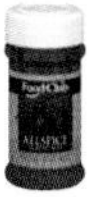

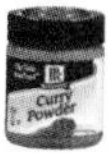

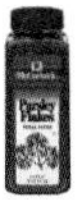

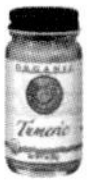

	C	F	Cb
Average all types, 1 tsp	5	0	1
All Purpose, 1 tsp	0	0	0
Allspice, ground	5	0	1
Chili Powder	8	0	1
Cinnamon, ground	6	0	2
Curry Powder	6	0	1
Garlic Powder	9	0	2
Nutmeg, ground	12	0	1
Onion Powder	7	0	2
Parsley, dried	4	0	1
Pepper, average	6	0	1
Saffron	2	0	0
Salt-Free Blends, 1 tsp	0	0	0
Tumeric, ground	8	0	1
Seeds: Fenugreek	12	1	2
Mustard, Poppyseed	15	1	1
Other varieties, average	7	0	1

Home-Popped Popcorn   C   F   Cb

	C	F	Cb
Popping Corn Kernels,			
2 Tbsp, 1 oz	110	1	26
(makes approximately 5 cups)			
Air-popped, without oil: Plain, 1 oz	110	1	22
1 cup, 0.2 oz	20	0	5
Oil-popped: Plain, 1 oz	145	8	16
1 cup, 0.4 oz	55	3	6
Popcorn Oil, 1 Tbsp	120	14	0

Microwave Popcorn

	C	F	Cb
Average all Brands: *Per 1 Cup Popped, Unless Indicated*			
Butter: Regular, 1 cup	35	2	4
Light, 1 cup	25	1	4
Act II Popcorn:			
Butter: 1 cup	25	1	4
4¹⁄₂ cups, 1 oz	130	6	19
94% Fat-Free Butter:			
1 cup	20	0.5	4
6¹⁄₂ cups, 1 oz	130	2	27
Butter Lovers: 1 cup	25	1	4
4¹⁄₂ cups, 1 oz	140	7	19
Xreme Butter: 1 cup	25	1	4
4¹⁄₂ cups	160	9	19
BodyKey *(Amway)*, Slim Popcorn,			
Sea Salt, 1 bag	110	7	10
Jolly Time:			
Blast O Butter, 1 cup	45	3	4
Crispy & Light Butter, 1 cup	25	1	4
Xtra Butter: 1 cup	40	2.5	4
4 cups	160	10	16
Newman's Own:			
Butter Flavor, Microwave:			
Regular, 3¹⁄₂ cups	130	5	18
Light, 3¹⁄₂ cups	120	4	19
Butter Boom, 3¹⁄₂ cups	130	5	18
Orville Redenbacher's: *Popped*			
Butter: 4 cups	170	12	17
Light, 6 cups	160	6	26
Movie Theater Butter, 5 cups	160	10	18
Ultimate Butter, 4¹⁄₂ cups	160	9	19
Naturals, Lime & Salt, 5 cups	220	15	21
Sweet & Savory: Caramel, 3 cups	170	8	26
Cheddar Cheese, 4¹⁄₂ cups	180	14	16
Pop Secret: *Per Cup*			
94% Fat-Free, Butter	20	0	3
Double Butter	40	2	3

Bagged Popcorn   C   F   Cb

	C	F	Cb
Average All Brands (Ready-to-Eat)			
Regular/Plain: ¹⁄₂ oz package	80	5	8
1 oz package	160	10	16
4 oz package	640	40	64
2 oz Box (store/airport)	320	16	32
3 oz Bag (9" high x 5" wide)	480	24	48
Caramel Popcorn,			
with nuts, 1 cup, 1.5 oz	230	12	39

Bagged Popcorn ~ Brands

	C	F	Cb
Boston's, Lite, 3¹⁄₂ cups, 1 oz	130	4.5	20
Cracker Jack: Original, 1 cup, 2 oz	240	4	46
Chocolate & Caramel, 1 cup, 2 oz	220	1	50
Crunch 'N Munch:			
Buttery Toffee: ²⁄₃ cup, 1.1 oz	150	5	24
1 cup, 1.65 oz	225	7.5	36
Caramel: ²⁄₃ cup, 1.1 oz	160	7	22
1 cup, 1.65 oz	240	10	33
12 oz box	1745	76	240
Fiddle Faddle:			
Average all varieties: 1 oz	120	2	24
1 cup, 2 oz	240	4	48
6 oz box	720	12	144
Popcorn Indiana:			
Kettlecorn:			
Original, 2 cups, 1 oz	130	5	21
Popcorn:			
Aged White Cheddar, 2.5 cups, 1 oz	150	9	14
Chicago Fair,			
Caramel & Cheese, 1 cup, 1 oz	140	6	20
Movie Theater, 2 cups, 1 oz	160	12	13
Seasalt, 3.5 cups, 1 oz	140	6	17
Poppycock:			
Bags: Cashew Lovers, ¹⁄₂ cup, 1 oz	150	6	20
Chocolate Lovers, ¹⁄₂ cup, 1.2 oz	160	7	22
Cannisters, Orig./Pecan Delight, av:			
¹⁄₂ cup, 1 oz	155	7	20
1 cup, 2 oz	310	14	40

Movie Theater Popcorn

	C	F	Cb
Small, (7 cups): Plain	385	21	44
with Butter (3 pumps, 0.8 oz)	570	42	44
Medium, (15 cups): Plain	825	45	94
with Butter (4 pumps, 1 oz)	1075	73	94
Large, (20 cups): Plain	1100	60	124
with Butter (6 pumps, 1.5 oz)	1485	102	124
Butter: 1 Pump, 0.3 oz	65	7	0
4 Pumps (2 Tbsp), 1 oz	250	28	0

Corn & Tortilla Chips   C F Cb

Average All Brands
Corn Chips:

	C	F	Cb
Average all types: 1 oz	150	8	18
8 oz bag	1200	64	144
Fritos, Original, 32 chips, 1 oz	160	10	15
Tortilla Chips: Average, 1 oz	140	7	18
(1 oz = approx. 12 chips or 13 strips)			
Doritos: Original, 1 oz	140	7	18
Nacho Chse; Salsa Verde, av., 1 oz	140	8	18
Popchips: Chili Limon, 1 oz	120	4	19
Nacho Cheese, 1 oz	130	5	18
Snyder's:			
El Restaurante, all flavors, 1 oz	150	8	17
Yellow Corn/White, av., 1 oz	135	5	21
Tostitos:			
Average all flav., 1 oz	145	7	19
Baked! Scoops, 1 oz	120	3	22
Utz: Multigrain, 1 oz	150	8	16
Baked, 1 oz	120	2	23
Other flavors, 1 oz	140	8	18

Potato Chips/Crisps

Average All Brands
Regular:

	C	F	Cb
Plain or flavored, (4 chips)	30	2	3
1 oz package (20 chips)	150	10	15
4 oz quantity	600	40	60
14 oz package	2100	140	210

Chips/Crisps ~ Brands

	C	F	Cb
Hippeas, Chick Pea Puffs,			
average all flavors, 0.78 oz	90	4	11
Lay's *(Fritolay):*			
Classics; Wavy Originals, 1 oz	160	10	15
Kettle Cooked, Original, 1 oz	150	9	17
Pringles:			
All Flavors: 1 oz	150	9	16
Large can, 6 oz	900	54	96
Stix, To Go Pak, Baked Cheese	80	3	10
Ruffles: Regular, av. all flavors, 1 oz	160	11	15
Reduced Fat, 1 oz	140	7	18
Simply7, Hummus/Lentil Chips,			
average all flavors, 1 oz	135	5	19
Sun Chips, Original, 16 crisps, 1 oz	140	6	18

Pretzels   C F Cb

Average All Brands
Hard-Baked Pretzels: *Each*

	C	F	Cb
1 oz quantity	110	1	23
Sticks, thin, 2¼" (9/oz)	12	0	3
Twists, thin, ¼" thick, (5/oz)	25	0	5
Dutch (2¾"x 2⅝"), 0.5 oz	55	1	11
Snyders, Sourdough, 0.8oz	100	0	22
Soft Pretzel Twists, average: *Each*			
Plain: Small, 2 oz	210	2	43
Medium, 4 oz	390	3.5	80
Large, 5 oz	485	4.5	100
Big Cheese, 1.8 oz	130	3	22
New York Street Vendors, 7 oz	660	6	135
Trader Joe's, Peanut Butter filled, 1 oz	140	8	14
Snyder's: Milk Chocolate Dips, 1 oz	140	6	19
White Creme Dips, 1 oz	130	6	19

Pretzels ~ Brands

	C	F	Cb
Flipz: Milk Choc, 8 pieces, 1 oz	130	5	20
White Fudge, 7 pcs, 1 oz	130	5	20
Rold Gold *(Frito-Lay):*			
Braided Twists,			
Honey Wheat (8), 1 oz	110	1	24
Pretzel, Sourdough (1)	90	1	19
Pretzel Thins (9), 1 oz	110	1	23
Rods (3), 1 oz	110	1	22
Tiny Twists (18), average, 1 oz	110	0	23
Sticks, 1 oz	100	0	23
Snyder's of Hanover:			
Butter Snaps (24), 1 oz	120	1	25
Choc Dipped Minis, av., 1 oz	135	6	20
Gluten Free Pretzel Sticks (30)	110	1.5	25
Pieces, average, 1 oz	140	8	16
Sticks (28), average, 1 oz	110	1	23
Thins (11), 1 oz	110	0	23
Twists (7), average,1 oz	120	2	24
Special K,			
Choc. Coated, av., all flavors, 1 oz	100	3.5	15
SuperPretzel:			
6 Count Soft, Original (1), 2.3 oz	160	1	34
Bites (5), 1.9 oz	140	0.5	32
Softstix, Cheese (2), 1.76 oz	130	3	22
Utz:			
Pretzels: Original; Extra Dark, 1 oz	110	1	21
Sourdough, Hard (1)	90	0	18

Snacks   C   F   Cb

Note: Actual weight of packaged snacks is usually 5-10% more than label Net Wt. For accuracy, weigh snack and allow extra calories, fat and carbs for any extra weight.

	C	F	Cb
Apple Chips (Seneca), av., 1 oz	**140**	7	20
Bagel Crisps (N.Y. Style), 6 crisps, 1 oz	**130**	6	17
Baguette Chips (Pillsbury), av., (21)	**130**	5	19
Banana Chips (T.Joe's), 13 chips, 1 oz	**160**	11	13
Beef Jerky (Jack Link's), av., 1 oz	**80**	1	5
Beef Sticks: (Slim Jim), Giant, 1 oz	**140**	11	4
Jack Link's, Original, 1.5 oz	**160**	13	2
Beet Chips (Rhythm), Sea Salt, 1oz	**130**	4	20
Trader Joes, 1.3 oz	**140**	0.5	29
BodyKey (Amway):			
Mixed Nuts & Pumpkin Seeds, 1 bag	**200**	16	8
Whole Grain Tortilla Chips, 1 bag	**210**	11	24
Bugles, Original; Nacho Cheese, 1 oz	**160**	9	18
Cheese Balls (Utz), 1 oz serving	**130**	7	16
Cheese Bites (Tr. Joes), 1 oz	**170**	12	0.5
Cheese Nips, 1.3 oz package	**170**	7	22
Cheese Puffs, average, 1 oz	**160**	10	15
Cheetos:			
Crunchy: Av. all flavors, 1 oz	**155**	11	13
4 oz package	**640**	40	60
Baked!; Fantastix, av., 1 oz	**130**	5	19
Simply Puffs, Wh. Cheddar, 1 oz	**150**	9	16
Cheez-It (Sunshine):			
Snack Mix: Classic, 1/2 cup, 1 oz	**140**	4.5	20
Double Cheese, 3/4 cup, 1 oz	**130**	5	19
Sriracha, 1/2 cup, 0.9 oz	**120**	5	17
Sweet & Salty, 1/2 cup, 1oz	**140**	5	21
Chester's: Fries, Flamin'Hot, 1 oz	**150**	8	17
Puffcorn, Cheese, 1 oz	**160**	11	14
Chex Mix, (General Mills),			
Traditional, 1 oz	**120**	3.5	22
Chicharrones ~ See Pork Skins			
Crackers (Tr. Joes), Mini Edamame (28)	**120**	2	21
Churros (Rubio's), Cinnamon, 2 oz	**240**	13	30
Combo, Crackers, av.,1/3 cup, 1 oz	**140**	6	18
Cool Cuts, Carrot & Ranch, 2.3 oz	**70**	5	5
Corn Chips ~ See Page 149			
Corn Nuts: Av all flav., 1 oz	**130**	4.5	20
1.7 oz bag	**210**	8	34
Corn Puffs/Twists, (32), 1 oz	**160**	11	15
Dunkin Stix (Dolly Madison), (3)	**490**	25	63
Edamame,			
Seapointe, Dry Roasted, 1 oz	**130**	4	11
Fritos: Corn Chips, all varieties, av., 1oz	**160**	10	15
Flavor Twists, Honey BBQ, 1 oz	**150**	9	16

Snacks (Cont)   C   F   Cb

	C	F	Cb
Fruit Snacks ~ See Page 102			
Funyuns, Onion Flavored, 1 oz	**130**	6	16
Goldfish, Crackers, av., 1 oz	**140**	5	20
Gold-n-Chees (Lance):			
Snack Crackers, 1.25 oz pkg	**160**	5	25
Snack Mix, 2.25 oz tube	**320**	17	36
Gripz (Sunshine), Mighty Tiny (1)	**120**	6	15
Flamin Hot Peanuts (Munchies), 1 oz	**180**	14	6
Kale Chips (Rhythm),			
Roasted Garlic & Onion, 1 oz	**160**	11	14
Trader Joes, average, 1 oz	**150**	10	9
Lance, Sandwich Crackers (6), av.	**200**	9	25
Munchies (Frito-Lay),			
Snack Mix, all flavors, 1 oz	**140**	7	18
Munchos (Fritolay), all flavors, 1 oz	**160**	10	16
Newtons:			
Single Serve: 2 oz pkg	**200**	4	40
Fat-Free, 2 oz package	**200**	0	46
Nutella, w/ Breadsticks/Pretzels (1)	**270**	14	35
Nutter Butter, Sandwich Cookies:			
1.87 oz Package	**250**	10	37
Bites, Go-Pak, 3.5 oz	**490**	21	74
Onion Rings (T.G.I. Friday), 1 oz	**140**	7	16
Oreo Cookies, all Creme Fillings:			
Double Stuf (2), 1 oz	**140**	7	21
Mini Bite Size: 1 oz	**130**	6	21
Go-Pak, 3.5 oz	**455**	21	74
Oreo Cakesters, Golden, Soft, 0.9 oz	**110**	5	16
Oriental Mix Rice Snacks, 1 oz	**125**	3.5	21
Peanut Butter Nuggets, (10), 1 oz	**140**	6	15
Pepitas, dried or roasted,			
1/4 cup, 1 oz	**155**	14	3
Pirate's Booty:			
Aged White Cheddar, 4 oz	**560**	24	72
Veggie, 4 oz bag	**560**	28	72
Pita Chips, (9), average, 1 oz	**130**	4	18
Plaintain Chips (Goya), 1 oz	**150**	8	19
PopCorners, Butter/Kettle, 1 oz	**125**	3.5	20
Popcorn ~ See Page 148			
Pork Cracklins, 1 oz	**160**	12	0
Pork Skins/Rinds: 1 oz	**160**	10	0
Baken-ets, Traditional, 0.5 oz	**80**	5	0
Mission, Chiccarones, 4 oz package	**640**	40	0
Potato Chips ~ See Page 149			
Potato Skins (TGI Friday),			
all flavors, 16 chips, 1 oz	**140**	8	15
Puffed Wheat,			
Sabritones, Chili & Lime, 1 oz	**140**	8	16
Pretzels ~ See Page 149			

Snacks (Cont)

	C	F	Cb
Rice Cakes:			
Lundberg, (1), average	80	0.5	17
Quaker: Plain, lightly salted (1)	35	0	7
Chocolate Crunch (1)	60	1	12
Rice Chips,			
Lundberg, average, 1 oz	140	7	18
Sandwich Crackers:			
Austin, Cheese Crackers:			
with Cheddar, 1.4 oz	190	10	23
with Peanut Butter, 1.3 oz	190	10	23
PB & J Flavored, 1.4 oz	190	8	26
Lance: Nip Chee, 6 pieces	190	9	24
Toasty, 6 pieces	180	9	21
Toast Chee, PB, 1.5 oz	220	1	25
Ritz Bits: Cheese (12), 1 oz Pkg	150	8	17
3 oz Pak	450	25	50
P'nut Butter: 1.5 oz pkg	210	11	24
Big Bag, 3 oz	420	22	48
Sesame Sticks, Salted,			
SunRidge Farm, 1 oz	170	12	14
Smart Puffs,			
Pirates Booty, 1 oz	140	7	16
Soybeans in Pods,			
AFC, ½ cup, 3.2 oz	90	5	3
Soy Crisps, average, 1 oz	120	3	17
Soy Nuts: Dry Roasted, ¼ cup, 1 oz	130	6	9
Choc-coated, 1 oz	140	7	13
Sun Chips,			
Fritolay, average, 1 oz	140	6	19
Takis: Crunchy Fajitas, 1 oz	140	8	16
4 oz package	560	32	64
Tings *(Robert's),* 2 oz bag	300	16	36
Toasted Chips *(Ritz),* av. all, 1 oz	130	5.5	20
Tortilla Chips,			
Garden of Eatin, Chili & Lime, 1 oz	140	7	18
Trail Mix (Nuts/Seeds/Dried Fruit):			
Regular, 3 Tbsp, 1 oz	140	9	13
Tropical, 3 Tbsp, 1 oz	130	7	16
Turkey Jerky: Teriyaki, 1 oz	80	1	8
Trader Joe's, Original, 1 oz	60	0.5	6
Veggie Crisps,			
Snyder's, 1 oz	140	6	18
Wheat Thins *(Nabisco),* av. all, 1 oz	135	5	21
Woats, Oatsnack, av., ¼ cup, 1 oz	120	5	17
Yogurt Pretzels, 1.5 oz	190	8	28
Yogurt Raisins, Vanilla,			
Sun-Maid, 1 oz	120	4.5	20

Fruit Snacks

	C	F	Cb
Betty Crocker: Fruit Gushers, 0.9 oz	90	1.5	21
Fruit by the Foot, 1 roll, 0.8 oz	80	1	17
Fruit Roll Ups, 1 roll, 0.5 oz	50	1	11
Fruit Flavored Shapes,			
all varieties, 0.9 oz	80	0	19
Sunkist:			
Fruit Lover's Trail Mix: B'fast Espresso, 1.5 oz	190	9	27
Other flavors, 1 oz	120	4	20
Fruit Snack Cups ~ See Page 102			

Vending Machines

	C	F	Cb
Bugles, Nacho Cheese, 1 oz	160	9	18
Cheese Balls *(Utz),* 1 oz	130	7	16
Cheetos, Crunchy, 1 oz	150	10	13
Cheeze-It, Snack Mix, 1.5 oz	195	6.5	30
Chester's, Flamin' Hot Fries, 1 oz	150	8	17
Choc Chip Cookies:			
Chips Ahoy, 1.2 oz	160	8	22
Famous Amos, (4), 1 oz	150	8	18
Grandma's, (1), 1.4 oz	200	10	25
Chocolate Bars:			
Hershey's, Milk Choc., 1.6 oz	220	13	22
Kit Kat, 1.5 oz	210	11	25
Snickers, 1.9 oz bar	250	12	33
Donut, plain cake, 1.4 oz	160	9	18
Doritos, av. all flavors, 1 oz	145	8	18
Fritos, Corn Chips, Orig., 1.8 oz	280	17	26
Fruit Pie,			
Hostess, Lemon, 4.5 oz	510	25	65
Granola/Cereal Bars, av., 1 oz	140	3	26
M & M's:			
Milk Chocolate, 1.7 oz	240	10	34
Peanuts, 1.8 oz	250	13	30
Oreo Cookies, 2 oz	270	11	41
Peanut Butter Cups,			
Reese's, 1.5 oz	210	12	24
Popcorn, plain, 1 oz	160	10	16
Pop Chips, 0.8 oz	100	3	16
Pork Skins, 1.5 oz	240	15	0
Potato Chips: 1 oz	150	10	15
Baked! *(Ruffles),* Orig., 1 oz	120	3	22
Potato Skins *(TGI Friday's),*			
all flavors, 1 oz	140	8	15
Pretzels *(Snyder's),* Olde Tyme, 1 oz	120	1	24
Raisins, 0.5 oz package	45	0	11
Rice Krispies Treat	90	2	17
Skittles, 2 oz	230	2.5	52
Starburst, Fruit Chews, Orig., 1.4 oz	130	0	31
Tortilla Chips, 1 oz	140	7	18

S Soups

Homemade & Restaurant

Restaurant & Take-Out: Average All Preparations: Per 8 fl.oz	C	F	Cb
Bean Medley	200	3	34
Beef Consomme	30	0	2
Borscht, with Sour Cream	130	8	14
Bouillabaisse	400	15	10
Chicken & Corn	290	14	20
Chicken & Wild Rice	80	4	9
Chicken Consomme	50	0	2
Chicken Curry	180	8	18
Chicken Jambalaya	160	7	8
Chicken Noodle	80	2	12
With Chicken	160	4	12
Chicken Soup	80	2	6
Chili with Beans	250	12	25
Clam Chowder	240	15	17
Corn & Crab	120	3	18
Corn Chowder	150	8	16
Cream of Broccoli	200	12	20
Cream of Potato	150	6.5	17
Cream of Mushroom	200	13	15
Fish Chowder	220	15	6
French Onion	420	15	25
Gazpacho	50	0	5
Lentil Soup	250	9	28
Lobster Bisque	320	15	10
Matzo Ball, with 1 large ball	180	7	24
Minestrone	125	2.5	20
Mulligatawny	300	15	8
Pea & Ham	240	10	25
Potato & Bacon	170	7	19
Pumpkin, Creamy	210	10	26
Shark Fin Soup	100	4	8
Spicy Shrimp Soup, 1 bowl	160	7	10
Split Pea Soup	180	2.5	30
Vegetable (Fat Free)	75	0	18
Vegetable Beef	80	2	10
Vichyssoise	200	9	15
Watercress	90	4	13

Other Soups ~ *See International & Fast-Foods Sections (Arby's, Au Bon Pain, Boston Market, Dunkin' Donuts, Denny's, Schlotzsky's, Sizzler, Souplantation, Sweet Tomatoes, Zoup!)*
Homemade Soups: *Calculate calories, fat and carbohydrates from recipe ingredients.*

Bouillon Cubes & Powders

Bouillon Cubes: *Average all types*	C	F	Cb
Regular, 1 cube	5	0	1
Extra Large, 1 cube	20	1	1
Powders, average, 1 tsp	10	0	1
Herb-Ox:			
Instant Broth & Seasoning,			
Beef, 1 envelope, 0.14 oz	5	0	1
Chicken, 1 envelope, 0.14 oz	5	0	1

Soup ~ Brands

Amy's:
Heat & Serve (Organic): *Per 1 Cup, Unless Indicated*

	C	F	Cb
Alphabet	80	0	16
Black Bean Vegetable	140	1.5	26
Chunky Vegetable	80	1.5	13
Carrot Ginger	200	13	18
Cream of M'shrm, ¾ cup	150	9	13
Lentil Vegetable	160	4	24
Rustic Italian Vegetable	190	8	24
Southwestern Vegetable	140	5	20
Split Pea	110	1	19
Thai Coconut, ½ can	160	11	12
Thai Curry Sweet Pot. Lentil	280	20	20
Tuscan Bean & Rice	160	4.5	25

Bertoli: *Per ½ Carton, 12 oz*
Meal Soups:

	C	F	Cb
Tomato Florentine & Tortellini with Chicken	420	20	37

Campbell's:
Chunky: *Per Cup, Unless Indicated*

	C	F	Cb
Baked Potato w/ Ched. & Bacon Bits	190	8	22
Baked Potato with Steak & Cheese	190	9	21
BBQ Seasoned Pork	170	1	29
Beef Burrito	170	6	19
Beef Rib R'st w/ Pot. & Herbs	110	1.5	17
Beer-n-Cheese, with Beef & Bacon	200	9	22
Chicken Corn Chowder	180	8	20
Chipotle Chicken & Corn Chowder	180	8	20
Classic Chicken Noodle	120	3	14
Creamy Chkn & Dumplings	170	9	14
Fajita Chkn w/ Rice & Beans	130	1	23
Grilled Chicken & Sausage Gumbo	140	3.5	21
Kickin' Buffalo-Style Chicken	150	7	15
Mushroom Swiss Burger	160	7	16
Philly-Style Cheesesteak	170	9	14

Hearty: Beef Barley

	C	F	Cb
Beef Barley	140	1	24
Chicken with Vegetables	80	1	13
Cheeseburger Soup	200	12	15
Italian Style Wedding	110	2.5	16

Campbell's (Cont):	C	F	Cb
Condensed Soup: *Per ½ Cup, 4 fl.oz*		
Broccoli Cheese	100	5	11
Beef Noodle	70	1.5	9
Beef with Vege & Barley	100	1	18
Cheddar Cheese	100	5	14
Chicken Gumbo	70	1.5	12
Cream of Asparagus	100	7	8
Cream of Celery	100	7	8
Cream of Mushr'm with Rstd Garlic	90	6	9
Cream of Onion	100	6	10
Green Pea	180	3	28
Old Fashioned Tom. Rice	125	1.5	25
Tomato	90	0	20
25% Less Sodium: Chicken Noodle	60	1.5	9
Cream of Mushroom	100	7	8
98% Fat Free: Broccoli Cheese	80	2	12
Cream of Celery	60	2.5	9
Cream of Mushroom	60	2	9
Soup on the Go: *Per Container*		
Cheesy Chicken Tortilla	100	4	13
Cheesy Potato with Bacon Flav.	130	6	16
Classic Tomato	140	0.5	32
Creamy Tomato	230	10	30
Creamy Tomato Parmesan Bisque	230	8	35
Healthy Request: *Per ½ cup, Unless Indicated*		
Cheddar Cheese	60	1	12
Cream of Chicken	70	2.5	9
New England Chowder, 1 cup	130	3	21
Savory Vegetable, 1 cup	110	0.5	22
Tomato	90	1.5	17
Tuscan-Style Lentil	140	0.5	25
Vegetable	90	1	19
Homestyle: *Per Cup*		
Butternut Squash Bisque	130	5	18
Chicken Noodle	90	2.5	10
Creamy Chicken & Herb Dumplings	160	9	14
Creamy Gouda Bisque with Chicken	190	11	16
Creole-Style Chicken w/ Beans & Rice	130	3	18
Italian Style Wedding	120	3.5	15
Mexican-Style Chkn Tortilla	130	2	20
Potato Broccoli Cheese	170	10	16
Southwest-Style White Chicken Chili	130	2	20
Vegetable Medley	90	0.5	18
Light: Baked Pot. w/ Bacon & Cheddar	100	3	15
Chicken & Dumplings	90	2.5	12
Creamy Chicken Alfredo	90	2	12
New England Clam Chowder	100	1.5	16

Campbell's (Cont):	C	F	Cb
Slow Kettle Style: *Per Container*		
Baked Potato with Smoked Bacon	390	26	33
Braised Beef Stew	300	9	34
Creamy Broccoli Cheddar Bisque	340	25	22
Fiesta Chicken Lime Tortilla w/ Chkn	190	3	28
Kickin' Crab & Sweet Corn Chowder	440	27	37
Portobello Mushr'm & Madeira Bisque	420	31	29
Roasted Red Pepper & Gouda Bisque	300	16	32
Tomato & Sweet Basil Bisque	510	28	58
Vegetarian Black Bean	420	3	77
Health Valley Organics: *Per Cup*		
40% Less Sodium:		
Chicken Noodle	80	2	11
Garden Vegetable	90	0	18
Creamed:		
Cream of Chicken	120	3	17
Cream of Mushroom	90	1.5	16
No Salt Added:		
Chicken & Rice	100	1.5	19
Chicken Noodle	80	2	13
Lentil	150	1.5	27
Minestrone	100	2	18
Split Pea	160	2.5	26
Tomato	110	2	22
Vegetable	90	2	15
Healthy Choice:		
Canned: *Per Cup*		
Chicken & Dumplings	150	3	22
Chicken Noodle	90	0.5	12
Chicken with Rice	110	3	15
Country Vegetable	110	0.5	21
Vegetable Beef	130	1.5	20
Imagine:		
Broths, Organic: *Per Cup*		
Beef Flavor	20	1	2
Free Range Chicken	20	0.5	2
Vegetable	20	0	4
Vegetarian, No-Chicken	15	0	2
Chunky Style, Organic: *Per Cup*		
Chicken & Dumplings	120	4.5	16
Ginger Miso	70	1.5	11
Italian Style Wedding	150	4.5	20
Italian Vegetables & Beans	130	1.5	25
Loaded Baked Potato	120	5	18
Potato Quinoa & Spinach	120	3.5	19
Soy-Ginger Chicken & Edamame	80	2	10
White Bean & Kale	110	1	21

Continued Nex Page...

Imagine (Cont):	C	F	Cb
Creamy: Per 8 fl.oz Cup			
Butternut Squash	100	1.5	21
Cauliflower & Potato	70	1	14
Garden Tomato	80	1	16
Potato Leek	90	2.5	18
Portobello Mushroom	80	2.5	12
Tomato; Tomato Basil	80	1	15
Kettle Cuisine: Per 8 fl.oz Cup			
Albondigas Meatball Soup	170	7	17
Beef, Barley & Vegetable	110	2	14
Broccoli Cheddar	320	24	15
Buffalo Chicken	250	15	14
Carrot Ginger	110	4	18
Chicken Tortilla	120	3	15
Chipotle Sweet Potato	140	7	20
Classic Gazpacho	60	1	10
Cream of Crab	290	22	15
Hot Honey & Butternut Squash	140	4	26
Lobster Bisque	270	18	18
Manhattan Clam Chowder	120	3	16
Minestrone	80	2	14
North Atlantic Haddock Chowder	260	17	14
Portuguese Kale with Linguica	200	7	21
Organic: Chickpea & Chicken	210	6	25
Tomato Cheddar	250	16	14
Knorr:			
Cubes: Per ½ Cube, 1 Cup, Prepared			
Beef; Chicken, average	15	1.5	1
Vegetable	20	1	1
Homestyle Stock: Per 1 Tsp			
Beef	10	0.5	1
Chicken	10	1	0.5
Lipton:			
Cup-a-Soup: Per Envelope			
Chkn Noodle, White Meat	50	1	8
Cream of Chicken	70	1.5	12
Recipe Secrets: Per 1 Tbsp Dry Mix			
Onion	20	0	4
Onion Mushroom	35	0	7
Savory Herb with Garlic	35	0	6
Manischewitz:			
Canned: Per 1 cup			
Broth, Chicken	15	0	2
Chicken Noodle	180	2	20
Glass Jar: Per 1 Cup			
Matzo Ball	120	5	15
Reduced Sodium	130	6	17
Matzo Ball in Broth	180	8	23
Reduced Sodium	180	8	21
Maruchan:			
Instant Lunch,			
average all flavors, 1 pkg	290	12	38
Ramen, all flavors, 1 pkg, 3 oz	380	14	52

Nissin:	C	F	Cb
Souper Meal: Per ½ of 4.3 oz Ctn			
Chicken Flavor, with Veggie Medley	280	13	37
Picante Shrimp Flavor, Hot & Spicy	290	13	37
Top Ramen, all flavors, 3 oz pkg	380	14	53
Pacific Foods:			
Condensed: Per ½ Cup			
Cream of Chicken	90	3.5	10
Cream of Mushroom	80	3.5	10
Hearty Organic: Per 1 Cup			
Butternut Squash Bisque	120	3	22
Cashew Carrot Ginger Bisque	140	6	22
Coconut Curry	200	9	28
Poblano Pepper & Corn Chowder	180	9	22
Rosemary Potato Chowder	170	8	22
Santa Fe Style Chicken	140	2.5	22
Spicy Black Bean & Kale	120	0	24
Split Pea & Uncured Ham	160	2	26
Vegetable Quinoa	110	2	20
Progresso:			
Broths: Beef, 1 cup	20	0	3
Chicken, 1 cup	10	0	1
Vegetable, 1 cup	5	0	1
Rich & Hearty: Per Cup			
Beef Pot Roast w/ Country Vegetables	110	1.5	17
Chicken & Homestyle Noodles	100	2	14
Creamy Roasted Chicken Wild Rice	120	4.5	15
Creamy Roasted Vegetable	140	6	19
Hearty Chicken Pot Pie	150	5	21
Lentil & Andouille Sausage	210	11	22
Minestrone w/ Italian Sausage	150	5	17
New England Clam Chowder	180	8	22
Tomato Florentine w/ Italian Sausage	160	6	20
Traditional: Per 1 Cup			
Cheese Tortellini	100	1	20
Chickarina	110	4	12
Chicken & Sausage Gumbo	110	2.5	17
Italian-Style Wedding	120	4	15
Manhattan Clam Chowder	100	2	17
Steak Burger & Country Vegetables	130	4	17
Vegetable Classic: Per 1 Cup			
Creamy Mushroom	150	10	11
Green Split Pea	160	2.5	29
Minestrone	100	2	20
Southwestern-Style Corn	110	2	21
Light: Per 1 cup			
Beef Pot Roast	80	1.5	12
Broccoli Cheese	120	6	11
Chicken Noodle	70	1	9
Vegetable	70	0	15

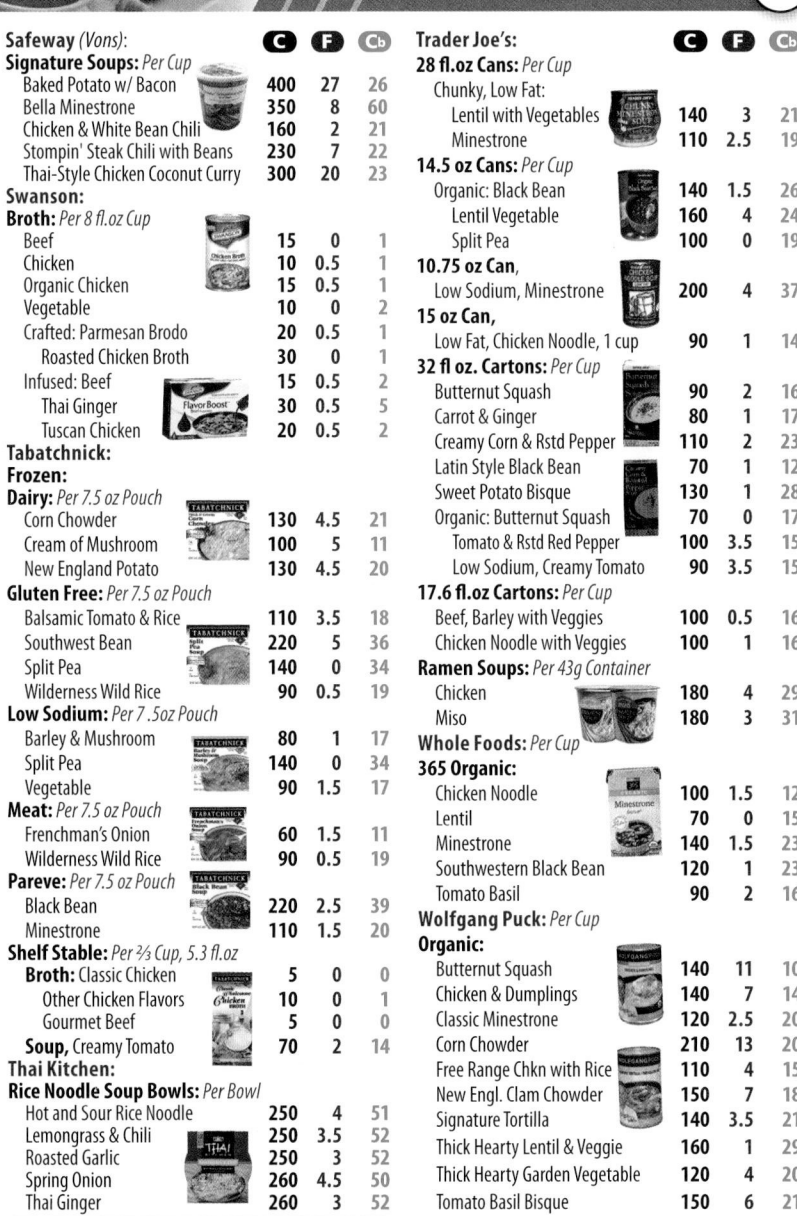

Safeway *(Vons)*:	C	F	Cb
Signature Soups: *Per Cup*			
Baked Potato w/ Bacon	400	27	26
Bella Minestrone	350	8	60
Chicken & White Bean Chili	160	2	21
Stompin' Steak Chili with Beans	230	7	22
Thai-Style Chicken Coconut Curry	300	20	23
Swanson:			
Broth: *Per 8 fl.oz Cup*			
Beef	15	0	1
Chicken	10	0.5	1
Organic Chicken	15	0.5	1
Vegetable	10	0	2
Crafted: Parmesan Brodo	20	0.5	1
Roasted Chicken Broth	30	0	1
Infused: Beef	15	0.5	2
Thai Ginger	30	0.5	5
Tuscan Chicken	20	0.5	2
Tabatchnick:			
Frozen:			
Dairy: *Per 7.5 oz Pouch*			
Corn Chowder	130	4.5	21
Cream of Mushroom	100	5	11
New England Potato	130	4.5	20
Gluten Free: *Per 7.5 oz Pouch*			
Balsamic Tomato & Rice	110	3.5	18
Southwest Bean	220	5	36
Split Pea	140	0	34
Wilderness Wild Rice	90	0.5	19
Low Sodium: *Per 7 .5oz Pouch*			
Barley & Mushroom	80	1	17
Split Pea	140	0	34
Vegetable	90	1.5	17
Meat: *Per 7.5 oz Pouch*			
Frenchman's Onion	60	1.5	11
Wilderness Wild Rice	90	0.5	19
Pareve: *Per 7.5 oz Pouch*			
Black Bean	220	2.5	39
Minestrone	110	1.5	20
Shelf Stable: *Per ⅔ Cup, 5.3 fl.oz*			
Broth: Classic Chicken	5	0	0
Other Chicken Flavors	10	0	1
Gourmet Beef	5	0	0
Soup, Creamy Tomato	70	2	14
Thai Kitchen:			
Rice Noodle Soup Bowls: *Per Bowl*			
Hot and Sour Rice Noodle	250	4	51
Lemongrass & Chili	250	3.5	52
Roasted Garlic	250	3	52
Spring Onion	260	4.5	50
Thai Ginger	260	3	52

Trader Joe's:	C	F	Cb
28 fl.oz Cans: *Per Cup*			
Chunky, Low Fat:			
Lentil with Vegetables	140	3	21
Minestrone	110	2.5	19
14.5 oz Cans: *Per Cup*			
Organic: Black Bean	140	1.5	26
Lentil Vegetable	160	4	24
Split Pea	100	0	19
10.75 oz Can,			
Low Sodium, Minestrone	200	4	37
15 oz Can,			
Low Fat, Chicken Noodle, 1 cup	90	1	14
32 fl.oz. Cartons: *Per Cup*			
Butternut Squash	90	2	16
Carrot & Ginger	80	1	17
Creamy Corn & Rstd Pepper	110	2	23
Latin Style Black Bean	70	1	12
Sweet Potato Bisque	130	1	28
Organic: Butternut Squash	70	0	17
Tomato & Rstd Red Pepper	100	3.5	15
Low Sodium, Creamy Tomato	90	3.5	15
17.6 fl.oz Cartons: *Per Cup*			
Beef, Barley with Veggies	100	0.5	16
Chicken Noodle with Veggies	100	1	16
Ramen Soups: *Per 43g Container*			
Chicken	180	4	29
Miso	180	3	31
Whole Foods: *Per Cup*			
365 Organic:			
Chicken Noodle	100	1.5	12
Lentil	70	0	15
Minestrone	140	1.5	23
Southwestern Black Bean	120	1	23
Tomato Basil	90	2	16
Wolfgang Puck: *Per Cup*			
Organic:			
Butternut Squash	140	11	10
Chicken & Dumplings	140	7	14
Classic Minestrone	120	2.5	20
Corn Chowder	210	13	20
Free Range Chkn with Rice	110	4	15
New Engl. Clam Chowder	150	7	18
Signature Tortilla	140	3.5	21
Thick Hearty Lentil & Veggie	160	1	29
Thick Hearty Garden Vegetable	120	4	20
Tomato Basil Bisque	150	6	21

Soybean Products | C | F | Cb
	C	F	Cb
Cheeses (Soy) ~ *See Page 78*			
Miso Soy Bean Paste:			
Cold Mountain: Light Yellow, 1 tsp	10	0	1
Mellow Red, 1 tsp	15	0	3
Red, 1 tsp	10	0	1
Miso Soup (dry mix):			
1 Tbsp., dry mix	35	1	5
1 cup, prepared	35	1	5
Natto, ½ cup, 3 oz	160	7	14
Okara (Tofu fiber residue), ½ c., 2 oz	47	1	8
Tempeh: 1 piece, 3 oz	180	8	12
Fried, 3 oz	250	14	14
Seitan *(Westsoy)*, Strips, 3 oz	120	2	4
Soybean Protein *(TVP)*, 1 oz	95	0	8
Soy Bean Paste, 1 tsp	10	0	2
Soy Beans ~ *See Page 160*			
Soy Drinks ~ *See Page 49*			

Tofu ~ Brands
	C	F	Cb
Azumaya Tofu:			
Extra Firm; Firm, av., 3 oz	70	4	2
Soft (Silken), 3.2 oz	45	2	1
House Foods: *Per 3 oz*			
Premium Tofu: Extra Firm	80	4.5	2
Firm	70	4	2
Medium Firm	60	3.5	2
Soft (Silken)	60	3	2
Organic Tofu: Firm	70	4	2
Extra Firm	70	3.5	2
Ethnic: Tokusen Kinugoshi, Extra Soft	80	4	3
Sukui; Soon (Extra Soft)	45	2	2
Yaki Tofu (Broiled)	90	5	2
Mori-Nu Tofu:			
Morinaga Silken:			
Soft, 3 oz, 1" slice	45	2.5	1
Firm, 3 oz, 1" slice	50	2.5	2
Extra Firm, 3 oz, 1" slice	50	2	1
Organic Silken, Firm, 3 oz, 1" slice	50	2.5	2
Lite, Firm, 3 oz, 1" slice	30	1	1
Nasoya: Extra Firm, 3 oz	80	4	3
Firm, 3 oz	70	3.5	2
Silken, 3.2 oz	45	2	1
Soft, 2.8 oz	60	3	1
Tofuplus:			
Extra Firm, 3 oz	80	4	2
Firm, 3 oz	70	3	2
Sprouted, Super Firm, 3 oz	100	5	3

Supplements
	C	F	Cb
Aloe Vera Juice, undiluted, 2 fl.oz	5	0	1
: Tablets, 2 tabs	4	0	0.5
Flakes, 1 heaping Tbsp, 0.3 oz	30	0.5	4
Powder, 1 heaping Tbsp, 0.5 oz	50	0.5	6
Calcium Chews: *CVS,* 1 chew	20	0	3
Trader Joe's, Chocolate,1 chew	20	1	3
Cod Liver Oil, 1 Tbsp	125	13	0
Fiber Choice, 2 tabs	15	0	4
Fiber,			
Fibersure, 1 heaping tsp	25	0	6
Fish Oil Capsules, (1), av.	10	1	0
Flax Oil:			
Capsules (2)	10	1	0
Barlean's, softgels (3)	110	11	0
Garlic Tablets/Capsules, each	3	0	0
Glowelle:			
Beauty Drink, 8 fl.oz	100	0	24
Powder Stick (1)	50	0	12
Lecithin Granules, 1 Tbsp	55	4	0.5
Metamucil, Powder:			
Orange (Smooth Texture),			
1 rounded Tbsp	45	0	12
Sugar-Free, 1 rounded tsp	20	0	5
Pink Lemonade, Sugar-Free,			
1 rounded tsp	20	0	5
Capsules: Heart & Digestive (6)	10	0	3
Strong Bones (5)	10	0	3
Meta, Fiber Wafers (2)	100	4.5	16
Protein, Powders, av., 1 oz	100	0.5	0
Seaweed: Dried, 1 oz	85	0.5	22
Soaked, drained, 1 oz	15	0.5	3
Spirulina, 1 tablet	2	0	0.5
Vitamins/Minerals: Tabs/Caps (1)	2	0	0
Vitamin E Capsules, each	5	0.5	0
Viactiv Chews, Choc. (1)	20	0.5	4

Cough & Pharmaceutical
	C	F	Cb
Antacids: Av., 1 tablet	4	0	1
Liquid, 1 Tbsp	6	0	1
Antacid Sodium Counts ~ *See Page 280*			
Cough/Cold Syrups:			
Regular: With sugar, 1 Tbsp	35	0	9
With alcohol, 1 Tbsp	46	0	9
Diabetic Tussin, Sugar Free, 1 T.	0	0	0
Cough Drops/Lozenges ~ *See Page 75*			
Sudafed, Syrup 1 tsp	14	0	3
Tylenol, Liquid: Child, 1 tsp	17	0	4
Extra Strength, 1 tsp	11	0	3

Sugar

	C	F	Cb
White Sugar, granulated:			
1 level teaspoon, 4g	15	0	4
1 heaping teaspoon, 6g	25	0	6
1 Tablespoon, 12g	50	0	12
1 ounce, 1 oz	110	0	28
1 cup, 7 oz	775	0	200
1 lb (16 oz)	1760	0	454
Single Portion Packages:			
1 stick	15	0	4
1 packet	15	0	4
1 cube	10	0	2.5
Brown Sugar: 1 Tbsp	50	0	13
1 ounce, 1 oz	110	0	28
1 cup, not packed, 5 oz	550	0	140
1 cup, packed, 7.8 oz	835	0	216
Powdered Sugar:			
Sifted, 1 cup, 3.5 oz	390	0	100
Unsifted, 1 cup, 4¼ oz	470	0	120
Coconut Palm Sugar, 1 tsp, 4g	15	0	4
Dextrose, 1 tsp	12	0	3
Fructose, powder, 1 tsp	12	0	3
Glucose Powder, 1 oz	110	0	27
Glucose Tablets, (1)	20	0	5
Palm Sugar, 3 Tbsp	45	0	11
Piloncillo, (Brown Sugar), 3oz	325	0	81
Turbinado Sugar, 2 Tbsp, 1 oz	110	0	27

Sugar Substitutes

Agave, 1 Tbsp, 0.7 oz	60	0	16
DiabetiSweet, 1 teaspoon	9	0	4.5
Note: Carb figure includes 4.5 g sugar alcohol			
Domino, Light, ½ tsp	5	0	2
Equal: Tablet (2)	0	0	0
Granular, 1 tsp	0	0	0
Packet (1)	0	0	0
Next, 1 packet	0	0	0
Nectresse, 1 packet	0	0	0
NutraSweet, 1 tsp	0	0	0
Splenda, Granulated No Calorie Sweetener:			
1 tsp	0	0	0
1 cup	95	0	24
Packets, all flavors	0	0	0
Sugar Blend,Orig/Brown, ½ cup	385	0	96
Stevia, single serving	0	0	0
Sugar Twin, 1 packet	0	0	0
Sweet 'N Low, 1 packet	0	0	0
Truvia, 1 packet	0	0	0
Walgreens, Wal-Sweet, 1 packet	0	0	0
Whey Low, 1 tsp	4	0	1

Syrups, Molasses, Agave

Syrups· Plain: *Average All Brands*
(Corn/Rice/Maple/Pancake/Sundae/Waffle)
Includes Aunt Jemima, Cary's, Karo, Hershey's,
Hungry Jack, IHOP, Log Cabin, Mrs Butterworth's

	C	F	Cb
Regular/Dark/Light Color:			
1 Tbsp, 0.5 fl.oz	55	0	14
¼ cup (4 Tbsp)	220	0	55
Single Portion, 1.5 oz pkg	170	0	42
Lite, 1Tbsp, 1 oz	25	0	6
Sugar-Free: 2 Tbsp, 1 oz	18	0	5
Maple Grove, Cozy Cottage, 2 Tbsp	10	0	3
IHOP, 4 Tbsp, 2 oz	20	0	7
Fruit Syrups, (IHOP), ¼ cup, 2 oz	200	0	52
Honey Cream Syrup, ¼ cup, 2 oz	220	0	55
Molasses: Dark/Light: 1 T, 0.7 oz	60	0	15
1 cup, 12 oz	975	0.5	252
Blackstrap, 1 Tbsp, 0.8 oz	47	0	13
Agave Nectar, av. all flavors,			
1 Tablespoon, 0.8 oz	60	0	15

Flavored Syrups/Ice Cream Toppings

Hershey's: *Per 2 Tbsp*			
Double Chocolate,	105	0	26
Other Flavors, average	90	0	23
Lite	45	0	12
Smuckers: *Per 2 Tbsp*			
Magic Shell, average all flavors	220	17	16
Spoonables: Reg., average all flavors	115	1	28
Sugar Free: Caramel; Hot Fudge	90	0	24
Strawberry	30	0	9
Note: Carb figures include 8g-17g sugar alcohol			
Sundae Syrups: Regular, av. all flavors	105	0	25
Sugar Free, average all flavors	90	0	24
Note: Carb figures includes 15g sugar alcohol			

Honey, Jam, Preserves

Average all Brands

Honey: 1 tsp, 0.23 oz	20	0	5.5
1 Tbsp, 0.7 oz	60	0	17
1 oz	85	0	24
½ cup, 6 oz	515	0	145
Single Portion, 0.5 oz package	45	0	12
Jams/Jellies/Marmalade/Preserves:			
Regular: 1 tsp, 0.3 oz	20	0	5
1 Tbsp, 0.8 oz	55	0	14
1 ounce, 1 oz	80	0	20
Single Portion, 0.5 oz pkg	40	0	11
Apple/Fruit Butters, 1 T., 0.6 oz	20	0	6
Fruit Spreads: Regular, 1 tsp	15	0	4
Low Sugar, 1 tsp	8	0	2
Jelly: Regular, average, 1 tsp	18	0	4.5
Imitation, Low Calorie, 1 tsp	1	0	1

Vegetables	C	F	Cb
Alfalfa Sprouts, 1/2 cup, 0.5 oz	5	0	0.5
Artichokes, Globe/French:			
1 medium, 4.5 oz	60	0	13
1 large, 5.7 oz	75	0	17
Artichoke Heart, plain, 2 pieces	15	0	3
Asparagus, raw/frozen:			
Cuts & Tips, 1/2 cup, 4.3 oz	20	0	3
Spears, 3 medium	10	0	2
Bamboo Shoots, cooked, 1/2 cup, 2 oz	7	0	1
Beans, Green/Snap/String:			
10 beans (4" long), 2 oz	20	0	4
Pieces, 1/2 cup, 3 oz	30	0	7
Dried Beans (Kidney, Brown, Lima, Navy, Pinto, White):			
Raw: 2 Tbsp, 1 oz	95	0.5	18
1 cup, 7 oz	665	3	126
Cooked: 1 oz	35	0	7
1/2 cup, 3 oz	105	0	21
Bean Sprouts, average, 1/2 cup, 2 oz	15	0	3.5
Beets (Beetroot):			
Raw, 1 beet (2" diam.), 4 oz	35	0	8
Cooked, 1 cup, slices, 3 oz	35	0	8
Canned ~ *See Page 161*			
Beet Greens, cooked, 1/2 cup, 2.5 oz	20	0	4
Bell Pepper ~ *See Peppers*			
Bitter Melon/Gourd, 1 cup, 1.5 oz	15	0	1.5
Blackeye Peas, cooked, 1/2 cup, 3 oz	100	0.5	18
Bok Choy (Chinese Chard), cooked, 3 oz	10	0	1.5
Breadfruit, 1/4 small fruit, 3 oz	100	0	26
Broadbeans (Fava Beans):			
Green, raw, (in pod): 4 pods (3.5 oz with shells, 1.2 oz beans)	30	0	6
1 cup beans, without shell, 4.5 oz	110	1	22
Mature Seeds: Raw, 1 cup, 5.3 oz	510	2.5	87
Cooked, 1/2 cup, 3 oz	95	0	17
Broccoflower, 1/5 head, 3.5 oz	35	0	7
Broccoli: Raw, chopped, 1 cup, 3 oz	30	0	6
3 Florets, 2.5 oz	25	0	5
1 Spear (5" long), 1.oz	10	0	2
1 Whole: Medium, 14 oz	135	1.5	26
Large, 21 oz	205	2	40
1 Head (no stalk), 11 oz	105	1	21
1 Stalk, small (5" long), 5.3 oz	50	0.5	10
Brocco Sprouts, 1/2 cup, 1 oz	15	0	2
Brussels Sprouts:			
Cooked, 1/2 cup, 2.8 oz	30	0.5	6
2 Sprouts, 1.5 oz	15	0	3
Butterbeans, cooked, 1/2 cup, 3 oz	90	0	16
Cabbage, average other flavors:			
Raw: 1 leaf, large, 1 oz	5	0	2
Shredded, 1 cup, 2.5 oz	15	0	4
1/2 large head (7" diam), 22 oz	150	1	35
Cooked, shredded, 1/2 cup, 2.5 oz	15	0.5	3.5

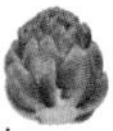
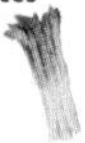

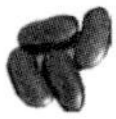
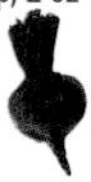
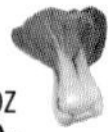
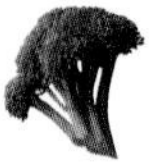
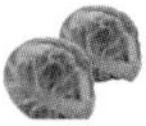
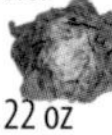

Vegetables (Cont)	C	F	Cb
Cactus Leaf (Nopales):			
1 leaf, 4.5 oz	20	0	4
1 cup (slices), 3 oz	15	0	3
Carrots, regular thick variety:			
1 small, 4 oz	45	0	11
1 medium, 6 oz	70	0	16
1 large, 8 oz	95	0	22
Chopped, 1 cup, 4.5 oz	50	0	12
Grated, 1 cup, 4 oz	45	0	11
Slices, 1 cup, 4.5 oz	50	0	12
Sticks (4"), 4-5, 1.5 oz	20	0	4
Long thin variety, 1 medium, 2.2 oz	25	0	6
Baby: Snack size, 3 medium, 1 oz	10	0	2.5
Snack Pack, 3 oz	30	0	7
Cassava, raw, 1 cup, 2.5 oz	330	0.5	78
Cauliflower, raw:			
Pieces, 1 cup, 3.5 oz	25	0	5
1/2 medium head, 10 oz	70	0	15
Cooked, 3 florets, 2 oz	10	0	2
Celeriac, 1/2 cup, raw, 2.8 oz	35	0	7
Celery: 1 large stalk, 11", 2.2 oz	10	0	2
4 Strips, thin sticks, 0.5 oz	5	0	1
Chopped, 1 cup, 3.5 oz	15	0	3
Chard (Swiss), 1/2 cup, cooked, 3 oz	20	0	3.5
Chayote Squash:			
1 medium, 7 oz	40	0	9
Pieces, 1 cup, 4.5 oz	25	0	6
Chickpeas, (Garbanzo Beans):			
Dry, 1 cup, 7 oz	730	12	121
Cooked, 1 cup, 5.8 oz	270	4	45
Chicory Greens, 1 cup, 1 oz	7	0	1.5
Chili Peppers ~ *See Peppers*			
Chinese Long Bean, slices, 1 cup, 3.2 oz	45	0	8
Chives, chopped, 1 Tbsp	1	0	0
Choy Sum, 3 oz	15	0	3
Cilantro, (Coriander), 1 cup	5	0	0.5
Collards, cooked, 1/2 cup, 3 oz	25	0	5
Corn, Yellow/White:			
Raw: Kernels, 1/2 cup, 3 oz	80	0.5	19
Ear (5"x 1 3/4"), 5.5 oz	155	1	37
Cooked: Kernels, 1/2 cup, 3 oz	77	0.5	18
Cob, small, 2.3 oz	60	0.5	14
Ear, large, 5.5 oz	120	1	28
Cress, garden, raw, 1 cup, 1.8 oz	15	0	3
Cucumber, average other flavors:			
Slices, 1/2 cup, 2 oz	10	0	2
Green, 1 medium (9"), 11 oz	45	0	11
Persian, 1 medium (8"), 6 oz	25	0	5
Daikon Radish, 1/2 cup, slices, 2 oz	9	0	2
Dandelion Greens, raw, 1/2 cup, 1 oz	10	0	2.5
Edamame, (Immature green soybeans):			
Shelled, 1/2 cup, 2.6 oz	110	5	8
With shells, 10 pods, 1.3 oz	30	1	3

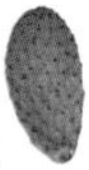
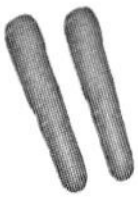
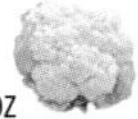
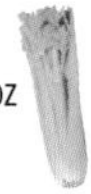
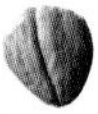
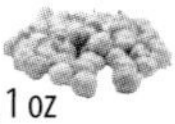
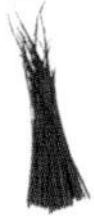
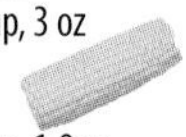
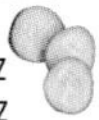
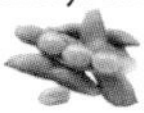

Vegetables (Cont)

	C	F	Cb
Eggplant, raw: 4 oz	30	0	7
1/2 cup, 1" pieces, 1.5 oz	10	0	2
1 slice, fried, 1 oz	75	4	10
Endive, Belgian/French: Raw,			
1 medium head (6"), 2.5 oz	12	0	3
Fennel, 1 cup, sliced, 3 oz	25	0	7
Gai Choy Cabbage, cooked, 1 cup, 6 oz	20	0	3
Gai Lan, (Chinese Kale), cooked, 1 cup	35	0.5	7
Garbanzo Beans ~ *See Chick Peas*			
Garlic, 1 clove	4	0	1
Ginger: 1/4 cup slices, 1 oz	20	0	5
Crystallized (sugared), 7 pieces, 1.5 oz	130	0	35
Horseradish, raw, 1 pod, 0.5 oz	5	0	1
Jerusalem Artichoke, raw, 1/2 cup	55	0	13
Jicama, raw, sliced, 1/2 cup, 2.3 oz	25	0	6
Kale, 1 cup, chopped, 2.5 oz	35	0.5	7
Kalettes, 1 cup, 2 oz	30	0	4
Kohlrabi, cooked, 1/2 cup, 1.8 oz	17	0	5
Leek, cooked, 1 whole, 4.5 oz	40	0	9
Lentils, green/brown: Dry, 1 oz	100	0.5	17
1 cup, 6.8 oz	675	3	115
Cooked, 1/2 cup, 3.5 oz	115	0.5	20
Lettuce: 1 cup, chopped/shredded, 2 oz	7	0	1
Butterhead, 2 leaves, 0.5 oz	2	0	0.5
Cos/Romaine, shredded, 1 cup	10	0	2
Iceberg: 1 outer leaf, 0.5 oz	2	0	0.5
1 medium head, 16 oz	75	1	16
Lima Beans, baby, cooked, 1/2 cup, 3 oz	105	0	20
Lotus Root, cooked, 10 slices, 3 oz	60	0	14
Mung Bean Sprouts, 1/2 cup, 2 oz	15	0	3
Mushrooms, average all varieties:			
Raw, diced/siced, 1 cup, 3 oz	20	0	3
Pieces, 1 cup, 1.3 oz	8	0	1
Fried/Sauteed, 6 oz	220	16	10
Grilled, pieces, 1/2 cup, 2.5 oz	20	0.5	4
Shitake, dried, 1 oz package	90	0	22
Mustard Greens, raw, 1/2 cup, 1 oz	7	0	2
Okra: Raw, 8 pods, 4 oz	30	0	7
Cooked, 1/2 cup, 2.8 oz	20	0	4
Onions, Raw: 1 small, 2.5 oz	30	0	7
1 medium, 4 oz	50	0	11
1 large, 5.5 oz	65	0	15
1 jumbo, 16 oz	190	0.5	46
Chopped: 1/2 cup, 3 oz	35	0	8
1 Tbsp, 0.4 oz	5	0	1
Slices: 1 cup, 4 oz	50	0	12
1 medium slice (1/8"), 0.5 oz	5	0	1
1 large slice (1/4"), 1.3 oz	15	0	4
Flakes, dried 1/4 cup, 0.5 oz	50	0	12
Rings, breaded & fried, 2 rings	80	5	9
Scallions, 1/2 cup, 2 oz	15	0	3
Spring, chopped, 1/2 cup, 2 oz	15	0	3

Vegetables (Cont)

	C	F	Cb
Parsley, chopped, 1/2 cup, 1 oz	10	0	2
Parsnip: 1 medium, 4 oz	85	0	20
Cooked, slices, 1/2 cup, 2.8 oz	55	0	13
Peas: Green, raw, 1/4 cup, 1.5 oz	30	0	5
With pods, 0.5 lb	70	0	13
Snow Peas, 10 pods, 1.2 oz	15	0	3
Split: Dry, hulled, 1 oz	100	0.5	17
Cooked, 1 cup, 7 oz	230	1	42
Peppers:			
Sweet, 1 medium, 4.2 oz	30	0	7
Bell: 1 medium, 4.2 oz	30	0	7
raw, chopped, 1/2 cup, 2.5 oz	20	0	5
2 rings (5" diam. x 1/4" thick)	3	0	1
Chili: Green/Red, 1.5 oz	20	0	5
Habanero, 1 only, 0.3 oz	10	0	2
Pigeon Peas, cooked, 1/2 cup, 3 oz	95	1	17
Pimientos, 3 medium, 3.5 oz	25	0	5
Poi, 1/2 cup, 4.2 oz	135	0	33
Potatoes:			
Raw (with skin):			
1 baby, 2 oz	45	0	10
1 small, 6 oz	135	0	30
1 medium, 8 oz	180	0	40
1 large, 12 oz	270	0	60
1 extra large, 16 oz	360	0	80
Baked, (no added fat), large, 10 oz (raw wt):			
Plain: With skin, 7 oz (cooked wt)	185	0	42
W/o skin, 5.5 oz (cooked wt)	145	0	34
With Skin/Toppings:			
With 2 tsp fat	270	8	58
With Grated Cheese, 1 oz	370	9	58
With Plain Yogurt, 2 Tbsp	260	1	60
With Sour Crm & Chives, 2 Tbsp	320	6	60
Mashed:			
With milk plus fat, 1/2 cup, 4 oz	120	4.5	18
KFC Style without gravy, 4 oz	90	3	15
Loaded (fat/cream/cheese/bacon):			
Side serving, 6 oz	180	9	22
Large serving, 12 oz	360	18	44
Potato Skins, baked w/ cheese topping,			
1/2 whole, 4 oz	240	13	22
French Fries: Small serving, 2.6 oz	250	13	30
Medium serving, 4 oz	380	20	47
Frozen, uncooked, 18 fries, 4 oz	165	5.5	28
Oven-heated, 18 fries, 4 oz	165	5.5	28
Take-Out, 1 cup, 5 oz	440	25	60
Au Gratin, 1/2 cup, 4.3 oz	160	9	14
Pancakes, 2 small, 2 oz	120	6.5	12
Puffs, fried, 4 puffs, 1 oz	55	2.5	8
Scalloped, 8.5 oz	220	9	26

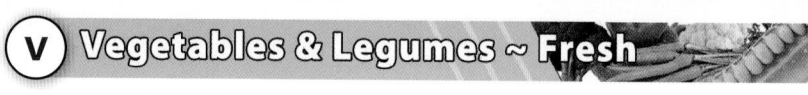

Vegetables (Cont)	C	F	Cb
Pumpkin:			
Raw, 1" cubes, 1 cup, 4 oz	30	0	7
Cooked:			
Baked, without fat, 4 oz	90	7	9
Mashed: 1 scoop, 2 oz	10	0	2
1/2 cup, 4.3 oz	25	0	6
Pumpkin Flowers, 1 cup, 1.2 oz	5	0	1
Purslane: Cooked, 1/2 cup, 2 oz	10	0	2
Raw, 1" cubes, 1 cup, 1.5 oz	5	0	1.5
Radicchio: 2 leaves, 0.5 oz	5	0	1
Shredded, 1 cup, 1.5 oz	20	0	4
Radishes: 1 small	0	0	0
10 medium/5 large, 1.6 oz	5	0	1
Slices, 1/2 cup, 2 oz	10	0	2
Rhubarb, raw, 1/2 cup, 2 oz	15	0	3
Rutabaga, cubes, cooked, 1/2 cup, 3 oz	30	0	7
Salsify, cooked, slices, 1/2 cup, 2.5 oz	50	0	11
Sauerkraut, 1/2 cup, 2.5 oz	15	0	3
Seaweed: Dried, 1 oz	5	0	2
Soaked, drained, 1 oz	15	0	4
Nori/Laver, dried, 6 sheets, 0.5 oz	35	0	5
Shallots, chopped, 1 Tbsp, 0.5 oz	5	0	1
Sorrel, raw, 1/2 cup, 4 oz	20	0	4
Soybeans: Dry, 1/2 cup, 3.3 oz	390	18	28
Mature, dry, 1 oz	120	5.5	9
Cooked, 1/2 cup, 3 oz	150	7.5	8
Soy Products/Tofu/Tempeh ~ *See Page 156*			
Spinach: Cooked, 1/2 cup, 3 oz	20	0	4
Creamed, average, 1/2 cup, 4.5 oz	190	15	8
Raw: 3 leaves, 1 cup, 1 oz	7	0	1
1 Bunch, 12 oz	80	1.5	12
Squash:			
Summer: Raw, 1/2 cup, 2.5 oz	10	0	2
Cooked, slices, 1/2 cup, 3 oz	15	0	3
Winter, cooked:			
Acorn: Cubes, 1/2 cup, 3.5 oz	35	0	9
1/2 medium (10 oz raw weight)	115	0	30
Butternut: Cubes, 1/2 cup, 3.5 oz	40	0	10
1/4 medium (9 oz raw weight)	115	0	30
Spaghetti, 1/2 cup, 1.8 oz	15	0	3
Succotash, cooked, 1/2 cup, 3.3 oz	110	1	23
Sweetcorn ~ *See Corn*			
Sweet Potatoes:			
Cooked with skin (w/o fat),			
1 medium, 4 oz	105	0	24
Without skin, mashed, 1/2 cup, 5.5 oz	125	0	29
Fries (Alexia, Julienne syle),			
approximately 12 pieces, 3 oz	140	5	24

Vegetables (Cont)	C	F	Cb
Swiss Chard, cooked, chopped, 1 c., 6 oz	35	0	7
Taro, cooked, 1/2 cup, 2.3 oz	95	0	23
Tomatoes: 1 small (2 1/4" diam.), 3 oz	15	0	3
1 medium (2 3/4" diameter), 5 oz	25	0	5
1 large (3 1/2" diameter), 8 oz	40	0.5	9
1 extra lge (4" diam.), 12 oz	60	0.5	14
Chopped, 1 cup, 6.5 oz	35	0.5	7
Tomatillo: 1 medium, 1.2 oz	10	0	2
1 lb quantity for recipe	135	4.5	27
Turnip: Cooked, 1/2 cup, 2.8 oz	15	0	4
Greens, cooked, 1/2 cup, 2.5 oz	15	0	3
Water Chestnuts: 5-6 nuts, 1 oz	56	0.5	13
Raw, slices, 1/2 cup, 2.3 oz	60	0	15
Canned, 1 oz	15	0	3
Watercress, 10 sprigs, 1 oz	3	0	0.5
Yams: Cooked, steamed, 1/2 cup, 2.5 oz	80	0	19
Baked:			
1 medium (6") 8 oz	265	0.5	63
1 large (9") 12 oz	400	0.5	94
Yardlong Bean, 1 pod, 0.5 oz	5	0	1
Yucca Root, raw, 1/2 cup, 3.5 oz	165	0	39
Zucchini: Raw, 1 medium, 7 oz	30	0.5	7
1 large, 12 oz	60	1	12
Cooked, slices,			
1/2 cup, 3 oz	15	0	4

Frozen Vegetables			
Birds Eye:			
Mixtures & Blends:			
Broccoli, Cauliflower & Carrots, 3 oz	35	0	5.5
Stir-Fry: Broccoli, 3.4 oz	35	0	6
Crisp Green Bean, 5.5 oz	60	0	11
Sugar Snap, 3.4 oz	40	0	7.5
Pure & Simple:			
Baby: Broccoli Florets, 1 cup, 3 oz	35	0.5	4.5
Gold & White Corn, 2/3 cup, 3.2 oz	105	1	22
Sweet Peas, 2/3 cup, 3 oz	80	0	14
Recipe Ready:			
Chopped Green Peppers & Onions, 2.8 oz	25	0	5
Southwest Blend, 3.3 oz	80	0.5	15
Sauced & Seasoned: *Per 1 Cup*			
Green Beans & Spaetzle,			
in Bavarian Sauce	95	4.5	10
Pasta & Veggies in Creamy Cheese Sauce	125	3	20
Steamfresh:			
Pure & Simple Blends:			
Baby Broccoli Blend, 1 cup	65	1.5	8
Baby Potato Blend, 3/4 cup	50	0	10
Brocc. & Cauliflower, 1 cup, 3.4 oz	30	0.5	4.5

Frozen Vegetables (Cont) · C · F · Cb

Green Giant:

	C	F	Cb
Mashed Cauliflowe: Original, 4.2 oz	80	5	7
Cheddar & Bacon, 4.2 oz	90	6	6
Riced Cauliflower/with Brocc., 3 oz	20	0	4
Roasted Veggies: Broccoli, 3 oz	30	0	6
Brussels Sprouts, 3 oz	30	0	6
Carrots, 3 oz	30	0.5	7
Cauliflower, 3 oz	20	0	3
Corn, 3 oz	120	1.5	25
Sautes:			
Fire Roasted, Prepared:			
Corn, Peppers & Onions, 1/2 cup	80	0.5	16
Root Veggies w/ Red Onions, 2/3 c.	60	0	14
Tri color Peppers, 1/3 cup	25	0	5
Zucchini, Carrots & Onions, 1/3 cup	20	0	4
Kits: Herb B'Nut Squash Medley, 4.3 oz	35	1	7
Chipotle Harvest, 1 cup prepared	280	3	25
Thai Coconut, 1 cup prepared	210	4	18
Steamers: Corn Niblets, 3 oz	90	1	19
Backyard Gr. Potatoes, 1/2 cup prep.	110	3	20
Creamed Spinach, 3.8 oz	70	2	9
Veggie Tots: Broccoli & Cheese, 3 oz	130	6	14
Brocolli; Cauliflower, 3 oz	110	4.5	15

Ore-Ida: *Per 3 oz Unless Indicated*

Fries:

	C	F	Cb
Bold & Crispy: Chili Cheese Crinkle	160	7	22
Garlic Black Pepper Steakhouse	180	8	25
Zesties, Seasoned	180	7.5	26
Zesty, Seasoned Curly	185	9	24
Classic: Golden Crinkles	120	4.5	19
Golden	130	3.5	21
Steak	110	3	19
Extra Crispy Easy, Golden Crinkles	170	6	25
Extra Crispy:			
Fast Food Fries	150	6	24
Golden Crinkles	160	7	22
Seasoned Crinkles	150	6	22
Premium: Crispers	230	14	23
Country Style French	130	4.5	20
Golden Twirls	150	6	23
Texas Crispers	150	7	20
Hash Browns: Golden Patties (1)	140	8	15
Potatoes O'Brien	60	0	13
Shredded Hash Browns Pattie (1)	70	0	16
Mashed Potato Bites:			
Four Cheese, 2.5 oz	180	10	18
Loaded Baked, 2.5 oz	170	10	18
Onion: Chopped, 3 oz	20	0	5
Gourmet Rings, 2.7 oz	185	9	24
Onion Ringers, 3 oz	180	10	21
Steam n' Mash, Cut Russet, 3.5 oz	70	0	16
Tater Tots, Reg., Crispy Crowns, av.	165	9	20

Canned/Bottled · C · F · Cb

Solids & Liquid

	C	F	Cb
Artichoke Hearts:			
Fancifoods: Plain, 1 oz (1)	8	0	1
Marinated, 1/4 bottle, 1 oz	25	1.5	2
Asparagus: Drained, 3 spears	10	0	1.5
Pieces, 1/2 cup, 4.3 oz	25	0.5	3
Bamboo Shoots, 1 cup, 4.5 oz	25	0	4
Bean Salad, 1/2 cup, 4.4 oz	90	0	20
Beans: Baked, 1/2 cup, 4.5 oz	120	0.5	27
Butter, 1/2 cup, 4.5 oz	90	0	16
Green, 1/2 cup, 2.5 oz	15	0	3
Italian, 1/2 cup, 4.5 oz	30	0	6
Kidney, 1/2 cup 3.5 oz	105	0.5	19
Lima, 1/2 cup, 4.5 oz	80	0	15
Pinto, 1/2 cup, 4.5 oz	105	1	18
Beets: Sliced, 1/2 cup, 3 oz	25	0	6
Crinkle/Pickled, 1/2 cup	80	0	20
Carrots: Sliced, 1/2 cup, 2.5 oz	20	0	4
Del Monte, Honey Glazed, 1/2 cup	75	0	18
Corn: Kernels, 1/2 cup, 4.5 oz	80	0.5	18
Creamed style, 1/2 cup, 4.5 oz	90	0.5	23
Garbanzo/Chick Peas, 1/2 c, 4.2 oz	145	1.5	27
Hearts of Palm, (1), 1.2 oz	7	0	1
Mushrooms: 1/2 cup, 2.5 oz	20	0	4
In Butter Sauce, 2 oz	20	1	2
Onions: Cocktail (1)	0	0	0
Pickled, 1 medium, 0.5 oz	10	0	2
Peas, 1/2 cup, 3 oz	60	0.5	10
Peppers: Hot Chili, Jalapeno (1), 1 oz	5	0	1
Red/Green, 1 oz	5	0	1
Sweet, undrained, 2.5 oz	13	0	3
Jalapeno, with liquid, 1/2 cup chopped	20	0.5	3
Fried, drained, 2 Tbsp, 1 oz	60	5	3
Salsa, average all varieties, 2 Tbsp	10	0	2
Sauerkraut, drained, 1 cup, 5 oz	25	0	6
Spinach, 1/2 cup, 3.5 oz	25	0.5	3.5
Succotash: Cream Style, 1/2 cup	100	0.5	23
w/ whole kernels, undrained, 1/2 cup	80	0.5	18
Sweetcorn ~ *See Corn*			
Sweet Potato, 1/2 cup, 3.5 oz	90	0	24
Tomatoes, Sundried: Nat., 5-6 pieces	20	0	5
In Oil, drained, 6 pieces, 0.5 oz	40	2.5	4
Tomato Products ~ *See Page 144*			
Vegetables, mixed, 1/2 cup, 4 oz	45	0	8
Yams: In Light Syrup, 1/2 cup, 4 oz	105	0	25
Candied, 1/2 cup, 5 oz	170	0	46
Zucchini, in Tomato Sauce, 1/2 cup, 4 oz	30	0	8

Quick Guide

	C	F	Cb
Yogurt: *Average All Brands: Per 8 oz Container*			
Plain Yogurt: Whole	140	8	10
Low-Fat	145	3.5	16
Fat-Free	125	0.5	17
Fruit Flavored: Whole	225	8	32
Low-Fat	230	3	43
Fat-Free, regular	215	0.5	43
Fat-Free, no sugar added	80	0	15
Yogurt Parfait/Deli Cups:			
With Fruit Pieces: ($^2/_3$ Yogurt + $^1/_3$ Fruit)			
Small, 8 oz cup	140	3	20
Large, 12 oz cup	210	4.5	30
With Fruit + Granola:			
Small, 8 oz cup (+ 0.75 oz Granola)	235	7	30
Large, 12 oz cup (+ 1.3 oz Granola)	400	13	58

Yogurt ~ Brands

	C	F	Cb
Activia:			
4 oz Containers: Fiber with Fruit, av.	100	1.5	19
Fruit/Fusion, average all flavors	90	2	15
Lactose Free, average	100	2	16
Light, nonfat, all flavors	60	0	10
Greek, nonfat, 5.3 oz Ctn:			
Regular, average all flavors	125	0	20
Almond Dream *(Non Dairy): Per 6 oz Ctn*			
Coconut	130	2.5	27
Mixed Berry; Strawberry	160	2.5	33
Plain	150	3	30
Vanilla	160	3	33
Alpina:			
Artisan Granolas: Plain, 6 oz	170	4.5	18
Blueberry, av., 6 oz	240	4	38
Strawberry; Vanilla, 6 oz	190	3.5	26
Greek, Non-Fat, av., 5.3 oz	125	0	19
Amande:			
Almond Milk Yogurt: Plain, 8 oz	170	9	19
Coconut, 6 oz	170	8	23
Fruit Flavors, 6 oz	150	6	23
Vanilla, 8 oz	220	8	26
Axelrod:			
32 oz Ctn: Regular Plain, 8 oz	160	8	15
Fat Free, Plain, 8 oz	130	0	19
6 oz Containers:			
Low Fat, Fruit flavors, av.	180	1.5	36
NonFat Vanilla	90	0	17
Brown Cow:			
Cream Top, On The Bottom: *Per 5.3 oz Ctn*			
Whole Milk: Apricot Mango	150	5	22
Cherry Vanilla; Strawberry, av.	160	5	25
Chocolate	170	5	26

	C	F	Cb
Brown Cow (Cont):			
Cream Top: *Per 5.3 oz Ctn*			
Whole Milk: Plain	110	6	9
Cherry Vanilla	160	5	25
Coffee; Vanilla, av.	150	6	19
Specialties: *Per 5 oz Ctn*			
Cafe Mocha	140	5	20
Marbled Chocolate Raspberry	150	5	22
Vanilla Salted Caramel	150	5	20
Cabot: *Per 8 oz Serving*			
Greek Style, 32 oz Ctn:			
Plain	310	22	12
Lowfat (2%): Plain	180	5	12
Honey	230	4.5	29
Strawberry; Van. Bean	240	4	34
Chobani Greek Yogurt: *Per 5.3 oz Ctn*			
Blended: Coconut	140	4	15
Coffee	160	2.5	22
Orange & Cream	140	4.5	15
Plain: Whole Milk, 1 cup	230	11	9
Non Fat	120	0	9
Flip: Almond Coco Loco	230	10	23
Coffee Brownie Bliss	180	4	24
Fruit On The Bottom:			
Apricot	140	2.5	18
Strawberry; Pomegranate	120	0	18
Smooth, Low-Fat:			
Fruit Flavors	120	1.5	16
Vanilla	120	2	15
Tots, Whole Milk, average	95	4.5	10
Coconut Dream *(Non Dairy): Per 6 oz Ctn*			
Plain	120	4	24
Berry varieties, aveage	135	3	28
Vanilla	120	3	28
Dannon:			
Activia ~ *See Activia*			
All Natural, Plain: Lowfat, 8 oz	150	3.5	19
Nonfat, 8 oz	120	0	18
Whole Milk, 8 oz	175	8	18
Creamy, Strawberry, 4 oz	70	0	14
Fruit On The Bottom, av, 5.3 oz	130	1.5	25
Lowfat: Coffee; Vanilla, av., 5.3 oz	140	2	24
Vanilla, 6 oz	130	2	21
Whole Milk, all flav., 5.3 oz	140	4.5	20
Fage: *Per 5.3 oz Ctn*			
Crossovers:			
Caramel with Almonds	230	10	20
Maple Syrup with Granola	190	6	20
Total Split Cups:			
5% Fat: Fruit Flav., av.	150	6	13
Honey	210	6	29
2% Fat, Fruit Flav., av.	125	2.5	14
0% Fat, Fruit Flavors	110	0	14

Yogurt Brands (Cont)   C   F   Cb

Fage (Cont):
Total, Plain: *Per 6 oz Container*

	C	F	Cb
5% Fat	190	10	6
2% Fat	140	4	6
0% Fat	90	0	5

Great Value *(Walmart):*
Greek, Fat Free:

	C	F	Cb
32 oz Ctn: Plain, 8 oz	120	0	9
Strawberry, 6 oz	140	0	22

Non Fat Light Greek: *Per 5 oz Container*

	C	F	Cb
Peach	80	0	9
Strawberry	90	0	8
Vanilla	90	0	10

Horizon Organic:
Whole Milk:

	C	F	Cb
32 oz Ctn: Plain, 8 oz	170	8	14
Vanilla, 8 oz	210	6	30
6 oz Ctn, average all flavors	170	5	25

Kemps,

	C	F	Cb
Light, 80 Calories, all flavors, 6 oz	80	0	15

La Yogurt: *Per 6 oz Container*

	C	F	Cb
Low Fat: Orig., Fruit Flavors, av.	155	1.5	30
Rich & Creamy, Fruit Flav., av.	180	1.5	35

LALA:

	C	F	Cb
32 oz Tubs, Plain, 8 oz	130	2.5	17
Singles, Fruit Flav., av., 6 oz	150	1.5	30

Lucerne:

	C	F	Cb
Greek Nonfat, Plain, 8 oz	130	0	14
Low-Fat, Strawberry	130	2	23
Light Nonfat, Vanilla, 6 oz	120	0	22
Fat Free, Plain, 8 oz	120	0	21

Mountain High: *Per 8 oz*
32 oz Containers:

	C	F	Cb
Whole Milk Original: Plain	170	7	15
Strawberry; Vanilla	200	7	28
Lowfat: Plain	130	2.5	16
Vanilla	170	2.5	28
Fat Free: Plain	110	0	16
Vanilla	160	0	30

Nancy's:
Natural Whole Milk: *Per 8 oz*

	C	F	Cb
Fruit flav., av	225	5	39
Honey	170	8	17

Organic Whole Milk: *Per 8 oz Container*

	C	F	Cb
Plain	180	8	16
with Fruit on Top, average	230	5	40
Organic Lowfat, Plain	140	3	16
Organic Nonfat: Plain	120	0	17
with Fruit On Top, average	155	0	28
Organic Soy: Plain, 6 oz	150	3	25
Plain, unsweetened, 6 oz	80	3.5	6

Oikos *(Dannon):*   C   F   Cb
Greek: *Whole Milk: Per 5.3 oz Ctn*

	C	F	Cb
Whole Milk: Coffee	160	4	20
Fruit flavors, av.	155	4	18
Mayan Chocolate	150	4.5	15
Non Fat: Plain, 5.3 oz	80	0	6
Fruit flavors, 5.3 oz	110	0	15
Protein Crunch, av., 5 oz carton	150	1	19
Triple Zero Greek, all flavors, 5.3 oz	120	0	14
O Organics: Blended Low-Fat, av. 8 oz	150	2	26
Greek, Plain, Nonfat, 5.3 oz carton	90	0	8

Siggi's:
Skyr: *Per 5.3 oz Unless Indicated*

	C	F	Cb
0%: Plain	90	0	6
Fruit Flavors, average	120	0	13
Vanilla	110	0	12
2%: Coconut	170	5	16
Fruit Flavors, average	140	2.5	14
4%: Fruit flavors, 4.4 oz	130	4.5	11
Fruit, no added sugar, av., 4.4 oz	115	4	10

Silk: *Per 5.3 oz Containers*

	C	F	Cb
Almond Yogurt: Plain	180	13	10
Fruit flavors, average	180	11	18
Vanilla	200	11	21
Soy Yogurt: Fruit flavors, av	140	3.5	21
Vanilla	140	3.5	20

So Delicious:
Cultured Coconut Milk:

	C	F	Cb
Plain, 8 oz	170	7	25
Blueb./Strawb. 5.3 oz	140	4	24
Chocolate, 5.3 oz	150	5	27
Vanilla, 8 oz	190	6	33
Unsweetened: Plain, 8 oz	110	7	10
Vanilla, 8 oz	110	7	12

Stonyfield Organic:
Double Cream:

	C	F	Cb
Madagascar Vanilla, 5 oz	150	8	19
Pacific Coast Strawberry, 5 oz	150	7	16

Fat Free Fruit On Bottom: *Per 5.3 oz*

	C	F	Cb
Blueberry	90	0	17
Chocolate Underground	110	0	22

Smooth & Creamy (32 oz Ctn):

	C	F	Cb
0% Fat: Plain, 8 oz	100	0	15
French Vanilla, 8 oz	150	0	27
Lowfat: Plain, 8 oz	110	2	14
Vanilla, 8 oz	150	2	25
Whole Milk, French Vanilla, 8 oz	200	7	27

Yogurt Brands (Cont)

	C	F	Cb
Trader Joes:			
Organic: Banana; Vanilla, 4 oz	100	3	14
Cream Top, Whole Milk, Plain, 8 oz	160	9	9
Low Fat, Fruit Flavors, 6 oz	145	2.5	25
Nonfat: Plain + Vit D, 8 oz	110	0	15
Strawb. + Vit D, 4 oz	90	0	17
Vanilla, 5.3 oz cup	120	0	16
European: Lowfat, Choc./Mocha, 5.3 oz	135	3	21
Smth & Crmy: Whole Milk, Plain, 8 oz	170	7	14
Nonfat, Plain, 8 oz	120	0	17
French Village: Cream Line, Plain, 8 oz	180	10	13
Nonfat: Apricot Mango/Strawb., 6 oz	130	0	25
32 oz Ctn, Plain, 8 oz	120	0	17
Greek, 2% Low Fat, Plain, 8 oz	170	4.5	10
Whole Milk: Plain, 8 oz	280	22	12
Apricot Mango; Honey, av., 8 oz	300	18	27
0% Non Fat: Plain, 8 oz	120	0	7
Fruit Flavors; Honey, 5.3 oz	120	0	17
Vanilla Bean, 5.3 oz	130	0	20
Goats Milk, Plain ¾ cup, 6 oz	100	4.5	7
Voskos:			
Original: Plain, 8 oz	280	20	15
Fruit On The Bottom, av., 6 oz ctn	140	0	19
Honey, 8 oz	290	14	32
Nonfat: Plain, 8 oz	140	0	9
Fig, 5.3 oz ctn	160	0	28
Average other Fruit Flavors, 5.3 oz	120	0	18
Wallaby Organic, Blended,			
Low-Fat, Fruit Flavors, average, 6 oz	140	2	18
Wegmans:			
Fruit On The Bottom, Lowfat:			
Blueberry, 6 oz	160	2	29
Average other Fruit Flavors, 6 oz	170	2	32
Greek, Non-Fat: Plain, 5.3 oz	80	0	5
Fruit flavors, av., 5.3 oz	120	0	16
Vanilla Flavored, 5.3 oz	100	0	13
Whole Foods (365):			
32 oz Ctn, Plain: Whole Milk, 8oz	160	9	13
Low-Fat, 8 oz	120	2	15
Fat-Free, 8 oz	120	0	17
6 oz Ctn: Blueberry Lemon	160	1.5	31
Peach Melba	140	1	27
Greek, 0% Nonfat, Plain, 6 oz			
YoCrunch: *Per 4 oz Container*			
Lowfat Vanilla Yogurt:			
with M&M's toppings	80	1	15
with Oreo Cookies toppings	80	1	16
with Snickers toppings	120	1.5	24
with Twix toppings	120	1.5	24

Yogurt Brands (Cont)

	C	F	Cb
Yoplait:			
Original, Fruit Flavors, av.	150	2	26
Greek:			
100%, average, 5.3 oz	100	0	11
Dippers, Rasp. Choc Chunk,			
w/ Choco-Drizzled Pretzels, 4.6 oz	240	5	38
Regular, fruit flavors, 5.3 oz	135	0	21
Whips: 2%, all flav., 4 oz	120	2	17
Fat Free, all flavors, 4 oz	100	0	15
Kids: Whole Milk, Strawb. Ban., 4 oz	110	3.5	14
Low Fat, average fruit flavors, 4 oz	100	0.5	20
Lactose Free, all flavors, 6 oz	150	2	25
Light: Fruit flavors, 6 oz	90	0	16
Thick & Creamy, 6 oz	100	0	19
Mix-Ins: Cherry Choc. Almond, 5.3 oz	200	8	26
Salted Caramel Pretzel, 5.3 oz	180	4.5	29
Very Berry Crisp, 5.3 oz	180	4	31
Thick & Creamy, all flavors, 6 oz	180	2.5	31
Trix, all flavors, av., 4 oz	100	0.5	20
Whips!: Chocolate, 4 oz	160	4	25
Fruit flavors, 4 oz	140	2.5	25

Yogurt Drinks & Probiotics

	C	F	Cb
Dannon:			
Activia, av. all flavors, 7 fl oz	165	3	27
DanActive, fruit flavors, 3.1 fl.oz	70	1	14
Danimals Smoothies,			
average all flavors, 3.1 fl.oz	60	0.5	10
Dan-o-nino, all flav., 3.1 fl.oz	70	0.5	15
Light & Fit, all flavors, 7 fl.oz	90	0	14
Glen Oaks, av. all flavors, 8 fl.oz	150	2.5	27
LaLa:			
5G Prot. Smoothies, average, 7 fl.oz	150	4	24
Greek Smoothies, all flav., 6.7 fl.oz	160	2.5	20
Lifeway Kefir:			
Whole Milk, Natural, 8 fl.oz	160	8	12
Lowfat: Plain, 8 fl.oz	110	2	12
Chocolate Truffle, 8 fl.oz	140	2	20
Other flavors, 8 fl.oz	140	2	20
Biokefir, Nonfat, all flavors, 3.5 fl.oz	60	0	11
Perfect 12, all flavors, 8 fl.oz	110	2	12
Protein 40g, all flavors, 8 fl.oz	160	0	20
With Oats, all flavors, 8 fl.oz	160	2	24
Stonyfield Organic,			
Smoothies, av. all flav., 6.5 fl.oz	110	1.5	18
Yakult:			
Regular, 2.7 fl.oz bottle	50	0	12
Light, 2.7 fl.oz	30	0	6

Cafeteria-Style Foods   **C** **F** **Cb**

Average All Preparations:

	C	F	Cb
Beef Stroganoff, 5 oz	195	13	7
Beef Stroganoff, with 4 oz noodles	350	14	36
Chicken Lasagna, 1 piece	300	11	32
Chicken Chop Suey, with 4 oz rice	245	4	37
Deep Dish Burrito, 7 oz	265	13	20
Ground Beef Casserole, 2 scps, 6 oz	245	13	17
Italian Meat Sce, for Spaghetti, 5 oz	150	9	9
with 5 oz Spaghetti	350	10	49
Lasagna, 1 piece	275	11	25
Meatloaf, 3 oz	205	13	4
Ranch Beans, 2 scoops, 6 oz	350	11	45
Red Beans & Rice, 7 oz	280	9	37
Scalloped Potato/Ham, 2 scoops, 6 oz	160	6	20
Stuffed Shells in Sauce, (1)	105	3	17
Swedish Meatballs, (3)	205	12	9
Sweet & Sour Pork/Rice, 9 oz	240	3	40
Swiss Steak, w/ Mushroom Gravy, 6 oz	280	11	4
Tator Tot Casserole, 2 scoops, 6 oz	260	15	20
Tenderloin Tips/Mshrm Gravy: 5 oz	210	13	3
With 5 oz noodles	395	15	38
Tuna Noodle Casserole, 2 scoops, 6 oz	180	6	17
Turkey Tetrazzini, 2 scoops, 6 oz	195	7	17
Vegetable Lasagna, 1 piece	250	13	21

Croissants

	C	F	Cb
Unfilled, medium 1.5 oz	180	10	21
Filled: With Ham (2 oz), garnish	280	14	24
With Ham (2 oz), Cheese (2 oz)	470	30	20
With Chick (2 oz) Cheese (2 oz)	470	30	20
With Turkey/Ham/Cheese (2 oz ea.)	580	36	20
Au Bon Pain: Ham & Cheese	390	21	35
Spinach & Cheese	290	17	28

7-Eleven ~ *See Page 236*

Bagels

	C	F	Cb
Plain: Large, 4 oz (without filling)	320	2	65
With 2 oz Cream Cheese	500	27	54
With 2 oz Lox (Smoked Salmon)	400	4	65

Also see Bagels Section ~ *Page 54*
Fast-Foods Restaurants ~ *Page 175*
Au Bon Pain ~ *Page 179*
Bruegger's ~ *Page 185*
Einstein Bros Bagels ~ *Page 199*

Sandwiches   **C** **F** **Cb**

No Spreads Unless Indicated:
Includes 2 Slices Bread ~ 3 oz

	C	F	Cb
BLT, (5 strips Bacon, 2 Tbsp Mayo)	600	40	46
Breaded Chicken & Garnish	540	28	46
Chicken Salad, with Mayo., 5 oz	580	30	49
Chopped Liver, Egg Mayonnaise	630	25	44
Corned Beef with Mustard, 5 oz	560	28	44
Egg Salad, with Mayonnaise	570	29	49
Egg Salad Club, with Bacon & Mayo,	780	53	49
Grilled Cheese, (3 oz)	540	30	44
Ham, (4 oz), Cheese (4 oz), & Mayo.	910	56	44
Lobster Salad, (4 oz), w/ Mayo.	530	25	45
Overstuffed Tuna Salad, (7 oz)	870	39	75
Philly Cheese Steak Sandwich	550	23	42
Reuben, (6 oz Beef/Pastrami,			
2 oz Cheese, 2 Tbsp Dressing)	920	60	28
Roast Beef, (4 oz), with Mustard	460	12	45
Roast Pork, (4 oz), with Apple Sauce	500	16	55
Shrimp Salad Club, w/ Bacon & Mayo	800	57	48
Sloppy Joe with Sauce, (7 oz)	600	30	45
Steak Sandwich, (5 oz cooked)	680	32	41
Triple Cheese Melt, (4 oz)	720	45	46
Tuna Salad, (5 oz), with Mayonnaise	610	30	49
Turkey Breast, (5 oz), w/ Mayo.	460	18	44
Turkey Breast, (5 oz,) with Mustard	360	7	44
Turkey Club, with Bacon & Mayo.	830	38	31
Vegetarian, with Avocado & Cheese	820	49	72

7-Eleven ~ *Page 236*
Schlotzsky's ~ *Page 237*
Subway ~ *Page 245*

Wraps & Roll-Ups

Average All Types
Meat/Chicken/Fish/Veggie:

	C	F	Cb
Small, approximately 9 oz	500	25	48
Regular, approximately 15 oz	830	40	80
Large, approximately 22 oz	1400	70	134

Fast-Foods Restaurants ~ *Page 175*
Au Bon Pain ~ *Page 179*
Sonic Drive-In ~ *Page 241*
Subway ~ *Page 245*
WAWA ~ *Page 254*

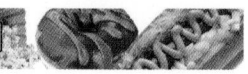

Fair & Carnival Foods   **C**   **E**   **Cp**

Barbeque Chicken/Meats:

Chicken, ¹/₂ chicken, 15 oz	740	24	34
Grilled Chicken Pita, with dressing	680	19	82
Teriyaki Chicken, on stick, w/ dress.	250	6	4
Pork Ribs, 18 oz	1360	68	21
Turkey Leg: Regular, 19 oz	1135	54	0
Caveman (2lb Turkey Leg, with 1lb Bacon)	2360	177	3
Bacon: Fried, on-a-stick, with syrup	230	16	5
Choc-covered Bacon, 4.5 oz dish	640	43	30
Beef Stew over Rice, 2 cups	440	14	61
Butter Balls, deep fried, 4 Balls	460	38	24
Cheese Curds, Breaded & fried, *Culver's*, 6.7 oz	670	38	54
Corn Dogs: Regular, 4 oz	250	14	23
Jumbo, 6 oz	375	21	36
Pretzel-Wrapped Dog	300	16	30
Papa Pup, on-a-stick	400	24	32
Pronto Pup, on-a-stick	170	9	16
Corn On The Cob, 8"(1), 16 oz	200	1	42

Finger Foods:

Artichoke, fried, 9 pieces	250	14	24
Chicken Nuggets, (6)	340	17	26
Chicken Strips, (4), 4.5 oz	445	21	33
Onion Rings, 3 rings	310	13	40
Onion Flower	1320	72	140
Shrimp, Fried, 10-12 pieces, 5 oz	555	30	36
Spam, deep-fried in batter, 2 pieces	330	24	18

Gator:

Big Gator, Nuggets/Hushpuppies	550	31	54
Stick Gator, 1 sausage	250	20	4

Greek:

Baklava, 2" square	245	13	32
Falafel, 11.6 oz	660	27	85
Greek Salad, 14 oz	520	48	17
Gyro, 7.5", 12 oz	680	40	55
Spanakopita, 8 oz	200	7.5	23

Hamburgers:

¹/₃ Pound Burger, 7.5 oz	670	41	26
Cheeseburger, 6 oz	550	36	25

Hot Dogs: *With Bun*

Regular: No extras	215	14	28
With Chili, 6 oz	450	32	32
With Chili & Cheese, 7.3 oz	500	36	31
¹/₃ Pound Hot Dog	550	41	31
Foot Long Hot Dog	470	26	41
Jumbo, Bratwurst/Kielbasa, average	800	60	28

Fair & Carnival Foods (Cont)

Mexican: **C**   **F**   **Cb**

Burrito, with Bean/Beef, 17 oz	1100	41	104
Carne Asada, 14.5 oz	820	44	58
Cheese Quesadilla, 1.8 oz	480	27	40
Chicken Taco, 3.3 oz	210	12	16
Fish Taco, 5 oz	270	13	31
Jalapeno Pepper, choc-covered (3)	270	15	31
Nachos with Cheese, 9" plate	860	59	70
Tamale, 3.5 oz	180	8	21
Taquito, 5 oz	370	17	43

Pizza:

Pizza Bread, Pepperoni, ¹/₂ loaf, 12 oz	1115	32	151
Pizza on-a-stick, 1 piece	535	28	55
Personal Pizza: *Per 7"*			
Cheese	670	24	80
Pepperoni	795	35	80
Ham & Pineapple	800	31	87

Potatoes & Fries:

Australian Battered Potatoes	1290	66	155
Baked Potato, 14 oz	435	0.5	100
Fries: French, 7 oz	560	24	79
Cheese Fries, 10 oz	645	38	62
Chili Fries, 10 oz	700	36	83
Curly Fries, 7 oz	620	30	78
Jamaican Jerk Fries, 7 oz	640	34	77
Sweet Potato, baked, 14 oz	405	0.5	97
Tornado, on-a-stick	210	15	18

Salads/Sides:

Chili, 1 cup	280	11	24
Cole Slaw, 5 oz	350	21	37
Pickle, whole (6")	30	0	8
Potato Salad, 5 oz	290	15	35

Sandwiches: *7¹/₂" Roll*

Ham, 11 oz	645	39	47
Hot Pastrami, 9 oz	760	17	62
Roast Beef, 11 oz	620	36	46
Philadelphia Cheese Steak, 13 oz	680	36	49
Turkey, 11 oz	665	24	65

Drinks:

Icee, 16 fl.oz	235	0	59
Shakes, average, 16 fl.oz	690	33	85
Slushies: Horchata, 16 fl.oz	280	8	50
Lemonade, 18 fl.oz	210	0	52
Orange Julius, 20 fl.oz	490	10	96
Strawberry Julius, 20 fl.oz	430	0	98
Soft Frozen Lemonade, 12 fl.oz	300	0	78
Smoothies, Berry Flavors, 16 fl.oz	350	1	80

Fair & Carnival Foods (Cont)

	C	**F**	**Cb**
Cakes· Pastries:			
Funnel Cake, Plain (1)	760	44	80
Toppings:			
Apple Cinnamon, 2 oz	85	3	16
Cinnamon & Sugar, 2 tsp	40	0	10
Strawberry & Cream, 2 oz	70	0	16
Cheesecake on-a-stick, 6 oz	655	47	56
Churro, (1), 9", 1.6 oz	170	8	22
Cream Puff, 4.3 oz	500	43	22
Fried Twinkie, (1)	420	34	45
Puff-on-a-Stick, (4), 8.6 oz	995	86	44
Strawberry Crepe, 4.3 oz	280	14	36
Twinkie Dog, (Sundae)	500	14	89
Candied Apple, 7 oz	330	0	80
Cookies:			
Sweet Martha, (1), 0.8 oz	90	4	14
Deep Fried: Oreos, tray (5)	890	48	108
Cookie Dough on stick, 3 pieces	670	32	89
Cotton Candy:			
Small, 1 oz	110	0	27
Large, 2.3 oz	250	0	62
Family Size, 5.5 oz	610	0	151
Dirt Dessert, 1 cup, 9.3 oz	405	12	69
Donuts, Jumbo Twist, (1), 7.5 oz	905	49	109
Fried Dough/FryBread:			
Plain: 7", 3.7 oz	390	19	47
9", 4³/₄ oz	510	25	61
Toppings: Cinnamon Sugar, 2 tsp	40	0	10
Butterscotch; Caramel, 2 Tbsp	115	0	29
Hot Fudge, average, 2 Tbsp	110	4	22
Cheese Powder, 2 tsp	70	3	2
Honey, 1 Tbsp, 0.8 oz	65	0	17
Fudge, 1.5 oz	200	11	25
Ice Cream & Frozen Treats:			
Deep-fried Klondike Bar, w/ syrup	430	16	18
Dippin' Dots Ice Cream, 6 oz cup	380	20	46
Frozen Banana, choc. coated, 5 oz	240	4	53
Frozen Yogurt, in sugar cone, 14 oz	475	2	94
Ice Cream: Small, sugar cone, 10 oz	775	42	83
Large, sugar cone, 14 oz	935	54	96
Sherbet, 8 oz	270	4	59
Snow Cone, with 3 oz syrup	270	0	68
Strawberry, Choc. Dipped, 1 piece	125	7	15
Popcorn:			
Plain: Small, 3 oz	450	24	48
Large, 6 oz	900	48	96
Kettle Corn: Small, 5 oz	600	15	110
Large, 10 oz	1200	30	220
Pretzels, Soft, 4.5 oz	340	2	70
S'more, on stick	275	16	27

Stadium Foods

	C	**F**	**Cb**
Burgers:			
Bacon Burger, 8.3 oz	470	25	34
Cheeseburger, 8.3 oz	450	23	33
Hamburger, 7.8 oz	400	19	33
French Fries, 6.4 oz	470	34	39
Fruit Cup, 6 oz	80	0	20
Hot Dogs:			
Chili Dog, 7.7 oz	520	29	45
Hot Dog, 6.4 oz	465	21	50
Jumbo Dog, 6 oz	440	25	38
Kraut Dog with Sauerkraut, 7.8 oz	490	27	41
Individual Pan Pizza (6"): *Per Pizza*			
BBQ Chicken	630	24	71
Cheese	630	27	71
Pepperoni	660	30	70
Nachos, 40 chips, with 4 oz cheese	1100	59	132
Sandwiches:			
Chicken: With Bacon, 8.3 oz	530	31	41
With Cheese, 8.3 oz	510	29	40
Without Cheese, 7.7 oz	460	25	40
Polish Sausage Sandwich, 7 oz	565	33	46
Snacks:			
Brownie, 2.5" x 4.5"	360	18	44
Cheese Sauce, 1.3 oz	100	8	4
Cheetos, 2.8 oz package	440	28	42
Chocolate Chip Cookie, 2.3 oz	280	12	40
Churro, (1), 10", 2 oz	210	10	26
Doritos, Nacho, 2.8 oz package	390	20	48
King Size Candy:			
Butterfinger, 3.8 oz	480	18	75
Nestle Crunch, 2.8 oz	390	21	85
Lay's, Chips, 2.8 oz package	440	28	42
Peanuts, in shell, 8 oz	930	80	24
Popcorn: Small (9 cup size)	575	35	56
Large (15 cup size)	950	58	93
Pretzel, Soft, Reg., 5.5 oz	490	3.5	101
Red Vines, 5 oz box	500	0	117
Snow Cone: With 3 oz syrup	270	0	68
With 6 oz syrup	540	0	136
Beverages:			
Orange Juice, 12 fl.oz	180	0	2
Beer:			
Heineken, 16 fl.oz	200	0	16
Miller: Draft, 16 fl.oz	195	0	17
Lite, 16 fl.oz	125	16	4
Jack Daniels, Punch, 12 fl.oz	235	0	34
Wine, White, 9 fl.oz	190	0	6
Soda, (with ¹/₂ ice), average:			
20 fl.oz	160	0	40
32 fl.oz	260	0	65
Starbuck's, Coffee, Frappuccino, 9.5 fl.oz	200	3	37

Restaurant & International Foods

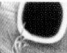

Asian & Chinese Dishes   C   F   Cb

Appetizers:

	C	F	Cb
Crab Cake, 2.3 oz	125	10	1
Dumplings: *Per Dumpling*			
Pork: Steamed	80	4.5	5
Fried	90	6	5
Vegetable, steamed	35	1	5
Egg Rolls, Mini, 3 rolls	100	3	11
Spring Roll:			
Small, 1.5 oz	85	4	9
Medium, 3 oz	170	8	17
Large, 5 oz	290	15	29
Wonton, 1 only	75	4	5
Soup: Egg Flower, bowl 12 oz	90	2	16
Hot & Sour Soup, bowl 12 oz	110	3.5	14
Rice: Plain,1 cup, 6.5 oz	320	2	66
2 Cups, 13 oz	640	4	132
Fried: 1 cup, 5 oz	365	11	55
Large dish, 16 oz	950	28	67
Noodles, Chinese Egg, cooked, 1 cup	200	4	37
Entrées & Mains: *Per Serving*			
Almond Chicken, 6 oz	270	10	21
BBQ Pork, 5.5oz	440	23	15
Beef in Black Bean Sauce, 8.5 oz	390	17	17
Broccoli Beef, 6 oz	370	21	13
Chicken & Broccoli, 5.5 oz	160	8	10
Chicken Skewers, 3 oz	210	9	18
Chop Suey:			
Chicken, 5 oz	140	9	2
Pork, 5 oz	170	12	3
Chow Mein, Beef/Chicken, 8 oz	390	12	59
Crab Puff/Rangoon, 1 dumpling	190	11	13
Crispy Fried Chicken, 8 oz	485	33	12
Egg Drop Soup: With Noodles, 1 cup	110	3	16
Without Noodles, 1 cup	60	3	4
Egg Foo Yung with Sauce, 1 cup	270	15	16
Kung Pao Chicken, 5.5 oz	240	15	12
Lemon Chicken, 5 oz	525	21	57
Lo Mein, stir-fried, 8 oz	705	42	49
Omelet, Chicken/Shrimp, 16 oz	990	82	10
Orange Chicken, 5.5 oz	500	27	42
Steamed Whole Fish,			
$^1/_2$ Sockeye Salmon	646	36	23
Sweet & Sour:			
Fish, 20 oz	1160	58	106
Pork, 5.5 oz	400	23	35
Vegetable Combo, with oil, 6 oz	367	5	66
Vegetables, Steamed, without oil, 6 oz	135	1	29
Sauces: Mandarin Sauce 1.5 oz	70	0	17
Potsticker Sauce, 1.5 oz	35	0	8
Bubble Tea, average, 12 fl oz	280	0.5	68
Fortune Cookie, each	32	0.5	7

Cajun & Creole   C   F   Cb

	C	F	Cb
Alligator, cooked, 4 oz	160	2	0
Baked Herb Chicken, 1 serving	850	53	2
Bouillabaisse	400	15	10
Cajun Fried Turkey, 1 serving	630	25	0
Cocktail Sauce, 2 Tbsp	30	0	6
Couche-Couche, $^1/_2$ cup	80	0	17
Crawfish Bisque, 1 serving	500	10	10
Crawfish, cooked, 2 oz	45	0.5	0
Creole Jambalaya,			
1 serving	550	30	15
Frog Legs, steamed (2)	45	0	0
Guinea Fowl, flesh, 4 oz, cooked	160	4	0
Hogshead Cheese, $^1/_4$ cup	80	5.5	0
Jambalaya, Shrimp & Crabmeat	520	14	12
Red Beans & Rice, 1 serving	400	17	52
Roasted Quail, with Bacon, on Toast	550	25	15
Remoulade Sauce, 2 Tbsp, 1 oz	110	11	2
Shrimp Creole, 1 serving	450	20	10
Stuffed Smothered Steak,			
with 1 cup Rice	890	50	50
Turtle, cooked, 3 oz	120	3	0

Canadian Foods

	C	F	Cb
Bagels, Montreal-Style:			
Plain, 100g/3.5 oz	300	2	60
Poppyseed, 100g/3.5 oz	310	4	58
Sesame, 100g/3.5 oz	320	6	56
Bannock: Plain 33g/1.2 oz	120	3	20
With currants/raisins, 85g/3 oz	215	9	32
Meals:			
Baked Beans in Maple Syrup,			
1 cup, 250g/8.8 oz	320	1	62
Donnairs (*Pizza Delight*):			
Famous, regular, 250g/8.8 oz	510	21	60
Super, regular, 310g/11 oz	685	34	62
Poutine:			
A&W, 330g/12 oz	610	33	58
Boston Pizza, regular, 400g/14 oz	610	30	67
Burger King, Classic, 330g/11.6 oz	680	36	72
Harvey's, 240g/8.5 oz	730	41	63
McDonald's, 1 serving	510	29	44
Swiss Chalet,			
Chalet -Style, 340g/12 oz	150	12	195
Shish Taouk:			
Chicken: 1 skewer, 200g/7 oz	270	25	9
Wrap, 455g/16 oz	1150	12	195
Tassot:			
Beef, 283g/10 oz	430	28	12
Goat, 100g/3.5 oz	360	36	9
Toutiere, 170g/6oz	600	42	35

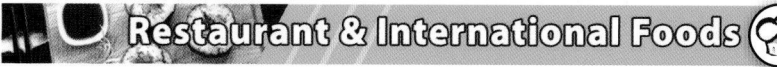

Canadian (Cont)   C   F   Cb

	C	F	Cb
Pastries:			
Beaver Tails:			
Cheese & Garlic, 80g/2.8 oz	390	30	28
Cinnamon & Sugar, 80g/2.8 oz	315	13	30
Butter Tart, mini, 1 tart	120	3	16
May West			
Original, 54g/1.9 oz	240	11	34
Nanaimo Bar, 56g/2 oz	270	16	30
Snacks: Maple Syrup Taffy, 40g/1.4 oz	130	0	33
Potato Chips: Dill Pickle Flav., 40g	160	10	15
Ketchup Flavor, 50g/1.8 oz	260	16	26

French Foods

	C	F	Cb
Blanquette d' Agneau, (Lamb Stew)	800	30	17
Brioche, 1 cake	280	14	34
Bouillabaisse	400	15	10
Coq au Vin, leg/thigh	700	28	31
Coquilles St. Jacques	320	13	36
Crème Brulée, 1 serving	460	40	21
Baguette, 3 slices, 2.2 oz	150	1	35
Creme Caramel, (Caramel Custard)	260	10	38
Crepe Suzette, 1x6" crepe with sauce	220	10	13
Duck a l'Orange, ¼ duck, 22 oz	970	44	19
Escargot, (Snails), in garlic butter (6)	200	10	4
Frog Legs, fried, 4 medium pairs	400	20	10
Lamb Noisettes, fried, 2 chops	500	40	1
Potage Creme Crecy, (Carrot Soup)	360	18	14
Salade Nicoise, (Tuna/Olives/Vegs)	450	13	14
Veal Cordon Bleu, (Veal/Ham)	650	25	18
Vichyssoise, (Potato /Leek Soup), 1 c.	200	9	15
Baguette & French Stick ~ *Page 54*			

German Foods

	C	F	Cb
Beef: Goulash with Veggies	520	20	46
Weiner Schnitzel, 1 medium	750	35	38
Chicken: Fried, Viennese-style	530	20	28
Livers with Apple/Onion, 6 oz	460	28	10
Herring, pickled: Rollmops, 4 oz	260	16	3
With Sour Cream, 4 oz	310	20	3
Pork, Sauerbraten (Pot Roast)	650	35	15
Sausage: Bratwurst, grilled, 6 oz	450	37	2
Hot Sausage Curry	300	7	6
Cakes:			
Black Forest, 1 slice	380	16	30
Bavarian Bread Dumpling, 3 small	330	10	28
Kugelhupf Cake, 1 large slice, 4 oz	400	23	40
Torte: Linzer (Almond/Raspb. Jam)	430	18	58
Sacher (Chocolate/Apricot Jam)	260	12	23

Greek Foods   C   F   Cb

	C	F	Cb
Baklava Pastry: Small	240	13	32
Large, 3.8 oz	400	21	45
Calamari, deep fried, 1 cup	300	13	17
Chicken Kebob Plate	345	13	8
Dolmades, 2 rolls, 6 oz	200	5	13
Galactobureko, 1 only			
(Filo, Custard, Pastry in Syrup)	360	15	48
Greek Chicken Salad	400	18	9
Gyros: 6" Pita, 8 oz	475	32	35
7½" Pita, 12 oz	680	40	55
Hummus & Pita, 4 oz	260	12	30
Kataifi, (Filo, Nut, Pastry in Syrup)	350	11	56
Moussaka: Small serving, 8 oz	350	22	22
Large serving, 16 oz	700	44	44
Soup, Avgolemono (Egg & Lemon			
with Chicken & Rice), 1 cup	85	6	5
Souvlaki, (Lamb), each, 2 oz	120	6	1
Stuffed Tomatoes, (2)	250	12	17
Taramosalata, 1 T., 0.5 oz	40	3	2
Tyropita, (Filo/Egg/Cheese Pastry)	350	26	31

Hawaiian

	C	F	Cb
Ahi Tuna, grilled w/o fat, 6 oz fillet	220	2	0
Chicken Long Rice, 1 cup, 7 oz	240	14	12
Gyoza, 1 only	55	2	6
Haupia, (Coconut Pudd.), 1 pce, (4"x 2½")	120	6	17
Hawaiian Sweet Bread, ½" slice, 2 oz	180	4.5	29
Kalua: Chicken, 4 oz	280	16	0
Pork, 4 oz	350	24	0
Kim Chee, (pickled cabbage), ½ cup, 4 oz	20	0	5
Kulolo, (Taro Pudding), 1 slice	125	5	19
Lau Lau:			
Chicken (1), 7 oz	280	21	3
Pork (1), 7 oz	320	26	5
Loco Moco, (rice/burger/egg/gravy)	650	27	63
Lomi Salmon, ¼ cup, 4 oz	20	1	2
Malasadas, (Donut), 2 oz	240	13	26
Manapua, (Char Siu Pork Bun), 2.3 oz	180	8	25
Poi ,(mashed cooked taro), 1 cup, 8.5 oz	270	0.5	65
Poke, average all types, 3 oz	90	1	0
Portuguese Sausage, 2 oz	180	15	2
Potato Salad, ½ cup, 5 oz	170	10	17
Shave Ice, *(Matsumoto),* all flavors:			
With Ice Cream, 1 large	300	4	64
With Beans, 1 large	290	0	72
Spam Musubi:			
With Regular Spam	265	11	34
(4 oz rice+1.3 oz Spam/7-Eleven Hawaii)			
Homemade, w/ Lite Spam (50% less fat)	220	5	34
Taro Pancake Mix, ⅓ cup (makes 2)	140	2	26

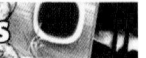

Hawaiian (Cont)   C F Cb

Plate Lunches:

	C	F	Cb
Chicken Katsu, (9 oz:) With Rice	1110	48	108
+ Macaroni Salad, ³/₄ cup	1360	68	123
or Tossed Salad + 2 T. French Dress.	1240	61	111
Hamburger, (5 oz): With Rice	710	24	81
Gravy + Macaroni Salad	1135	49	112
Mahi Mahi, (7 oz): With Rice	650	12	90
+ Macaroni Salad + Tartar Sce	1150	58	109
or Macaroni Salad, w/o Tartar ce	935	34	108
or Tossed Salad + 3 Tbsp Fr. Dress.	815	27	96
or Tossed Salad, without dressing	670	12	93
Teri Beef, (5 oz): With 2 scoops Rice	790	23	94
+ Macaroni Salad, ³/₄ cup	1095	47	113
or Tossed Salad, without dressing	800	23	95

Indian & Pakistani

Per Serving, Meat dishes allow 4 oz meat/serving

	C	F	Cb
Aloo Samosa, each	155	12	12
Alu Gosht Kari, (Meat/Potato Curry)	600	40	23
Chicken Korma	500	35	6
Chicken Pilaf	700	53	50
Chicken Tikka	260	16	2
Chicken Vindaloo	400	20	8
Chapati/Roti, 7" diameter, 1 piece	60	0.5	11
Dahl, (Lentil Puree):			
1 cup, without oil	230	1	37
1 Tbsp Tadka (oil topping)	120	13	0
Dhakla, (Lentil Dish), 1" square, 1 oz	105	5	13
Dhansak, ¹/₂ cup	105	3.5	11
Gosht Kari	460	25	17
Lamb Pilaf	520	35	40
Lassi, (Sweet or Mango), 1 cup, 8 oz	160	4	24
Masala Gosht, (Beef/Tomato/Gravy)	400	25	18
Mulligatawney Soup	300	15	8
Murgh Tikka, 1 cup	300	4	7
Naan Flatbread, 2 oz	160	3.5	29
Pappadum, 1 large/2 small	50	3	5
Pesrattu, (Lentil Crepe), 9", 2.6 oz	130	5	15
Pork Vindaloo Curry, without Rice	620	47	3
Rajmah, 1 cup	225	5	35
Rogan Josh,			
without Rice/Potatoes	500	30	3
Shahi Korma, (Braised Lamb)	430	28	3
Tandoori Chicken:			
Breast	260	13	5
Leg/Thigh portion	300	17	6

Italian Dishes   C F Cb

Entrees:

	C	F	Cb
Baked Ziti: Small	370	27	32
Regular	575	42	49
Breadstick, 2 oz piece	120	2.5	25
Broccoli Fettucine Alfredo, regular	815	23	125
Bruschetta, 2 slices	380	17	53
Calzones, av. all varieties	840	34	101
Cannelloni, 1 tube, 6 oz	280	15	18
Cheese Breadstick, 2.4 oz piece	180	8	20
Cheese Ravioli, with sauce	495	17	65
Chicken Alfredo	775	29	82
Chicken Parmigiana, 11 oz	520	22	16
Chicken Scallopine, dinner	1110	71	68
Eggplant Parmigiana	900	39	78
Fettucine Alfredo: Lunch, 9 oz	885	65	63
Dinner, 15 oz	1475	108	104
Linquine & Seafood, dinner	1130	71	79
Manicotti Formaggio	800	38	57
Meat Lasagne:			
Small, 10 oz	440	23	39
Large, 16 oz	700	36	60
Meat Ravioli	725	22	102
Minestrone Soup, 1 bowl	110	2	18
Penne Rustica: Lunch	1300	71	76
Dinner	1540	80	101
Ravioli, over-stuffed, average	990	67	57
Panini Sandwich:			
Chicken, 16 oz	900	38	81
Meats, average, 18 oz	940	39	81
Vegetarian, 15 oz	750	31	83
Pizza, Ready To Eat ~ *See Page 135*			
Spaghetti & Meatballs:			
With Tomato Sauce: Kids	500	20	58
Medium/Lunch	1080	63	89
Large/Dinner	1430	81	119
With Meat Sauce: Kids	550	25	56
Medium/Lunch	1300	79	84
Large/Dinner	1700	103	110
Veal Marsala, dinner	1320	66	132
Veal Parmigiana, dinner	1270	65	116
Vegetable Primavera	610	8	116
Salad,			
Caprese , 11 oz	445	34	10
Desserts:			
Gelato: Vanilla (Milk Base), ¹/₂ cup	200	15	18
Choc. Hazelnut (Milk), ¹/₂ cup	370	29	26
Water Base, ¹/₂ cup	100	0	25
Lemon Ice,	180	0	45
Tiramisu, 1 piece, 5 oz	400	29	30

Further listings ~ *See Fast-Foods Section*

Japanese

Food	C	F	Cb
Sashimi: (Sliced Raw Seafood/Beef)			
Ika (Squid), 4 oz	105	2	0
Hamachi (Yellowtail), 4 oz	165	6	0
Maguro (Yellowfin Tuna), 4 oz	120	1	0
Niku (Beef), 5 oz	200	10	0
Saba (Mackerel), 4 oz	160	7	0
Suzuki (Sea Bass), 4 oz	110	0.5	0
Tako (Octopus), 4 oz	95	1	0
Sushi Rice: Cooked, 1 Tbsp	25	0	5
1 cup, 5.3 oz	380	3	82
Sushi (Maki) Rolls: *Per Piece*			
Average all types (California Rolls; Cream Cheese with Crab; Eel; Salmon; Shrimp; Tuna; Yellowtail; Vegetable)			
Small (1.2" diam. x 1.2" high), 0.8 oz	25	0.5	3.5
Medium (1³/₄" diam. x 1³/₄" high), 1.6 oz	50	1	7
Large (2¹/₄" diam. x ⁷/₈" high), 2 oz	60	1.5	9
Sushi Packs: *Per Pack*			
Average all types: 6 large pieces	370	5	55
9 medium pieces	360	6	60
12 small pieces	265	3	45
Futomaki (thick roll), 6 pieces	380	5	72
Hand Roll (Cone), 4 oz	120	2	18
Inari (rice filled soybean pocket), 4 pces	420	9	73
Sushi-Nigiri, (fish on rice), average all varieties, 1 piece	70	0.5	12
Sushi Plate, Assorted: 6 pieces	420	3	36
Combination (Sushi & Sushi Rolls) 2 Sushi + 6 small & 3 medium rolls	400	7	72
Dipping Sauces: Average, 2 Tbsp	30	0	7
Ginger Vinegar Dressing, 2 Tbsp	20	0	5
Edamame: (young green soybeans):			
Boiled beans (no pods), 4 oz	160	7	12
Steamed (in pods), 4 oz	60	3	5
Katsu-don, Pork with Rice	1100	39	141
Miso Soup, with Tofu pieces, 1 cup	85	3	11
Sake Wine, (16% alcohol), 3 fl.oz	115	0	7
Seaweed Salad, 1.5 oz	20	2	0
Sukiyaki, (Beef/Tofu/Veggies), 8 oz	400	24	32
Tempura:			
3 large shrimp & veggies	320	18	25
1 shrimp only	60	4	3
Teppan Yaki, (Steak, Seafood & Veggies), 10 oz serving	470	30	15
Teriyaki: Beef, 4 oz	350	25	4
Chicken, 4 oz	260	9	7
Salmon, medium, 6 oz	270	8	3
Yakatori, 1 skewer, 2.5 oz	140	5	1

Kosher/Deli Foods

Food	C	F	Cb
Bagel/Bialy, 1 small, 2 oz	160	2	32
Beiglach, (Cheese Knish)	350	17	35
Blintzes: Average, 1 only	120	1	25
With Sour Cream & Preserves	370	10	30
Borscht, (Without Sour Cream): 1 cup	85	3	14
Diet/Reduced Calorie, 1 cup	30	1	7
Cabbage Roll, (meat/rice), 5 oz	170	6	21
Chicken Broth: 1 cup	80	8	0
With vegetables	100	8	5
With noodles	150	9	16
Lowfat, plain, 1 cup	25	1	0
Cholent, 1 medium serving, 1 cup	350	16	48
Chopped Liver: 1 serving, 3 oz	110	6	5
With Egg Salad, ¼ cup	100	7	3
Farfel, dry, ½ cup	90	0.5	21
Gefilte Fish Balls:			
Regular, 2 oz	55	2	4
With Jelled Broth	80	2	6
Cocktail size, 1 oz	30	1	2
Sweet: Medium, 2 oz	65	2	4
With Jelled Broth	95	2	9
Hallah, (Yeast Bread), 1 slice, 1 oz	85	2	14
Herring: Smoked, 2 oz	120	8	0
In Sour Cream, 2 oz	150	10	0
Kasha, cooked, ½ cup	100	0.5	20
Kipfel, (Vanilla/Almdond Cookie), 1 pce	60	2	7
Knaidlach ~ *See Matzo Balls*			
Knish: Kasha/Potato, 1 only	130	4	22
Cheese, 1 only	350	17	35
Kreplach, beef, 1 piece	40	1	6
Kugel, potato/noodle, 1 serving	300	20	25
Latkes, (Potato Pancake): 2 oz	200	11	22
3 Latkes w/ Sour Cran Apple Sauce	750	25	95
Lochshen: Plain, 1 cup	130	2	26
Pudding, 1 cup	380	13	48
Lox, (Smoked Salmon), 2 oz	65	2	0
Mandelbrot, (Almond Bread), 1 slice, ¼" thick	45	2	5
Matzo, 1 oz board	110	0.5	21
Matzo Balls: 2 small, or 1 large, 2"	90	3	12
Extra large ball, 3"	180	6	24
Matzo Ball Soup:			
Cup w/ 2 small or 1 large ball	150	5	27
Bowl w/ Chkn & Noodles	325	13	34
Jerry's Deli, large bowl	560	17	56
NY Cheesecake, 4 oz	350	24	26
Pierogi, potato/cheese, 1 piece	90	4	11
Reuben S'wich, w/ ½ lb Corned Beef	920	60	28
Schmaltz, (Rend'd Chicken Fat), 1 T.	90	10	0

Updated Nutrition Data ~ www.CalorieKing.com
Persons with Diabetes ~ See Disclaimer (Page 22)

Restaurant & International Foods

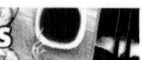

Korean Food	C	F	Cb
Bibimbab, (Veg. & Beef on Rice), 1 cup	565	15	89
Bulgogi, (Barbeque Beef), 3.5 oz	325	12	15
Galbi (Short Ribs), 16 oz	975	61	16
Gujeolpan, (Pancake with Meat & Vegetables), 1 cup with 1 pancake	340	11	39
Japchae, (Noodle w/ Veggies & Meat), 1¼ cups	365	19	34
Sides:			
Kimchee, (Cabbage Relish), ½ cup	30	0	6
Namool, (Assorted Vegetables), 1 cup	125	6.5	9
Soups: *Per Serving*			
Muguk, (Radish & Chive Soup), 6 oz	105	7	6
Samgyetang, (Ginseng Chkn Soup):			
Without Chicken Skin, 1 cup	520	11	60
With Chicken Skin, 1 cup	725	35	60
Yuk Gae Jang,			
(Spicy Beef Soup), 1¼ cups	180	13	5

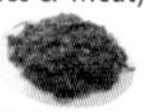

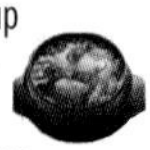

Lebanese/Middle East	C	F	Cb
Baba Ghannouj, 2 Tbsp, 1 oz	70	6	2
Baklava, (Pastry, Nuts, Syrup), 1 pastry, 1¾ oz	245	18	18
Cabbage Rolls, (Cabb. Leaf, Meat, Rice), 1 roll, 3 oz,	100	3	12
Cous Cous, (Semolina, Milk, Fruit, Nuts), 1 cup	400	21	43
Falafel, (Chick Pea Fritter), Fried, 1 medium, 1 oz	60	4	4
Hummus, ¼ cup, 2.2 oz	105	3	5
Fried Kibbi, (Wheat, Meat Pinenuts), 1 piece, 3 oz	180	8	15
Kafta, (Ground Lamb, Ssge on Skewer), 1 skewer, 1.5 ozoz	85	5	2
Kibbeh Naye, (raw Lamb, Bulgur & Spice) 1 cup, 9 oz	450	18	28
Lebanese Omelet, 1 serving, 4 oz (Egg, Spinach, Pinenuts, Onion)	200	12	13
Pilaf, (Rice, Onion, Raisins, Apr., Spice) 1 cup	400	11	60
Shawourma, (Spit-Roast Beef), 4 oz serving	280	15	2
Shish Kabob, 1 stick, 2.5 oz	130	7	2
Spinach Pie, 1 piece, 3.5 oz	290	21	20
Sweet Almond Sanbusak, (Pastry, Almonds, Spices), 1 piece	200	15	11
Tabouli, 1 serving, 4 oz	125	7	13
Tahini Sauce, average, 1 Tbsp	90	8	2

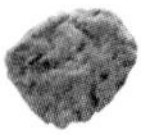

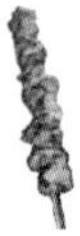

Mexican	C	F	Cb
Burritos *(Taco Bell):* Bean	370	10	56
Supreme Beef	420	16	53
Chili, plain, ¼ cup	90	6	8
Chili con Carne: With Beans, 1 cup	310	17	15
Without Beans, 1 cup	370	28	10
Chimichangas, Beef, 5 oz	400	19	43
Chorizo Sausage, 2 oz	265	23	0
Churro, (1), 1.5 oz	150	8	18
Corn Chips, ½ cup, 1 oz	160	10	17
Enchilada, average	330	10	49
Fajitas, Chicken	200	7	20
Guacamole, average, 2 Tbsp, 1 oz	45	4	2
Horchata: *(Don Jose),* 1 cup, 8 fl.oz	140	4	25
Cacique, 1 pint bottle, 16 fl.oz	320	7	62
Margarita, with 1.5 oz Tequila	160	0	6
Masa, (Pre-mixed for Tamales), 1 oz	80	5	9
Menudo:			
With Hominy, 1 cup	240	9	19
Without Hominy, 1 cup	170	9	2
Nachos: With cheese, peppers, 1 portion, 6-8 nachos, 7 oz	600	33	60
With cheese, beans, beef, peppers, 1 portion, 6-8 nachos, 9 oz	570	31	56
Del Taco: Regular, 4 oz	300	19	30
Macho Nachos, 17 oz	1000	56	94
Taco Bell, BellGrande®, 10.8 oz	780	40	84
Nopal Cactus Salad, 1 cup	130	9	11
Papas Fritas, (1), 6 oz	325	18	40
Piloncillo, (Brown Sugar):			
1 Tbsp, 0.5 oz	50	0	13
Cone, small, 3", 3 oz	325	0	81
Quesadilla, Cheese	490	28	39
Queso Fresco, ¼ cup	80	4.5	8
Refried Beans, ¾ cup, 6 oz	160	3	26
Rice Pudding, (Arroz Con Leche), 4 oz	140	3	24
Soup, Black Bean, 1 bowl	200	3	34
Tacos *(Taco Bell):*			
Crunchy: Regular	170	10	12
Supreme	200	12	15
Soft: Crispy Potato	270	13	31
Grilled Steak	250	14	19
Taco Salad with Salsa	840	52	85
Taco Sauce, average, ¼ cup	15	0	3
Taco Shell, regular	50	2	8
Tamales, Beef/Chicken, av. 4.5 oz	250	11	27
Taquitos, Beef & Cheese, 4.5 oz	330	15	36
Tostada *(Taco Bell)*	250	10	29
Tortilla, Corn, 6" diameter	70	1	14
Tortilla Chips, 1 oz	150	8	18
Soup, Black Bean, 1 bowl	200	3	34

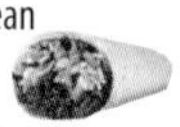

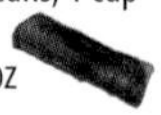

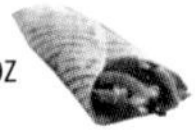

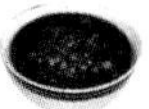

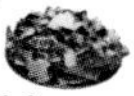

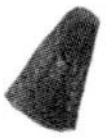

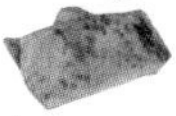

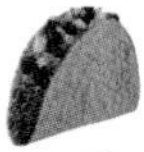

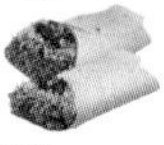

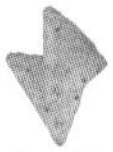

Extra Food Listings ~ See Fast Food Section
(Examples: Del Taco, Taco Bell, Taco Cabana, Taco Time)

Mexican (Cont)   **C** **F** **Cb**

Breads:

	C	F	Cb
Bolillos, 1 roll, 3.5 oz	240	4	42
Mexican Cornbread, 4" square	210	11	19
Pan de Leche, 1 roll, 1.3 oz	110	2.5	20
Telera, 2 oz	150	1.5	19

Cakes, Cookies, Pastries Pan Dulce:

	C	F	Cb
Banderilla, 1 piece	140	10	8
Bigotes, 7"	570	22	44
Capirotada, (Bread Pudding), 10 oz	810	38	107
Cinnamon Cookies, 2	125	8	13
Concha, av. all varieties:			
Small (3" diameter), 2.5 oz	250	8	38
Medium (4" diameter), 3.5 oz	350	11	53
Large (5" diameter), 5.5 oz	550	18	84
Cream Puff, with Custard, 4.3 oz	255	14	25
Cuernos, (Horns), 3 oz	340	17	41
Donut, large, 4", 3.5 oz	440	21	58
Elotes, 3.5 oz	450	24	51
Empanadas, average all varieties:			
Medium, 3 oz	300	14	42
Large, 4 oz	400	19	56
Fiesta Cookie, (1), 2.3 oz	280	8	47
Galletas Mixtas:			
Small, 1 oz	100	2.5	16
Medium, 2 oz	200	5	32
Large, 3 oz	300	7.5	48
Guayaba, 3.3 oz	360	14	53
Jelly Roll, (1), 3.3 oz	240	4	46
Mantecadites, 4.5 oz	670	42	64
Mini Cupcake, (1), 1.8 oz	180	8	25
Muffins/Nino Enbuelto, large, 6 oz	465	11	48
Nuez, 3.3 oz	380	17	52
Ojo de Buey, 4 oz	360	15	55
Orejas, 1 medium, 3 oz	310	15	38
Pan Dulce, 1 bun	330	10	45
Panquecitos, 2.5 oz	260	11	36
Piedras, 4 oz	470	15	76
Polvorones: Small, 1.5 oz	180	9	24
1 large, 3 oz	370	18	48
Pound Cakes, mini, 3.5 oz	380	16	52
Puerquitos, 3.5 oz	350	12	55
Rebanadas, 3.5 oz	390	18	51
Roles De Canela, (Cinn. Roll) 4.5 oz	490	15	81
Roscas, 1 piece, 2.8 oz	360	18	44
Semitas (Bimbo), 1 piece, 2.2 oz	210	6	33
Sopapillas, (flaky pastry puffs): 1 piece	100	7	10
With Honey & Cream	200	14	18
Strawberry Crema Roll, 2.5 oz slice	240	5	45

Extra Food Listings ~ *See CalorieKing.com*

Polish   **C** **F** **Cb**

	C	F	Cb
Cabbage Rolls, w/ Sour Cream, 2 small	220	10	30
Chicken Casserole, w/ Mshrms, 1 cup	520	27	5
Kielbasa, (Sausages, Onions, fried), 2 large	350	28	2
Meatballs, in sour cream, 3 x 1½" balls	300	16	11
Pierogi, Fruit/Vegetables, 3" ball	80	2	15
Pork Goulash, (Pork/Vegetable Stew)	550	21	38
Pot Roast, with Vegetables	630	21	28

Soul Foods

	C	F	Cb
Breakfast Sausage, fried, 2 patties	250	17	0
Brunswick Stew, 1 cup, 8.5 oz	320	14	19
Cornbread, homemade, 3 oz	200	7.5	28
Fatback, 0.5 oz	110	11	0
Ham Hock, pickled, 3 oz	200	12	0
Hog Maw, 1 oz	70	4.5	0
Hominy, cooked, ¾ cup	110	0.5	25
Hush Puppies, 5 pieces	260	12	35
Kale, cooked, ½ cup	20	0.5	4
Opossum, roasted, without bone, 3 oz	190	9	0
Oxtail, cooked, without bone, 2 oz	85	4.5	0
Pig's Ear, ¼ ear	50	3	0
Pig's Foot, ½ foot	70	4.5	0
Pig's Tail, ⅛ tail	115	10	0
Poke Salad, cooked, ½ cup	16	0.5	3
Pork Brains, braised, 3 oz	115	8	0
Pork Chitterlings, simmered, 3 oz	260	25	0
Pork Cracklings, 0.5 oz	80	6	0
Pork Neck Bones, cooked, no bone, 2 oz	100	4.5	0
Pork Skin, 1 cup	70	4.5	0
Pork Tongue, ⅓ tongue	75	5.5	0
Sousemeat, 1 oz	60	4.5	0
Succotash, ½ cup	80	1	17
Sweet Potato Pie, ⅛ of 9" pie	250	12	34
Tripe, 2 oz	55	2	0
Vienna Sausage:			
2 small, 1 oz	90	8	1
1 small, 0.5 oz	45	4	0.5

OLD McDONALDS FARM
128 FOR PEOPLE WHO WANT BETTER
Brooklyn

Restaurant & International Foods

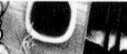

Spanish

C **F** **Cb**

	C	F	Cb
Arroz Abanda, (Fish with Rice)	340	8	31
Arroz Con Pollo, (Rice/Chkn Salad)	500	23	50
Clams Marinara, 8 clams	330	16	22
Cochifrito, (Lamb with Lemon/Garlic)	650	25	5
Cochinillo Asado, (Rst Suckling Pig), 2 slices	300	15	3
Cocido Madrileno, (Madrid-Style Boiled Dinner)	450	27	18
Flan de Leche, (Caramel Custard)	325	9	52
Fritadera de Ternera, (Sauteed Veal)	450	27	2
Gazpacho, 1 bowl	60	0	15
Mole Poblano, 1/2 cup	205	14	16
Paella a la Valenciana, (Chicken & Shellfish Rice)	900	42	70
Pollo a la Espanola, (Chicken)	475	30	4
Ternera al Jerez, (Veal with Sherry)	660	29	6
Zarzuela, (Fish & Shellfish Medley)	530	27	40

Thai Foods

	C	F	Cb
Appetizers: Satay Pork, 1 oz	100	4	2
Spring Roll, 1.3 oz	110	6	13
Soups, Tom Yam (Hot & Sour): Spicy Shrimp/Seafood:			
1 cup	100	4	6
1 bowl	160	7	10
Vegetarian, 1 cup	50	0	11
Curries: Chicken with Ginger, 1 cup	390	34	4
Thick Red Curry with Beef, 1 cup	600	50	7
Thai Chicken Curry, 1 cup	340	23	4
Massaman Curry, 1 cup	680	57	8
Green Curry with Pork, 1 cup	480	44	5
Pad Thai, large serving, 18 oz	990	38	125
Fish: Steamed with Spicy Thai Sce	450	8	46
Crispy Fried, 5 oz	290	15	9
Spicy Chicken, stir-fry	450	22	14
Spicy Garlic Tofu, stir-fry	340	18	18
Sticky Thai Rice: Plain 1 cup, 6 oz	170	0.5	36
With Coconut & Sesame Seeds, 1 cup	880	28	120
Stir-fried Rice Noodles, 1 cup 5.5 oz	270	9	40
Stir-fried Vegetables, 1 cup	100	3	18
Salads: Green Papaya Salad	160	0	40
Spicy Prawn, 9 shrimp	170	3	15
Thai Beef Salad, 1 serving	260	9	15
Thai Chicken, 1 serving	330	9	17
Thai Noodle, 1 serving	410	13	45
Satay Chicken & Peanut Sauce, 1 satay stick	390	24	20
Sauce, Peanut Satay, 1/2 cup, 4 oz	160	10	13

Vietnamese

C **F** **Cb**

	C	F	Cb
Banh Cuon, (Steam Rice w/ Pork), 1 roll	105	7	8
Bo Nuong, (Beef Satay), 2 sticks	265	9	4
Bo Xao Dau Phong, (Ginger Beef with Onion, Fish Sce)	750	30	10
Ca Chien Gung, (Whole Snapper/Ginger)	600	16	6
Canh Chay, (Vegetable/Tofu Soup)	80	3	13
Cari Chicken, 1 cup	475	29	16
Cari Chicken, with Rice Noodle, 1 cup curry & 1 cup noodles	660	29	60
Cari Chicken, with Steamed Rice, 1 cup curry & 1 cup rice	650	29	55
Cuu Xao Lan, (Curried Lamb and Veggies in Coconut)	900	40	80
Ga Chien, (Crisp Chick + Plum Sauce)	900	40	105
Ga Nuong, (Chicken Satay + Sauce)	240	10	4
Ga Xao Rau, (Marinated Chicken Braised with Vegetables)	800	26	100
Gio Lua, (Lean Pork Pie), 1/6 of pie	245	12	0
Goi Cuon, (Cold Spring Rolls), 1 roll	60	1	7
Rau Cai Xao Chay, (Stir Fried Veggies)	400	15	65
Thit Bo Vien, (Beef Balls), 6 balls	225	14	2
Thit Heo Goi Baup Cai, (Spicy Cabb. Rolls with Pork), 1 roll	200	7	11
Soup: *Per Bowl, 1/2 Cup* Bun Bo Hue, (Hot & Spicy Soup):			
Without Pork Feet	340	9	35
With Pork Feet	830	45	35
Chicken & Rice Noodle Soup	400	3	55
Pho Bo, (Beef Noodle Soup)	410	7	59
Pho Ga, (Chicken Noodle Soup)	460	6	58
Pho Tai, (Rare Beef & Noodle Soup)	440	7	73
Salad, Goi Du Du, (Green Papaya), 1/2 cup	155	3	29
Sauce, Nuoc Cham (Hot Sauce)	5	0	1

Gourmet & Miscellaneous

	C	F	Cb
Ants Eggs/Larvae, 1 Tbsp	20	0	0
Ants, chocolate coated, 3 Tbsp	140	7	2
Bee Maggots, canned, 3 Tbsp	65	2	0
Caviar, black/red, 1 Tbsp	40	3	0
Caterpillars, canned, 2 oz	60	2	0
Frog Legs, fried, 1 pair (large)	125	7	0
Haggis, boiled, 4 oz	350	24	22
Locusts, roasted, 1 oz	35	1	0
Silkworms, raw, 1 oz	60	2	0
Snails in garlic butter, 6 large	200	10	4
Snake, roasted, 4 oz	160	6	0

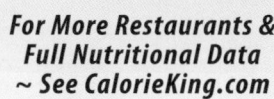

Fast - Foods & *Restaurants*

For More Restaurants & Full Nutritional Data ~ See CalorieKing.com

Fast - Foods & *Restaurants*

A&W® (Sept '18)
California Restaurants Only

	C	F	Cb
Burgers: Cheeseburger	400	21	39
Double Cheeseburger	455	26	40
Hamburger	340	16	39
Bacon Cheeseburger: Original	440	25	41
Double	645	41	42
Papa Burger	550	33	43
Sandwiches:			
Crispy Chicken	550	25	52
Fish	575	29	58
Grilled Chicken: 1 tender	400	15	40
2 Tenders	475	13	51
Grilled Chicken Club	490	22	40
Chicken Tenders, breaded, 3 pcs	260	9	5
Corn Dog Nuggets, 10 pieces	350	17	40
Hot Dogs: Plain	310	19	23
Coney Chili Dog	340	20	26
Coney Cheese Dog	380	23	28
Footlong Hotdog	460	34	21
Fries/Sides: Cheese Curds, 5 oz	570	40	27
Chili Cheese Fries, 7 oz	410	17	52
French Fries:			
Small/Kids, 2.5 oz	200	8	29
Regular, 4 oz	310	13	45
Large, 5.5 oz	430	17	61
Onion Rings, 7-9 rings	350	16	45
Dipping Sauces: Per 1.25 oz			
BBQ	90	0	22
Honey Mustard	140	11	10
Papas, Regular/Spicy	170	15	8
Spicy Ketchup	60	0	15
A & W Root Beer: Small, 16 fl.oz	220	0	58
Regular, 20 fl.oz	270	0	72
Large, 32 fl.oz	440	0	116
Famous Floats:			
A&W Root Beer Float:			
16 oz Cup	330	5	70
20 oz Cup	350	5	77
32 oz Cup	640	10	136
Diet Root Beer, 16 oz	170	5	30
Freeze:			
A&W Root Beer: 16 oz	370	8	68
32 oz	820	18	150
Diet Root Beer, 16 oz	260	8	39
Polar Swirls: Oreo/M&M's, av. 12 oz	605	23	92
Reese's, 12 oz	615	29	82
Shakes:			
Chocolate/Vanilla, av., 16 oz	590	18	97
Strawberry, 16 oz	670	29	90
Soft Serve: Includes Cone			
Small, 4 oz	200	5	32
Regular, 5.5 oz	260	7	41
Sundaes: Choc./Strawberry, av.	310	8	50
Caramel/Hot Fudge, av.	345	10	54

Applebees® (Sept '18)

Appetizers: As Served	C	F	Cb
Boneless Wings, plain	680	35	52
Dressings: Bleu Cheese	220	22	3
Classic Buffalo; Ranch, av.	190	19	4
Sauces: Honey BBQ	230	0.5	55
Sweet Asian Chili	250	2	55
Brew Pub Pretzels & Beer Chse Dip	1080	45	133
Brisket Quesadillas	910	58	62
Cheeseburger Eggrolls	980	60	77
Chips & Salsa	630	27	89
Crunchy Onion Rings	1120	59	133
Grilled Chicken Wonton Tacos	500	20	50
Mozzarella Sticks	910	50	79
Salsa Verde Beef Nachos	1770	117	109
Spinach & Artichoke Dip	950	57	89
Burgers: Without Sides			
Classic	750	46	44
Quesadilla	1300	92	49
All Day Brunch	1160	76	61
The American Standard	990	66	47
Triple Bacon	1180	81	48
Whisky Bacon	1220	79	72
Chicken: As Served, without Choice of Extra Sides			
Bourbon Street Chicken & Shrimp	640	31	41
Cedar Grilled Lemon Chicken	570	25	47
Chicken Tenders Platter, small	1150	66	101
Chicken Wonton Stir Fry	790	19	107
Classic Chicken Parmesan	1430	59	147
Fiesta Lime Chicken	1110	57	96
Grilled Chicken Breast	190	4	1
Handhelds: Without Sides			
BBQ Brisket Tacos	1160	67	108
Chicken Fajita Rollup	1090	65	67
Clubhouse Grille S'wch	1080	61	77
Zesty Chicken Sandwich	870	52	68
Pasta: As Served			
4-Cheese Mac & Chse,			
w/ Honey Pepper Chkn Tenders	1420	52	171
Spin. & Artichoke Gr. Chkn Cavatappi	950	40	87
Three-Cheese Chicken Cavatappi	1150	60	88
Seafood: As Served, without Choice of Extra Sides			
Cedar Salmon w/ Glaze	350	10	28
Double Crunch Shrimp	1320	74	129
Shrimp Wonton Stir Fry	650	13	108

176

Applebees® cont... (Sept '18)

Steaks & Ribs: W/out Sauce or Sides

	C	F	Cb
6 oz USDA Sirloin	200	8	1
8 oz USDA Sirloin	280	12	1
Double Glazed Baby Back Ribs			
Full Rack	860	65	1
Half Rack	430	32	0
Riblets:			
Small	940	54	62
Large	1360	81	77
Ribs Sauce:			
Honey BBQ/Texas Style BBQ, av:			
Full rack	155	1	36
Half rack	80	0.5	18
Salads: Per Regular, with Dressing			
Crispy Chicken & Cornbread	1400	94	78
Grilled Chicken & Cornbread	1090	70	53
Oriental Grilled Chicken	1290	85	84
Pecan Crusted Chicken	1280	74	108
Southwestern Steak Salad	990	64	65
Fries & Sides: As Served			
4-Cheese Mac & Cheese	440	21	40
Baked Potato	410	26	40
Loaded	500	33	40
Classic Fries	430	20	57
Four-Cheese Mac& Cheese	410	16	44
Garlic Mashed Potatoes	250	11	35
Garlic Mashed Potatoes, loaded	410	24	36
Garlicky Green Beans	190	15	11
Steamed Broccoli	90	8	6
Wood-Fired Grilled Veggies	150	12	9
Soup:			
Chicken Tortilla	160	7	17
Chili	410	25	16
French Onion	330	18	22
Loaded Potato	390	33	13
New England Clam Chowder	190	13	12
Portsmith Clam Chowder	160	7	18
Tomato Basil	180	11	16
Desserts:			
Apple Chimi Cheesecake	1000	38	151
Blue Ribbon Brownie	1520	65	211
Chocolate Chip Cookie Sundae	1260	49	191
Hot Fudge Sundae Shooter	410	20	51
Triple Choc. Meltdown	980	52	125

Arby's® (Sept '18)

Sandwiches:

	C	F	Cb
Beef 'n Cheddar: Classic	450	20	45
Double	630	32	48
Half Pound	740	39	48
Roast Beef: Classic	360	14	37
Double	510	24	38
Half Pound	610	30	38
Buttermilk Chicken:			
Buffalo Chicken	550	26	52
Chicken Bacon & Swiss	660	33	55
Chicken Cordon Bleu	700	36	52
Crispy Chicken	560	27	52
Signature: Loaded Italian	680	40	49
Reuben	680	31	62
Roast Beef Gyro	550	29	48
Smokehouse Brisket	600	35	42
Turkey Gyro	470	20	48
Turkey:			
Grand Turkey Club	480	24	37
Roast Turkey & Swiss	710	28	79
Roast Turkey, Ranch & Bacon	800	34	79
Wraps: Roast Turkey & Swiss	520	27	39
Roast Turkey, Ranch & Bacon	620	34	39
Sliders: Buffalo Chicken	290	13	31
Chicken Tender 'n Cheese	290	12	30
Ham 'n Cheese	230	9	22
Jalapeno Roast Beef 'n Cheese	240	11	21
Roast Beef 'n Cheese	240	11	21
Chicken Tenders: 3 pieces	360	17	28
5 pieces	600	28	47
Dipping Sauces: Buffalo, 1 oz	10	1	2
Honey Mustard, 1 oz	140	13	5
Ranch, 1 oz	100	11	2
Curly Fries: Small, 4.5 oz	410	22	49
Medium, 6 oz	550	29	65
Large, 7 oz	650	35	77
Loaded Curly Fries, 8.2 oz	700	46	57
Snacks:			
Jalapeno Bites:			
5 pieces, no sauce	290	17	31
8 pieces, no sauce	470	27	50
Mozzarella Sticks: 4 pieces	440	23	37
6 pieces	650	35	56
Potato Cakes: 3 pcs	370	21	35
4 pieces	490	28	46
Steakhouse Onion Rings, 5 rings	420	21	52

continued next page...

Fast - Foods & *Restaurants*

Arby's® cont... (Sept '18)

Salads: Without Dressing

	C	F	Cb
Chopped Farmhouse:			
Crispy Chicken	430	24	26
Roast Turkey	230	13	8
Side Salad	70	5	4
Dressings: *Per 1.5 oz Packet*			
Balsamic Vinaigrette	130	12	4
Buttermilk Ranch	210	22	2
Dijon Honey Mustard	180	16	8
Light Italian	20	1	2
Kids Menu: Chicken Tenders (2)	240	11	19
Curly Fries, 2.75 oz	250	13	29
Roast Beef 'n Cheese Slider	240	11	21
Breakfast: *Per Serving*			
Biscuits: Bacon, Egg & Cheese	480	29	38
Ham, Egg & Cheese	470	25	39
Sausage, Egg & Cheese	640	45	39
Croissants: Bacon, Egg & Cheese	440	27	29
Ham, Egg & Cheese	420	23	30
Sausage, Egg & Cheese	590	44	30
Sourdoughs:			
Bacon, Egg & Cheese	490	23	46
Ham, Egg & Cheese	470	19	47
Sausage, Egg & Cheese	640	39	47
Wraps: Bacon, Egg & Cheese	500	27	42
Ham, Egg & Cheese	440	22	42
Sausage, Egg & Cheese	630	41	42
Sauces: Arby's, 0.5 oz	15	0	3
Bronco Berry, 1 oz	60	0	15
Cheddar Cheese, 1.5 oz	50	3.5	4
Horsey, 0.5 oz	60	5	3
Marinara, 1 oz	20	0	4
Spicy Three Pepper, 0.5 oz	25	1	3
Tangy BBQ, 1 oz	40	0	9
Turnovers: Apple	430	18	65
Cherry	390	13	65
Iced Tea, Unsweetened	5	0	1
Juice, Capri Sun Fruit Juice, 6.5 oz	80	0	21
Shakes: *Per Small*			
Chocolate; Jamocha	545	18	88
Vanilla	450	17	67
Sodas: *Without Ice*			
Dr Pepper, Small	180	0	48
Mist Twist, Small	190	0	50
Mountain Dew, Small	200	0	54
Pepsi, Small	180	0	49

Atlanta Bread Co® (Sept '18)

Breakfast Bagel Sandwiches:

	C	F	Cb
Egg & Cheese	410	13	54
Egg, Cheese & Ham	470	16	54
Egg, Cheese & Turkey Sausage	520	20	55
Side, Breakfast Potatoes	170	9	20
Paninis: Chicken Pesto	680	25	80
Cuban	670	24	76
Hot Pastramki	870	57	49
Sandwiches: Chicken Salad	680	37	51
Gourmet Grilled Cheese	860	48	78
Roast Beef	490	15	55
Roasted Turkey	460	14	58
Veggie	430	17	59
Salads: *Without Dressing or Bread*			
Balsamic Blue	630	45	43
Caesar	630	58	20
Chardonnay Brie, half	130	8	9
Chopstix Chicken	750	41	70
Salsa Fresca Salmon	280	11	23
Sides: Edamame	150	4.5	14
Black Beans & Corn	190	9	24

Au Bon Pain® (Sept '18)

Bagels: Per Bagel

	C	F	Cb
Asiago Cheese, 3.6 oz	300	7	46
Cinnamon Raisin, 3.1 oz	370	6	71
Everything, 3.2 oz	250	2	50
Honey Sprouted Grain, 3.6 oz	250	1.5	53
Plain Bagel, 3.1 oz	230	1	49
Sesame Seed Bagel, 3.2 oz	250	2.5	50
Whole Wheat Skinny , 1.6 oz	90	1	21
Breakfast Sandwiches:			
2 Eggs on a Bagel	380	11	50
with Bacon	430	15	50
with Cheese	430	16	50
Egg Whites, Cheddar w/ Skinny Bagel	210	7	22
Signature Farmhouse Omelet	520	22	56
Smoked Salmon Wasabi	370	9	54
Fruit Cup, Large, 12 oz	140	0.5	36
Yogurt Parfait:			
Blueb. Yogurt & Wild Blueb. 10.2 oz	380	10	68
Greek Van. Yog. & Wild Blueb., 10.2 oz	340	8	47
Greek Van. Yog. & Strawberry,11.3 oz	340	8	48
Oatmeal, Classic Medium, 12 oz	260	5	47
Sandwiches: *Per Whole Sandwich*			
Cafe: BLT	470	22	52
Black Angus Roast Beef & Cheddar	580	22	62
Herb Chicken Salad	470	13	58
Tuna Salad	480	12	59
Turkey & Swiss	670	28	65
Signature: Turkey Club	600	25	53
Chipotle Turkey & Avocado	700	33	60

Au Bon Pain® cont... (Sept '18)

Harvest Hot Bowls:

	C	F	Cb
Mayan Chicken	550	10	84
Mediterranean Chicken	690	28	75
Roasted Vegetarian	650	33	75
Teriyaki Steak	600	9	96
Mac. & Cheese, medium, 12 oz	880	43	92
Soups: Chicken Gumbo, 12 fl.oz	200	9	23
Chicken Noodle, 12 f.loz	120	2.5	15
Clam Chowder, 12 fl.oz	350	20	32
French Onion, 12 fl.oz	110	5	15
Harvest Pumpkin, 12 fl.oz	230	13	24
Lobster & Corn Bisque, 12 fl.oz	280	16	25
Minestrone, 12 fl.oz	180	6	24
Vegetarian Chili, 12 fl.oz	260	2	46
Salads: Without Dressing			
Chicken Caesar Asiago	280	10	20
Chicken Cobb, w/ Avocado	430	26	15
Harvest Turkey	380	15	32
Vegetarian Deluxe	260	13	26
Dressings: Bals. Vinaigrette, 1.5 oz	80	7	5
Caesar, 1.5 oz	190	19	3
Ranch, 1.5 oz	180	19	4
Cake, Cookies, Croissants, Danish : Per Item			
Cake, Iced Carrot, 4.2 oz	430	23	52
Cookies:			
Chocolate Chip, 2.8 oz	370	18	54
Oatmeal Raisin, 2.2 oz	290	11	46
Croissants: Almond, 4 oz	500	31	48
Apple & Cinn., 3.4 oz	220	8	35
Chocolate, 4 oz	470	25	55
Ham & Cheese Croissant	410	21	25
Danish: Cherry, 4.6 oz	400	15	58
Sweet Cheese, 4.7 oz	410	20	50
Muffins: Blueberry, 4.9 oz	480	25	59
Double Choc. Chunk, 4.7 oz	580	30	66
Raisin Bran, 4.7 oz	430	12	75
Palmier, 2.6 oz	380	20	46
Pecan Roll, 6 oz	740	42	86
Beverages: Caffe Latte, 16 fl.oz	140	7	12
Caramel Macchiato, 16 fl.oz	270	7	43
Hot Chocolate, 16 fl.oz	350	12	51
Raspberry Iced Tea, 24 fl.oz	180	0	50
Strawberry Smoothie, 16 fl.oz	290	0	68

Extra Menu Items ~ See CalorieKing.com

Auntie Anne's® (Sept '18)

Pretzels: With Butter

	C	F	Cb
Cinnamon Sugar	470	12	84
Jalapeno	330	5	63
Original	340	5	65
Pepperoni	480	16	65
Roasted Garlic & Parm.	380	8	68
Sour Cream & Onion	380	8	68
Sweet Almond	390	6	74
Dipping Sauces:			
Caramel, 1.5 oz	130	3	23
Cheese, 1.4 oz	90	8	2
Hot Salsa, 1.4 oz	90	8	2
Light Cream Cheese, 1.25 oz	80	6	1
Marinara, 2 oz	45	1	7
Melted Cheese, 2 oz	150	12	6
Sweet Glaze, 1.4 oz	130	0	32
Sweet Mustard, 1.25 oz	60	2	10
Pretzel Dogs: Original	360	20	33
Cheese	370	20	33
Jalapeno & Cheese	370	20	34
Jumbo	610	29	67
Mini Pretzel Dogs (8)	510	29	45
Beverages: Per 16 fl.oz			
Frozen Lemonade Mixer,			
Blue Raspberry; Strawberry, av.	235	0	60

Back Yard Burgers® (Sept '18)

Black Angus Burgers: On White Bun

	C	F	Cb
Back Yard: *Without Cheese*			
Classic Burger	580	28	48
Double Classic	860	46	48
Black Jack Burger	660	38	43
Black & Bleu Burger	760	46	45
Chipotle Burger	810	48	55
Mushroom Swiss Burger	660	37	43
Chicken Sandwiches: On White Bun			
Blackened Chicken, w/out cheese	610	27	49
Black Jack Chicken Club	700	37	46
Grilled Chicken, w/out cheese	450	12	45
Hawaiian Chicken, w/out cheese	520	12	63
Specialties:			
Breaded Chicken Tender Basket,			
w/out Toppings, Sauce or Bread	540	36	27
Veggie Burger, without cheese	420	11	67
Turkey Burgers: On White Bun			
Classic, w/out cheese	530	28	41
Club	650	38	42
Wild	600	34	43

continued next page ...

Fast - Foods & Restaurants

Back Yard Burgers® cont... (Sept '18)

Fries:

	C	F	Cb
Chili Cheese Fries, seasoned, reg.	790	59	52
Seasoned Fries: Regular, 4.5 oz	480	36	38
Large, 6 oz	640	47	50
Sweet Potato Fries, regular, 6 oz	450	29	40
Waffle Fries: Kid's, 4.5 oz	620	42	49
Regular, 6 oz	820	56	66
Sides: Back Yard Chili	310	18	15
Creamy Coleslaw	200	16	11
Loaded Baked Potato	420	21	45
Panko Onion Rings, regular, 4 oz	340	13	47
Salads: Without Dressing			
Back Yard Salad: w. Grilled Chicken	350	10	21
with Blackened Chicken	450	21	22
Cranberry Pecan Chicken	660	30	52
Side Salad	140	6	14
Dressings: Bleu Cheese	220	24	1
Gorgonzola Vinaigrette	170	15	6
Honey Mustard	240	23	7
Ranch, Homestyle	150	15	2
Dessert/Cobblers: Apple/Cherry	390	16	58
Apple/Cherry Cobbler A La Mode	540	24	78
Ice Cream, A La Carte	150	8	20
Milk Shakes: With Whole Milk & Whipped Topping			
Chocolate	750	35	100
Chocolate Oreo	850	40	115

Baja Fresh® (Sept '18)

Baja Bowls: With Black Beans

	C	F	Cb
Carnitas	680	18	92
Chicken	700	22	82
Shrimp	660	20	83
Steak	690	22	82
Veggie	540	14	90
Burritos: With Standard Components			
Baja: with Carnitas	800	41	63
with Chicken	820	46	53
with Steak	810	45	53
Bean & Cheese: With Pinto Beans			
Carnitas	1060	40	113
Chicken	1080	44	103
Steak	1070	44	103
Mexicano: With Black Beans			
Chicken	800	27	94
Steak	790	26	94
Ultimo: Carnitas	950	45	88
Chicken	970	50	78
Steak	960	50	78
Nachos: Regular Size, with Black Beans			
Carnitas	1110	56	106
Chicken	1150	60	101
Steak	1140	60	101

Baja Fresh® cont... (Sept '18)

Fajitas: With Pinto Beans

	C	F	Cb
Chicken: with Corn Tortillas	1060	39	121
with Flour Tortillas	1250	44	146
Shrimp: with Corn Tortillas	990	35	123
with Flour Tortilla	1180	41	148
Steak: with Corn Tortillas	1050	38	121
with Flour Tortilla	1240	44	146
Wahoo: with Corn Tortillas	990	35	121
with Flour Tortillas	1180	40	146
Tacos: With Standard Toppings			
Americano, Soft Taco: Carnitas	220	9	21
Chicken	230	11	19
Wahoo, Crispy Taco	250	15	24
Baja, meat varieties, average	160	6	17
Salads: Without Dressing			
Baja Ensalada: with Carnitas	300	9	28
with Chicken	260	11	18
with Shrimp	280	12	19
with Steak	250	11	17
Tostada: Carnitas & Pinto Beans	1010	48	99
Chicken & Black Beans	1020	53	86
Shrimp & Pinto Beans	1000	51	90
Steak & Black Beans	1020	52	86
Sides: Guacamole, 8 oz	310	27	19
Rice & Black Beans, 17 oz	550	11	90
Rice & Pinto Beans, 17 oz	570	11	95
Tortilla Chips, 5 oz	710	28	99
Tortilla Chips & Guacamole	1020	55	119

For Complete Nutritional Data ~ see CalorieKing.com

Baskin Robbins® (Sept '18)

Cones:

	C	F	Cb
Cake	25	0	5
Fresh-Baked Waffle	160	3.5	29
Sugar	45	0.5	9
Ice Creams: Per 4 oz Scoop			
Classic Flavors: Cherries Jubilee	220	11	26
Chocolate Chip	250	16	23
Chocolate	240	14	26
Jamoca Almond Fudge	260	15	28
Mint Chocolate Chip	250	16	23
Old Fashioned Butter Pecan	260	18	20
Oreo Cookies 'n Cream	260	15	27
Peanut Butter 'n Chocolate	300	20	25
Pistachio Almond	270	19	21
Pralines 'n Cream	270	14	32
Reese's P'nut Butter Cup	300	17	32
Rocky Road	270	15	29
Rum Raisin	240	11	29
Vanilla	240	16	21
Very Berry Strawberry	200	11	24
Wild 'n Reckless Sherbet	130	2	25

Updated Nutrition Data ~ www.CalorieKing.com
Persons with Diabetes ~ See Disclaimer (Page 22)

Baskin Robbins® cont... (Sept '18)

Ice Creams (Cont): Per 4 oz Scoop

	C	F	Cb
Seasonal Flavors: Black Walnut	270	18	21
Chocolate Fudge	240	15	27
Creole Cream Cheese	230	13	24
Strawberry Cheesecake	250	13	28

Grab-N-Go: Per 1.3 oz Cookie

Dark Chocolate Chunk Cookie	170	7	26
Double Fudge Cookie	160	6	26
Peanut Butter 'n Chocolate Cookie	160	7	23
White Chunk Macadamia Cookie			

Ice Cream Quarts: Per ½ Cup

Ice Cream Quarts:			
Chocolate	170	9	21
Mint Chocolate Chip	170	10	18
Vanilla, 2.6 oz	170	10	17

Soft Serve:

Cups: Vanilla: Kid's, 3 oz	110	4.5	14
Regular, 6 oz	230	9	29
Large, 9 oz	340	14	43
Parfaits: M&M's, Regular	820	32	119
Oreo, Regular	710	28	104
Snickers, Regular	730	24	114

31 Below' Mix-In: Per 16 oz Medium Cup

Butterfinger	850	34	120
Choc. Chip Cookie Dough	870	32	129
Heath	910	46	111
M&M's	1000	40	139
Oreo	720	29	99
Reese's PB Cup	910	45	109

Sundaes:

Banana Royale	680	33	90
Brownie	810	42	99
Chocolate Chip Cookie Dough	1100	47	160
Made with Snickers	1060	43	155
Two Scoop	570	33	63
Warm Brownie	810	42	99

Beverages: Per Medium, 24 fl.oz

Blasts: Caramel Cappuccino	790	25	130
Mocha Cappuccino	610	22	97
Fruit Blast: Mango	500	1.5	123
Strawberry Citrus	350	0	89
Tropical	370	0.5	93
Milk Shakes: Chocolate Chip	1030	54	117
Mint Chocolate Chip	1030	55	117
Smoothie: Mango Banana	620	2	149
Strawberry Banana	520	1	126
Tropical Banana	540	1.5	130

Big Apple Bagels® (Sept '18)

Bagels:

	C	F	Cb
Asiago Melt; Swiss Melt	370	6	65
Cinnamon Sugar	370	2	78
Fruit Varieties, average	330	3	66
Plain or Salt	320	2	64

Cream Cheese: Per 1.5 oz

Plain/Veg./Scallion, average	130	12	2
Plain, Lite	100	9	2
Strawberry	130	11	5
Walnut Raisin	140	12	5

Muffins: With Whole Egg

Mini: Blueberry	90	4.5	12
Cinnamon Swirl Cheesecake	90	5	9
Lemon Poppyseed	90	4.5	12
Large: Blueberry	590	28	78
Chocolate Cheesecake, 6 oz	650	38	70

Breakfast Sandwiches: Per Sandwich

French Toast w/ Egg: on BAB Bagel	1020	55	107
On MFM Bagel	1060	55	117

Salads: With Dressing

Caesar, with Caesar Dressing	450	34	19
Chicken Club, with Ranch Dressing	760	59	18
Mediterranean Bread Salad, with Balsamic Vinaigrette	740	41	63

Beverages: Per Medium, 16 fl.oz

Hot Chocolate	440	12	71
Mocha; White Chocolate Latte, av	380	8	66
Vanilla Creme Latte	310	8	50

Biggby Coffee® (Sept '18)

Hot Drinks: Per Tall, 16 fl.oz, without Whipped Cream

	C	F	Cb
Caffe au Lait: with 2% Milk	100	4	9
with Non-Fat Milk	65	0	9
with Soy	90	3	11
Caffe Latte: with 2% Milk	175	7.5	16
with Non-Fat Milk	115	0	16
with Soy	160	5	19
Cappuccino: with 2% Milk	95	3	11
with Non-Fat Milk	70	0	10
with Soy	95	3	11
Chai Latte: with 2% Milk	315	9	51
with Non-Fat Milk	255	0	51
Dark Hot Chocolate: w/ 2% Milk	320	9	50
with Non-Fat Milk	260	1.5	50

Frozen Creme Freeze: Per 20 fl.oz, with 2% Milk, Whipped Cream & Sugar, without Reduced Calorie

Avalanche Latte	640	19	108
Banana Chip	750	20	135
Coconut Creme	640	19	110
Mellow Mochanut	645	19	109

BJ's Restaurant® (Sept '18)

Shareable Appetizers: Full Order	C	F	Cb
Ahi Poke	320	10	24
Chicken Lettuce Wraps	500	21	43
Mozzarella Sticks	810	39	76
Root Beer Glazed Ribs	450	16	63
Sliders	880	32	97
Wings, Bone In, 10 pieces	750	57	6
Handcrafted Burgers: *With French Fries*			
Bacon Cheeseburger	1380	84	97
Bacon Guacamole Deluxe	1590	98	103
Classic Burger	1250	71	98
Crispy Jalapeno Burger	1380	81	106
Portobello Swiss Burger	1430	81	105
Brunch: Avocado Toast	410	20	47
Buttermilk Pancakes, short stack	910	31	143
Calif. Scramble, w/ sourdough	1210	69	90
Enlightened Veggie Omelette, with Fruit	270	9	24
Enlightened Entrees: *Includes Menu Set Sides*			
Cherry Chipotle Glazed Salmon	580	26	39
Lemon Thyme Chicken	630	19	52
Mediterranean Chicken Pita Tacos	670	20	79
Quinoa Bowls: Fresh Atl. Salmon	790	44	47
Roasted Chicken	650	28	47
Seared Ahi Salad	570	31	42
Vegetarian Pita Tacos	550	17	81
Pasta: *Includes Garlic Knot*			
Deep Dish Ziti	1400	91	99
Gr. Chicken Alfredo	1380	69	129
Italiano Vegetable Penne	800	38	92
Jumbo Spaghetti & Meatballs	1600	82	161
Shrimp & Asparagus Penne	870	38	94
Pizza, Deep Dish: *Per Slice, 1/8 Med. Pizza*			
BBQ/Buffalo Chicken, average	310	10	35
California Supreme	280	12	33
Classic Combo; Pepp. Extreme, av.	335	17	32
Spicy Hawaiian Chicken	350	15	36
Sweet Pig; Vegetarian, average	265	10	34
Pizza, Tavern-Cut: *Per Slice (1/12 Pizza)*			
Brewhouse; Italian Market	110	6	9
Garlic Chicken Pesto	100	5	9
Spicy Pig/Old Country Tomato, av.	80	4	10
Sandwiches: *With French Fries*			
Barbeque Pulled Pork	1600	82	172
California Chicken Club	1280	66	90
Slow Roasted Turkey Club	1660	111	104
Ribs & Steaks: *Without Sides, with Sauce*			
Baby Back Pork Ribs, half rack, with BBQ Sauce	710	34	75
Classic Rib-eye	1080	67	5
Prime Rib Dinner	110	106	6
Top Sirloin	500	32	2
Soups: Chicken Tortilla, Bowl	280	12	30
Clam Chowder: Bowl w/ crackers	440	26	33
Sourdough Loaf, w/ crackers	1470	42	219

BJ's Restaurant® cont...(Sept '18)

Salads: With Dressing & Toppings	C	F	Cb
BBQ Chicken Chopped Salad	930	48	64
Caesar Salad	810	64	44
Derby-Style Chicken Cobb Salad	940	69	20
Honey-Crisp Chicken Salad	1370	103	77
Santa Fe Salad, w/out protein	980	57	55
Sides: Broccoli	40	0	6
Classic Baked Potato	590	28	70
French Fries	350	19	40
Garlic GreenBeans	70	4	7
Rice Pilaf	230	6	39
White Cheddar Mashed Potatoes	330	18	33
Desserts: Baked Beignet	630	25	91
Monkey Bread Pizookie	1260	56	177
Salted Caramel Pizookie	1360	55	200
Soda Floats, average all flavors	510	19	79

For Complete Nutritional Data ~ see CalorieKing.com

Blimpie® (Sept '18)

Cold Deli Subs:	C	F	Cb
Per Regular, 6" White Sub, with Standard Menu Board Toppings			
Blimpie Best	470	17	54
Club; Ham & Swiss	430	14	54
Roast Beef & Provolone	460	14	53
Tuna	460	21	41
Turkey & Provolone	480	22	48
Wraps: Chicken Caesar	570	28	50
Southwestern; Buffalo Chicken, av.	590	31	53
Hot Deli Subs: *Per Regular White Sub with Standard Menu Board Toppings Unless Indicated*			
BLT	510	27	48
Meatball Parmigiana	740	38	59
Philly Cheesesteak	570	28	49
Salads: *Regular, without Dressing*			
Buffalo Chicken	180	8	9
Garden	40	0	8
Grilled Chicken	160	5	6
Ultimate Club	310	16	11
Dressings: Creamy Caesar, 1.5 oz	210	23	2
Creamy Italian, 1.5 oz	240	26	1
Thousand Island	200	19	6
Soups: *Per 8.6 oz*			
Chicken Noodle	210	4	29
Cream of Broccoli with Cheese	190	11	15
Cream of Potato with Bacon	190	9	24
New England Clam Chowder	170	3	28
Vegetable Beef with Barley	100	3	14
Breakfast:			
Biscuits: Bacon, Egg & Cheese	410	22	37
Sausage, Egg & Cheese	560	36	37
Bluffin, Egg & Cheese	240	8	29
Burritos: Ham, Egg & Cheese	570	27	51
Sausage, Egg & Cheese	710	43	50
Sandwich, Grilled Bacon	520	23	49

Bob Evans® (Sept '18)

Burgers: *Low Calorie*

	C	F	Cb
Big Farm Burgers: Hamburger	630	33	49
Bacon Cheeseburger	840	50	51
Steakhouse	1070	71	53
Three Cheese Burger	780	44	50

Sandwiches: *Low Calorie*

Farmboy	650	37	46
Farmhouse Gr. Chkn	820	40	56
Farmouse Fried Chicken	880	49	73

Slow Roasted:

Ham & Cheese	910	42	76
Pot Roast	840	50	51
Turkey Bacon Melt	640	32	48

Dinners: *Low Calorie Option with Set Menu Items*

Beef: Country Fried Steak	920	52	86
Black Angus Chopped Steak	920	64	53
Blackened USDA Choice Sirloin	920	53	55
USDA Choice Sirloin	1030	64	55

Chicken:

Grilled Breast: Farm	570	23	48
Wildfire	600	23	54
Homestyle, Fried Chicken Tenders	1020	54	94
Seafood: Gr. Salmon Fillet	740	41	48
Biscuit Breaded Fried Shrimp	860	46	88
Potato Crusted Flounder	640	31	61
Wildfire Grilled Salmon Fillet	790	41	61
Slow Roasted Entrees: Pot Roast	920	55	65
Turkey & Dressing	1090	52	112

Comfort Classics: *Low Calorie, with Set Menu Items*

Chicken Pot Pie	1370	86	117
Slow-Roasted Meatloaf	1000	57	87
Slow-Roasted Pot Roast	920	55	65
Slow-Roasted Turkey & Dressing	1090	52	112

Sides: Baked Potato

Baked Potato	330	12	51
Loaded	570	32	53
Bread & Celery Dressing	340	15	42
Broccoli, with Butter	110	10	5
Coleslaw	200	14	19
French Fries	330	14	47
Glazed Baby Carrots	90	4.5	13
Green Beans with Ham	30	1.5	4
Hash Browns	220	12	28
Golden Brown Home Fries	250	17	24
Mac & Cheese	250	12	25
Mashed Potatoes w/ Chicken Gravy	210	14	19

Sauces: *Per 1 oz Ramekin*

A.1.	50	0	13
Bob Evans Wildfire	50	0	13
Honey Mustard	120	11	5
Ranch	100	10	0.5
Sriracha-Avocado Mayo	160	18	0.5

Salads: *Regular Size High Calorie, with Set Menu Items*

Chicken Cobb Chicken, w/ dressing	1400	85	80
Farmhouse Garden Chicken, w drssng	1150	68	103

Bob Evans® cont... (Sept '18)

Soups: *Per Bowl, with 2 Saltine Crackers*

	C	F	Cb
Cheddar Baked Potato	390	21	32
Chicken N Noodles	290	15	26
Hearty Beef Vegetable	230	5	36
Tomato Basil	340	16	42

Breakfast:

Farm-Fresh Eggs: *High Calorie, with Set Menu Items*

Big Egg Breakfast	1350	99	69
Country Fried Steak & Eggs	1500	102	105
Farmers Choice	1820	95	199
Homestead	1500	111	83
Rise & Shine	1280	94	68
Sirloin Steak & Eggs	1470	102	70

3 Egg Omelets: *Low Calorie, with Set Menu Items*

Border Scramble	830	50	54
Veggie	850	58	53
Western	740	43	52

French Toast: *High Calorie, with Set Menu Items*

Brioche	830	25	134

Hotcakes: *Low Calorie, with Set Menu Items*

Cinnamon Supreme	1170	29	192
Double Blueberry	1190	25	206
Double Chocolate	1210	30	202

Sausage Selection: *Low Calorie, with Set Menu Items*

Sausage Gravy Bowl	830	49	82
Sunshine Skillet	770	51	51

Breakfast Sides: Banana Nut Bread

Banana Nut Bread	420	22	37
B'Milk Biscuit (2), with Butter	520	31	53
Country Gravy, cup	20	0.5	3
English Muffin, with Butter	150	3	25
Fresh Fruit Dish	60	0	14
Golden-Brown Fries	250	17	24
Grits, bowl	390	32	25
Hardwood Smoked Bacon, 1.4 oz	190	14	0.5
Hickory Smoked Ham, 3.5 oz	100	2.5	2
Sausage Links (3)	190	16	0
Sausage Patties (2)	320	26	2
Shredded Hash Browns	220	12	28
Sourdough Toast, with butter, 3.4 oz	280	8	45
Steel Cut Oats, low calorie, set add ins	200	3	39
Turkey Sausage Links (2)	140	7	2
Wheat Toast with Butter, 2 slices	170	6	24

Kid's: *With Set Menu Items*

Lil' Farmer's, 1 Bacon Strip; 1 ssg. av.	530	28	58
Plenty of Pancakes, low calorie	460	13	78
Sunny Scrambles	240	15	13

Dessert: Coconut Cream Pie, 1 slice

Coconut Cream Pie, 1 slice	590	36	63
French Silk Pie, 1 slice	650	43	59
Peanut Butter Brownie Bites (8)	880	40	120

183

Fast - Foods & Restaurants

Bojangles® (Sept '18)

Biscuit:	C	F	Cb
Plain	340	17	40
Bacon, Egg & Cheese	480	28	42
Cajun Filet	550	27	55
Country Ham	450	24	40
Gravy Biscuits	460	23	51
Sausage	540	35	40
Sausage & Egg	580	38	40
Smoked Sausage	490	29	41
Steak	570	35	49
Biscuit Add Ons: American Cheese	45	3.5	1
Egg	45	3	0
Chicken: Breast (1)	280	13	10
Leg (1)	100	5	5
Thigh (1)	240	17	9
Wing (1)	100	7	5
Homestyle Tenders, 4 pieces	500	24	41
Supremes, 4 pieces	390	19	29
Sandwiches:			
Cajun Filet: Regular	650	30	65
Club	740	40	70
Grilled Chicken: Regular	470	22	41
Club	570	30	42
Pulled Pork BBQ	460	21	48
Fixins': Per Individual Size, Unless Indicated			
Bo-Tato Rounds, medium	370	19	45
Cole Slaw	170	11	20
Green Beans	40	0	8
Macaroni & Cheese	260	13	29
Mashed Potatoes 'N Cajun Gravy	120	4.5	14
Seasoned Fries: Small	250	16	37
Medium	340	21	50
Picnic size	610	38	90
Salads: Without Dressing or Croutons			
Chicken Supreme	450	24	31
Garden	160	10	10
Grilled Chicken	290	14	11
Sweets: Bo-Berry Biscuit (1)	470	23	61
Cinnamon Twist (1)	370	21	41
Sweet Potato Pie	370	24	35

Boston Market® (Sept '18)

Sandwiches: Per Whole Sandwich on White Sub Roll	C	F	Cb
All-White Chkn Salad, w/out Chse	830	48	61
Meatloaf Carver	960	49	84
Roasted Turkey Carver	810	44	61
Rotisserie Chicken Carver	730	33	61
Individual Meals: Without Sides or Corn Bread			
Meatloaf, regular	470	33	17
Rosemary lemon Half Chicken	640	37	9
Rotisserie Half Chicken	500	24	1
Rotisserie Prime Rib	630	47	0
St Louis Style BBQ Ribs, half rack	860	64	23

Boston Market® cont...(Sept '18)

Salads: Entree Size, with Dressing	C	F	Cb
Chicken Caesar	430	28	15
Southwest Santa Fe, 13.7 oz	500	29	28
Sides: Corn Bread	160	3	31
Creamed Spinach	200	14	10
Fresh Steamed Veggies	60	3.5	7
Fresh Vegetable Stuffing	220	10	28
Green Beans	80	4.5	7
Macaroni & Cheese	260	9	34
Mashed Potatoes	240	10	32
Rotisserie Potatoes	180	4	33
Southwest Rice	170	6	26
Sweet Corn	120	3.5	20
Sweet Potato Casserole	450	12	85
Soup, Chicken Noodle	240	9	20
Kid's: Without Sides or Corn Bread			
Meatloaf	240	16	9
Turkey	80	2.5	0
White Chicken, 1 breast, 1 wing	270	11	0
Sauce: Beef or Chicken Au Jus/Gravy	10	0	2
Horseradish	60	3	6
Tartar Sauce	45	4.5	1
Zesty BBQ	40	0	10
Desserts: Apple Pie, 1 slice	430	21	59
Chocolate Brownie (1)	340	14	53
Chocolate Cake, 1 slice	570	33	66
Chocolate Chunk Cookie (1)	370	18	53

For Complete Nutritional Data ~ see CalorieKing.com

Boston Pizza® Canada (Aug '18)

Starters:	C	F	Cb
Medit. Hummus & Veggie Platter	1010	45	125
Oven Roasted Wings, 12.5 oz	780	50	9
Spinach & Artichoke Dip, 14.7 oz	850	66	36
Burgers: Dble Bacon BBQ Burger	1110	78	60
Most Valuable Burger	1040	77	49
Pepperoni & Bacon Pizzaburger	1160	75	68
Pastas: Full Order, without Garlic Toast			
Boston's Lasagna	790	23	107
Montréal Smoked Meat Spagh.	890	16	142
Pesto Chicken Bowtie	1220	46	143
Pizza: Per 8" Individual Pizza			
Classic Crust: Boston Royal	780	26	97
Deluxe	770	27	92
Hawaiian	700	19	100
Pepperoni	750	28	89
Thin Crust: The Meateor	540	25	51
Bacon Double Cheeseburger	530	23	53
New Thin Crust Pizzas: Per Slice of Medium Pizza			
Cherry Bomb Margherita, 2.47 oz	150	6	17
Fiesta Chicken, 2.86 oz	200	11	18
Potato Bianca, 3.2 oz	170	5	24

Boston Pizza® Canada cont... (Sept '18)

Sandwiches: Without Sides

	C	F	Cb
Big Dipper	1320	71	117
Boston Brute	800	24	108
Chipotle Chicken Club	950	40	86
Montreal Smoked Meat	910	59	40
Steak Sandwich	1010	50	105
Salads: Full Order with Dressing			
Crispy Chicken Pecan	1160	88	44
Roasted Beef & Peach	550	32	56
Desssert:			
NY Cheesecake	600	32	76
The Panookie, with ice cream	940	44	127

For Complete Nutritional Data ~ see CalorieKing.com

Braum's® ~ see CalorieKing.com

Bruegger's® (Sept '18)

Bagels:

	C	F	Cb
Blueberry, 4.1 oz	310	2	63
Cinnamon Sugar, 4.1 oz	320	2	63
Everything, Whole Wheat, 4.1 oz	280	2.5	55
Jalapeno Cheddar, 5.5 oz	440	9	75
Plain, 4.1 oz	300	2	60
Rosemary Olive Oil, 4.1 oz	330	6	59
Cream Cheese: Per 1.5 oz			
Bacon Scallion, Jalapeno, av.	140	12	5
Honey Walnut	150	12	8
Light Herb Garlic/Plain	100	6	4
Plain	130	11	6
Smoked Salmon	150	13	3
Breakfast Bagel S'wiches: With Standard Toppings			
Egg & Cheese	430	18	63
Egg White, Cheese & Bacon	460	12	64
Plain Bagel: Smoked Salmon	460	10	66
Sriracha Egg	650	30	70
Western	670	34	67
Deli Sandwiches: With Standard Toppings			
BLT on Wheat Bread	610	44	38
Chicken Breast on Plain Bagel	550	6	81
Garden Veggie on Plain Bagel	360	2	72
Ham on Wheat Bread	470	10	67
Deli Classics: With Standard Toppings			
Cheese & Tomato, on rye	690	35	63
Harvest Turkey, on Ciabata	700	24	83
Pastrami & Swiss Melt,on Rye	530	31	62
Tarragon Chkn Salad, on Wheatberry	530	30	44
Turkastrami Melt, on Rye	650	21	77
Signature & Classic Sandwiches: With Standard Toppings			
Herby Turkey/Sesame Bagel	570	15	75
Leon. da Veggie/Asiago Parm. Bgl	490	14	70
Sm. Salmon Egg Salad/Pumpnkl Bgl	570	21	64
Turkey Chipotle Club/Evrythng Bread	810	45	66

Bruegger's® cont... (Sept '18)

Café Salads: Without Dressing

	C	F	Cb
Blue Apple, 7 oz	360	18	30
Chicken Caesar, 7.7 oz	200	8	14
Pastrami Cobb, 10.3 oz	280	16	15
Dressings: Balsamic Vinaig., 1 oz	60	6	3
Caesar, 1 oz	80	7	2
Ranch	90	10	1
Dessert:			
Chocolate Chunk Brownie, 3.3 oz	440	22	55
Cheesecake Brownie, 3.1 oz	340	18	43
New York Coffee Cake, 5.1 oz	590	29	77

For Complete Menu & Data ~ see CalorieKing.com

Burgerville® (Sept '18)

Burgers: With Standard Ingredients

	C	F	Cb
American Colossal	540	29	40
American ½ lb Colossal	790	47	40
Double Cheeseburger	490	28	31
Original: Hamburger	340	17	31
Cheeseburger	380	21	31
Pepper Bacon Cheeseburger	670	40	37
Tillamook Cheeseburger	600	34	38
Chicken Tenders, (3), with Fries	770	43	71
Sandwiches: With Standard Menu Components			
Deluxe Gr. Chicken, on Kaiser Bun	550	25	42
Deluxe Crispy Chkn, on Kaiser Bun	780	43	67
Halibut Fish, without Cheese, on Plain Bun	460	27	40
Turkey, without Cheese, on Sesame Seed Bun	450	19	40
French Fries: Small, 2.8 oz	220	11	28
Regular, 5 oz	400	19	50
Large, 6.5 oz	510	25	65
Salads: Full Size, Without Dressing			
Grilled Chicken Club	170	9	4
Smoky Blue Cheese	150	6	17
Wild Smoked Salmon & Hazelnuts	170	11	5
Dressing: Balsamic Vinaigrette	180	18	5
Blue Cheese	180	18	2
Honey Mustard	200	19	8
Ranch	190	20	2
Breakfast: With Standard Menu Components			
B'fast Platter, Bacon, Engl. Muffin	760	45	63
Burger, w/ Pepp. Bacon, Chedd. Chse	470	27	27
Burrito, Ssg Patty & Chedd Cheese	690	45	40
Ice Cream Sundaes: With Whipped Cream			
Caramel	390	19	50
Hot Fudge	390	19	51
Triple Berry	350	18	41

Burger King® (Sept '18)

Whopper Sandwiches:

	C	F	Cb
Whopper	660	40	49
without Mayo	500	22	49
with Cheese & Mayo	740	46	50
Bacon & Cheese Whopper	790	51	50
Double Whopper Sandwich	900	58	49
With Cheese	980	64	50
Whopper Jr	310	18	27

Flame Broiled Burgers:

	C	F	Cb
Bacon Cheeseburger	300	15	27
Bacon Double Cheeseburger	370	20	27
Bacon King Sandwich	1150	79	49
Cheeseburger	270	12	27
Double Cheeseburger	350	18	27
Extra Long Cheeseburger	590	34	45
Hamburger	240	10	26
Homestyle Cheeseburger	550	27	48

Grilled Dogs: Classic Dog

	C	F	Cb
Classic Dog	310	16	32
Chili Cheese Dog	330	19	28

Chicken Sandwiches:

	C	F	Cb
Crispy Chicken Jr.	450	30	34
Crispy Chicken Sandwich	670	41	54
Grilled Chicken Sandwich	470	19	39
Original Chicken Sandwich	660	40	48
Spicy Crispy Chicken Jr.	390	21	37

Chicken Nuggets: 4 pieces

	C	F	Cb
4 pieces	170	11	11
6 pieces	260	16	16
10 pieces	430	27	27
Chicken Fries, Regular, 9 pieces	280	17	20

Dipping Sauces: BBQ

	C	F	Cb
BBQ	40	0	11
Buffalo	80	8	2
Chicken Fry	140	13	6
Ranch; Zesty Onion Ring, av.	145	15	2
Big Fish S'wich	510	28	51
Veggie Burger: M'Star	390	15	42
Without Mayo	310	7	42

French Fries: Small, 4.3 oz

	C	F	Cb
Small, 4.3 oz	320	14	44
Medium, 5.8 oz	380	17	53
Large, 7 oz	430	19	60

Onion Rings: Small

	C	F	Cb
Small	320	16	41
Medium	410	21	53
Large	500	25	64

Garden Fresh Salads:
Bacon Cheddar Ranch Chicken:

	C	F	Cb
Crispy, w/ Dressing	710	50	34
Grilled, w/ Dressing	620	41	18

Garden Grilled Chicken:

	C	F	Cb
Crispy, without Dressing	440	25	31
Grilled, without Dressing	340	15	16
Garden Side Salad, w/o Dressing	60	4	3
Dressing, Ken's Ranch, 1.5 oz pkt	260	28	2

Burger King® cont... (Sept '18)

Breakfast:

	C	F	Cb
Biscuits: Bacon, Egg & Cheese	380	23	29
Ham, Egg & Cheese	370	21	30
Sausage	390	25	28
Sausage, Egg & Cheese	510	35	29
Burrito, Egg-Normous Burrito	910	55	73

Croissan'wich:

	C	F	Cb
Bacon, Egg & Cheese	340	18	30
Egg & Cheese	300	15	30
Fully Loaded	610	40	31
Ham, Egg & Cheese	330	16	31

King Croissan'wich:

	C	F	Cb
with Double Sausage	700	51	31
with Ham & Sausage	530	34	31
with Sausage & Bacon	580	39	31
French Toast Sticks: 5 pieces	380	18	49
with 1 oz Breakfast Syrup	500	18	79

Hash Browns: Small, 3 oz

	C	F	Cb
Small, 3 oz	250	16	24
Medium, 6 oz	500	33	48
Large, 8 oz	670	44	65
Oatmeal, Orig. Maple Flavored	170	3	32
Platters: Pancakes & Sausage	610	31	72
Ultimate Breakfast	1190	66	123

Sweets:

	C	F	Cb
Cinnamon Roll	280	11	41
Chocolate Chip Cookie (1)	165	8	24
Pies: Dutch Apple	340	14	51
Hershey's Sundae	310	19	32
Reese's P'nut Butter	310	19	31
Snickers	300	16	36
Sundaes: Caramel	290	6	53
Chocolate Fudge	280	7	47
Vanilla Soft Serve, in cone	190	4.5	32

Shakes: Chocolate

	C	F	Cb
Chocolate	610	16	103
Chocolate Oreo	610	19	99
Oreo	730	21	121
Strawberry	640	15	113
Vanilla	580	15	98
Smoothies: Strawb. Ban.,16 fl.oz	310	1	71
Tropical Mango, 16 fl.oz	370	0	86
Beverages: Frappe, av., 16 fl.oz	405	16	62

Coca Cola/Sprite: With 50% Ice

	C	F	Cb
Value, 15 fl.oz	140	0	39
Small, 20 fl.oz	190	0	51
Medium, 30 fl.oz	290	0	77
Large, 40 fl.oz	380	0	102
Minute Maid Orange Juice, 10 fl.oz	140	0	33
Icee, Coke/Fanta Cherry, 16 oz	140	0	38
Iced Coffee: Regular, 16 oz	150	8	19
Vanilla, 16 oz	190	8	28
Sweet Tea, 20 oz	120	0	35

186

Updated Nutrition Data ~ www.CalorieKing.com
Persons with Diabetes ~ See Disclaimer (Page 22)

Captain D's Seafood® (Sept '18)

From The Grill: W/out Sides, Rice or Breadsticks

	C	F	Cb
Blackened Tilapia	210	7	1
Grilled Wild Salmon	230	10	2
Grilled Whitefish & Shrimp Skewer	280	11	3
Lemon Pepper Whitefish Fillet	180	8	1
Shrimp Skewers (2)	200	6	2

Other Favorites:

	C	F	Cb
Cheese Sticks, 1order	500	32	35
Jalapeno Poppers, 1 order	510	36	40

Seafood:

	C	F	Cb
Butterfly Shrimp (6)	360	27	24
Popcon Shrimp	490	27	48
Stuffed Crab, 1 piece	140	10	11

Side Dishes:

	C	F	Cb
Baked Potato, plain, (1)	210	0	48
Coleslaw, 1 order	180	13	15
French Fries, 1 serving	330	22	28
Hushpuppy (1)	80	4	9
Dessert, Chocolate Cake, 1 order	300	11	49

Caribou Coffee® (Sept '18)

Without Whipped Cream Unless Indicated

Hot Coffees: Per Medium

	C	F	Cb
Classic: Coffee Of The Day, 2% Milk	90	3.5	9
Cappuccino, with 2% Milk	110	4.5	10
Espresso, 4 oz	0	0	0
Latte, with 2% Milk	180	7	17
Macchiato, with 2% Milk	20	1	1

Hot Chocolate: Per Medium, with Whipped Cream

	C	F	Cb
Milk Chocolate, 2% Milk	600	36	50

Specialty, Mint Condition Mocha,

	C	F	Cb
Milk Choc., 2% Milk, Wh. Crm, med	630	34	68

Cold Beverages: Per Medium, Without Whipped Cream

Blended Fruit & Yogurt Smoothies:

	C	F	Cb
Mango Orange Key Lime	420	5	106
Strawberry Banana	360	0	87

Classics: Iced Americano

	C	F	Cb
Iced Americano	5	0	0
Iced Latte, with 2% Milk	110	4.5	10
Iced Mocha, Milk Choc., 2% Milk	250	7	33

Coolers: Chocolate, Milk Chocolate

	C	F	Cb
Chocolate, Milk Chocolate	660	24	93
Coffee	350	7	72
Vanilla	430	6	93

Specialty Blended Cooler:

	C	F	Cb
Caramel High Rise	540	12	107
Mint Condition, Milk Chocolate	590	9	114
Turtle Mocha, Milk Chocolate	700	15	127
Vanilla White Mocha, White Choc.	600	9	121

Carl's Jr.® (Sept '18)

California menu only. Please check instore for further nutritional information.

Charbroiled Burgers:

	C	F	Cb
Famous Star with Cheese	670	37	57
Super Star with Cheese	920	56	59
Teriyaki Burger	660	29	71
The Big Carl	920	58	56
Western Bacon Cheeseburger	750	35	75
Double	1010	55	76
½ lb Thickburgers: Original $6	980	69	59
Guacamole Bacon	1200	89	51
Lettuce Wrapped	630	55	9

Chicken Sandwiches:

	C	F	Cb
Bacon Swiss Crispy Chicken Fillet	770	41	58
Big Chicken Fillet	650	33	55
Charbroiled: BBQ Chicken	390	7	50
Chicken Club	590	27	46
Santa Fe Chicken	550	25	45
Spicy Chicken Sandwich	490	29	43

Chicken Tenders, hand breaded,

	C	F	Cb
5 pieces, without Sauce	440	21	21

Chicken Stars,

	C	F	Cb
6 pieces, without Sauce	270	15	19

Breakfast:

	C	F	Cb
Bacon & Egg Burrito	570	35	32
Breakfast Burger, Single	730	43	47
Grilled Cheese & Sausage S'wich	660	43	43
Hash Brown Nuggets: Small, 3.8 oz	350	23	32
Medium, 4.2 oz	390	26	36
Large, 6 oz	560	37	52
Loaded B'fast Burrito	760	48	46
Steak & Egg Burrito	630	36	37

Fries: CrissCut Fries, 5 oz

	C	F	Cb
CrissCut Fries, 5 oz	450	29	42
Natural Cut: Small, 3.5 oz	300	15	39
Medium, 6 oz	430	21	55
Large, 6.5oz	460	22	59
Fried Zucchini, 5 oz	380	23	39
Onion Rings, 4.5 oz	530	28	61

Salads: Without Dressing

	C	F	Cb
Charbroiled Chicken Salad	280	9	19
Garden, Side	140	7	15

Dressings: Per 2 oz Package

	C	F	Cb
Blue Cheese	310	34	2
House	210	23	5
Low-Fat Balsamic	20	1	3

Dessert: Choc. Chip Cookie, 2.5 oz

	C	F	Cb
Choc. Chip Cookie, 2.5 oz	330	17	43
Chocolate Cake, 3 oz	290	11	46
Strawberry Swirl Cheesecake, 3.5 oz	320	17	3

Malts: With Ice Cream

	C	F	Cb
Oreo Cookie	780	40	94
Other flavors, average	765	36	99

Shakes: With Ice Cream

	C	F	Cb
Oreo Cookie	710	39	79
Vanilla; Chocolate; Strawberry, av.	695	35	85

Carvel® (Sept '18)

Carvelanche:	C	F	Cb
Oreo/M&M'S, av: Small, 12 oz	595	30	70
Regular, 16 oz	875	47	102
Large, 24 oz	1310	70	153
Classic Sundaes: Per Small, 12 oz			
Caramel	700	36	84
Hot Fudge	540	30	60
Strawberry	610	34	67
Sundae Dashers: Per Regular, 16 oz			
Banana's Foster	1020	31	176
Fudge Brownie	1170	60	147
Mint Chocolate Chip	1230	64	157
Peanut Butter Cup	1420	86	134
Strawberry Shortcake	730	38	91
Ice Cream:			
Chocolate/Vanilla, average:			
Junior Cup, 4.5 oz	260	14	28
with Carvelite	175	4	30
Small Cup, 7.5 oz	430	24	47
with Carvelite	285	6	52
Medium Cup, 9.5 oz	550	30	60
with Carvelite	360	8	65
Thick Shakes: Per 16 oz			
Chocolate; Vanilla, av.	650	29	90
Strawberry	600	31	70

Charley's Grilled Subs® (Sept '18)

Subs: Per Regular			
Bacon 3 Cheese Steak	840	43	58
Chicken Buffalo/Teriyaki, av.	735	30	62
Chicken California	800	40	56
Italian Deli Deluxe	860	48	61
Pepperoni Steak	890	49	58
Philly Cheesesteak	780	38	58
Philly Chicken, with Provolone	600	18	55
Turkey Cheddar Melt	790	33	65
VeggieDelight	500	15	69
Salads: Without Dressing			
Fresh Garden	35	0	7
Grilled Chicken; Steakhouse, av.	130	3	8
Fries: Original	400	22	46
Cheese Gourmet	550	31	62
Ultimate Gourmet	790	54	61
Breakfast:			
Hashbrowns	280	18	27
Omelet Platter: Bacon, Egg & Chse	830	52	55
Sausage, Egg & Cheese	990	69	55
Steak, Egg & Cheese	860	50	55
Sandwiches: Bacon, Egg & Chse	490	26	36
Sausage, Egg & Cheese	650	44	36
Steak, Egg & Cheese	520	25	36
Toast, 2 slices	130	2	24

For Complete Menu & Data ~ see CalorieKing.com

Cheesecake Factory® (Sept '18)

Cheesecake: Per Slice	C	F	Cb
Original	800	n/a	62
Godiva Chocolate	1230	n/a	97
Reese's P.B. Chocolate Cake	1480	n/a	153
White Chocolate Raspb. Truffle	1120	n/a	88
Small Plates & Snacks: Ahi Tartare	260	n/a	19
Beets with Goat Cheese	360	n/a	31
Crispy Crab Bites	350	n/a	11
Crispy Cuban Roll	770	n/a	49
Dynamite Shrimp	570	n/a	40
Fried Zucchini	530	n/a	30
Loaded Baked Pot. Tots	950	n/a	56
Stuffed Mushrooms	470	n/a	15
Glamburgers & Sandwiches: Without Sides			
American Cheeseburger	1280	n/a	75
Bacon-Bacon Burger	1590	n/a	74
Classic Burger	1380	n/a	64
Crispy Shrimp S'wich	1330	n/a	102
Grilled Turkey Burger	1070	n/a	67
Kobe Burger	1380	n/a	83
Mushroom Burger	1400	n/a	69
Smokehouse BBQ Bgr	1380	n/a	97
Veggie Burger	1220	n/a	113
Glamburger Sides: French Fries	470	n/a	72
Green Salad	190	n/a	8
Sweet Potato Fries	470	n/a	72
Fish & Seafood:			
Fish & Chips	1550	n/a	118
Shrimp Scampi	1900	n/z	130
Sthrn Fried Catfish	1380	n/a	96
Pasta: Four Cheese	1210	n/a	106
with Chicken	1490	n/a	106
Fettuccine Alfredo with Chicken	2660	n/a	130
Louisiana Chicken Pasta	2510	n/a	162
Specialties: Baja Chicken Tacos	1500	n/a	165
Cajun Chicken "Littles"	2030	n/a	222
Chicken Bellagio	2010	n/a	153
Chicken Enchiladas	1380	n/a	106
Chicken with Lemon Couscous	1440	n/a	72
Crispy Chkn Costoletta	2590	n/a	102
Eggplant Parm.	1430	n/a	131
Factory Burrito Grande	1670	n/a	148
Famous Factory Meatloaf	1630	n/a	117
Grilled Fish Tacos	1500	n/a	165
Grilled Steak Tacos	1530	n/a	157
White Chicken Chili	570	n/a	36
Salads: Includes Dressing			
Caesar	1320	n/a	34
Santa Fe	1730	n/a	104
Seared Tuna Tataki	540	n/a	17

n/a = not available

Updated Nutrition Data ~ www.CalorieKing.com
Persons with Diabetes ~ See Disclaimer (Page 22)

Chick-fil-A® (Sept '18)

Breakfast:	C	F	Cb
Bagel, Chicken, Egg & Cheese	480	18	51
Biscuits: Plain, buttered	300	13	41
Bacon, Egg & Cheese	420	21	40
Chicken	450	21	50
Egg White Chicken Grill	300	7	31
Sausage, Egg & Cheese	600	40	41
Bowl, Hash Brown Scramble	450	28	19
Burrito, Hash Brown Scramble	450	22	34
Chick-n-Minis, 4 pieces	350	14	39
Hash Browns, 2.7 oz	240	16	23
Parfait, Greek Yogurt, fruit topping	240	8	29
Chick-fil-A Sandwiches: Without Sauce			
Chicken	440	19	40
Deluxe	500	23	42
Grilled Chicken	310	6	36
Grilled Chicken Club	430	16	37
Spicy Deluxe	540	25	43
Cool Wrap, Grilled Chicken, without sauce	360	14	30
Chicken: Without Dipping Sauce			
Chick-n-Strips, breaded, 4 count	470	23	29
Nuggets: Breaded, 8 count	260	12	9
Grilled, 8 count	140	3.5	2
Salads: Without Dressing			
Cobb, with Breaded Ckn Nuggets	510	28	28
Grilled Market, with Chick-n-Strips	560	28	47
Spicy Southwest, w/- Grilled Filet	450	19	37
Dressings: Avocado Lime Ranch	310	32	3
Creamy Salsa	290	31	3
Garlic & Herb Ranch	280	29	2
Light Italian	25	1.5	3
Sauces: BBQ Sauce	45	0	11
Honey Mustard Sauce	45	0	11
Polynesian Sauce	110	6	13
Sweet & Spicy Sriracha Sauce	45	0	10
Sides: Fruit Cup, medium	50	0	12
Chicken Noodle Soup, small bowl	130	3.5	15
Side Salad, with toppings	160	11	12
Superfood Side Salad, with toppings:			
Small	150	9	18
Large	190	9	25
Waffle Potato Fries: Med.	360	18	43
Large	460	24	56
Dessert: Chocolate Chunk Cookie	350	16	50
Icedream Cone, large	260	6	45
Frosted Coffee, large	300	7	51
Milkshakes: Chocolate, large	720	26	108
Cookies & Cream, large	750	31	107
Vanilla, large	620	25	86

Chili's® (Sept '18)

For The Table: As Served	C	F	Cb
Bottomless Tostada Chips w/ Salsa	910	45	113
Classic Nachos: Beef	1640	108	57
Chicken	1480	95	57
Southwestern Eggrolls	800	41	82
Texas Cheese Fries, full order	1860	127	97
Triple Dipper: *Serving for One*			
Big Mouth Bites	780	54	40
Original Chicken Crispers	510	33	22
Baby Back Ribs: Full Rack, without Sides			
Dry Rub	1480	107	30
Original BBQ	1430	106	21
Honey Chipotle BBQ	1480	106	35
House BBQ	1440	107	21
Burgers: Without Side Fries			
Classic Bacon Beef	1020	72	77
Oldtimer, with Beef Burger	890	55	47
Southern Smokehouse Beef	1270	80	77
Crispers & More: As Served, with Set Sides			
Cajun Pasta with Grilled Chicken	1180	53	111
Original Tempura	1350	67	127
Fresh Mex: As Served			
Bacon Ranch ChickenQuesadilla	1740	131	69
Chicken Enchiladas	960	52	56
Chipotle Chicken Bowl	1000	50	79
Ranchero Chicken Tacos	940	51	48
Lighter Choices: As Served			
Ancho Salmon	630	30	42
Grilled Chicken Salad	430	23	22
Mango Chile Chicken	490	19	49
Margarita Grilled Chicken	630	16	67
Sirloin (6 oz), w/ Grilled Avocado	420	21	23
Sandwiches: Without Fries			
Bacon Avocado Chicken	1130	59	74
Buffalo Chicken Ranch	880	48	69
CA Turkey Club	1090	64	86
Steaks: As Served			
Classic Sirloin, 6 oz	680	37	41
Classic Ribeye	1050	64	40
Country-Fried Steak	1290	67	121
Sides: As Served			
Homestyle Fries	420	17	60
Loaded Mashed Potatoes	380	23	32
Mexican Rice	160	4.5	27
Spiced Panko Onion Rings	390	19	48
Salads: As Served			
Boneless Buffalo Chicken	970	66	44
Caribbean with Seared Shrimp	600	25	80
Quesadilla Explosion	1400	93	81
Sweet Stuff: Per Slice			
Cheesecake	720	43	73
Molten Chocolate Cake	1150	61	142

For Complete Menu & Data ~ see CalorieKing.com

Chipotle® (Sept '18)

	C	F	Cb
Tortillas:			
Burrito Size Flour Tortillas (1)	320	9	50
Taco Size: Crispy Corn Tortilla (3)	200	9	29
Soft Flour Tortillas (Taco), (3)	250	8	40
Meal Components: Barbacoa, 4 oz	170	7	2
Black/Pinto Beans, average, 4 oz	130	1.5	22
Brown Rice, 4 oz	210	6	36
Carnitas, 4 oz	210	12	0
Cheese, 1 oz	110	8	1
Chicken, 4 oz	180	7	0
Fajita Vegetables, 2.5 oz	20	0	5
Guacamole, 3.5 oz	230	22	8
Lettuce, 1 oz	5	0	1
Sofritas, 4 oz	150	10	9
Steak, 4 oz	150	6	1
Condiments:			
Queso, 2 oz	120	8	4
Salsa: Chili Corn, 3.5 oz	80	1.5	16
Green Tomatillo, 2 oz	15	0	4
Red Tomatillo, 2 oz	15	0	4
Sour Cream, 2 oz	110	9	2
Extras, Chips, serving, 4 oz	540	25	73

Chuck E. Cheese® (Sept '18)

	C	F	Cb
Appetizers:			
Cheesy Breadsticks (1)	170	11	13
French Fries, 7 oz	380	12	59
Parmesan Breadstick (1)	240	10	30
Sandwiches & Wraps: Per Half Sandwich/Wrap			
BBQ Chicken Ciabatta	270	9	30
Italian Ciabatta	320	17	25
Wraps: Chicken Caesar	400	20	29
Club	470	30	28
Specialty Pizzas: Per Medium Slice			
BBQ Chicken	210	9	24
Cali Alfredo; Meat Combo	200	10	19
Super Combo	190	9	19
Vegetarian	160	6	19
Traditional Wings:			
Small: with BBQ or Sweet Chili Sauce	450	27	17
with Lemon Pepper Sauce	400	27	4
Desserts: Apple Pie Pizza, whole	440	7	89
Churros (4)	560	21	90

Church's Chicken® (Aug '18)

	C	F	Cb
Chicken: Per Serving			
Original: Breast, 1 piece	250	14	9
Leg, 1 piece	150	8	6
Thigh, 1 piece	360	27	12
Wing, 1 piece	290	18	8
Spicy: Breast, 1 piece	280	17	12
Leg, 1 piece	160	9	9
Thigh, 1 piece	380	25	21
Wing, 1 piece	350	20	19
Tender Strips, average, 1 piece	100	5	5
Sides: Per Regular Serving			
Baked Macaroni & Cheese, 4.7 oz	210	12	19
Cole Slaw, 4.2 oz	170	11	16
Dinner Roll (1), 1.7 oz	60	1	11
French Fries, 2.6 oz	210	9	29
Honey Butter Biscuits (1), 2.2 oz	230	15	25
Jalapeno Cheese Bombers (4)	220	11	24
Mashed Potatoes & Gravy, 4.5 oz	110	1	24
Okra, 3.4 oz	260	15	30
Sauces: BBQ, pkt	45	0	11
Creamy Jalapeno, pkt	120	13	2
Honey Mustard/Ranch, av., pkt	140	15	2
Dessert, Apple Pie	270	13	37

Cici's Pizza® (Sept '18)

	C	F	Cb
Adventurous Taste Pizzas: Per Slice			
BBQ Pork	200	7	27
Zesty Ham & Cheddar/Veggie, av.	170	6	23
Deep Dish Pizza, 1 slice	170	6	21
Flatbread, Spinach Alfredo, 1 slice	140	7	14
Traditional Pizzas: Per Slice			
Alfredo; Spinach Alfredo	160	5	22
Beef; Pepperoni & Jalap; Ssg, av.	190	7	24
Wings: BBQ (5)	260	12	16
Buffalo (5), average	215	13	4
Garlic Parmesan (5)	270	18	5
Sides: Chicken & Pasta Soup, 8 oz	90	2.5	13
Pasta with Alfredo Sauce, 7 oz	315	12	53
Dessert: Brownie	140	6	21
Cinnamon Roll	130	1.5	20
Lemon Creme Bar	170	7	25
Pizzas, average, 1 slice	130	3	23

Cinnabon® (Sept '18)

	C	F	Cb
Cinnabon Classic Roll (1)	880	37	127
MiniBon Roll (1), 3.4 oz	350	15	51
Bites: Cinnabon Classic (4)	430	17	60
Caramel Pecan Bites (4)	580	29	73
Centre of The Roll Classic (1)	750	33	106
Chillata: Oreo Cookies & Cream	870	40	118
Double Chocolate Mocha	360	13	59
Strawberries & Cream	710	33	96

Updated Nutrition Data ~ www.CalorieKing.com
Persons with Diabetes ~ See Disclaimer (Page 22)

Claim Jumper® (Sept '18)

Appetizers: As Served

	C	F	Cb
Southwest Eggrolls	1190	53	114
Three Cheese Potatocakes (3)	1075	71	80

Burgers & Sandwiches: Without Sides

Grilled Cobb Sandwich	1210	78	78
Widow Maker Burger	1370	87	84

Calzones: Specialty

	1430	80	137
Traditional	1350	66	140

Meals: As Per Menu Description

Favorites: Country Fried Steak	2030	107	189
Giant Stuffed Chicken Baker	990	34	118
Meatloaf & Mashed Potatoes	1300	75	117
Pasta: Black Tie Pasta	1535	84	126
Parmesan Crusted Chicken	975	47	83
Pizza: Calif. Works, Classic Crust	1295	64	127
Steakhouse, Flatbread	820	47	65
Specialties: BBQ Baby Back Pork Ribs,			
Full Rack	1745	111	111
Roasted Tri-Tip with Demi Glaze	800	47	19
Seafood: Atlantic Salmon, Blcknd	715	42	48
Tilapia Bianca, with Shrimp,			
Artichoke Hearts & Sauce	1165	80	56

Entree Salads: Without Dressing or Bread

Calif. Citrus Chkn, Charbroiled	865	53	58
Seared Ahi Spinach	515	24	31

Soups: Per Bowl

New England Clam Chowder	525	45	23
Potato Cheddar	710	61	31
Sweets: Choc. Motherlode Cake	2770	144	340
Italian Lemon Cake	1240	62	158

Coldstone Creamery® (Sept '18)

Ice Cream:

	C	F	Cb
Amaretto: Like it	340	21	36
Love it	550	33	57
Gotta have it	820	49	85
Chocolate: Like it	330	20	34
Love it	520	31	54
Gotta have it	780	47	81

Hot Stone:

Brownie A La Cold Stone, 11.5 oz	1070	50	148
Choc. Lava Meltdown, 11.5 oz	980	47	127
Hot For Cookies, 7.9 oz	730	39	91

Sorbet:

Strawberry Mango Banana:

Like it, 5 oz	210	0	54
Love it, 8 oz	340	0	87
Gotta have it, 12 oz	510	0	130

Cosi® (Sept '18)

Bowls: W/ Set Menu Components

	C	F	Cb
Adobo Chicken with Avocado	680	21	99
Thai Curry Chicken	740	22	101
Thai Curry Tofu	740	26	103

Soups:

Chicken Noodle: Bowl	150	4	18
Cup	100	3	12
Macaroni & Cheese: Bowl	990	56	82
Cup	680	39	56
Medit.Lentil: Bowl	320	19	30
Cup	210	13	20
Tomato Basil: Bowl	600	47	30
Cup	400	31	20
Turkey Chili: Bowl	360	7	67
Cup	240	5	45

Salads: With Menu Set Dressing

Cobb	740	56	20
Greek	535	47	20
Signature	620	45	40

Breakfast:

Santa Fe Wrap, 8.8 oz	470	29	30
Spinach Florentine Wrap, 7.3 oz	380	22	28
Squagel (Plain) S'wich Cosi Club	560	21	64
Dessert: Blondie Brownie, 2.25 oz	280	14	36
Chocolate Chunk Brownie, 2.25 oz	300	16	39
Chocolate Croissant, 3 oz	360	16	46
Chocolate Hazelnut Muffin, 4 oz	550	35	33

Cousins Subs® (Sept '18)

Subs: Per 7.5", Standard Toppings

	C	F	Cb
Grilled To Order:			
Chicken Bacon Cheddar	640	24	53
Chkn Bacon MushroomSwiss	760	34	59
Chkn Cheese Steak	590	20	52
Classics:			
Club, with Mayo	680	39	50
Italian Special, with Oil	830	48	52
Tuna with Mayo	650	36	51
Deli Fresh:			
Ham & Provolone, with Mayo	630	32	51
Roast Beef & Cheddar, with Mayo	740	37	52
Turkey Breast with Mayo	550	25	53

Soup: Per Cup

Beef Steak with Noodles	105	3.5	12
Cheddar Cauliflower	110	5	13
Chicken Noodle	110	3	16
Cream of Potato	170	8	21
New England Clam Chowder	150	2.5	25

For Complete Nutritional Data ~ see CalorieKing.com

Culver's® (Sept '18)

ButterBurgers:	C	F	Cb
Original: Single	390	17	38
Double	560	30	38
Triple	730	43	38
Cheddar:			
Single	470	24	38
Double	720	44	38
Culver's Bacon Deluxe:			
Single	610	36	42
Double	850	56	42
Culver's Deluxe:			
Single	570	35	41
Double	810	52	42
Mushroom & Swiss, Single	500	26	40
Sourdough Melt, Single	480	24	39

Sandwiches:	C	F	Cb
Beef Pot Roast	410	13	40
Crispy Chicken	460	14	57
Grilled Reuben Melt	660	37	43
North Atlantic Cod Filet	600	33	50
Pork Tenderloin	630	25	72

Sides:	C	F	Cb
Green Beans, reg.	130	9	9
Chili Cheddar Fries	690	32	80
Crinkle Cut Fries, reg.	360	14	53
Mashed Potatoes & Gravy, regular	130	1	25
Wisconsin Cheese Curds, 5.3 oz	510	25	51

Dinners: With Fries, Cole Slaw, Dinner Roll & Butter & Accompanying Sauce

	C	F	Cb
Butterfly Jumbo Shrimp, 6 pieces	1090	54	129
North Atlantic Cod, Fried, 2 pieces	1480	98	108

Soup:	C	F	Cb
Broccoli Cheese	220	12	17
Chicken Noodle	100	2	15
Potato with Bacon	240	10	28

Salads: Without Dressing	C	F	Cb
Chicken Cashew w/ Gilled Chicken	450	24	14
Cranberry Bacon Bleu, with Grilled Chicken	360	14	14
Garden Fresco with Grilled Chicken	360	14	15
Side Salad	50	2	5

Kid's Meals:	C	F	Cb
Corn Dog	240	14	23
Chicken Tenders, Breaded, 2 pieces	270	12	21
Grilled Cheese Sourdough Sandwich	360	16	39

Dressings: Chnky Bleu Chse, 1.8 oz	310	33	2
French Dressing, 1.8 oz	190	13	19
Ranch, 1.75 oz	180	19	2
Sesame Ginger, 2 oz	70	0	16

Culver's® cont... (Sept '18)

Concrete Mixers: No Toppings	C	F	Cb
Chocolate, regular	700	36	88
Cookie Dough, regular	1010	56	113

Sundaes: Per 2 Scoops	C	F	Cb
Banana Split	1065	60	122
Caramel Cashew	1000	51	121
Fudge Pecan	1040	64	107
Turtle	1040	62	112

Beverages: Chocolate Malt, reg.	850	38	114
Chocolate Shake, reg.	820	38	108
Strawberry Malt, reg.	760	38	92
Strawberry Shake, reg.	730	38	86

D'Angelo® (Sept '18)

Burgers: Without Condiments	C	F	Cb
Regular	450	18	45
Cheeseburger	480	21	46
Steak #9	830	34	83
Western Bacon Cheddar	780	42	51

Deli Sandwiches: Per Medium, with Standard Toppings on Italiab Sub	C	F	Cb
Cranberry Pecan Chicken Salad	980	58	78
Roast Beef & Cheese	750	38	76
Tuna Salad	950	68	61

Wraps: Per Medium, with Standard Toppings, on Tortilla Wrap	C	F	Cb
Buffalo Chicken	1020	62	58
Chicken Caesar	1090	63	68
Cobb BLT	700	31	78

Fresh Entree Salads: With Dressing, without Pokket			
Entree: Caesar	630	53	26
Greek	240	13	17
Grilled Topped:			
Chicken Cobb	800	58	26
Steak Cobb	870	64	26
Steak Greek	780	62	20

Soup: Per Bowl	C	F	Cb
Beef Stew	330	12	34
Extreme Broccoli & Cheddar	370	28	18
Main Lobster Bisque	540	43	24
New England Clam Chowder	480	27	46

For Complete Menu & Data ~ see CalorieKing.com

Dairy Queen® (Sept '18)

Burgers:	C	F	Cb
Cheeseburger: Original	370	18	31
Deluxe	460	24	39
GrillBurgers: ¼ lb Bacon Cheese	630	36	42
½ lb Cheese	800	49	42
½ lb Flame Thrower	970	68	39
¼ lb Mushroom Swiss	590	36	37

Updated Nutrition Data ~ www.CalorieKing.com
Persons with Diabetes ~ See Disclaimer (Page 22)

Dairy Queen® cont... (Sept '18)

Sandwiches:

	C	F	Cb
Artisan Bakes!:			
Chicken Bacon Ranch	500	20	45
Kansas City BBQ PulledPork	430	15	69
Turkey BLT	580	28	45
Chicken Strip Baskets: *Without Beverage*			
4 pieces, with Country Gravy	1000	49	103
6 piece, with Country Gravy	1250	61	121
Hot Dogs: Regular	340	20	28
Chili Cheese	420	26	28
Snack Melts: Buffalo Chicken	290	16	21
Chicken Bacon BBQ	280	11	27
Salads: *Without Dressing*			
Chicken BLT:			
Crispy Chicken	400	21	28
Grilled Chicken	270	11	10
Side Salad	25	0	5
French Fries, regular, 4 oz	290	13	39
Onion Rings, 4 oz	360	16	48
Breakfast: Bacon Biscuit S'wich	420	26	19
Chicken & Gravy	420	21	29
Country Platter:			
with Bacon	1150	73	55
with Ham	850	42	60
Ham Biscuit Sandwich	350	18	19
Pancake Platter with Sausage	510	21	60
Desserts: *Per Medium*			
Blizzard Treats: Banana Split	580	16	97
Butterfinger	720	25	109
Cookie Dough	1040	41	151
Heath	870	37	119
Oreo Cookies	780	29	117
Reese's Peanut Butter Cups	750	32	102
Salted Caramel Truffle	1040	48	142
Turtle Pecan Cluster	900	48	105
DQ Dipped Cone, Chocolate, med.	460	22	59
DQ Sundaes: Caramel	430	11	73
Hot Fudge	430	15	66
Strawberry	330	10	53
Bakes, Hot:			
Fudge Stuffed Cookie	640	33	80
Triple Chocolate Brownie	540	25	74
Shakes: Caramel	750	25	115
Chocolate	710	23	110
Strawberry	620	23	87
Vanilla	660	23	97
Add Malt	80	1	18
Moo Latte: *Per Medium, with Whipped Topping*			
Caramel	570	17	96
Mocha	580	22	88
Vanilla	530	16	90

Daphne's Greek Cafe® (Sept '18)

Califonia Menu Only. Check Instore for Latest Information

Starters:

	C	F	Cb
Fire Feta & Warm Pita	340	17	39
Hummus & Warm Pita	320	12	47
Classic Pita Sandwiches: *Without Tzatziki Sauce*			
with Chicken	410	16	41
with Crispy Shrimp	410	17	48
with Falafel	640	17	96
with Gyro	680	45	49
Plates: *Without Pita or Tzatziki Sauce*			
Cali-Greek Bowls:			
with Crispy Shrimp	930	38	117
with Falafel	1160	39	165
with Grilled Chicken	930	37	109
with Grilled Shrimp	1060	46	91
Mediterranean Veggie	1300	56	161
Surf & Turf	690	25	85
Classic Greek Salads: *W/ Dressing, w/o Pita & Sauce*			
Crispy Shrimp	440	31	25
Falafel	670	31	74
Grilled Chicken	440	30	18
Add, Pita & Tzatziki	130	3	21
Sides: Cucumber-Tomato Salad	120	11	5
Fire Roasted Vegetables	70	3	12
French Fries	440	22	55
Greek Salad, small	140	12	7
Lemon Chicken Soup	280	12	37
Moroccan Carrot Salad	180	13	15
Pita Chips	220	6	36
Pita Bread	190	3	36
Seasoned Rice	360	8	68
Tabouli	220	15	20

Davanni's® (Sept '18)

Hot Hoagies: Per Half, with 6" White Bun & Standard Toppings

	C	F	Cb
Assorted	490	30	39
Cheese	500	31	39
Chicken & Bacon, w/ Honey Mustard	505	22	46
Chicken Parmigiana	445	16	40
Club	495	27	40
Pastrami	470	27	40
Roast Beef	470	25	39
Southwestern Chicken	535	26	43
Tuna Melt	645	44	42
Turkey Bacon Chipotle	565	33	39
Pasta: *As Served, with Garlic Toast*			
Chicken Florentine, half portion	570	23	56
Lasagna, half portion	625	43	37

continued next page...

Davanni's® cont... (Sept '18)

Pizzas: Per 1/8 of Medium Pizza

	C	F	Cb
Five Meat: Thin Crust	255	13	19
Traditional Crust	305	13	30
Solo, Thin Crust	655	36	44
Veggie: Thin Crust	220	10	19
Traditional Crust	275	10	30
Works: Thin Crust	265	14	19
Traditional Crust	315	15	30

Del Taco® (Sept '18)

Breakfast:

	C	F	Cb
Burritos: Breakfast	430	21	38
Half Pounders: Bacon	640	36	38
1/2 lb Chorizo/Steak, av.	510	26	39
Hash Brown Sticks, 5 pieces	230	17	18
Tacos: Bacon	230	14	15
Chorizo	240	15	16
Carne Asada Steak	240	13	16
Egg & Cheese	190	11	15

Burgers: Without Fries

Bacon Double Del Cheeseburger	740	51	35
Del Cheeseburger	470	28	34
Double Del Chseburger	690	47	35

Crinkle Cut Fries: Kids, 3 oz

	160	10	17
Small, 4 oz	210	13	22
Medium, 6 oz	320	19	34
Macho, 8.8 oz	470	28	49
Chili Cheddar Fries, 10.5 oz	570	35	42

Burritos: 1/2 lb Bean & Cheese, av.

	460	10	69
Classic Gr. Chicken	530	33	40
Del Beef	500	24	40
Del Combo	540	17	64
Epic: Carne Asada	750	24	90
Chipotle Chicken Avocado	950	48	91
Grilled Chicken Avocado	840	36	90
Macho Combo	950	37	100

Loaded Nachos,

Carne Asada/Chicken, av.	970	46	100

Platos: Per Plate

2 Street Tacos:

Beer Battered Fish	1060	45	139
Carne Asada Steak	960	35	127
Grilled Chicken	940	35	127
Carne Asada Wet Burrito	1300	48	150
Chicken Verde, Wet Burrito	1220	48	154

Quesadillas: Mini Bacon

	170	9	14
Cheddar	460	26	31
Chicken/ Cheddar orSpicy Jack, av.	550	31	35

Del Taco® cont... (Sept '18)

Tacos:

	C	F	Cb
Beer Battered Fish	230	12	26
Chicken Street	170	7	20
Del Taco: Crunchy Beef	310	20	14
Soft Meat	300	18	17
Grilled Chicken	210	12	16

Salads: Without Dressing

Chicken, Bacon Avocado	590	46	23
Mexican Chopped Chicken	510	23	39
Signature Taco	550	29	38

Sides:

Bean & Cheese Cup, 7.8 oz	320	3.5	52
Carne Aada Fries, 12.5 oz	810	59	46
Cheddar Potato Poppers, 4 pieces	240	14	20

Denny's® (Sept '18)

Breakfast:

	C	F	Cb
Favorites: *With Hash Browns, without Bread*			
Country Fried Steak, 11 oz	520	33	38
Grand Slamwich, 19 oz	1290	82	87
Moons Over My Hammy, 17 oz	950	60	57
Omelettes:			
Ham & Cheese Omelette, 13 oz	780	54	20
Loaded Veggie	620	44	24
Philly Cheesesteak	880	64	25
Ultimate	850	68	20
Skillets:			
Bourbon Chkn, 20 oz	870	39	68
Fit Fare Veggie, 17 oz	370	16	40
Smoky Gouda Prime Rib & Broccoli	530	37	33
Slams: *Without Bread*			
All American, w/ Hash Browns, 15 oz	930	74	19
Fit Slam, 15 oz	420	11	56
French Toast, without Egg, 11 oz	860	53	65
Lumberjack, without Egg, 19 oz	970	49	96
Pancakes: *Without Hash Brown, Egg & Meat*			
Blueberry	460	11	80
Dulce De Leche Crunch	1220	35	207
Peanut Butter Cream	990	47	122
Salted Caramel & Banana	1140	27	207
Sides: Bacon Strips (4)	210	16	2
Buttermilk Biscuit (2)	470	26	54
Cheddar Cheese Hash Browns,5 oz	250	18	15
English Muffin, w/out Margarine	130	1	25
Grilled Ham, 3 oz slice	90	3	1
Hash Browns, 1 serve	170	12	15
Hearty Breakfast Sausage (1)	350	31	5
Oatmeal, w/ Milk & Br. Sugar, 10 oz	240	2	45
Red Skinned Potatoes, 4 oz	200	8	26
Wheat Toast, with Margarine	230	11	29

Denny's® cont... (Sept '18)

Appetizers:	C	F	Cb
Bacon Cheddar Tots, with Sour Cream (10)	580	34	54
Chicken Strips: with Buffalo Sauce	700	30	68
with Sweet & Tangy BBQ Sauce	760	21	106
Italian Sampler, 21 oz	1250	71	96
Loaded Nacho Tots (10)	990	63	66
Mozzarella Cheese Sticks, w/o Sce	560	22	60
Zesty Nachos: Half Size, 15 oz	880	56	68
Full size, 25 oz	1670	108	131

Lunch Burgers & Sandwiches: *Without Sides*			
Burgers: Bacon Gouda	1090	68	58
Bacon, Avocado Cheeseburger	1000	66	53
Bourbon Bacon	910	52	58
Slamburger, without Egg	860	51	52
Spicy Sriracha	920	55	55
Sandwiches: Cali Club	820	48	55
Club	830	39	74
The Grand Slamwich	1120	71	72
The Super Bird	600	28	43

Lunch Sides:			
Bacon & Cheddar Tots (6), without Sour Cream	300	15	31
Bacon Strips (2)	100	8	1
Caesar Salad, 6 oz	280	22	15
French Fries, 4 oz	400	22	46
Garden Salad, w/out Dressing, 7 oz	170	9	19
Hash Browns, 1 serving	170	12	15
Seasoned Fries, 5.5 oz	490	26	57

Dinners: *Without Sides or Bread*			
Brooklyn Spag. & M'balls, 20 oz	990	48	86
Chicken Strips, 7 oz	490	17	53
Country Fried Steak, w/ Gravy, 10 oz	560	34	35

Melts: *Without Sides*			
Chicken Philly	760	40	57
Pot Roast Melt	870	46	54
Prime Rib Philly	910	52	62
Sirloin Steak, 8 oz	360	15	1
T-Bone Steak, 13 oz	490	30	0
Tilapia Ranchero, 9 oz	300	12	6
Wild Alaska Salmon	350	23	1

Dinner Sides: Broccoli, 3 oz	25	0	4
Fresh Sauteed Zuchini & Squash, 3 oz	70	6	3
Fresh Steamed Zucchini &Squash, 3 oz	15	0	3
Garlic Toast/dinner Bread, 2 pieces	190	7	25
Red-Skinned Potatoes: Plain, 4 oz	200	8	26
Mashed, without gravy	120	5	17
Sweet Petite Corn, 5 oz	210	13	20
Whole Grain Rice, 5 oz	240	2.5	48

Denny's® cont... (Sept '18)

Salads: *Without Bread*	C	F	Cb
Avocado Chicken Caesar, with Caesar Dressing, 15 oz	730	59	10
Cobb Salad: *Without Dressing*			
without Meat, 13 oz	430	30	20
with Fried Chicken Strips, 18 oz	800	43	59
with Grilled Chicken, 18 oz	630	39	20
with Prime Rib, 15.5 oz	560	38	23
House Salad: *Without Dressing*			
without Meat	190	9	19
with Fried Chicken Strips, 15 oz	560	22	58
with Grilled Chicken, 15 oz	390	18	19
with Prime Rib, 12.5 oz	320	17	22
with Wild Alaskan Salmon, 16 oz	540	32	20

Soups: *Without Bread*			
Chicken Noodle: Cup	260	10	28
Bowl	390	15	43
Loaded Baked Potato: Cup	360	24	25
Bowl	470	31	36
Vegetable Beef: Cup	200	11	27
Bowl	310	16	40

Condiments: Pico de Gallo, 2 oz	15	0	3
Sour Cream, 1 oz	45	4	1
Tomato Sauce, 1.5 oz	25	1	3
Whipped Margarine, 0.5 oz	40	4.5	0

Dressings: *Per 1.5oz*			
Blue Cheese	160	16	2
Caesar	250	26	1
French	130	8	2
Honey Mustard	180	15	12
Ranch	200	21	1
Thousand Island	160	16	7

Sauces: *Per 1.5 oz*			
Bourbon	110	0	26
Buffalo	70	7	1
Sweet & Tangy BBQ	110	0	30

Desserts: *As Served*			
Caramel Apple Pie Crisp, 13 oz	760	26	126
Chocolate Lava Cake	700	34	85
New York Style Cheesecake, plain	500	34	42

Beverages:			
Hot Chocolate, 8 oz	190	3	37
Iced Tea, Sweetened, 12 oz	160	0	40
Lemonade Iced Tea, 12 oz	80	0	21
Mango Lemonade, 15 oz	210	0	57
Strawb. Lemonade, 12 oz	210	0	55
Milk Shakes: Chocolate, 16 oz	870	43	111
Vanilla, 16 oz	800	43	97
Smoothie: Groovy Mango, 15 oz	340	0	86
Strawberry Banana Bliss, 15 oz	330	0.5	82

For Complete Nutritional Data ~ see CalorieKing.com

Dippin' Dots® (Sept '18)

Flavored Ices: Per ½ Cup, 3 oz

	C	F	Cb
Rockin' Cherry with Popping Candy	130	0.5	30
Other varieties	100	0	26

Frozen Yogurt: Per ½ Cup

YoDots: Cookies 'N Cream	130	3	25
Cookie Dough	130	2.5	26
Cotton Candy	100	1.5	20
Strawberry Cheesecake	100	0	21

Ice Cream: Per ½ Cup

Banana Split	160	8	20
Choc. Chip Cookie Dough	230	11	32
Mint Chocolate	170	8	21
Strawberry	160	8	18

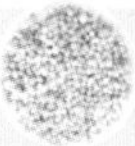

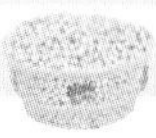

Donatos Pizza® (Sept '18)

Pizzas: Per Slice

	C	F	Cb
Hand Tossed Signature Pizzas: Per Slice of 14" Pizza			
Chicken Spinach Mozzarella	290	11	30
Founder's Favorite	320	13	32
Mariachi Beef	300	12	33
Mariachi Chicken	230	6	33
Serious Meat	340	15	32
The Works	270	12	26
Thick Crust Signature Pizzas: Per Slice of 14" Pizza			
Bourbon BBQ Bacon	160	7	18
Chicken Spinach Mozzarella	150	7	14
Double Bacon Pepperoni	200	10	16
Founders Favorite	180	8	16
Margherita	160	8	14
Serious Meat	190	9	16
The Works	170	8	17

Oven Baked Subs:

Big Don: Italian Sub, Marinara	600	25	62
Chicken Bacon Cheddar	770	38	61
Fresh Vegy	490	19	62
Ham & Smoked Prov.	560	21	61
Hot Chicken	830	42	72
Meatball	800	36	70
Stromboli: Deluxe	860	33	95
Pepperoni	980	45	94
Three Meat	970	42	94

Salad: Entree Size, with Menu Set Dressing

Chicken Caprese	390	25	17
Chicken Harvest	600	37	42
Italian Chef	500	43	11

Wings: Per 6 pieces, without Dipping Sauce

Boneless Chkn: Mild/Hot Sce, av.	395	22	25
Asian Sauce	450	17	51
BBQ	410	16	43

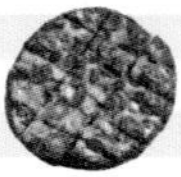

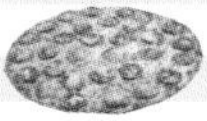

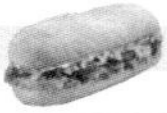

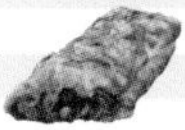

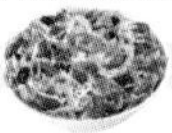

For Complete Nutritional Data ~ see CalorieKing.com

Domino's® (Sept '18)

Regular Pizzas Use Regular Cheese Base

	C	F	Cb
12" Hand Tossed: Per Slice, ⅛ Pizza			
Bacon, Beef, & Sausage	290	14	27
Beef, Green Pepp., On. & Mshrm	210	7	27
Black Olives, Green Peppers, Onions, Mushrooms, Tomatoes	200	7	27
Ham & Pineapple	200	6	28
Pepperoni	220	9	26
Pepperoni & Sausage	250	11	26
Sausage	240	11	26
Sausage, Beef & Pepperoni	270	14	26
14" Brooklyn: Per Slice, ⅙ Pizza			
Beef, Green Pepp., On. & Mshrm	270	11	29
Black Olives, Green Peppers, Onions, Mushrooms, Tomatoes	260	10	29
Ham & Pineapple	270	10	31
Pepperoni	290	14	28
Pepperoni & Sausage	340	19	28
Sausage	330	18	28
14" Thin Crust: Per Slice, ⅛ Pizza			
Bacon, Beef & Sausage	300	19	19
Beef, Green Pepp., On. & Mshrm	200	10	19
Black Olives, Green Peppers, Onions, Mushrooms & Tomatoes	190	9	19
Ham & Pineapple	200	9	20
Pepperoni	210	12	18
Pepperoni & Sausage	250	16	18
Sausage	240	15	18
12" Specialty Handmade Pan: Per Slice, ⅛ Pizza			
Cali Chicken Bacon Ranch	370	21	30
Deluxe	310	16	30
Memphis BBQ Chicken	330	16	33
Spinach & Feta	300	15	29
12" Specialty Hand-Tossed: Per Slice, ⅛ Pizza			
Buffalo Chicken	260	12	26
Deluxe	230	10	27
ExtravaganZZa	280	13	28
MeatZZa	270	13	27
Ultimate Pepperoni	270	13	26
14" Specialty Thin Crust: Per Slice, ⅛ Pizza			
Buffalo Chicken	260	15	17
Cali Chicken Bacon Ranch	320	21	18
Honolulu Hawaiian	250	13	20
Memphis BBQ Chicken	260	14	22
Wisconsin 6 Cheese	250	14	18

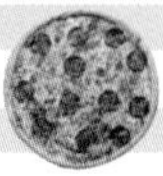

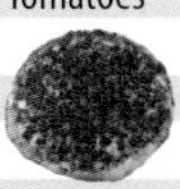

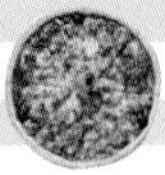

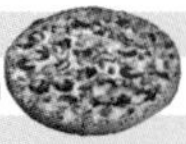

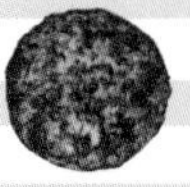

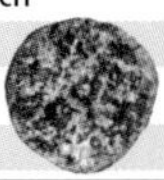

Domino's® cont... (Sept '18)

Chicken Wings: W/out Sauce	**C**	**F**	**Cb**
Barbecue, 4 wings	240	13	18
Hot, 4 wings	200	13	8
Chicken Dipping Cups: *Per 1.5 oz Container*			
Blue Cheese	200	21	2
Kicker Hot	45	3.5	2
Ranch	200	21	2
Sweet Mango Habanero	60	0	17
BreadBowl Pasta: Per 1/2 Bowl			
Chicken Alfredo, 10.5 oz	690	25	91
Chicken Carbonara, 11.6 oz	730	28	92
Italian Sausage Marinara, 11.85 oz	730	27	96
Pasta Primavera, 11 oz	660	24	91
Oven Baked Sandwiches: Per Sandwich			
Buffalo Chicken with Blue Cheese	840	42	74
Chicken Bacon Ranch	880	44	72
Chicken Parmesan	760	30	74
Italian	820	40	72
Mediterranean Veggie	700	28	76
Philly Cheese Steak	640	24	74
Sweet & Spicy Chicken Habanero	800	32	84
Pasta In Dish: Chkn Alfredo, 11.9 oz	620	30	60
Chicken Carbonara, 13 oz	690	35	63
Italian Sausage Marinara, 13.5 oz	690	34	70
Pasta Primavera, 11.9 oz	550	27	61
Salads: Per Serving without Dressing			
Chicken Caesar	210	7	15
Classic Garden	200	9	17
Salad Dressings: Per 1.5 oz Package			
Caesar Dressing	210	23	2
Italian	160	17	4
Light Balsamic Dressing	90	9	5
Ranch Dressing	200	21	2
Bread Side Items:			
Garlic Bread Twists2.4 oz	220	11	27
Parmesan Bread Bites, 2.4 oz	220	10	27
Spin. & Fetta Stuffed Cheesy Bread, 1.9 oz	160	7	17
Stuffed Cheesy Bread, 1.9 oz	150	7	17
Bread Dipping Sauces: Per Container			
Garlic, 1 oz cup	250	28	0
Marinara, 2 oz cup	30	0	6
Cinnamon Bread Twists, 2.6 oz	250	12	31
Sweet Icing, Dipping Cup	230	4	51
Dessert: Choc. Lava Crunch Cake	350	17	47
Marbled Cookie Brownie	190	9	25

Dunkin' Donuts® (Sept '18)

Bagels: Per Bagel	**C**	**F**	**Cb**
Plain	310	1	64
Cinnamon Raisin	320	1	66
Everything	340	3	67
Multigrain	350	7	63
Sesame Seed	350	5	65
White Cheddar Twist	390	8	64
Donuts: Apple 'n Spice	260	14	29
Apple Crumb	320	15	42
Bavarian Kreme	270	15	30
Bismark	490	24	65
Boston Kreme	300	16	37
Buttered	410	20	55
Chocolate Butternut	410	20	54
Chocolate Frosted Cake	350	19	40
Chocolate Headlight	330	18	39
Coconut	390	20	48
Coffee Roll	390	18	51
Double Chocolate	350	20	39
French Cruller	220	13	23
Glazed	260	14	30
Glazed Jelly	310	14	42
Jelly	280	14	34
Lemon	260	15	29
Maple Frosted	280	15	32
Maple Vanilla Creme	360	20	43
Old Fashioned Cake	290	19	28
Peanut	450	26	48
Powdered	320	19	33
Sour Cream	350	17	47
Strawberry Frosted	280	15	32
Sugared	230	14	22
Vanilla Creme	330	20	35
Muffins: Blueberry, Regular	460	15	76
Chocolate Chip	550	21	83
Coffee Cake	590	24	87
Corn	460	16	72
Munchkins: Cinnamon	60	3.5	7
Glazed	70	4	7
Glazed Chocolate	70	3.5	8
Jelly	70	4	9
Old Fashioned	60	3.5	6
Powdered	60	3.5	7
Other Bakery Items:			
English Muffin	180	2	34
Plain Croissant	340	18	38
Regional Sandwiches:			
Grilled Cheese	430	24	37
Grilled Cheese, with Bacon	490	29	37
Grilled Cheese, with Ham	460	25	38

continued next page...

Dunkin' Donuts® cont... (Sept '18)

Breakfast:

	C	F	Cb
Hash Browns, 6 pieces	140	8	17
Oatmeal,			
Brown Sugar Flavored Oatmeal, with Dried Fruit Topping	310	2	66
Plain Bagels:			
Bacon, Egg & Cheese	520	18	67
Egg & Cheese	460	13	67
Ham, Egg & Cheese	490	14	67
Sausage, Egg & Cheese	680	33	68
Big N' Toasted, with Toast	620	38	41
Biscuit, Chicken	490	23	49
Croissants: Bacon, Egg & Cheese	560	35	41
Egg & Cheese	500	31	40
Ham, Egg & Cheese	530	32	41
Sausage, Egg & Cheese	710	51	41
English Muffins:			
Bacon, Egg & Cheese	390	19	37
Ham, Egg & Cheese	340	15	37
Sausage, Egg & Cheese	550	34	37
Wake-Up Wraps:			
Bacon, Egg & Cheese	210	13	15
Egg & Cheese	180	10	14
Ham, Egg & Cheese	190	11	15
Turkey Sausage	240	14	15

Hot Beverages: Per Medium Size

	C	F	Cb
Chocolate: Original	330	10	59
Mint	300	10	52
Dunkaccino	350	15	52

Cold Beverages: Per Medium, 24 fl.oz

Coolatta:

	C	F	Cb
Cotton Candy	350	0	92
Pineapple; Watermelon, av.	360	0	93

Iced Latte: *Per Medium, 24 fl.oz, with Whole Milk without sugar*

	C	F	Cb
Butter Pecan Swirl	340	9	54
Maple Pecan Swirl	350	9	56
Mocha Swirl	350	10	54
Peppermint Mocha Swirl	360	10	60
Pumpkin Swirl	340	9	53

Iced Macchiato: *Per Medium, 24 fl.oz, with Whole Milk*

	C	F	Cb
Caramel Swirl	290	6	49
Cookie Dough Swirl	330	9	52
Girl Scouts Coconut Caramel	350	59	54
Pistachio Swirl	340	9	53

Eat 'N Park® (Sept '18)

Breakfast:

	C	F	Cb
Bananas Foster French Toast, 2 slices	440	6	88
Omelettes: Ham & Cheese	665	47	6
Meat Lover's	760	58	6
Pancakes:			
Buttermilk (2)	325	3	65
Blueberry (2)	335	3	68
Scramblers:			
All-American with Bacon	605	27	58

Appetizers

	C	F	Cb
Chicken Quesadilla	1030	62	62
Fried Cheese Sticks	590	35	41
Fried Ravioli	895	59	66
Mac 'n Cheese Bites	950	74	55

Burgers: Without Sides

	C	F	Cb
Black Angus:			
American Grill	705	45	32
Bacon Cheeseburger	755	46	37
Classic Cheeseburger	710	41	39
Mushroom & Onion Cheeseburger	750	43	41
Superburgers: Black Angus	1040	69	28
Original	680	42	38

Sandwiches: With Menu Set Ingredients

	C	F	Cb
Bacon Turkey Swiss	625	33	37
Buffalo Chicken Wrap, with Ranch	825	47	60
Chargrilled Chicken	475	16	41
Classic Grilled Cheese	720	37	70
Hot Turkey	500	7	74
Reuben	1020	72	45
Shredded Pot Roast	540	31	28
Turkey Club	850	46	48
Whale of a Cod Fish	930	35	96

Dinners: Without Sides

	C	F	Cb
Baked Chicken Parmigiana:			
with Marinara Sauce	955	39	97
with Meat Sauce	1105	50	93
Baked Lemon Sole, 2 fillets	305	21	1
Chicken Fillets, 5 pieces	545	27	29
Fisherman's Platter	1020	53	75
Nantucket Cod	390	27	8
Pasta Noodles w/ Marinara Sauce	665	9	124
Pasta Noodles with Meat Sauce	835	22	120
Smothered Ground Sirloin Steak	445	27	8
Whale of a Cod	625	30	39

Continued Next Page....

Updated Nutrition Data ~ www.CalorieKing.com
Persons with Diabetes ~ See Disclaimer (Page 22)

Eat 'N Park® cont... (Sept '18)

Salads:	C	F	Cb
Buffalo, w/ Gr. Chkn, w/o Drssng	595	28	34
Eat'n Park, w/ Rib-Eye, w/o Drssng	665	36	30
Greek, w/ Gr. Chicken, w/ Dressing	380	19	17
Grilled Chkn & Strawb., w/ Dressing	510	25	35
Sides: Baked Potato	190	0	44
Broccoli	40	0	8
Carrots	40	1	9
Coleslaw	120	8	12
Cheese Fries	505	29	55
French fries	350	17	47
Mac'n Cheese	215	3	38
Mashed Potatoes	110	6	13
Onion Rings	165	9	20
Pasta: with Alfredo Sauce	445	14	63
with Marinara Sauce	340	4	65
Soup Bowls: Chicken Noodle	275	8	34
Clam Chowder	450	21	52
Cream of Broccoli	275	10	36
Farmsource Vegetable	120	3	22
Desserts:			
Ice Cream, 2 scoops	295	16	33
Pies: Apple Pie, 1 slice	395	14	65
Blackberry Pie, 1 slice	430	14	72
Coconut Cream Pie, 1 slice	475	23	59
Dutch Apple Pie, 1 slice	405	16	65
Molten Lava Cake	210	7	35
Sundaes: Caramel, 2 scoops	475	19	73
Oreo	560	24	80

Edo Japan® (Sept '18)

Bento Box: Without Teriyaki Sauce	C	F	Cb
Beef Yakisoba, 20.3 oz	840	29	102
Chicken Yakisoba, 20.5 oz	790	24	102
Sizzling Shrimp, 22 oz	790	15	122
Sukiyaki Beef, 20.3 oz	880	27	120
Teriyaki: Without Teriyaki Sauce			
Beef & Shrimp, 17 oz	660	18	82
Sukiyaki Beef, 14.8 oz	580	15	80
Soup: Per 33 oz Bowl			
Beef Udon	580	17	72
Chicken Udon	550	13	72
Maki Sushi: Per 6 Pieces			
California Roll, 7.6 oz	430	17	61
Spicy Tuna Roll, 6.5 oz	300	2.5	54
Nigiri Sushi: Per 1 Piece			
Ebi (Steamed Prawn), 1.7 oz	70	0.5	12
Salmon Sashimi, 0.7 oz	30	1.5	1

Einstein Bros® (Sept '18)

Bagels:	C	F	Cb
Bagels: Asiago Cheese	300	4	54
Blueberry	290	1	59
Chocolate Chip	300	3.5	58
Cinnamon Sugar	320	6	59
Garlic	280	2	57
Honey Whole Wheat	260	3	49
Onion	270	1.5	55
Potato	280	4	52
Sesame	290	2.5	56
Gourmet Bagels:			
Apple Cinnamon	450	9	83
Green Chile	390	12	54
Power Protein	350	6	64
Six-Cheese	370	10	53
Spinach Florentine	370	12	53
Bagel Dogs:			
Original	530	26	57
Asiago	580	29	57
Egg Sandwiches: 1 Egg Classic on Plain Bagel			
Applewood Bacon & Spinach	470	16	55
Cheddar Cheese	410	11	57
Ham & Swiss	450	12	57
Turkey Sausage & Cheddar	470	17	56
Signature Egg Sandwiches: 2 Eggs			
Bacon & Spin. on Spin. Florentine	810	49	57
Chorizo Sunrise	920	57	62
Farmhouse	790	38	65
French Toast Egg	780	36	78
Santa Fe	640	28	61
Salads: Without Dressing			
Chicken Caesar	210	6	18
Strawberry Chicken	220	6	24
Tostinis: BBQ Chicken	530	12	68
Buffalo Chicken & Bacon	620	22	60
Italian Chicken	680	31	62
Roasted Veggie	500	20	63
Turkey Club	690	32	62
Wraps: Santa Fe	710	39	60
Turkey Club Mex	740	42	57
Cream Cheese: Per 1.2 oz Schmear			
Reduced Fat:			
Garlic Herb/Garden Veggie	110	9	5
Honey Almond; Strawberry, av.	120	8	10
Plain	120	12	2
Onion and Chive	120	10	4
Smoked Salmon	110	10	4
Sweets: Blueberry Muffin, 4 oz	420	20	57
Cinnamon Twist, 3.4 oz	360	16	50
Snickerdoodle Cookie, 2.9 oz	420	20	59

El Pollo Loco® (Sept '18)

Starters: Per Small Serving	C	F	Cb
Chicken Tortilla w/ Tortilla Strips	210	9	19
without Tortilla Strips	140	5	10
Bowl: Original Pollo, 18.1 oz	610	10	87
Double Chicken, 24.7 oz	930	30	93
Burritos:			
Chicken Avocado, 17.9 oz	950	53	74
Chicken Fajita, 17.1oz	870	38	84
Chipotle Chicken Avocado	920	41	89
Ranchero Chicken	930	45	86
Flame-Grilled Chicken: Skin On			
Breast; Thigh, av.	220	12	0
Leg; Wing, av.	90	4.5	0
Stuffed Quesadillas:			
Chicken Avocado	960	61	59
Chicken Fajita Avocado	910	54	63
Salads: Without Dressing			
Classic Chicken	240	8	19
Mexican Chicken Cobb	520	25	38
Tacos:			
Crunchy Chicken, 4.6 oz	230	11	19
Grande: Avocado & Chicken, 6.4 oz	340	20	20
Avocado Shrimp, 6.2 oz	320	18	20
Taco al Carbon: Chicken, 3.2 oz	160	6	18
Shrimp, 3 oz	160	7	17
Tostada Salads: With Shell, without Dressing			
Chicken,17.3 oz	860	42	77
Double Chicken, 21.6 oz	1030	50	82
Under 500 Calories: Without Dressing			
Black Bean Bowl, Chicken, 18.7 oz	480	12	57
Chicken Avocado Tortilla Wrap	480	20	46
Double Chicken Avocado Salad	380	15	15
Dressings: Creamy Cilantro: 3 oz	320	35	2
Light Creamy Cilantro, 1.5 oz	70	5	5
Ranch, 1.5 oz	230	24	2
Sides: Black Beans, 6 oz	140	1	24
Cole Slaw, 4 oz	130	10	9
Cut Corn with Red Peppers, 5 oz	160	5	24
Gravy, 1 oz	10	0	2
Macaroni & Cheese, 6 oz	310	19	24
Mashed Potatoes, 5 oz	110	1.5	23
Pinto Beans, 6 oz	200	4	29
Condiments:			
Pico de Gallo, 1.5 oz	15	1	2
Salsa: Avocado, 1.5 oz	30	2.5	2
House; Roja, av.,1.5 oz	10	0	2
Sour Cream, 1.3 oz	80	7	1
Dessert, Two Cinnamon Churros	320	22	30

Fatburger® (Sept '18)

Burgers: Without Extras	C	F	Cb
Burgers: Small	400	21	37
Medium	590	31	46
Large	850	41	69
Turkeyburger	480	21	50
Veggieburger	510	20	60
Hot Dogs: Without Extras			
Chili Cheese	480	27	35
Regular Hot Dog	320	15	32
Sandwiches: Without Extras			
Chicken: Crispy	560	27	53
Grilled	430	14	42
Fish	560	31	55
Fries: Fat Fries	380	18	47
with Chili	480	24	52
with Chili & Cheese	590	33	53
Skinny Fries	390	15	58
with Chili Cheese	600	30	64
Add-Ons: American Cheese, 1 slice	70	5	1
Cheddar Cheese, 1 slice	110	9	1
Mayonnaise, 1 serving	90	10	1
Relish, 1 serving	20	0	5
Sides: Chili Cup	200	11	10
with Cheese & Onions	320	20	12
Onion Rings	540	29	64
Shakes: Chocolate	910	45	115
Cookies & Ice Cream	1180	59	163
Maui-Banana	940	44	126
Peanut Butter	950	53	114
Strawberry; Vanilla, average	885	44	112

For Complete Nutritional Data ~ see CalorieKing.com

Fazoli's® (Sept '18)

Oven-Baked Pasta: Per Serving	C	F	Cb
Baked Ziti	570	19	71
Chicken Broccoli Penne	800	35	74
Chicken Parmigano	690	21	91
Penne Romano	750	37	72
Penne with Creamy Basil Chicken	840	43	70
Spicy Sausage Penne	740	37	72
Classic Pastas: Chicken Fett. Alfredo	810	25	107
Fettuccine Alfredo	690	22	104
Spagh. with Marinara	510	3.5	108
Spaghetti with Meatballs	470	14	70

Continued Next Page....

Fazoli's® cont... (Sept '18)

Samplers: Per Serving	C	F	Cb
Classic Sampler	820	25	120
Spicy Sampler	1110	42	129
Ultimate Sampler Platter	1050	30	163
Signature Pasta:			
Chicken Carbonara	80	29	112
Three Cheese Tortellini Alfredo	840	34	78
Ultimate Pasta: Fettuccine	900	33	110
Spaghetti	920	37	116
Submarinos:			
Meatball da Vinci	920	56	65
Primo Italiano	840	45	60
Turkey Club Classico	720	34	56

For Complete Nutritional Data ~ see CalorieKing.com

Firehouse Subs® (Sept '18)

Hot Subs: Per Medium White Sub, Standard Toppings and Dressings	C	F	Cb
Ham	760	38	69
Roast Beef	740	37	53
Turkey	680	35	58
Veggie	720	45	60
Specialty: Club on a Sub	770	40	63
Engineer	690	35	59
Hero	800	38	63
Hook & Ladder	720	36	62
Italian	940	58	65
Meatball	840	50	61
Sides, Chili, Bowl	300	16	26

Under 500 Calorie Salads:

Canadian Chopped: With Light Italian Dressing			
with Grilled Chicken	410	24	18
with Honey Ham	460	26	29
Firehouse Chopped: Without Dressing			
with Grilled Chicken	260	8	15
with Ham	310	10	27
with Turkey	220	7	15
Italian, w/ Grilled Chkn, w/o drssng	380	21	14

Five Guys® (Sept '18)

Burgers: Without Toppings or Sauce	C	F	Cb
Bacon Burger	920	50	39
Cheeseburger	980	55	40
Hamburger	840	43	39
Little Burgers: Bacon Burger	620	33	39
Bacon Cheeseburger	690	39	40
Hamburger	540	26	39

Five Guys® cont... (Sept '18)

Burger Sauces & Toppings:	C	F	Cb
Sauce: A.1	15	0	3
BBQ Sauce	50	0	15
Ketchup; Relish, average	20	0	5
Mayo	110	11	0
Toppings: Lettuce & Tomato	11	0	3
Cheese, 1 slice	70	8	0.5
Grilled Onions	10	0	2
Grilled Mushrooms	20	0	4
Hot Dogs: Bacon	600	42	40
Cheese	590	41	41
Sandwich, BLT	600	34	42
Fries, medium, 14.5 oz	955	41	131

Flame Broiler® (Sept '18)

Bowls: With White Rice	C	F	Cb
Beef	620	11	74
Chicken	600	14	68
Chicken & Veggie	510	14	49
Half & Half	610	13	71
The Works	520	13	52
Plates: With White Rice			
Beef	840	18	94
Rib	1100	44	95
The Works	700	19	63

Freshens® (Sept '18)

Smoothies: 100% Juice	C	F	Cb
Blended Fruit Classics: Per 20 fl.oz			
Bangin' Berry	370	0	90
Caribbean Craze; Maui Mango	330	0	81
Jamaican Jammer; Or. Sunrise	320	2	70
Peach On The Beach	280	3	61
Purple Reign	320	0	79
Tropical Therapy	480	6	109
Wild Strawberry	340	0	87
Peanut Butter Protein	500	12	76
Crepes: Buffalo Chicken	410	22	25
Chicken Caesar	600	44	25
Chipotle Ranch Turkey Melt	520	31	25
Denver, with Bacon	520	29	27
Honey Mustard Chicken	460	22	36
Pesto Chicken	490	29	27
Southwest Chicken	580	33	36
Rice Bowls: Buffalo Chicken	600	22	69
Florence	450	12	62
KC BBQ	590	11	90
Mexican	710	29	83
Power Protein	670	27	70
Spicy Korean	520	8	89
Salad: Buffalo Chicken	480	27	29
Grilled Chicken Caesar	520	37	26
Roadhouse BBQ Chicken	420	17	42
Strawberry & Kale	490	15	56

Godfather's Pizza® (Sept '18)

Golden Crust Pizza: Per Slice	C	F	Cb
Cheese: Medium, 1/8 pizza	210	8	25
Large, 1/10 pizza	230	10	27
Combo: Medium, 1/8 pizza	280	13	27
Large, 1/10 pizza	310	15	29
Super Combo: Medium, 1/8 pizza	310	16	27
Large, 1/10 pizza	360	18	30
Mozza-Loaded:			
All Meat Combo: Medium, 1/8 pizza	360	19	28
Large, 1/10 pizza	400	22	31
Original Crust Pizza:			
BLT: Mini, 1/4 pizza	220	11	19
Medium, 1/8 pizza	370	18	32
Jumbo, 1/12 pizza	500	25	42
Buffalo Chicken: Mini, 1/4 pizza	170	7	18
Medium, 1/8 pizza	270	9	32
Jumbo, 1/12 pizza	380	14	41
Super Taco Pie: Mini, 1/4 pizza	220	10	22
Medium, 1/8 pizza	370	17	36
Jumbo, 1/12 pizza	450	20	46
Thin Crust Pizza:			
BBQ Chicken: Medium, 1/8 pizza	210	9	21
Large, 1/10 pizza	240	11	23
Pepperoni: Medium, 1/8 pizza	210	10	21
Large, 1/10 pizza	270	16	18
The Don: Medium, 1/8 pizza	280	17	16
Large, 1/10 pizza	350	19	25
Sides:			
Breadstick, Golden, av., 1 oz	80	3	11
Cheesestick, average, 1.2 oz	100	5	11
Chicken Wings: Bone-In, Buff., 3 oz	190	14	2
Breaded Hot Wing, full order, 8 oz	920	54	38
Garlic Bread: 1 piece	160	9	17
with Cheese, 1 piece	200	12	17
Potato Wedges, 3 oz	140	7	18

Gold Star Chili® (Sept '18)

Burritos & Burrito Bowls:	C	F	Cb
Chili Burrito	840	42	81
Grilled Chicken Bowl	510	33	30
Coneys: Cheese	300	18	21
Plain	210	11	21
Mustard & Onion	230	11	23
Ways, Oringinal Chili:			
Regular: 2-Way	410	12	56
3-Way	760	41	56
4-Way	830	41	70
5-Way	850	41	74
Super, 5-Way	1160	53	111
Chili Bowls, Original:			
Plain, 8 oz	200	11	12
Beans & Onions, 8 oz	290	12	30

Gold Star Chili® cont...(Sept '18)

Double Deckers: With White Bread	C	F	Cb
Ham & Bacon	1080	80	46
Ham & Turkey	760	46	46
Turkey & Bacon	1070	78	46
Salads: Full Salad, without Dressing			
BBQ Chicken	490	24	36
Harvest Chicken	340	16	25
Fries: French, regular	460	19	67
Cheese	810	48	68
Chili Cheese	840	51	64
Garlic Parmesan	870	62	71
Vegetarian Chili	540	24	71

Golden Corral® (Sept '18)

Breakfast:	C	F	Cb
Corned Beef Hash, 1/2 cup	230	15	14
Hash Brown Casserole, 1/2 cup	100	3.5	14
Sausage & Egg Burrito	320	19	22
Scrambled Eggs, 1/2 cup	180	14	2
Hot Buffet: Without Sides			
Beef: Pot Roast, 1/2 cup	160	7	8
Roast, flat, 3 oz	180	10	1
Smoked Beef Short Ribs, 3 oz	180	10	1
Steak, Smothered Chopped, 5.9 oz	290	18	4
Chicken: Breast, Grilled, 2 oz	90	2.5	0
Fried Chicken, 3 oz	240	15	6
Orange Chicken, 6 oz	390	5	40
Smoked White Meat Chicken, 3 oz	150	6	0
Fish: Baked, 3 oz	150	8	1
Fried Catfish, 3 oz	180	10	12
Pork: Chops, Southern Style, 3 oz	230	16	8
Sweet & Sour, 6 oz	220	11	18
Sides: BBQ Baked Beans, 1/2 cup	160	1	35
Fried Okra (10)	110	7	10
Creamed Spinach, 1/2 cup	170	12	10
Fried Cubed Potatoes, 1/2 cup	160	9	19
Red Bliss Potatoes, 1/2 cup	80	2	13
Salad Buffet: Per 1/2 Cup Unless Indicated			
Caesar, without dressing, 1 cup	110	8	8
Chicken	250	22	3
Coleslaw	110	9	6
Potato	150	5	26
Seafood	140	10	9
Spinach, 1 cup	15	0	2
Tuna	190	12	4
Dressings: Balsamic Vinaig., 2 Tbsp	15	0	3
Caesar, 2 Tbsp	150	15	2
Ranch, 2 Tbsp	110	12	2

Updated Nutrition Data ~ www.CalorieKing.com
Persons with Diabetes ~ See Disclaimer (Page 22)

Fast - Foods & *Restaurants*

Great American Bagel Co® (Sept '18)

Bagels:

	C	F	Cb
Asiago Cheese	520	16	72
Cheddar Herb	390	8	66
Cinnamon Raisin	380	3.5	76
Jalapeno Cheddar	370	7	63
Plain	360	4	71
Spinach Tomazzo	640	20	86
Tomazzo	520	13	77

Paninis: *On Regular Baguette*

Chicken Pesto	770	35	70
Ham & Swiss	600	26	58
Philly Beef	920	40	92
Turkey Club	680	29	67

Sandwiches: *Asiago Omelet*

	720	29	80
BLT	550	17	72
Chicken Parmigiana	740	22	81
Ham	460	9	71
Roast Beef	465	9	71
Turkey	435	5	72

Cream Cheese Filling: *Per 1 oz*

Plain	100	10	1
Strawberry; Vegetable, average	90	8	4

Pastries:

Cookies: Chocolate Chunk, 4 oz	110	3.5	19
Oatmeal Raisin, 4 oz	120	5	18
Muffins: Banana Nut, 4.25 oz	430	18	61
Blueberry, 4.25 oz	430	16	64

Green Burrito® (Sept '18)

Burritos:

	C	F	Cb
Bean & Cheese	660	25	76
Green: Chicken	930	38	96
Steak	940	38	96
Grilled, Beef; Chicken; Steak, av.	840	33	89

Specialties:

Quesadillas: Cheese	640	34	53
Chicken	780	40	56
Steak	790	39	56
Rice, Bean & Chips Platter	340	10	51
Super Nachos, average	735	44	53
Taco Salad, Chicken; Steak	875	53	60

Tacos:

Crunchy Beef Taco	210	12	16
Soft Chicken Taco	250	12	18
Sides: Chips, 2 oz	300	17	35
Cilantro lim Rice, 3.4 oz	90	5	21
Guacamole, 2.7 oz	100	8	5
Pinto Beans, 3.7 oz	90	1.5	13

(The) Great Steak® (Sept '18)

Breakfast Sandwiches:

	C	F	Cb
Bacon, Egg & Cheese	550	31	38
Sausage, Egg & Cheese	660	42	38
Steak, Egg & Chse	540	27	38

Burgers:

Bacon Cheeseburger	1050	72	45
Cheeseburger	840	54	45
Hamburger	730	46	44
Philly Cheeseburger	780	48	44

Sandwiches: *Regular Sie*

Bacon Cheddar Cheesesteak	590	23	55
Buffalo Chicken Philly	750	38	61
Chicagoland Cheesesteak	610	24	59
Chicken Bacon Ranch	820	44	60
Great Steak Cheesesteak	790	45	55
Ham Delight	780	44	64
Orig. Philly Cheesesteak	510	17	55
Pastrami Philly	800	46	57
Reuben Philly	710	37	56
Super Steak Cheesesteak	800	45	57
Turkey Philly	750	42	57
Ultimate Chicken Philly	800	44	60
Veggie Delight	490	19	61
Wisconsin Inside-Out	530	26	50

Baked Potatoes:

Bacon & Cheese	440	23	36
Broccoli & Cheese	250	6	45
The Great Potato: Chicken	460	19	49
Ham	450	19	52
Steak	470	20	46
Turkey	430	17	48
The King	540	32	38

Fries:

Bacon Ranch: Regular	650	42	51
Large	1520	91	139
Great Fry: Kids	270	13	36
Regular	370	18	48
Large	930	40	132
King Fry, regular	480	27	52

Salads: *Without Dressing*

Great Salad: Chicken	370	22	16
Ham	360	22	19
Steak	390	23	17
Turkey	350	20	19
Salad Dressings: Mayo, reg., 1 oz	200	22	0
Ranch, 1 oz	150	16	2
Thousand Island, 1 oz	130	12	4
Sauce: BBQ, 1 oz	50	0	12
Buffalo, 1 oz	10	0	1
Honey Mustard, 1 oz	40	1	7
Teriyaki, 1 oz	25	0	3

203

Haagen-Dazs® (Sept '18)

Classic Flavors: Per 1/2 Cup

	C	F	Cb
Banana Peanut Butter Crisp	340	23	25
Belgian Chocolate	330	21	30
Brownies a La Mode	280	16	28
Butter Pecan	300	22	20
Caramel Cone	320	20	28
Cherry Vanilla	290	17	29
Choc. Chip Cookie Dough	290	17	30
Chocolate Chocolate Chip	300	19	26
Chocolate Peanut Butter	330	22	25
Coffee; Green Tea	250	17	20
Cookies and Cream	250	16	22
Dulce de Leche	270	16	28
Espresso Chocolate Cookie Crumble	310	21	25
Honey Salted Caramel Almond	290	18	26
Mint Chip	280	18	25
Pineapple Coconut	230	13	25
Rocky Road	290	17	29
Rum Raisin	250	16	22
Sea Salt Caramel Truffle	300	17	32
Strawberry	240	15	22
Vanilla Bean	270	17	25
Vanilla Swiss Almond	290	19	24
Vanilla Tangerine & Shortbread	290	18	26
White Chocolate Raspberry Truffle	280	16	31
Gelato, Sea Salt Caramel, 1/2 cup	250	17	20

Sorbet: Per 1/2 Cup

	C	F	Cb
Mango	150	0	38
Orchard Peach	140	0	34
Raspberry; Zesty Lemon, average	115	0	29

Ice Cream Bars/Cones ~ See Page 109

Hardee's® (Sept '18)

Burgers:

	C	F	Cb
All Natural Grass Fed, 11 oz	780	49	56
Cheeseburgers: 1/4 lb	440	23	37
1/3 lb	640	33	56
2/3 lb	970	59	57
Double, 5.7 oz	380	19	33
Small, 4.5 oz	300	13	33
Hamburger, Small, 4.2 oz	250	9	32
Thickburgers: 1/4 lb	530	35	34
Original: 1/3 lb	780	48	56
2/3 lb	1100	73	57
Bacon Cheese: 1/3 lb	850	54	54
2/3 lb	1170	79	55
Double, 2/3 lb	1130	77	58
Frisco: 1/3 lb	840	55	46
2/3 lb	1150	80	47
Mushroom 'N' Swiss:			
1/3 lb	680	38	53
2/3 lb	1000	63	54

Hardee's® cont... (Sept '18)

Sandwiches:

	C	F	Cb
Chicken: Big Chicken Fillet, 11 oz	710	36	64
Charbroiled: BBQ, 7.8 oz	350	6	46
Chicken Club	560	28	38
Spicy Chicken	440	23	44
Hot Ham 'N' Cheese: Regular	290	11	29
Big	530	20	51
Roast Beef: Regular	310	14	28
Big	500	23	48

Chicken Tenders: Without Sauce

Hand Breaded:

	C	F	Cb
3 pieces, 4.5 oz	260	13	13
5 pieces, 7.5 oz	440	21	21
Chili Dog, Jumbo	390	26	23

Fried Chicken Pieces:

	C	F	Cb
Breast, 5.2 oz	370	15	29
Leg, 2.4 oz	170	7	15
Thigh, 4.3 oz	330	15	30
Wing, 2.3 oz	200	8	23

Sides:

	C	F	Cb
Beer Battered Onion Rings	410	24	45
Coleslaw, 4 oz	270	22	17
Crispy Curls:			
Small, 4.1 oz	360	18	46
Medium, 5.36 oz	470	23	60
Large, 6.5 oz	570	28	72
Green Beans, 4.7 oz	40	1.5	5
Mashed Potatoes & Gravy, 5 oz	90	1	17
Side Salad, w/out Dressing, 6.7 oz	120	7	7

Fries & Onion Rings:

	C	F	Cb
Beer Battered Onion Rings, 4.5 oz	410	24	45
Natural Cut Fries:			
Kid's, 3 oz	240	12	31
Small, 3.7 oz	300	15	47
Medium, 5.9 oz	490	24	63
Large, 6.5 oz	530	26	69

Kids Meals: Includes Kid's Fries, w/out Drink

	C	F	Cb
Cheeseburger	520	23	62
Chicken Tenders	400	19	37
Hamburger	470	20	61
Hotdog	570	34	50

Updated Nutrition Data ~ www.CalorieKing.com
Persons with Diabetes ~ See Disclaimer (Page 22)

Hardee's® cont... (Sept '18)

Better For You Options:

	C	F	Cb
Low Carb It: ⅓ lb Thickburger	440	35	9
Breakfast Bowl	660	52	10
Charbroiled Chicken Club S'wich	340	22	13
Trim It, Charbr. BBQ Chkn S'wich	190	3.5	24
Veg It: Egg & Cheese Biscuit	410	23	38
Thickburger, hold the Patty	550	33	58
Side Salad, without dressing	120	7	7

Breakfast:

Low Carb Bowl	660	52	10

Breakfast Burritos:

Loaded	580	30	46

Made From Scratch Biscuits:

Bacon, Egg & Cheese	610	38	46
Bacon, Swiss, Cheese & Egg	840	54	56
Biscuit 'N' Gravy	620	39	57
Chicken Fillet	650	41	53
Cinnamon 'N' Raisin	320	14	46
Country Ham	500	30	44
Country Fried Steak	640	42	52
Jelly	460	26	52
Loaded Omelet	620	39	57
Monster	880	61	48
Pork Chop 'N' Gravy	590	33	49
Smoked Sausage	620	43	44
Sausage and Egg	690	48	46
Smoked Sausage, Egg & Cheese	790	57	48
Platter: with Bacon	900	57	64
with Ham	880	43	75
with Sausage	1070	72	76
Sandwich, Frisco Breakfast	450	19	45
Sunrise Croissant	450	28	30

Breakfast Sides: Grits, 5 oz

	110	4.5	17
Hash Rounds: Small, 2.9 oz	260	15	23
Medium, 4.2 oz	370	22	33
Large, 5.8 oz	510	30	45

Desserts:

Apple Turnover, w/out Cinnamon Sugar	270	13	35
Chocolate Chip Cookie (2), 2 oz	240	10	36
Freshed Baked (1), 2 oz	290	15	35

Single Scoop Ice Cream:

Vanilla: Bowl, 4 oz	240	13	27
Sugar Cone, 4.4 oz	300	14	37

Ice Cream Shakes:

Choc.; Strawb., av., 14 oz	705	34	86
Vanilla, 14 oz	700	33	86

Hissho Sushi® (Sept '18)

Starters: With White Rice

	C	F	Cb
Chicken Gyoza, 4 oz	180	6	20
Pork Gyoza, 4 oz	230	11	23
Spring Rolls: Regular	185	4	30
Ocean	180	2	29
Squid Salad, 4 oz	95	2	7

Maki Rolls: With White Rice

Rolls: Blazing California, 7 oz	405	12	65
California, 7 oz	295	3	59
Dynamaite Roll, 7 oz	470	13	66
Eel, 7 oz	375	1	69
Hissho Healthy, 6 oz	210	1	46
Nippon Favorite, 6 oz	300	4	45
Philadelphia, 7 oz	385	12	60
Snow Crab, 7 oz	295	3	55
Spicy, 7 oz	430	11	62
Sushicado,7 oz	290	3	54
Veggie Roll, 7 oz	275	2	57

Specialty Rolls: Per 7 oz Roll Unless Indicated

Caterpillar	480	5	84
Living Color	370	5	51
Mango Tango	420	10	58
Salmon Lover	720	32	63
Sriracha Party	540	14	77
Tempura Shrimp, 9 oz	665	19	108
TNT	545	14	71
Wasabi Crunch	550	19	76

Hot Dog on a Stick® (Sept '18)

Menu Items:

	C	F	Cb
American Cheese on a Stick	260	16	20
Beef Hot Dog on a Bun	330	21	25
Turkey Hot Dog on a Stick	240	12	27
Veggie Dog on a Stick	200	6	26
Pepperjack Cheese on a Stick	260	15	22
French Fries: Small, 7.2 oz	500	29	57
Regular, 14.4 oz	1000	59	113

Beverages: Per Regular Size, 16 fl.oz

Lemonade: Original	150	0	38
Cherry	210	0	52
Lime	230	0	57

Hungry Howie's Pizza® (Sept '18)

Counts may vary in Florida.

	C	F	Cb
Specialty Pizza: *12" Pizza, Per ⅛ Slice*			
BBQ Chicken, Butter Crust	240	8	30
Buffalo Chicken, Ranch Crust	210	8	25
Works, Cajun Crust	310	16	26
Veggie, Ranch Crust	200	6	27
Subs: *Per Regular 8" Sub, with Set Menu Toppings*			
Italian	660	23	81
Ham & Cheese	590	15	68
Steak, Cheese & Mushroom	610	18	81
Turkey Club	660	18	80
Veggie	610	19	83
Wings, Boneless, Buffalo, 3 pieces	280	11	21
Salads: *Regular Size, without Dressing*			
Antipasto	360	22	17
Chef	310	18	17
Garden	130	2.5	23
Greek	260	10	24
Dressings: *Per 1 oz*			
Creamy Italian	120	12	2
Greek	110	11	2
Ranch	140	14	1
Thousand Island	140	14	4

In-N-Out Burger® (Sept '18)

	C	F	Cb
Burgers:			
Hamburger: with Onion	390	19	39
w/ Mstrd & Ketchup, w/o Spread	310	10	41
Protein Style w/ Lettuce Wrap, without Bun	240	17	11
Cheeseburger: with Onion	480	27	39
w/ Mstrd & Ketchup, w/o Spread	400	18	41
Protein Style w/ Lettuce Wrap, without Bun	330	25	11
Double Double: with Onion	670	41	39
w/ Mstrd & Ketchup, w/o Spread	590	32	41
Protein Style w/ Lettuce Wrap, without Bun	520	39	11
French Fries, 4.5 oz	395	18	54
Drinks: Milk, 10 fl.oz	180	6	18
Coca-Cola, 16 fl.oz	195	0	54
Dr Pepper; 7-Up, av., 16 fl.oz	200	0	53
Lemonade, 16 fl.oz	180	0	40
Root Beer, 16 fl.oz	220	0	60
Shakes:			
Chocolate, 15 fl.oz	590	29	72
Strawberry, 15 fl.oz	590	27	81
Vanilla, 15 fl.oz	580	31	67

IHOP® (Sept '18)

	C	F	Cb
Pancakes:			
Belgian Chocolate (4)	1060	50	140
Double Blueberry (4)	620	17	102
NY Cheesecake (4)	920	35	130
Orig. Buttermilk (3)	430	17	57
Red Velvet (4)	680	17	117
Toppings: Glazed Strawberries	50	0	13
Peaches	60	0	14
Raspberry	70	0	18
Griddle Faves: *With Set Toppings*			
French Toast: Original	740	36	84
Bananas Foster Brioche	1000	49	123
Brioche, Plain	710	35	82
Strawberry Banana	850	31	121
Waffle, Belgian	590	30	69
Crepes: *With Set Toppings*			
Banana with Nutella	960	45	120
Chicken Florentine	900	53	48
German Crepes	680	34	76
Strawberries & Cream	780	32	105
Swedish	660	30	80
Omelettes: *Without Pancakes or Sides*			
Big Steak	1150	78	47
Chicken Fajita	960	63	24
Garden	830	66	16
Spicy Poblano	1100	83	31
Spinach & Mushroom	890	69	21
Combos: *With Two B'Milk Pancakes & Hash Browns*			
Country Fried Steak, w/ Ssg Gravy	1540	99	121
Sirloin Tips, w/ Gr. Onions & Mshrms	1030	123	87
Smokehouse, with 2 Poached Eggs	1200	84	70
T-Bone Steak (12 oz), w/ 3 Fried Eggs	1060	54	59
Burgers: *Without Sides*			
Bacon Cheeseburger	780	48	40
Cheeseburger Sliders	1100	67	73
Hamburger	620	37	39
Sandwiches: *Without Sides*			
Double BLT	670	42	42
Philly Cheese Steak Stacker	860	43	64
Roasted Turkey	850	43	59
Spicy Chicken Ranch	730	40	60
Sandwich Sides: French Fries	320	15	41
Hash Browns	280	18	28
Onion Rings	480	26	56
Entrees: *With Menu Set Sides, w/out Garlic Bread*			
Country Fried Steak & Country Gravy	1050	68	79
Pot Roast	850	44	66
Sirloin Steak Tips	760	105	70
Tilapia Florentine	680	42	34
55+ Lunch: *Without Soup or Salad*			
BLT Sandwich, on White Bread	410	25	29
Grilled Cheese S'wich, on Sourdough	720	38	63

For Complete Menu & Data ~ see CalorieKing.com

Updated Nutrition Data ~ www.CalorieKing.com
Persons with Diabetes ~ See Disclaimer (Page 22)

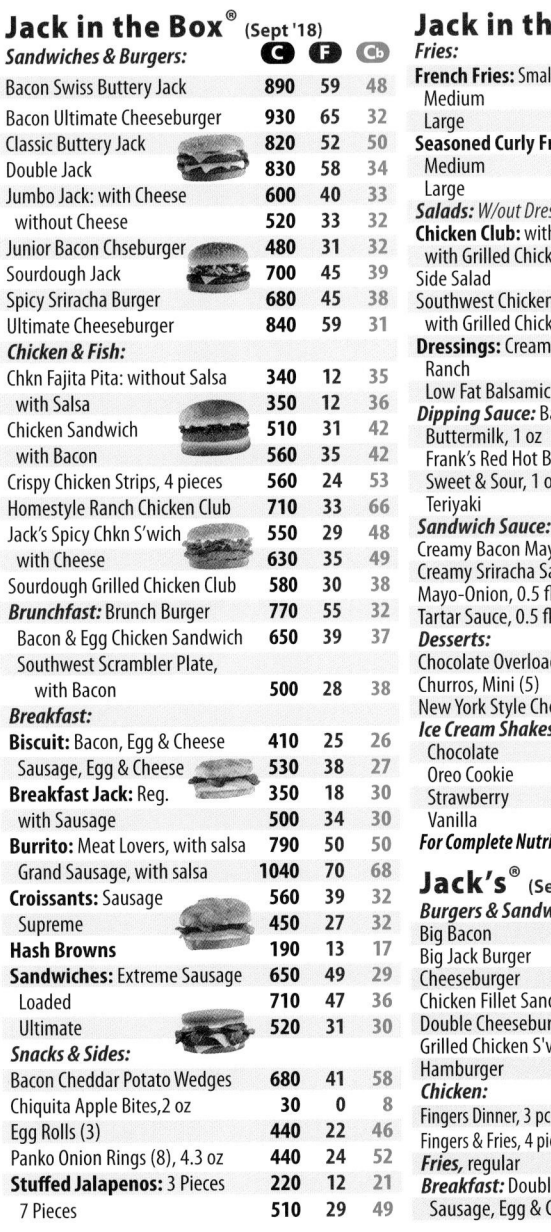

Jack in the Box® (Sept '18)

Sandwiches & Burgers:

	C	F	Cb
Bacon Swiss Buttery Jack	890	59	48
Bacon Ultimate Cheeseburger	930	65	32
Classic Buttery Jack	820	52	50
Double Jack	830	58	34
Jumbo Jack: with Cheese	600	40	33
without Cheese	520	33	32
Junior Bacon Chseburger	480	31	32
Sourdough Jack	700	45	39
Spicy Sriracha Burger	680	45	38
Ultimate Cheeseburger	840	59	31

Chicken & Fish:

	C	F	Cb
Chkn Fajita Pita: without Salsa	340	12	35
with Salsa	350	12	36
Chicken Sandwich	510	31	42
with Bacon	560	35	42
Crispy Chicken Strips, 4 pieces	560	24	53
Homestyle Ranch Chicken Club	710	33	66
Jack's Spicy Chkn S'wich	550	29	48
with Cheese	630	35	49
Sourdough Grilled Chicken Club	580	30	38
Brunchfast: Brunch Burger	770	55	32
Bacon & Egg Chicken Sandwich	650	39	37
Southwest Scrambler Plate,			
with Bacon	500	28	38

Breakfast:

	C	F	Cb
Biscuit: Bacon, Egg & Cheese	410	25	26
Sausage, Egg & Cheese	530	38	27
Breakfast Jack: Reg.	350	18	30
with Sausage	500	34	30
Burrito: Meat Lovers, with salsa	790	50	50
Grand Sausage, with salsa	1040	70	68
Croissants: Sausage	560	39	32
Supreme	450	27	32
Hash Browns	190	13	17
Sandwiches: Extreme Sausage	650	49	29
Loaded	710	47	36
Ultimate	520	31	30

Snacks & Sides:

	C	F	Cb
Bacon Cheddar Potato Wedges	680	41	58
Chiquita Apple Bites, 2 oz	30	0	8
Egg Rolls (3)	440	22	46
Panko Onion Rings (8), 4.3 oz	440	24	52
Stuffed Jalapenos: 3 Pieces	220	12	21
7 Pieces	510	29	49

Jack in the Box® cont... (Sept '18)

Fries:

	C	F	Cb
French Fries: Small	300	14	40
Medium	430	20	58
Large	550	25	75
Seasoned Curly Fries: Small	280	16	30
Medium	430	25	46
Large	480	28	52

Salads: W/out Dressing/Toppings

	C	F	Cb
Chicken Club: with Crispy Chicken	510	28	36
with Grilled Chicken	370	20	11
Side Salad	20	0	4
Southwest Chicken,			
with Grilled Chicken Strips	350	15	27
Dressings: Creamy Southwest	190	19	3
Ranch	250	25	5
Low Fat Balsamic Vinaigrette	25	1.5	3

Dipping Sauce: Barbecue, 1 oz

	C	F	Cb
Barbecue, 1 oz	40	0	10
Buttermilk, 1 oz	110	11	2
Frank's Red Hot Buffalo, 1 oz	10	0	1
Sweet & Sour, 1 oz	40	0	10
Teriyaki	50	1	11

Sandwich Sauce:

	C	F	Cb
Creamy Bacon Mayo, 0.7 fl.oz	120	13	1
Creamy Sriracha Sauce, 0.8fl.oz	120	13	1
Mayo-Onion, 0.5 fl.oz	90	10	0
Tartar Sauce, 0.5 fl.oz	50	4.5	2

Desserts:

	C	F	Cb
Chocolate Overload Cake	300	7	57
Churros, Mini (5)	350	18	42
New York Style Cheesecake	310	17	32

Ice Cream Shakes: 16 fl.oz, with Whipped Topping

	C	F	Cb
Chocolate	780	28	103
Oreo Cookie	800	43	95
Strawberry	760	38	97
Vanilla	680	38	78

For Complete Nutritional Data ~ see CalorieKing.com

Jack's® (Sept '18)

Burgers & Sandwiches:

	C	F	Cb
Big Bacon	800	57	36
Big Jack Burger	720	47	43
Cheeseburger	440	23	38
Chicken Fillet Sandwich	560	29	46
Double Cheeseburger	680	43	38
Grilled Chicken S'wich	410	17	35
Hamburger	400	19	38

Chicken:

	C	F	Cb
Fingers Dinner, 3 pce w/ Biscuit Only	950	56	82
Fingers & Fries, 4 piece	720	32	60
Fries, regular	260	16	27
Breakfast: Double Gravy Biscuit	950	58	90
Sausage, Egg & Cheese Biscuit	630	46	34

Fast - Foods & *Restaurants*

Jamba Juice® (Sept '18)

Freshly Squeezed Juice: 16 fl.oz	C	F	Cb
Orange Berry Antioxidant	200	1	48
Purely Carrot	130	0.5	30
Purely Orange	220	1	52
Tropical Kick-Start	210	1	50
Smoothies: Per Small			
Classic: Banana Berry	280	1	67
Mango-A-Go-Go	300	1.5	69
Peach Pleasure	280	1	65
Razzamatazz	290	1	67
Strawberry Surf Rider	320	1	78
Strawberries Wild	260	0	62
Fruit & Veggie: Apple 'n Greens	250	1	60
Berry UpBEET	240	1	52
Greens 'n Ginger	330	1	83
Protein: Chocolate	370	6	53
Cookies 'n Crème	480	15	59
PB & Banana	490	22	44
Super Blend:			
Apples 'N Charge	410	15	52
Green Up 'N Go	250	10	30
PB 'N Jealous	380	14	47
Tasty Bites:			
Artisan Flat Bread: *Per Flatbread*			
Four Cheese	330	13	37
Sweet 'n Spicy	330	11	38
Baked Goods: *Per Item*			
Apple Cinnamon Pretzel	380	4	76
Cheddar Tomato Twist	240	4.5	41
Sourdough Parmesan Pretzel	410	10	67
Sweet Belgian Waffle	320	15	42
Breakfast Wraps: Spinach 'n Chse	240	8	30
Turkey Sausage 'n Cheese	320	16	29
Steel-Cut Oatmeal: *With Soymilk*			
Plain	180	2.5	35
Add: Apple Cinnamon	70	0	16
Banana	50	0	13
Blueberries	10	0	2
Brown Sugar Crumble	40	1	8
Clover Honey	30	0	9
Strawberries	5	0	1
Toasted Bistro Sandwiches:			
Ham, Jarlsberg & Dijon	290	8	33
Roast Chicken, Cheddar & Honey Dijon	290	7	34
Three Cheeses	330	14	32
Energy Bowls: Per 16 fl.oz			
Acai Primo	490	10	99
Chunky Strawberry	590	17	96
Fruit & Greek Yogurt	390	4	62
Island Pitaya	470	8	100

Jersey Mike's Subs® (Sept '18)

Cold Subs: Per Regular, on White, without Vinegar, Oil or Mayo Unless Indicated	C	F	Cb
#1 BLT, with Mayo	780	48	67
#2 Jersey Shore Favorite	550	14	69
#3 American Classic	540	14	68
#5 Super Sub	570	15	70
#6 Roast Beef & Provolone	700	23	66
#7 Turkey Breast & Provolone	530	12	66
#8 Club Sub with Mayonnaise	860	45	69
#9 Club Supreme w/ Mayonnaise	930	48	68
#10 Albacore Tuna	800	43	70
#13 Original Italian	680	25	71
#14 Veggie	660	28	68
Hot Subs: Per Regular on White Roll			
#15 Meatball & Cheese	800	41	71
#17: Chicken Philly	700	23	69
Steak Philly	640	22	69
#18 Grilled Chicken Parmesan	620	18	64
#19 BBQ Beef	780	18	96
#20 Reuben	670	24	75
#42: Chipotle Chicken, with Mayo	990	53	72
#43: Chipotle Steak, with Mayo	920	52	71
#55: Big Kahuna Chkn	760	27	70
#56: Big Kahuna Steak	690	26	70
Signature Wraps: Flour/Spinach/Tomato Tortilla			
Baja	680	26	63
Buffalo Chicken	840	43	64
Caesar	650	28	57
Turkey Honey Mustard	560	20	63
Salads: Without Dressing			
Chef, 16 oz	250	10	16
Feta with Chicken, 16.7 oz	340	9	17
Gorgonzola, with Chicken, 17.8 oz	580	26	36
Mike's, 10.26 oz	60	0	13
Soup: Boston Clam Chowder, bowl	190	9	22
Cream of Broccoli, bowl	140	9	13
Vegetable, Beef & Barley, bowl	140	4.5	17
Wisconsin Cheese, bowl	340	24	24
Dressings: Per 2 Tbsp, 1 oz			
Caesar	150	15	2
Chipotle Mayo	180	20	0
Golden Italian	110	11	3
Ranch	120	12	2
Russian	160	16	4
Desserts: Choc Chip Cookie, 1.5 oz	190	9	26
Blondie Brownie, 4 oz	520	30	59
Drinks: Mountain Dew, 22 oz	310	0	84
Mug Root Beer, 22 oz	300	0	79
Tropicana Fruit Punch, 22 oz	310	0	77

Jimmy John's® (Sept '18)

Subs: (8") Figures Based on
French Bread w/ Standard Toppings & Mayo, Unless
Indicated

	C	F	Cb
#1 Pepe	625	30	59
#2 Big John	535	22	56
#3 Totally Tuna, without mayo	710	34	62
#4 Turkey Tom	505	20	57
#5 Vito with Italian Vinaigrette	655	31	60
#6 Vegetarian	695	40	61
JJBLT	615	31	56

Giant Club Sandwiches: Figures Based on French
Bread w/ Menu Set Ingredients

	C	F	Cb
#7 Smoked Ham Club	810	32	82
#8 Billy Club	830	33	79
#9 Italian Night	950	46	82
#10 Hunter's Club	850	35	77
#11 Country Club	800	31	80
#12 Beach Club	860	40	81
#13 Gourmet Veggie Club	1020	58	82
#14 Bootlegger	710	23	77
#15 Club Tuna w/o drssng	890	43	82
#16 Club Lulu	710	27	77
#17 Ultimate Porker	720	28	78

Plain Slims: Figures Based on French Bread without
Toppings, Dressing or Mayo

	C	F	Cb
Slim 1 Ham & Provolone Cheese	570	13	76
Slim 2 Roast Beef	480	6	73
Slim 3 Tuna Salad	660	23	75
Slim 4 Turkey Breast	450	3	74
Slim 5 Salami Capicola & Cheese	660	23	75
Slim 6 Double Provolone	610	21	75

Sides:

	C	F	Cb
Jimmy Chips: Average	150	9	16
Thinny, 1 oz	130	5	20
Cookies: Chocolate Chunk, 3 oz	410	19	56
Raisin Oatmeal, 3 oz	370	13	57
Jumbo Kosher Dill Pickle, 6.9 oz	20	0	4

Johnny Rockets® (Sept '18)

Starters:

	C	F	Cb
Fries: Regular	570	27	74
Bacon Cheese	830	44	82
Cheese	790	44	83
Chili Cheese	1050	65	90
Sweet Potato	590	31	75
Onion Rings	970	56	105
Sweet Potato	520	23	73

Johnny Rockets® cont... (Sept '18)

Original Hamburgers:

	C	F	Cb
Hamburger #12	740	46	48
Original Burger	670	40	49
Rocket: Single	680	40	46
Double	950	59	46
Route 66	760	48	47
Smoke House: Single	790	42	60
Double	1140	68	61
Streamliner	460	15	71
Chicken Tenders,BBQ Sauce	790	32	76
Chicken Philly Cheese Steak,			
with American Cheese	660	24	58
Hot Dogs: Rocket Dog	610	26	77
Rocket Chili Dog	830	53	56

Philly Cheese Steaks: *Without Substitutions*

	C	F	Cb
Beef	810	41	60
Chicken	730	27	59

Melts: *Standard, without substitutions*

	C	F	Cb
BBQ Chicken	1100	58	87
Patty Melt, ⅓ lb	850	47	60

Sandwiches: *Without Substitutions*

	C	F	Cb
BLT, on Sourdough	670	36	60
Chicken Club, on Sourdough	1050	51	91
Grilled Chicken, on Wheat Bun	610	30	47
Grilled Cheese, on Sourdough	740	42	63

Salads: *Without Dressing*

	C	F	Cb
Crispy Chicken Club	450	26	21
Grilled Chicken Club	420	23	10
Garden Salad	140	9	6

Breakfast: *Standard, without Subsititutions*

	C	F	Cb
Pancakes: B'milk (2) with Sausage	1090	71	93
B'milk (2), with Bacon	760	36	93
Scramblers: Bacon Denver	1210	91	50
Biscuits, Sausage & Gravy	1350	99	49
Country Sausage & Gravy	1530	121	59

Shakes:

	C	F	Cb
Banana; Strawberry, average	810	43	90
Butterfinger	960	52	107
Chocolate	900	44	112
P'nut Butter Banana	1170	71	107
Strawb. Oreo Crumble	970	50	114

For Complete Menu & Data ~ see CalorieKing.com

KFC® (Sept '18)

Chicken On The Bone: Per Piece	C	F	Cb
Original Recipe: Breast, 6 oz	390	21	11
Drumstick, 1.87 oz	130	8	4
Thigh, 3.7 oz	280	19	8
Whole Wing, 1.5 oz	130	8	3
Extra Crispy: Breast, 6.3 oz	530	35	18
Drumstick, 1.9 oz	170	12	5
Tenders, 1 order	140	7	8
Thigh, 3.5 oz	330	23	9
Whole Wing, 1.7 oz	170	13	5
Kentucky Grilled: Breast, 4.6 oz	210	7	0
Drumstick, 1.4 oz	80	4	0
Thigh, 2.5 oz	150	9	0
Whole Wing, 1 oz	70	3	0
Spicy Crispy: Breast, 5.2 oz	350	20	11
Drumstick, 1.6 oz	130	8	5
Thigh, 2.8 oz	270	20	10
Whole Wing, 1.2 oz	120	8	5
Go Cups: Chicken Littles	570	28	60
Exta Crispy Tenders	540	27	50
Fiery Buff. Hot Wings	480	25	49
HBBQ Hot Wings	540	25	61
Hot Wings	480	25	43
Popcorn Nuggets	570	32	53
Popcorn Nuggets: Kids	290	19	19
Large	620	39	49
Wings: Easch, without Dipping Sauce			
Fiery Buffalo, Hot	70	4	5
Honey BBQ, Hot	90	4	9
Hot	70	4	3
Dipping Sauces & Condiments: Per 0.9 oz Container			
Buttermilk Ranch Sauce	100	10	2
Colonel's Buttery Spread	35	4	0
Creamy Buffalo Sauce	70	7	2
Finger Linkin' Good; Honey Mstrd, av.	125	11	6
Honey Sauce	30	0	8
Ketcup	30	0	8
Lemon Juice	5	0	1
Strawberry Jam	35	0	9
Summertime BBQ Sauce	40	0	9
Sweet & Tangy Sauce	45	0	12
KFC Famous Bowls & Pot Pie:			
Chicken Pot Pie, 14 oz	720	41	60
Famous Bowl:			
Snack Size, 7 oz	270	13	27
Large	720	34	79
Sandwiches: Includes Mayo			
Chicken Littles	300	15	27
Crispy Twister	630	34	53
Georgia Gold	530	31	38
Nashville Hot	530	33	38

KFC® cont... (Sept '18)

Salads: W/out Dressing or Croutons	C	F	Cb
Caesar, Side	40	2	2
House Side Salad	15	0	3
Dressings & Add-Ins:			
Creamy Parmesan Caesar, 2 oz	260	26	4
Light Italian, 1 oz	15	0.5	2
Original Ranch Fat Free, 1.5 oz	35	0	8
Croutons, Parm. Garlic, 1 pouch	60	3	8
Homestyle Sides: Per Single Portion			
BBQ Baked Beans, 4.5 oz	240	1.5	43
Biscuit, 2 oz	180	8	22
Coleslaw, 4.2 oz	170	12	14
Corn on the Cob, 2.5 oz	70	0.5	17
Macaroni & Cheese, 4.8 oz	160	7	20
Mashed Potatoes, with Gravy, 5 oz	120	4	18
Potato Wedges, 3.8 oz	270	13	34
Sweet Kernel Corn	80	0.5	20
Desserts:			
Apple Turnover, 2.9 oz	230	10	32
Cafe Valley: Choc. Chip Cake, 1 slice	300	15	39
Mini Choc. Chip Cake (1)	300	12	49
Cafe Valley Lemon Cake, 1 slice	220	10	30
Chocolate Chip Cookie (1)	160	8	22
Oatmeal Raisin Cookie (1)	150	6	22
Oreo Cookies & Creme Pie	270	13	35
Reese's Peanut Butter Pie, 2.6 oz	300	17	33
Beverages:			
7-Up; Dr Pepper; Mug Root Beer, average			
12 fl.oz	140	0	35
16 fl.oz	190	0	46
20 fl.oz	240	0	58
Code Red Mountain Dew: 12 fl.oz	170	0	46
16 fl.oz	230	0	62
20 fl.oz	290	0	77
30 fl.oz	430	0	116
Dole: Classic Lemonade, 20 fl.oz	150	0	39
Strawberry Lemonade, 20 fl.oz	170	0	45
Mountain Dew: 12 fl.oz	160	0	44
16 fl.oz	220	0	59
20 fl.oz	270	0	73
30 fl.oz	410	0	110
Tropicana Fruit Punch: 12 fl.oz	170	0	45
16 fl.oz	230	0	60
20 fl.oz	280	0	75

Kilwins® ~ see CalorieKing.com

Kolache® ~ see CalorieKing.com

Updated Nutrition Data ~ www.CalorieKing.com
Persons with Diabetes ~ See Disclaimer (Page 22)

Krispy Kreme® (Sept '18)

Doughnuts:	C	F	Cb
Original Glazed:			
Regular	190	11	22
Mini size (3)	250	13	30
Apple Fritter	350	19	42
Chocolate Iced: Cake	340	19	40
Custard Filled	300	15	37
Glazed	240	11	33
with Sprinkles	250	11	36
Kreme Filling	350	19	41
Cinnamon Apple Filled	270	15	31
Cinnamon Bun	270	16	29
Cinnamon Sugar	190	11	21
Cruller: Glazed	240	15	25
Chocolate Iced Glazed	260	10	40
Double Dark Chocolate	370	20	46
Dulche De Leche	300	16	35
Glazed: with Kreme Filling	340	19	40
Lemon Filled	290	14	36
Maple Iced	240	11	34
Sour Cream Cake	300	15	40
Strawberry Iced	240	11	33
Powdered Cake	310	19	32
Powdered Strawberry Filled	270	15	30
Powdered Lemon Kreme	290	17	32
Doughnut Holes:			
Glazed Blueberry Cake (4)	180	7	28
Original Glazed (5)	210	12	25
Hot: Chocolate, w/ 2% Milk, 12 oz	390	14	57
Mocha Latte, w/ Skim Milk, 12 oz	260	4.5	42
Frozen Coffees: *With Whipped Cream*			
Caramel, 12 fl.oz	350	11	58
Mocha, 12 fl.oz	330	11	52
Vanilla Latte, 12 fl.oz	330	10	54
Frozen Lemonade, 12 fl.oz	200	0	52
Iced Lattes: *Per 12 fl.oz with Skim Milk*			
Caramel Latte, with wh. cream	310	8	52
Hazelnut	160	0	32
Iced Mocha, skim milk, 12 fl.oz	250	7	38
Skinny Iced Lattes: *With Skim Milk*			
Caramel, 12 fl.oz	160	1.5	29
Vanilla, 12 fl.oz	70	0	12

For Complete Menu & Data ~ See CalorieKing.com

Krystal® (Sept '18)

Krystals:	C	F	Cb
Original	130	6	15
Angus Bacon & Cheese	450	23	40
Bacon Cheese; Double	190	10	16
Cheese	150	8	15
Triple	240	15	16
Chik, regular	280	16	23
Pups: Chili Cheese Pup	230	14	16
Corn	250	17	18
Regular	160	9	21
Fries:			
French Fries: Small	140	9	14
Medium	240	15	24
Large	300	19	30
Loaded: Chili Cheese Fries	670	47	40
Junk Yard	800	59	42
Wings: Bone in (12)	1170	90	36
Boneless: with Buffalo Sauce (12)	970	49	70
with BBQ Sauce (12)	1080	47	103
Breakfast:			
Plates: *With Three Eggs*			
Bacon & Biscuit	480	30	29
Bacon & Toast	330	19	16
Sausage & Biscuit	520	36	28
Sausage & Toast	370	24	16
Sandwiches: Bacon on Toast	300	13	30
Krystal Sunrisers (2)	420	32	15
Sausage on Toast	340	19	29
Sausage Gravy Biscuit	370	21	41
Scramblers:			
Original: with Bacon	300	19	17
with Sausage	340	24	16
Low-Carb Scrambler,			
with Sausage	360	34	2
Sides: Grits, bowl	210	5	36
Kryspers (5)	240	18	21
Dessert, Apple Turnover	290	18	31
Coca-Cola:			
Small	190	0	52
Medium	230	0	65
Large	350	0	98
Hand-Spun Shakes: *Regular*			
Chocolate	650	18	114
Strawberry	560	17	92
Vanilla	510	17	80
Sundaes: Choc.; Strawb., av.	310	8	57
Oreo	350	13	54

For Complete Menu & Data ~ see CalorieKing.com

LaRosa's Pizzeria® (Sept '18)

	C	**F**	**Cb**
Classic Pizzas:			
Hand Tossed: *Per Slice, 1/8 of 12" Medium Pizza*			
Chicken Bacon Ranch	340	17	30
Double Pepperoni	290	13	30
Garlic Chicken	280	12	30
Hawaiian	290	11	33
Zesty BBQ Chicken	290	10	35
Traditional: *Per Slice, 1/12 of 14" Large Pizza*			
Chicken Bacon Ranch	290	18	19
Double Pepperoni	240	13	19
Hawaiian	240	12	22
Zesty BBQ Chicken	240	11	24
Deluxe Pizzas:			
Hand Tossed: *Per Slice, 1/8 of 14" Large Pizza*			
Buddy Deluxe	510	25	47
Meat Deluxe	580	30	47
Original Deluxe	490	23	47
Veggie Deluxe	360	11	49
Pan: *Per Slice, 1/8 of 14" Large Pizza*			
Buddy Deluxe	520	27	47
Meat Deluxe	590	32	47
Original Deluxe	510	25	47
Veggie Deluxe	370	13	49
Specialty Calzones: Standard Toppings, w/out Sauce			
Philly Chicken	820	26	108
Philly Cheese Steak	870	33	106
Three Meat	1070	52	106
Pasta Dinner: Without Bread, Soup or Salad			
Lasagna, with Meat Sauce	1100	63	83
Ravioli: Cheese, with Pasta Sauce	750	29	89
Meat, with Pasta Sauce	730	26	89
Ziti: Chicken Alfredo	1180	57	121
Sausage Pelucci w/ Spag. Sce	1040	42	136
Fresh Salad: Without Dressing or Breadstick			
Antipasto For One	420	30	14
Crispy Chicken	500	27	36
Grilled Chicken	290	12	15
JoJo BLT	150	9	9
Tossed Garden Salad	160	9	12
Tuna Plate	420	27	16
Salad Dressings: Per 2 oz Cup			
Bleu Cheese	280	30	2
Honey French	250	19	18
Italian	320	34	4
Soup: With 2 Packets Saltine Crackers			
Baked Onion	230	10	27
Minestrone	140	4	24

LaRosa's Pizzeria® cont... (Sept '18)

	C	**F**	**Cb**
Appetizers:			
Cheesy Flatbread, w/ Pizza Sauce	1470	89	116
Fried Mozz. Chse Stick (5), Pizza Sce	630	35	46
Garlic Fries, w/ Ranch Dressing	900	62	77
Onion Twists, w/ Diablo Sauce	1110	72	107
Rondo: Pepperoni, w/ Pizza Sauce	1260	67	115
Spinach, with Pizza Sauce	1215	67	107
Wings, with Sauce: BBQ (5)	440	35	12
Diablo (5)	510	43	9
Garlic-Romano (5)	640	60	2

La Salsa Fresh Mexican® (Sept '18)

	C	**F**	**Cb**
Breakfast:			
Burritos: Chicken	660	30	56
Steak	700	36	55
Huevos Ranchero Platter: Chicken	500	14	59
Chorizo	610	27	61
Steak	550	20	58
Taco	200	10	14
Burritos: Without Chips			
Black Beans & Cheese:	720	37	62
with Carnitas	820	41	62
with Grilled Chicken	810	40	63
California Steak, w/ Black Beans	830	39	81
Grande, Black Beans,			
with Carnitas/Chicken/Steak, av.	760	30	79
Pinto Beans & Cheese: Plain	810	37	79
with Chicken	910	40	80
with Steak	970	49	80
Overstuffed Burrito:			
with Carnitas	860	35	56
with Grilled Chicken	860	32	59
with Steak	980	49	58
Platters:			
Enchiladas:			
Pinto Beans: Carnitas; Chicken, av.	985	53	59
Cheese	850	49	58
Steak	1070	63	59
Three Pepper Fajita Flour Tortilla:			
Black Beans: Carnitas	700	29	55
Chicken	690	27	58
Steak	820	44	57
Taquitos & Quesadillas:			
Pinto Beans: Carnitas; Chicken, av.	1600	76	134
Cheese	1470	72	129
Steak	1660	84	134
Tacos: Without Chips			
Baja Grilled Fish	260	12	23
Baja Shrimp	250	9	23
Guadalajara Carnitas	300	17	22

Updated Nutrition Data ~ www.CalorieKing.com
Persons with Diabetes ~ See Disclaimer (Page 22)

La Salsa® cont... (Sept '18)

Favorites: Without Chips

	C	F	Cb
Classic Quesadillas: Carnitas	980	58	59
Cheese	880	54	59
Chicken	980	57	60
Steak	1040	65	60
Fire Roasted Bowls:			
Black Beans: Carnitas	510	18	54
Chicken	500	16	55
Steak	570	25	55
Nachos:			
Black Beans: with Carnitas	1150	56	93
with Chicken	1150	54	95
with Steak	1210	63	94
Pinto Beans:			
with Carnitas	1190	56	101
with Chicken	1170	54	98
with Steak	1230	63	98
Stuffed Fajitas: Carnitas	930	49	59
Cheese	830	45	59
Chicken	930	48	60
Steak	990	57	60

Little Caesars® (Sept '18)

14" Pizza: Per Slice, 1/8 Pizza

	C	F	Cb
Specialty Classic Round:			
3 Meat Treat	330	16	31
Hula Hawaiian, ham/bacon, av.	275	9	35
Italian Sausage	270	11	31
Ultimate Supreme	300	13	32
Veggie	270	10	32
Hot-N-Ready:			
Classic Pizza:			
Cheese	250	8	31
Pepperoni	280	11	31
Deep Deep Dish: Cheese	320	11	39
Pepperoni	350	14	40
Caesar Wings: *Per 8 Wing*			
BBQ	640	40	32
Buffalo, Mild	560	40	0
Garlic Parmesan	720	56	8
Oven Roasted	560	40	0
Caesar Dips: *Per 1.5 oz Container*			
Buffalo Ranch	230	24	3
Buttery Garlic, 0.5 oz	380	42	0
Cheezy Jalapeno	210	22	3
Ranch	250	26	3
Bread: Crazy Bread, 1 stick	100	3	15
Ital; Pepp. Chse Bread	135	6	15
Crazy Sauce, for Bread	45	0	10

Lone Star Steakhouse® (Sept '18)

Appetizers: Per Serving

	C	F	Cb
Lone Star Wings, mild, 3.5 oz	305	20	5
Spin. & Artichoke Dip, 3.5 oz	160	13	4.5
Texas Rose, 3.5 oz	285	19	25
Meals: *Without Sides, Toppings & Sauce*			
Chopped Steak, 9.6 oz	710	52	0
NY Strip, 9.6 oz	525	28	0
Texas Ribeye, 12.5 oz	710	40	5.5
Ribs Combo:			
Baby Back Ribs, with Chicken	740	30	46
Seafood:			
Fried Shrimp Entree, 11.7 oz	865	40	97
Grilled Shrimp: 3.5 oz	60	2	5.5
11 oz	190	7	17
Sweet Bourbon Salmon: 6oz	240	11	0
9 oz	360	16	0
Burgers:			
Bubba, 15.7 oz	1085	57	67
Swiss & Mushroom, 15.2 oz	845	38	53
Salads: *Per Serving, Includes Dressing*			
Dinner, Caesar, 6.3 oz	145	11	8
Grilled Chicken Caesar	480	24	19
Lettuce Wedge	395	34	10
Sides: *Per Serving*			
Garlic Mashed Potatoes, ½ cup	130	5	19
Steak Fries, 8 oz	610	26	86
Texas Seasoned Rice, 8 oz	100	3.5	14

Long John Silver's® (Sept '18)

Chicken,

	C	F	Cb
Chicken Tenders, 1 piece 2.1 oz	150	7	11
Sandwiches & Tacos:			
Baja Fish Taco	410	21	40
Crispy Fish Sandwich	400	16	44
Seafood:			
Baked Cod, 1 piece, 6 oz	160	1	1
Battered: Alaskan Pollock,			
1 piece, 3.2 oz	200	10	16
Cod, 1 piece, 3 oz	190	11	9
Shrimp, 3 pieces, 1.5 oz	100	7	5
Crab Cake, 1 cake, 2.2 oz	280	15	26
Snack Box: Breaded Clam Strips	340	20	35
Popcorn Shrimp, 3 oz	210	9	24

Continued Next Page....

Fast - Foods & *Restaurants*

Long John's® cont... (Sept '18)

Sauces & Condiments:

	C	F	Cb
Dipping Sauces: BBQ, 1 oz	40	0	10
Cocktail, 0.9 oz	20	0	4
Honey Mustard, 1packet	60	6	2
Ketchup, 1 pouch	30	0	8
Louisiana Hot Sauce, 1 tsp	0	0	0
Malt Vinegar, 0.5 oz	0	0	0
Marinara, 1 oz	15	0	4
Sweet Thai Chili, 1 oz	60	0	14
Tartar, 0.5 oz packet	40	4	3
Sides: Baked Potato, 12 oz	295	0	67
Breaded Mozzarella Sticks (3)	370	23	24
Brocc. Cheese Soup, 1 bowl, 7.4 oz	220	18	8
Clam Chowder, 1 bowl, 8 oz	230	16	16
Cole Slaw, 4 oz	170	11	18
Corn	160	8	9
Crumblies, 1 oz	170	12	13
Fries, 3.7oz	350	17	44
Hushpuppy, 2 pups, 1.5 oz	150	7	19
Jalapeno Cheddar Bites (5), 1 oz	240	16	18
Rice, 5 oz	180	1	37

For Complete Menu & Data ~ see CalorieKing.com

Macaroni Grill® (Sept '18)

Tappas & Antipasti:

Per Whole Appetizer as Served

	C	F	Cb
Calamari Fritti	760	55	33
Goat Cheese Peppadew Peppers	350	11	56
Loaded Fries	1020	74	68
Mac & Cheese Bites w/ Truffle Dip	920	70	44
Spicy Ricotta Meatballs	530	39	14
Meals: With Menu Set Sides			
Carne: Fig Marsala Pork Chop	1000	66	35
Grilled Lamb Chops	790	63	19
Rosemary Ribeye	1430	120	18
Chicken: Caprese	560	22	40
Marsala	790	32	61
Scaloppine	1110	74	51
Under a Brick	1590	145	20
Pasta: Eggplant Parmesan	1340	90	103
Fettuccine Alfredo	1040	59	86
Lasagna Bolognese	1110	67	69
Mom's Ricotta Meatballs:			
with Bolognese	1260	73	88
with Pomodoro	1100	62	84

Macaroni Grill® cont... (Sept '18)

Meals (Cont): Per Whole Entree

	C	F	Cb
Pasta (Ctnd):			
Mushroom Ravioli	930	66	53
Penne Rustica	1060	52	82
Truffle Mac &Cheese	1060	89	24
Seafood: Lobster Ravioli	920	74	36
Parmesan-Crusted Sole	1330	94	94
Artisan Pizzas: Per Whole Meal, as Served			
Cheese	1170	41	146
Farmhouse	1330	56	146
Margherita	1140	41	146
Pepperoni	1360	57	146
Kids: Chkn Tenders w/ Broccolini	860	45	67
Macaroni & Cheese	540	31	44
Pepperoni Pizza	630	25	72
Spaghetti & Meatballs,			
with Pomodoro Sauce	660	37	48
Salads: Includes Dressing			
Bibb & Blue, entrée	520	42	17
Caesar, with Chicken, entrée	650	41	16
Steak & Greens	950	71	32
Side: Florentine	300	22	22
Fresh Green	190	16	11
Dessert: Gelato, Vanilla	310	13	42
Homemade Choc. Cake	940	58	101
Lemon Passion	740	45	77
New York Style Cheesecake	690	41	70
Tiramisu	600	39	54

Manhattan Bagel® (Sept '18)

Bagels: Per Bagel

	C	F	Cb
Plain	320	1	68
Californian: Blueberry, 3.8 oz	300	1	65
Chocolate Chip, 3.8 oz	290	2.5	58
Cinnamon Raisin, 4 oz	290	1	63
Egg, 3.6 oz	300	5	54
Everything; Poppy, av., 3.7 oz	275	2.5	56
Pumpernickel, 3.6 oz	240	1.5	53
Gourmet: Asiago, 4.4 oz	370	5	68
Blueberry Glaze, 4.6 oz	370	1	83
Super Cinnamon, 4.6 oz	370	1	81
Garlic	340	1	74
Honey Whole Wheat	250	1	56
Jalapeno Cheddar	320	1.5	67
Poppy Seed	340	2.5	68
Salt	320	1	68
Cream Cheese: Plain, 1.3 oz	120	12	2
Lox, 1.25 oz	110	11	4
Scallion, 1.3 oz	140	12	5

Manhattan Bagel® cont... (Sept '18)

Breakfast:

	C	F	Cb
Bagel Sandwich: *On Plain Bagel*			
Egg & Cheese	480	13	69
Egg Bacon & Cheese	620	25	70
Egg, Pork Roll & Cheese	710	31	71
Wrap, Ranchero, with Bacon	780	44	58
Grilled Lunch Sandwiches:			
Chelsea Chicken, on Asiago Roll	760	31	75
East Side Reuben, on Marble Rye	730	40	56
Steak Roll: Bronx Bomber	430	14	49
Manhattan Cheesesteak	620	25	60
SoHo Chicken Caesar Wrap	550	23	53
Thintastic: Avocado BLT	440	23	49
Turkey	330	6	47
Soup: Chicken Noodle	250	7	30
Cream of Broccoli	320	18	27

Marie Callender's® (Sept '18)

Appetizers: With Menu Set Items

	C	F	Cb
Crispy Chicken Tenders, 12.9 oz	870	47	72
Crispy Green Beans, 10.5 oz	810	52	75
Mozzarella Sticks, 8.6 oz	690	42	46
Burgers and Sandwiches: With Fries, w/out Cheese			
Original Burger	1290	87	84
Frisco Chicken Breast	1290	81	95
Meatloaf on Cheese Sourdough	1250	78	96
Roasted Turkey Croissant Club	1450	97	95
Main Meals: With Menu Set Sides			
Comfort Classics:			
Chicken & Broccoli Fettuccine	1090	49	98
Home-Style Meatloaf Dinner	610	35	34
Delightful Dishes:			
Avocado Shrimp Stack	590	33	53
Chicken Street Taco	440	13	51
Mahi Mahi Cabo Taco	570	23	53
From The Grill:			
Cajun Salmon & Jumbo Shrimp	1280	63	115
St. Louis BBQ Ribs & Shrimp Skewer	800	47	39
Pies, Chicken Pot Pie, w/out sides	1140	79	70
Salads: Includes Dressing			
Calif. Waldorf Chicken with Mango	740	40	73
Crunchy BBQ Chicken	1060	56	90
Traditional Caesar, with Chicken	700	43	28
Sides: Cornbread, w/ Honey Spread	340	21	33
French Fries, 4 oz	380	20	45
Loaded Mashed Potatoes, 6.2 oz	340	23	23
Macaroni & Cheese, 6.4 oz	230	9	26
Soups: Per Bowl			
Chicken Tortilla	230	10	26
Clam Chowder	270	13	22
Hearty Vegetable	90	3	13
Split Pea & Ham	220	13	17

Marie Callender's® cont... (Sept '18)

Breakfast: With Menu Set Items

	C	F	Cb
Classics: Croissant Sandwich	1100	70	76
Eggs Benedict: California	1210	67	126
Traditional	1060	54	110
Hearty Man's Combo	1540	80	155
Tremendous Ten, with Bacon	1350	61	155
Griddle Greats: Belgian Waffles	600	19	99
Buttermilk Pancakes (3)	670	28	92
Lemon Blueberry Pie Pancakes	550	11	101
Old Fashioned French Toast	830	31	123
Omelettes: BTA	1610	84	161
Oh My	1710	87	156
Spanish	1550	78	166
Quiche: Bacon, 1 slice	990	79	45
Ham, 1 slice	1030	83	39
Desserts: Per Slice Unless Indicated			
Pies: Apple	570	28	78
Banana Cream, with Meringue	510	24	66
Chocolate Cream, with Meringue	570	25	77
Coconut Cream with Meringue	590	29	75
Traditional NY Style Cheesecake	810	59	56

For Complete Nutritiona Data ~ see CalorieKing.com

Max & Erma's® (Sept '18)

Shareables: As Served

	C	F	Cb
Baja Fish Taco: Crispy	1120	43	134
Grilled	760	28	84
Chicken Fajita Quesadilla	820	54	51
Potato Skins	1990	91	232
Spinach Dip	710	46	13
Wings with Blue Cheese Dressing:			
Cherry Cola BBQ	2090	120	118
Sweet Chili	1840	120	54
Burgers: Without Fries			
Cola BBQ Bacon	1320	80	93
Garbage, 6 oz	1650	118	60
Sauteed Mushroom & Swiss	1200	85	53
Tortilla	1260	84	61
Salads: Entrée Size, w/ Dressing, w/out Breadstick			
3rd Street	127	11	41
Grilled Chicken Santa Fe	1160	83	46
Village	430	37	14
Sides: Baked Potato	220	0	51
Creamy Coleslaw	160	12	14
Fresh Fruit Salad	90	0	23
Mashed Potatoes	290	11	43
Seasoned Fries	360	17	49
Dessert:			
Banana Cream Pie	820	38	111
Chocolate Cake a la Mode	1650	83	216

For Complete Menu & Data ~ See CalorieKing.com

McAlister's Deli® (Sept '18)

Sandwiches:

	C	F	Cb
Black Angus Club	840	43	73
California Turkey Reuben	950	46	81
Four Cheese Griller	760	38	66
French Dip	520	15	43
Grilled Chicken Club	830	37	78
Harvest Chicken Salad	730	48	56
Horseradish Roast Beef Cheddar	680	30	70
McAlister's Club	810	39	78
Reuben	900	41	76
Smoky Pepper Jack Turkey	780	36	72
Sweet Chipotle Chicken	630	15	77
The Italian	760	39	49
The Veggie	700	35	84

Mellow Mushroom® (Sept '18)

Burger:

	C	F	Cb
Ritz Burger	125	87	57
Calzones:			
Chicken & Cheese	1330	42	152
Steak & Cheese	1360	48	152
Hoagies, Whole: Chicken &Chse	1030	46	93
Italian	1230	72	91
Meatball	780	27	85
Mushroom Club	1300	74	96
Steak & Cheese	1100	59	91
Tofu	940	49	92
Munchies: Cheese Bread	870	42	84
Magic Mushroom Soup	350	24	15
Meatball Trio	330	22	11
Roasted Red Potatoes	150	3	27
Spinach & Artichoke Dip	790	47	67
Tomato Bisque	290	22	18
Wings: BBQ (10)	700	35	41
Sweet Thai Chili (10)	780	33	60
Pizzas: Per Medium Slice			
Buffalo Chicken; Holy Shitake Pie	475	25	44
Funky Q Chicken; House Special, av.	445	17	47
Kosmic Karma; Mega-Veggie, av.	385	15	48
Salads: Per Regular Size			
Caesar, with Caesar Dressing	800	70	29
Greek, with Feta, without Dressing	290	17	17
Dressings: Ranch, 1 oz	130	14	2
Balsamic Vinaigrette, 1 oz	90	8	5
Caesar, 1 oz	160	17	0.5
Desserts: Choc Chunk Cookie	600	29	83
Oatmeal Raisin Cookie	480	17	75
Peanut Butter Cookie	580	32	65

Extra Menu Items ~ See CalorieKing.com

McDonald's® (Sept '18)

Beef Burgers/Sandwiches::

	C	F	Cb
Bacon Smokehouse	840	45	62
Double Bacon Smokehouse	1130	67	63
Big Mac Burger	540	28	45
Cheeseburger: Single	300	12	33
Double	430	21	35
Triple	520	28	35
Hamburger	250	8	31
McDouble: Original	380	18	34
Bacon	450	23	34
Pico Guacamole	580	33	41
Sweet BBQ Bacon	700	38	52
Quarter Pounder: with Cheese	530	27	41
Double, with Cheese	770	45	40
Chicken Sandwiches: On Artisan Roll			
Aritsan Grilled Chicken	380	6	45
Bacon Smokehouse:			
Artisan Grilled Chicken	750	31	62
Buttermilk Crispy Chicken	920	45	81
Buttermilk Crispy Chicken	630	29	64
Classic Chicken	510	24	49
McChicken, on regular bun	410	22	39
Filet-O-Fish Sandwich	390	19	38
Chicken McNuggets:			
4 pieces	180	11	11
6 pieces	270	16	16
10 pieces	440	27	26
Sauces: Per Packet			
Creamy Ranch	110	12	1
Siganture	100	9	3
Spicy Buffalo	30	3	1
Sweet 'N Sour; Tangy BBQ	50	0	11
French Fries: Kids, 1.3 oz	110	5	15
Small, 2.6 oz	230	11	29
Medium, 3.9 oz	340	16	44
Large, 5.9 oz	510	24	66
Ketchup, packet	10	0	2
Breakfast:			
Big Breakfast: with Reg. Biscuit	750	49	53
with Hotcakes	1350	65	155
Biscuits: Regular			
Bacon, Egg & Cheese	450	24	40
Sausage	460	30	36
Sausage with Egg	530	34	38
Steak, Egg & Cheese	530	30	40
Burrito, Sausage	300	16	26
Fruit 'N Yogurt Parfait	150	2	30

McDonald's® cont... (Sept '18)

Breakfast (Cont):

	C	F	Cb
Fruit & Maple Oatmeal:			
with brown sugar	310	4	62
w/out brown sugar	260	4	49
Hash Browns, (1), 2 oz	150	9	16
Hotcakes: Plain (3)	330	8	56
with Syrup and Whipped Butter	600	16	102
McGriddles:			
Bacon, Egg & Cheese	420	18	45
Sausage	430	24	42
Sausage, Egg & Cheese	550	32	45
McMuffins: Egg	300	12	30
Egg White Delight	280	10	29
Sausage	400	25	29
Sausage with Egg	470	30	30

Happy Meals:

	C	F	Cb
Chicken McNuggets (4):			
+Apple Slices + 1% Low Fat Milk	295	13	27
+Apple Slices + Fat Free Choc Milk	325	11	38
+ Go-Gurt Strawb Yog. & Apple Jce	310	12	30
Hamburger:			
+Apple Slices + 1% Low Fat Milk	365	11	47
+Apple Slices +Fat Free Choc Milk	395	8	58
+ Go-Gurt Strawb Yog. & Apple Jce	380	9	60
Cheeseburger:			
+Apple Slices + 1% Low Fat Milk	415	15	49
+ Apple Slices & Fat-Free Choc Milk	445	12	60
+ Go-Gurt Strawb Yog. & Apple Jce	430	13	62

Mighty Kid's Meal:

	C	F	Cb
Chicken McNuggets (6):			
+ Apple Slices+ Fat Free Choc Milk	415	16	43
+ Go-Gurt Strawb Yog. + Apple Jce	400	17	45

Salads: Without Dressing

	C	F	Cb
Bacon Ranch: Grilled Chicken	320	14	9
Buttermilk Crispy Chicken	490	28	28
Southwest: Grilled Chkn, w/ glaze	350	11	27
B'milk Crispy Chicken, wih glaze	520	25	46
Side Salad	15	0	3

Salad Dressings: Per Package

	C	F	Cb
Newman's Own: Ranch, 2 fl.oz	200	17	11
Low-Fat: Balsamic Vinaig., 1.5 fl.oz	35	1.5	3
Family Recipe Italian, 1.5 fl.oz	50	1.5	8
Snacks: Apple Slices	15	0	4
Yoplait Go-Gurt, Strawberry, 1 tube	50	0.5	8

Desserts & Shakes:

	C	F	Cb
Baked Apple Pie, 2.6 oz	230	10	33
Cookies: Choc. Chip, (1)	170	7	23
Oatmeal Raisin (1), 1 oz	140	5	22

McDonald's® cont... (Sept '18)

Desserts & Shakes (Cont):

	C	F	Cb
Pie, Strawberry & Creme	290	15	34
McFlurry: M&M Candies, regular	630	22	96
Oreo Cookies, 12 fl.oz	510	17	80
Soft Serve: Kiddie Cone	45	1	5
Vanilla Cone	200	5	32
Sundaes:			
Hot Caramel, 6.4 oz	380	12	61
Hot Fudge, 6.3 oz	380	14	53
Strawberry, 6.3 oz	310	10	50
Milk: 1% Low-Fat, 8 fl.oz	100	2.5	12
Fat-Free Chocolate Milk, 8 fl.oz	130	0	23
Juice, Apple, box	35	0	9

Soda: With Ice, approximately 30%

	C	F	Cb
Coca-Cola or Sprite, average:			
Extra Small, 12 fl.oz cup	110	0	30
Small, 16 fl.oz cup	150	0	40
Medium, 21 fl.oz cup	215	0	56
Large, 30 fl.oz cup	290	0	75
Dr Pepper:			
Extra Small, 12 fl.oz cup	120	0	32
Small, 16 fl.oz cup	170	0	46
Medium, 21 fl.oz cup	210	0	58
Large, 30 fl.oz cup	290	0	79
Powerade, Mountain Berry Blast:			
Extra Small, 12 fl.oz cup	70	0	16
Small, 16 fl.oz cup	90	0	22
Medium, 21 fl.oz cup	120	0	31
Large, 30 fl.oz cup	170	0	42
Sweet Tea, medium	110	0	28

McCafe:

	C	F	Cb
Frappes: With Whipped Topping			
Caramel; Mocha, average:			
Small	420	17	60
Medium	510	21	72
Large	670	27	96
Shakes:			
Chocolate: 12 fl.oz cup	530	15	87
16 fl.oz cup	630	18	103
22 fl.oz cup	850	23	141
Vanilla: 12 fl.oz cup	490	14	79
16 fl.oz cup	590	17	95
22 fl.oz cup	800	22	131
Smoothies, all flavors:			
Small, 12 fl oz cup	200	0.5	45
Medium, 16 fl oz cup	245	1	56
Large, 22 fl oz cup	340	1	77

...cont next page

McDonald's® cont... (Sept '18)

McCafe:

	C	F	Cb
Hot Chocolate: With Whipped Cream & Toppings			
Whole Milk: Small, 12 fl oz	370	14	51
Medium, 16 fl oz	440	16	61
Nonfat Milk: Small, 12 fl oz	290	4	52
Medium, 16 fl oz	340	4	62
Iced Coffee: With Liquid Sugar & Light Cream			
Regular: Small, 16 fl.oz	140	5	24
Medium, 22 fl.oz	170	5	30
Large, 30 fl.oz	240	7	44
Caramel: Small, 16 fl.oz	140	5	23
Medium, 22 fl.oz	190	7	31
Iced Mocha: W/ Whole Milk, Syrup, Whipped Cream & Toppings			
Small, 16 fl.oz	290	11	40

Mimi's Cafe® (Sept '18)

Breakfast:

	C	F	Cb
Benedicts: W/ Roasted Potatoes			
Original	825	49	57
Smoked Salmon	755	44	57
Omelets: With Roasted Potatoes			
Bacon Avocado	920	65	30
Hickory-Smoked Ham & Cheese	675	45	27
Mushroom Bacon & Brie	775	56	28
Smoked Salmon	555	35	24
Griddle: With Eggs, any Style			
Brioche French Toast	755	34	75
Cinnamon Roll French Toast	880	41	96
Malted Berry Waffles	585	28	61
Lunch & Dinner: Without Side Choices			
Burgers: Brioche Cheeseburger	775	41	56
Hickory Bacon Cheddar	945	50	68
Mushroom & Brie	890	51	51
The French Quarter	1285	90	48
Craft Sandwiches:			
Chicken Cordon Bleu	1060	45	96
Roasted Turkey Club	1050	62	74
West Coast Reuben	1320	75	97
Entrees:			
Chicken Pot Pie	860	56	60
Beef Pot Roast	460	31	13
French Pot Roast	515	32	22
Quiche Lorraine	690	43	50
Roasted Chicken Crepes	455	37	15
Sides: Broccoli	115	9	5
Coleslaw	250	23	7
French Fries	120	3	22
Garlic Spinach	70	4	4
Mashed Potatoes	130	4	21
Mushroom Steak Topper	175	16	5
Roasted Potatoes	150	5	23

Mr. Goodcents® (Sept '18)

Cold Subs:

Per 8" Wheat Bread Sub with Standard Toppings

	C	F	Cb
Centsable	590	29	62
Garden Veggie	510	17	48
Goodcents Original	660	36	61
Oven Roasted Chicken Breast	490	18	60
Penny Club	500	19	61
Pepperoni	840	56	58
Tuna Salad	630	33	65
Toasted Sub: Per 8" Wheat Bread Sub with Standard Toppings			
Chicken Bacon Ranch	710	31	57
Meatball	720	28	69
Pasta:			
With Alfredo Sauce	840	40	103
With Marinara Sauce	640	18	107
Chicken Alfredo	970	43	104
Chicken Parmesan	810	23	109
Garlic Bread, 1 piece, 2 4 oz	290	12	44
Soup: Per 16 oz Bowl			
Broccoli Cheese	360	28	16
Chicken Homestyle Noodle	140	4	20
Potato with Bacon	420	28	36

Mr. Hero® (Sept '18)

7" Subs & Burgers:

	C	F	Cb
Burgers: Cheeseburger	720	50	44
Romanburger	805	56	46
Chicken Subs:			
Chicken Bacon Ranch	590	29	43
Chicken Philly	510	22	45
Deli Subs: Per 7" Sub with Menu Board Toppings			
Italiano	550	26	54
Original Italian	520	27	50
Tuna 'N Cheese	670	53	45
Turkey	330	2.5	49
Steak Subs: Baja Fire	625	36	44
Hatta Potatta	720	45	53
Hot Buttered Cheesesteak	580	31	42
Sicilian Parm	710	46	40
Zesty Bacon & Swiss	670	41	39
Sides: Per Regular Size			
Mozzarella Sticks	525	34	36
Onion Petals	545	36	52
Potato Waffer Fries	360	27	29
Desserts: Oreo Cheesecake	270	18	24
Snickers Cheesecake	270	18	23
Strawb. Swirl Cheesecake	250	17	21

Updated Nutrition Data ~ www.CalorieKing.com
Persons with Diabetes ~ See Disclaimer (Page 22)

Mrs Fields Cookies® (Sept '18)

Brownies: Per 2.15 oz Brownie

	C	F	Cb
Butterscotch Blondie	260	10	38
Double Fudge; Pecan Fudge, av.	265	14	33
Special Walnut Fudge & Blondie	260	13	35
Toffee/Walnut Fudge, average	265	14	33

Brownie Bites:

	C	F	Cb
Butterscotch Blondie (3)	200	8	29
Double/Toffee Fudge (3)	200	10	27

Coffee Cake,

	C	F	Cb
Chocolate Chip, small, 2.35 oz	240	11	30

Bite Size Nibblers Cookies:

	C	F	Cb
Cinnamon Sugar (3)	180	8	25
Peanut Butter (3)	170	9	19
Semi-Sweet Chocolate (3)	170	8	23
Triple Chocolate (3)	160	8	22
White Chunk Macadamia (3)	180	9	22
Cookies: Butter; Debra's Special (1), av.	200	8	28
Cut Out (1)	280	11	44
Oatmeal, Raisins and Walnuts (1)	200	9	27
Peanut Butter (1)	200	12	24
Semi-Sweet: Chocolate (1)	210	10	29
with Walnuts (1)	220	11	28
Triple Chocolate (1)	210	10	28
White Chunk Macadamia (1)	230	12	28

Muffins: Per 1.9 oz

	C	F	Cb
Blueberry	190	9	24
Chocolate Chip	200	10	26

For Complete Nutritional Data ~ see CalorieKing.com

My Favorite Muffin® (Sept '18)

Muffins: Per Large Muffin

	C	F	Cb
Large: Blueberry	590	36	60
Boston Cream Pie	740	33	105
Chocolate Chip	790	39	100
Carrot Cake	850	42	112
Deep Dish Apple Pie	560	22	85
Lemon Poppy Seed	670	32	90
Pumpkin Spice	600	26	86
Strawberry Cheesecake	580	31	67

Nathan's Famous® (Sept '18)

Burgers:

	C	F	Cb
Super Cheeseburger, 5 oz	960	67	48
Cheesesteak, Original Philly, 10.5 oz	680	33	52

Chicken:

	C	F	Cb
Sandwiches: Grilled Chicken, 8.2 oz	470	21	43
Krispy Chicken, 8.5 oz	660	37	58
Tenders, Krispy, 3 pieces, 6.3 oz	520	31	32
Wings, Original Buffalo, 10.5 oz	690	49	34

Nathan's Famous® cont... (Sept '18)

Hot Dogs: With Natural Casings

	C	F	Cb
Original, 3.5 oz	280	18	24
Chili, 5.5 oz	400	27	30
Chili Cheese, 6.5 oz	460	31	33
Hot Dog Nuggets, 3.5 oz	350	28	20
Corn Dog, on a stick, 3.2 oz	380	21	39

Fries::

	C	F	Cb
Bacon Cheese, regular, 10 oz	710	51	46
Crinkle Cut: Cheese, regular, 9 oz	570	38	46
French, regular, 7.5 oz	510	34	42

New York Fries® ~ See CalorieKing.com

Ninety Nine® (Sept '18)

Standout Starters: As Served

	C	F	Cb
Boneless Wings & Skins Sampler	1890	125	107
Mozzarella Moons	870	52	63
Outrageous Pot. Skins	1470	101	84

Burgers: Without Sides

	C	F	Cb
Bacon & Cheese	960	63	48
Black Bean	550	16	78
Vermont Cheddar	1100	76	52
West Coast Turkey	800	48	42

Sandwiches & Wraps: Without Sides

	C	F	Cb
Honey BBQ Chicken Wrap	850	33	100
Triple Decker Turkey Club S'wich	700	31	58

Meals: Served with Set Sides Unless Indicated

	C	F	Cb
Balsamic Grilled Chicken	500	18	31
Chicken Parmigiana	1390	47	179
Fish & Chips	1570	105	107
New Orleans Shrimp w/ Rice Pilaf	960	61	73
Orig. Crispy Chkn Tenders & Drssng	1080	68	65
Prime Rib: 12 oz, without sides	670	39	3
18 oz, without sides	940	53	3
Top Sirloin Steak, without sides	290	19	0

Gluten Sensitive Salads: With Caesar Dressing

	C	F	Cb
Chicken Heat of Caesar	790	55	7
Salmon Heart of Caesar	1030	78	7

Sides:

	C	F	Cb
Baked Potato with Sour Cream	310	8	52
Double Bleu Iceberg Wedge	460	42	11
French Fries	1040	64	107
Honey Butter Bisc., w/ Honey Butter	230	11	29
Pasta: with Butter	740	28	104
with Marinara	660	10	124
Perfect Coleslaw	150	12	10
Russet Mashed Potatoes	260	11	36

Dessert,

	C	F	Cb
Towering Midnight Fudge Cake	790	40	96

Noodles & Company® (Sept '18)

Noodles & Pasta: Regular Size

	C	F	Cb
Alfredo MontAmore	1410	84	110
Buttered Noodles	760	35	98
Japanese Pan Noodles	660	16	111
Mushroom Stroganoff	810	36	104
Pad Thai	1240	70	131
Penne Rosa, w/ Parmesan/Feta	720	25	102
Pesto Cavatappi, w/ Feta	750	32	93
Spaghetti	620	17	97
Spaghetti & Meatballs	980	46	104
Spicy Korean Beef Noodles	1000	30	140
Steak Stroganoff	1100	53	109
Thai Green Curry, with Shrimp	840	23	131
Wisconsin Mac & Cheese	980	38	119

Salads: Per Regular Size

	C	F	Cb
Grilled Chicken Caesar	400	26	18
Napa Market, with Chkn	600	45	24
The Med, with Chicken	370	15	33

Soups: Per Regular Size

	C	F	Cb
Thai Chicken	370	22	31
Tomato Basil Bisque	430	28	37

Extras: Cheesy Garlic Bread (3)

	C	F	Cb
Cheesy Garlic Bread (3)	350	13	44
Potsticker (6), with sauce	380	10	54
Side Caesar Salad	80	6	5
Wisconsin Mac & Cheese, side	270	12	31

Dessert: Chocolate Chunk Cookie

	C	F	Cb
Chocolate Chunk Cookie	490	22	69
Rice Crispy	540	19	87
Snoodledoodle Cookie	460	13	88

O'Charley's® (Sept '18)

Appetizers: As Served

	C	F	Cb
Chicken Tenders, Chipotle	1160	40	107
Nashville Deviled Eggs	720	61	24
Spicy Jack Cheese Wedges (7)	720	48	44
Top Shelf Combo Platter	1880	132	74

Burgers: Without Sides

	C	F	Cb
Better Cheddar Bacon	1000	68	49
Classic Cheeseburger	930	61	47

Chicken & Pasta: With Sides Unless Indicated

	C	F	Cb
Chicken Tenders & Fries	1410	85	74
Chicken Tender Dinner: Buffalo	1070	64	31
Chipotle	1040	40	77
Nashville Hot	1260	87	44
Garlic Shrimp Pasta	950	43	104
New Orleans Cajun Chicken Pasta	1170	61	99
Peach Chutney Chkn, w/out Sides	470	8	69

O'Charley's® cont... (Sept '18)

Classic Combos: Without Sides

	C	F	Cb
Steak & Chicken Tenders, 6 oz	1030	67	26
Steak & Gr. Atlantic Salmon, 6 oz	750	33	5
Steak & Half Rack Baby Back Ribs	890	49	48

Ribs & Steak: Without Sides

	C	F	Cb
Baby Back: Regular	1220	62	95
Carolina Gold	1220	62	96
Nashville Hot	1540	110	63
Slow Roasted Prime Rib: 8oz	830	70	3
12 oz	1140	95	3
16 oz	1460	120	4
Steak: Bacon & Bourbon Glazed Filet	640	42	28
Barrel House Pork Chops	820	45	62
Filet Mignon, w/ Garlic Butter	580	47	1
Grilled Top Sirloin, 6 oz	270	18	0
Louisianna Sirloin	600	43	3
Slow Roasted Prime Rib, 8 oz	830	70	3

Sandwiches: Without Sides Unless Indicated

	C	F	Cb
BLTC, with Fried Egg	930	59	56
Carolina BBQ Chicken	650	22	74
Classic French Dip	1020	55	79
Club Sandwich	950	85	91
Nashville Hot Chicken, with Fries	2000	101	119

Seafood! Favorites: Without Sides Unless Indicated

	C	F	Cb
Grilled Blackened Atl. Salmon, 9 oz	500	31	3
Grilled Salmon Bowl	990	70	44
Hand Battered Fish & Chips	1420	92	85
Hand Breaded Catfish, w/ Fries & Slaw	1720	124	103

Sides: Baked Potato (1)

	C	F	Cb
Baked Potato (1)	200	1	50
Broccoli, 5 oz	110	8	6
French Fries, 6 oz	400	24	40
Loaded Baked Potato, 1 portion	490	27	53
Sweet Potato Fries, 1 portion	280	19	27

Salads: Per Full Salad, with Dressing

	C	F	Cb
California Chicken	1020	67	71
Classic Cobb	1140	92	36
Sthrn Fried Chicken	1550	110	48
Sthrn Pecan Chicken Tender	1550	106	95

Signature Soup: Per Bowl

	C	F	Cb
Chicken Harvest	210	13	20
Chicken Tortilla	190	7	20

Desserts: Country Apple Pie, 1 slice

	C	F	Cb
Country Apple Pie, 1 slice	630	35	77
Double-Crust Cherry Pie, 1 slice	600	35	69
French Silk Pie, 1 slice	580	43	49
Goo Goo Crunch	1450	93	155
Ooey Gooey Caramel Pie, 1 slice	640	39	76
Southern Pecan Pie, 1 slice	730	45	78

For Complete Menu & Data ~ see CalorieKing.com

Old Spaghetti Factory® (Sept '18)

Appetizers: As Served

	C	F	Cb
Shrimp, Spinach & Artichoke Dip	590	40	39
Sicilian Garlic Cheese Bread	1220	78	97
With Bacon	1450	95	97

Entrées, Lunch/Dinner:

Classics:

Spaghetti: w/ Clam Sauce, 15 oz	810	31	107
with Marina Sauce, 15 oz	560	5	108
with Meat Sauce, 15 oz	650	11	108
with Sicilian Meatballs, 21 oz	1040	36	115

Factory Favorites:

Chicken Parmigiana, 18 oz	750	29	70
Spinach & Cheese Ravioli, 11 oz	470	16	63
Spinach Tortellini, w/ Alfredo Sce	940	56	86

Managers Favorites:

Marinara: Clam, 15 oz	690	18	107
Meat, 15 oz	600	8	108
Mushroom, 16.5 oz	610	10	109

Signature Selection:

Chicken Picatta	1150	76	63
Crab Ravioli, 11 oz	810	45	73
Spaghetti Vesuvius, 17.2 oz	850	29	112

Olive Garden® (Sept '18)

Appetizers:

Calamari	870	56	67
Sauce: Marinara	45	2.5	6
Ranch	210	21	3
Spicy Calabrian Chicken Tenders	900	67	19
Spicy Shrimp Scampi Fritta	560	37	34

Entrées:

Lunch: Chicken Piccata	350	21	11
Fettuccine Alfredo Mini Pasta Bowl	650	45	47
Lasagna Classico	640	36	39
Ravioli di Portobello	570	31	52
Spag. & Meat Sce Mini Pasta Bowl	360	12	51

Dinner:

Eggplant Parmig.	1060	54	113
Fettuccini Alfredo	1010	56	97
Five Cheese Ziti al Forno	1220	71	103
Grilled Chicken Parmigiana	760	29	54
Lasagna Classico	930	53	56
Ravioli di Portobello	820	46	73
Tour of Italy	1520	96	92

Desserts:

Black Tie Mousse Cake	750	50	76
Tiramisu	470	27	54
Warm Apple Crostata	630	29	83
Zeppoli, without sauce	810	28	119

On the Border® (Sept '18)

Appetizers: As Served

	C	F	Cb
Border Sampler	2180	147	116
Fajita Quesadillas:			
Chicken	1190	82	59
Steak	1280	97	56

Burritos: Without Bean, Rice or Sauce

Classic Chicken Tinga	640	32	41
Classic Ground Beef	820	49	44

Chimichangas: Without Beans, Rice or Sauce

Chicken Tinga	840	46	57
Ground Beef	990	58	66

Enchiladas: Without Bean and Rice

Ranchiladas	1180	73	43
Suizas	760	43	52

Salads: W/out Dressing

Fajita: Chicken	410	19	24
Steak	490	27	27
Grande Taco Salad: Chkn Tinga	710	46	49
with Ground Beef	830	57	51

Tacos: Without Beans and Rice

Brisket Tacos (2)	850	42	80
Grilled Fish Taco Del Mar	300	11	30
Southwest Chicken Taco (3)	1510	105	84

Soup: Chicken Tortilla, 1 cup	310	18	22
1 Bowl	510	26	44

Sides: Black Beans	220	2	38
Cilantro Lime Rice	180	2	37
Corn Tortillas (3)	130	2.5	33
Mexican Rice	220	6	37
Refried Beans	240	8	30

Dressings: Per Serving

Ranch	230	24	2
Smoked Jalapeno Vinaigrette	250	24	8

For Complete Nutritional Data ~ see CalorieKing.com

Orange Julius® (Sept '18)

Julius Originals: Per Medium Size

	C	F	Cb
Berry Pomegranate	430	0	108
Mango Pineapple	450	0	112
OrangeBerry	340	0	85
Strawberry Banana	530	8	118

Premium Fruit Smoothies: Per Medium Size

OrangeBerry	340	0	83
Pomegranate Berry	380	1	90
Strawberry	300	0.5	71
Sunshine Orange	360	0	84

Light Smoothies: Per Medium Size

OrangeBerry Xtreme; Strawberry	210	0	56
Strawberry Banana	210	0	58
Tripleberry	210	0.5	55
Boost, Banana, Small drink	30	1	7

Outback Steakhouse® (Sept'18)

Aussie-Tizers: Per Regular Size, with Selected Dressing/Sauce

	C	F	Cb
Alice Springs Chicken Quesadillas	1620	98	91
Aussie Cheese Fries: Small	1160	83	70
Large	1770	117	124
Bloomin' Onion	1950	155	123
Crab Cakes	800	66	22
Kookaburra Wings, medium/hot	1440	126	14
Seared Peppered Ahi, large	390	22	19
Steakhouse Quesadilla, regular	1590	107	78
Volcano Shrimp	960	73	55

Forkless Features: Without Sides

	C	F	Cb
Crispy Chicken Sandwich	880	52	69
Outback Burger, without Cheese	710	43	42
Steakhouse Philly S'wich	1030	61	54
The Bloomin' Burger	1160	83	58

Chicken & Ribs:

	C	F	Cb
Alice Springs Chicken & Fries, 5 oz	920	50	73
Baby Back Ribs & Fries, full order	1280	75	78
Grilled Chkn On The Barbie, 8 oz, with Fresh Mixed Veggies	520	16	6
Parmesan-Herb Crusted Chicken, with Mixed Veggies	670	33	30
Queensland Chicken & Shrimp Pasta	1210	55	98

Signature Steaks: Without Sides

	C	F	Cb
Melbourne Porterhouse, 18 oz	910	64	4
Outback Centre Cut Sirloin: 6 oz	210	7	0
9 oz Sirloin	320	10	0.5
Ribeye, 10 oz	540	35	0
Victoria's Filet Mignon, 6 oz	240	9	0

Straight From The Sea: Without Sides

	C	F	Cb
Bacon Bourbon Salmon, 10 oz	650	42	6
Hallibut Fish & Chips	1030	43	104
Tilapia, w/ Pure Lump Crab Meat	520	27	8

Entree Salads:

Aussie Cobb Salad, without dressing:

	C	F	Cb
with Crispy Chicken	840	52	47
with Grilled Chicken	530	27	19

Brisbane Caesar, with dressing:

	C	F	Cb
with Grilled Chicken	580	37	24
with Grilled Shrimp	580	38	26
Steakhouse, with dressing	940	59	50

Side Salads: With Dressing

	C	F	Cb
Blue Cheese Pecan Chopped	620	48	34
Blue Cheese Wedge	530	43	27
Caesar	280	24	12
House: with Blue Cheese Vinaig.	370	29	20
with Caesar Dressing	300	25	14
with Creamy Blue Cheese	350	31	13
with Honey Mustard	330	27	24
with Thousand Island	360	31	18

Outback Steakhouse® cont... Sept'18)

Soups:

	C	F	Cb
Baked Potato: Cup	280	17	23
Bowl	520	32	47
Chicken Tortilla Soup: Cup	170	9	13
Bowl	260	14	21
Clam Chowder: Cup	360	22	23
Bowl	710	44	47
French Onion	420	29	21

Sides:

	C	F	Cb
Aussie Fries	410	17	57
Baked Potato, with all toppings	390	12	58
Broccoli & Cheese	390	31	16
Fresh Seasonal Mixed Veggies	160	10	17
Grilled Asparagus	60	4	4
Loaded H'style Mashed Potatoes	300	20	21
Steakhouse Mac & Cheese	850	52	64
Sweet Potato, with all toppings	410	11	72

Kid's Menu: Without Sides or Drink

Entrees:	C	F	Cb
Boomerang Cheeseburger	600	36	40
Chicken Fingers	470	29	28
Grilled Cheese-A-Roo	580	21	77
Grilled Chicken on the Barbie	160	3.5	0
Junior Ribs, BBQ Sauce	300	21	2
Mac-A-Roo 'N Cheese	510	19	65

Desserts: Per Whole Dish

	C	F	Cb
Chocolate Thunder	1500	101	138
Double Chocolate Mini Parfait	590	39	54
NY Style Cheesecake, w/ Choc. Sce	1080	73	92
Triple Layer Carrot Cake	1290	68	174

For Complete Menu & Data ~ see CalorieKing.com

Panda Express® (Sept'18)

Appetizers:

	C	F	Cb
Chicken Egg Roll (1), 2.75 oz	200	10	20
Chicken Potsticker (3), 3.3 oz	160	6	20
Cream Cheese Rangoon (3), 2.4 oz	190	8	24
Crispy Shrimp (3), 1.8 oz	130	6	13
Veggie Spring Rolls (2), 3.4 oz	190	8	27

Entrées:

Beef:	C	F	Cb
Beijing Beef, 5.6 oz	470	26	46
Broccoli Beef, 5.4 oz	150	7	13
Shanghai Angus Steak, with String Beans, 6.4 oz	310	19	17

Chicken Breast:	C	F	Cb
String Bean, 5.6 oz	190	9	13
Sweet & Sour, 5.5 oz	300	12	40
SweetFire, 5.8 oz	380	15	47

Updated Nutrition Data ~ www.CalorieKing.com
Persons with Diabetes ~ See Disclaimer (Page 22)

Panda Express® cont... (Sept '18)

Entrees (Cont):

	C	F	Cb
Shrimp: Crispy Shrimp (6), 3.5 oz	260	13	26
Honey Walnut Shrimp, 3.7 oz	360	23	35
Vegetables: Eggplant Tofu, 6.1 oz	340	24	23
Country Style Bean Curd, 5.7 oz	190	12	14
Hot Szechuan Tofu, 5.5 oz	140	8	10
Mixed Vegetables, 4.3 oz	35	0	8
Sides: Chow Mein, 9.4 oz	510	20	80
Fried Rice, 9.3 oz	520	16	85
Steamed White Rice, 8.1 oz	380	0	87
Soup, Hot & Sour: Cup, 12.2 oz	120	5	14
Bowl, 17.4 oz	170	6	20
Dessert, Choc Chip Chunk Cookie	160	7	25

Panera Bread® (Sept '18)

Bagels:

	C	F	Cb
Asiago Cheese	330	6	55
Cinnamon Crunch	430	7	82
Breakfast Sandwiches, Grilled:			
Bacon, Egg & Cheese on Brioche	460	25	32
Sausage, Egg & Cheese on Brioche	550	34	33
Steak & Egg on Everthing Bagel	550	19	59
Bowls, Vegan Lentin Quinoa Broth	280	7	47
Sandwiches: Per Full Sandwich			
Bacon Turkey Bravo on Tomato Basil	630	24	57
Ham & Swiss, on Whole Grain	730	32	68
Mediterranean Veggie on Tomato Basil	440	13	65
Roasted Turkey & Avocado BLT, on Sourdough	640	33	50
Tuna Salad, on Black Pepper Foccacia	660	35	57
Flatbread, BBQ Chicken (1)	400	185	37
Panini, Frontega Chicken on Focaccia	750	24	85
Pasta:			
Chicken Tortellini Alfredo, 2 cups	750	39	68
Mac & Cheese:			
Small	470	30	36
Bread Bowl	1140	35	166
Salads: Full Size, with Dressing, without Bread			
Asian Sesame w/ Chkn	410	21	25
Chicken Caesar	450	27	17
Fuji Apple with Chicken	570	35	36
Greek	390	36	11
Strawberry Poppyseed with Chkn	340	13	31

Panera Bread® cont... (Sept '18)

Soups: Per Cup, without Bread

	C	F	Cb
Baked Potato	220	13	22
Broccoli Cheddar	230	13	19
Crm of Chkn & Wild Rice	180	10	18
New England Clam Chowder	370	25	27
Vegetarian Creamy Tomato	200	9	25
Cakes & Brownies:			
Cinnamon Crumb Coffee Cake, 1 slice	510	28	61
Double Fudge Brownie (1)	520	22	80
Cookies: Chocolate Chipper (1)	380	19	51
Oatmeal Raisin with Berries (1)	340	13	54
Pastries & Sweets:			
Bear Claw (1)	550	31	59
Cobblestone (1)	560	12	102
Pecan Roll (1)	720	46	69
Muffin: Apple Crunch	450	12	80
Pumpkin Muffin	580	22	90
Muffie, Chocolate Chip	320	14	46

Papa Gino's® (Sept '18)

Appetizers: Per Serving

	C	F	Cb
BBQ Chicken Tenders, 5.2 oz	360	18	33
Buffalo Chicken Tenders, 5.4 oz	390	25	22
Cheese Breadsticks, 3.75 oz	230	8	30
Chicken Tenders, 8.8 oz	350	20	24
Burgers: Cheeseburger, 6.7 oz	570	32	37
Classic Double, 12.8 oz	1040	67	43
Hamburger, 6.3 oz	520	28	35
French Fries: Small, 5 oz	470	24	66
Large, 13.7 oz	680	33	99
Pasta:			
Mac & Cheese, 17.8 oz	1040	60	87
Ravioli, 12.4 oz	560	21	67
Spaghetti & Meatballs, 19.8 oz	780	28	109
Pizzas:			
Thin Crust: *Per Slice, ⅛ Large Pizza*			
Boss BBQ Chicken	320	12	38
Cheese	230	7	32
Crispy Buffalo, w/ Blue Cheese	360	16	36
PapaRoni	340	16	32
Pepperoni	280	11	32
Super Veggie	250	8	35
Works	330	14	34
Subs: Per Small Sub			
BLT	690	35	67
Italian	590	24	64
Meatball Parmesan	790	38	79
Steak & Cheese	610	30	61
Super Steak	650	31	59
Tuna	730	39	64
Turkey Club	600	22	67

Papa John's® (Sept '18)

Pizzas:

Original Crust (14"): *Per ⅛ of Large 14" Pizza*

	C	F	Cb
BBQ Chicken & Bacon	340	11	45
Buffalo Chicken	380	17	40
Cheese	290	10	38
Grilled Chicken & Bacon	270	7	37
John's Favorite	390	20	36
Pepperoni	320	13	38
Pepperoni & Sausage	360	17	38

Thin Crust (14"): *Per ⅛ of Large 14" Pizza*

BBQ Chicken & Bacon	270	12	27
Buffalo Chicken	300	18	22
Cheese	210	11	20
Grilled Chicken & Bacon	190	8	19
John's Favorite	320	22	18
Pepperoni	250	14	20
Pepperoni & Sausage	310	20	20

Wings: *Per 8 Wings, with Dipping Sauce*

BBQ	880	57	20
Honey Chipotle	900	57	27
Spicy Buffalo	840	58	8
Chicken Poppers: 5 Poppers	270	10	21
10 Poppers	530	21	42
15 Poppers	800	31	64

Sides:

Breadsticks (2)	300	4	54
Garlic Parm (2)	340	10	54
Cheesesticks(10"), 1.2 oz	90	4	10
Desserts: Chocolate Chip Cookie	200	10	27
Double Chocolate Chip Brownie	240	12	34

Papa Murphy's® (Sept '18)

Pizzas:

Original Crust: *Per ¹⁄₁₂ of Family Size Pizza*

	C	F	Cb
BBQ Chicken	340	13	37
Chicken Garlic	330	15	30
Cowboy	370	19	32
Garden Veggie	270	11	33
Gourmet Vegetarian	320	16	32
Hawaiian	270	10	33
Murphy's Combo	350	18	33
Papa's Favorite	350	17	33
Pepperoni	300	14	31
Rancher	320	14	32
Thai Chicken	340	12	40

Stuffed Pizzas: *Per ¹⁄₁₆ of Family Size Pizza*

5 Meat	460	18	52
Big Murphy	450	18	53
Chicago Style	450	18	52
Chicken and Bacon	440	17	51

Papa Murphy's® cont... (Sept '18)

Pizzas (Cont):

Salads: *Per Whole Salad, w/out Dressing or Croutons*

	C	F	Cb
Caesar	100	5	7
Club	270	16	12
Garden	190	11	13
Italian	270	19	11
Mediterranean	320	17	23

Desserts:

Chocolate Chip Cookie, 1 slice	170	11	34
Cinnamon Wheel, 2 slices	250	7	42
S'mores Dessert Pizza, 2 slices	260	7	44

Pei Wei Asian Diner® (Sept '18)

Shareables: *Without Sauce*

Crab Wontons (4)	340	20	26
Korean BBQ Tacos (2)	520	23	51
Traditional Edamame	320	13	20
Vegetable Spring Rolls (4)	460	20	52
Sauces: Soy	15	0	2
Sweet Chile, 2 oz	140	0	34
Thai Peanut Dipping Sauce, 2 oz	230	15	20

Hand-Rolled Sushi Rolls: *Per 4 Rolls*

Mango California	190	5	28
Spicy Tuna Roll	180	6	22
Teriyaki Crunch	180	3	39
Wasabi Crunch	140	2.5	32

Rice Bowls: *Without Side Choices*

Fried White Rice:

Chicken, regular	1030	25	140
Steak, regular	1100	34	145
Veggies & Tofu, regular	1110	33	154

Pei Wei Original:

Shrimp, regular	790	33	107
Steak, regular	1210	54	150

Sesame:

Chicken, regular	860	40	75
Shrimp, regular	680	33	69
Steak, regular	1010	55	91

Salad Bowls: *With Dressing*

Ahi Aavocado	770	41	78
Asian Chopped Chicken	750	44	47
Asian Chile Lime Chicken	920	43	79
Soup: Hot & Sour, bowl	180	6	15
Thai Wonton, bowl	160	4.5	22

Pepe's Mexican® ~ see CalorieKing.com

Updated Nutrition Data ~ www.CalorieKing.com
Persons with Diabetes ~ See Disclaimer (Page 22)

Perkins® (Sept '18)

Breakfast: *Without Side Choices*

	C	F	Cb
Classic: Cntry Fried Steak & Eggs	740	45	47
Hearty Man's Combo	800	69	11
Steak Medallions & Eggs	530	28	8
Eggs Benedict	760	45	61

Perfect Platters: *Without Extras*

	C	F	Cb
Belgian Waffle	630	28	51
Brioche French Toast	730	33	68
Cinn. Roll French Toast	810	45	73
French Toast	620	32	53
Strawberry Pancake	930	39	123

Omelets: *Without Optional Sides*

	C	F	Cb
Everything	550	40	14
Farmers	660	54	8
Granny's Country	970	47	98

Syrups & Toppings:

	C	F	Cb
Apricot Syrup, 2 oz	120	0	30
Glazed Blueberries, 6 oz	200	0	51
Glazed Strawberries, 6 oz	140	0	36
Pancake/Twinberry Syrup, 2 oz, av.	130	0	33
Sugar Free, 2 oz	10	0	3

Side Choices:

	C	F	Cb
Bacon, 4 slices	140	12	0
Biscuits (2), Jumbo, with butter	650	36	68
Blueberry Muffin, with butter	650	33	81
Eggs (2)	170	13	2
English Muffin, with butter	230	11	28
Fresh Cut Fruit, 4 oz	70	0	19
Ham, grilled, 5.6 oz	160	4.5	6
Hash Browns, 4.3 oz	210	13	22
Homestyle Potatoes, 6.8 oz	210	3	40
Oatmeal, with butter blend, 2% Milk & Brown Sugar	390	15	57
Potato Pancakes (2), w/out extras	280	17	27
Sausage Patties (2)	380	38	1
Smoked Sausage, 4.1 oz	380	34	8
Sticky Bun, with butter	790	41	98
White Toast (2), with butter	310	16	34
Whole Wheat Toast (2), w/ butter	310	13	38

Burgers: *Without Side Choices*

	C	F	Cb
A-1 BBQ Bacon	1160	69	78
A-1 Tangler	1150	58	80
Classic Burger	920	62	49
Classic Cheeseburger	1080	74	51

Perkins® cont... (Sept '18)

Sandwiches: *W/out Side Choices*

	C	F	Cb
Chicken Strips Melt, on S'dough	1290	80	88
Country Club Melt, on S'Dough	990	57	64
Reuben Melt	1090	61	79
Roast Beef & Swiss	730	50	33
Turkey & Avocado BLT	700	39	47

Lunch & Dinners: *Without Sides*

Fork Worthy Entrées:

	C	F	Cb
Chicken Strips Dinner	800	43	59
Country Fried Steak Dinner	570	32	45
Fish 'n Chips, with Tartar Sauce	1290	85	97
Grilled Garlic Tilapia & Shrimp	550	20	57
Jumbo Shrimp	290	8	36
Steak Medallions & Mushrooms	480	29	6
Turkey & Dressing, w/- Cranb. Sce	510	20	39

Sides:

	C	F	Cb
Apple Sauce, 3 oz	40	0	9
Baked Potato,with Sour Cream	300	12	42
Buttered Corn	150	8	17
French Fries, 7 oz	570	36	56
Green Beans & Bacon, 4 oz	45	2.5	4
Herb Rice Pilaf, 6.5 oz	270	6	50
H'style Seasoned Potato, 6.8 oz	210	3	40
Macaroni & Five Cheese, 5.2 oz	300	16	26
Mashed Potatoes & Gravy, 8.6 oz	240	9	34
Sauteed Spinach, 4 oz	70	3.5	4
Tater Tots	470	28	47

Soups: *Per Bowl, Includes Crackers*

	C	F	Cb
Chicken Noodle	260	6	37
Loaded Potato; Tomato Basil	460	26	46
Tomato Basil	460	26	46

Salads: *With Set Dressing Unless Indicated*

	C	F	Cb
Chopped Cobb, w/out Dressing	510	30	18
Honey Mstrd Chkn Crunch	980	63	63
Southwest Avocado	820	50	61

Dessert:

Muffins: *Includes Whipped Butter Blend*

	C	F	Cb
Apple Cinnamon	630	33	76
Banana Nut	790	46	85
Blueberry	650	33	81

Pies: *Per Slice*

	C	F	Cb
Caramel Apple, 7.2 oz	500	22	68
Cherry	580	27	75
Lem. Meringue, 7 oz	500	17	80
Southern Pecan, 5.5 oz	670	33	86
Wildberry, no sugar added, 7 oz	470	27	50

Peter Piper Pizza® (Sept '18)

Appetizers:	C	F	Cb
Bone In Wings (10), without sauce	1160	97	0
Boneless Wings, 10 oz, without sauce	880	58	47
Cheddar Bacon Roll (1)	350	18	34
Garlic Cheese Bread, 3.25 oz	390	17	45
Handmade Breadsticks, with Marinara Sauce (6)	1190	31	199

Dipping Sauces:			
BBQ	240	0	60
Buffalo	120	9	6
Ranch	320	36	2
Sweet Chili	200	0	46
Xtra Hot Buffalo	90	6	5

Signature Pizzas:

Original Crust: *Per ⅛ of Large 14" Pizza*

	C	F	Cb
5 Meat Supreme	360	15	39
California Veggie	290	9	41
Cheese	320	11	39
Chicago Classic	330	13	40
Hearty Hawaiian	310	9	41
New York 3 Cheese w/ Pepperoni	390	18	39
Pizza Mexicana	390	18	39
Spinach Alfredo	350	15	37
The Werx	310	11	40
Veggie Harvest	300	9	42

Original Crust: *Per 1/12 of Extra Large 16" Pizza*

	C	F	Cb
5 Meat Supreme	350	16	34
California Veggie	250	8	35
Cheese	280	10	34
Chicago Classic	300	12	35
Hearty Hawaiian	270	8	36
New York 3 Cheese w/ Pepperoni	390	18	39
Pizza Mexicana	340	15	34
Spinach Alfredo	310	14	32
The Werx	290	11	34
Veggie Harvest	260	8	36

Salads: *Small Size, without Dressing*

	C	F	Cb
Caesar, with Croutons	320	14	35
Mandarin Cranberry	150	6	26

Dessert:			
Cinnamon Crunch, small slice	380	9	69
Vanilla Soft Serve: Cone	200	6	35
Cup	180	6	31

P.F. Chang's® (Sept '18)

Street Fare:	C	F	Cb
Cauliflower Tempura	680	45	64
Chang's BBQ Spare Ribs	810	22	37
Chang's Chicken Lettuce Wraps	660	27	67
Chang's Vegetarian Lettuce Wraps	570	28	53
Crispy Green Beans	990	77	68
Dynamite Shrimp	640	48	34
Edamame with Kosher Salt	400	17	25
Northern Style Spare Ribs	710	21	12
Tempura Calamari & Vegetables	960	73	60

Entrées:

Beef: *Per Whole Meal, without Rice*

	C	F	Cb
A La Sichuan	690	33	55
Beef with Broccoli	670	33	46
Mongolian	770	42	39
Wok Fired Filet Mignon	1140	72	72

Chicken: *Per Whole Dish, without Rice*

	C	F	Cb
Chang's Spicy	840	31	79
Crispy Honey Chkn	1120	60	87
Korean Fried Chicken	1380	74	94
Kung Pao	960	58	46
Orange Peel Chkn	840	31	79
Sesame Chicken	870	36	74

Seafood: *Per Whole Meal, without Rice*

	C	F	Cb
Chang's Lobster & Shrimp Rice	1060	46	112
Crispy Honey Shrimp	1020	55	79
Kung Pao Shrimp	760	52	40
Oolong Chilean Sea Bass	560	35	30
Orange Peel Shrimp	560	22	66
Salt & Pepper Prawns	500	22	37
Walnut Shrimp with Melon	1340	107	70

Vegetarian: *Without Rice*

	C	F	Cb
Buddha's Feast, steamed	260	4	32
Ma Po Tofu	920	59	57
Stir-Fried Eggplant	530	34	57
Thai Harvest Curry	1060	73	72

Noodles & Rice:

	C	F	Cb
Fried Rice: Combo	1200	35	160
with Beef	1140	33	155
with Chicken	1100	26	159
with Pork	1190	37	161
with Shrimp	1030	24	158
Long Life Noodles & Prawns	1040	37	130

Updated Nutrition Data ~ www.CalorieKing.com
Persons with Diabetes ~ See Disclaimer (Page 22)

P.F. Chang's® cont... (Sept '18)

Noodles & Rice (Cont):

	C	F	Cb
Lo Mein: Beef	980	31	127
Chicken	950	24	130
Combo	1050	33	132
Pork	1030	35	133
Shrimp	880	21	130
Vegetables	760	13	135
Hokkien Street Noodles	1280	20	224

Market Sides: Per Serving

	C	F	Cb
Brown Rice	250	2	53
Chili Garlic Green Beans	530	40	39
Sichuan-Style Asparagus	450	34	31
White Rice, 6 oz	290	0	65
Wok-Charred Brussels Sprouts	350	28	25
Wok'd Spinach w/ Garlic	140	6	15
Salad: Asian Caesar	410	30	21
Mandarin Crunch	730	46	71
Vietnamese Noodle	800	6	166
Dessert: Banana Spring Rolls	940	35	149
Chocolate Dome	610	43	61
New York Style Cheese Cake	940	61	80
The Great Wall of Chocolate	1700	71	259

Pita Pit® ~ See CalorieKing.com

Pizza Hut® (Sept '18)

Hand-Tossed Style: Per ⅛ of Medium 12" Pizza

	C	F	Cb
Cheese	210	8	26
Chicken-Bacon Parmesan	230	9	25
Meat Lover's	280	15	25
Pepperoni	220	10	25
Pepperoni Lover's	270	13	26
Supreme	240	11	26
Ultimate Cheese Lover's	230	10	25
Veggie Lover's	200	7	26

Original Pan: Per ⅛ of Medium 12" Pizza

	C	F	Cb
Cheese	260	12	28
Meat Lover's	320	18	28
Pepperoni	260	13	27
Pepperoni Lover's	320	17	28
Supreme	280	14	28
Ultimate Cheese Lover's	280	14	27
Veggie Lover's	240	10	29

Rectangle Slices: Per Slice, ⅛ of Pizza

	C	F	Cb
Backyard BBQ Chicken	260	9	34
Buffalo Chicken	240	8	32
Cheese	240	10	29
Pepperoni	250	11	28
Veggie Lovers	220	8	29

Pizza Hut® cont... (Sept '18)

Personal Pan: Per ¼ of 6" Pizza

	C	F	Cb
Backyard BBQ Chicken	180	6	25
Meat Lover's	210	12	17
Pepperoni	150	7	17
Pepperoni Lover's	180	9	17
Supreme	170	9	17
Ultimate Cheese Lover's	170	8	17
Veggie Lover's	140	5	18

Thin 'n Crispy: Per ⅛ of Medium 12" Pizza

	C	F	Cb
Backyard BBQ Chicken	210	7	27
Cheese	180	7	22
Chicken-Bacon Parmesan	220	10	21
Hawaiian Chicken	180	5	24
Meat Lover's	260	14	22
Pepperoni	200	9	22
Pepperoni Lover's	250	13	22
Supreme	210	9	23
Ultimate Cheese Lover's	210	10	21
Veggie Lover's	170	6	24

Pastas, Tuscani: Per Whole Pan

	C	F	Cb
Creamy Chicken Alfredo	890	49	74
Meaty Marinara	820	36	85
Sides: Baked Bone Out Wing (1)	60	2	4
Breadstick (1), without sauce	140	4.5	19
Buffalo Chicken Nachos	1110	50	132
Cheesy Dip 'N Cheese	660	36	78
Fried Onion Rings, with Ketchup	860	50	93
Garlic Bread, 1 piece	140	8	15
Stuffed Garlic Knot	80	2.5	10
Stuffed Pizza Roller	230	10	27

Salad: Entree Size, without Dressing

	C	F	Cb
Asian	330	15	24
BLT	400	26	26
Chicken Caesar	470	25	27
Harvest	470	19	48
Zesty Italian	370	22	30
Dressing: Blue Cheese, 1.5 oz	200	21	2
Buttermilk Ranch, 1.5 oz	200	22	2
Honey French,1.5 oz	190	15	13
Desserts: Hot Cinnamon Apple Pie	170	9	22
Hershey's: Tstd S'mores Cookie (1)	240	10	33
Triple Choc. Brownie, ⅛ square	380	16	56
New York Style Cheesecake, slice	840	57	69

Pizza Ranch® (Sept '18)

Figures based on West Coast Outlets **C** **F** **Cb**

Pizza:

Original Crust: *Per Slice, 1/10 of Medium Pizza*

	C	F	Cb
Bacon Cheeseburger	180	7	20
BBQ Chicken	170	6	20
Bronco	200	8	19
Buffalo Chicken	190	9	18
California Chicken	190	9	18
Chicken Bacon Ranch	230	12	18
Chicken Broccoli Alfredo	170	7	19
Macaroni & Cheese	210	9	22
Prairie (Veggie)	170	6	20
Roundup	190	8	20
Stampede	200	9	20
Sweet Swine	170	6	20
Texan Taco	220	9	27

Thin Crust: *Per 1/10 Slice of Medium Pizza*

	C	F	Cb
BBQ Chicken	150	7	12
Bronco	180	10	12
California Chicken	170	10	11

For Complete Menu & Data ~ see CalorieKing.com

Pollo Tropical® ~ See CalorieKing.com

Popeye's® (Sept '18) **C** **F** **Cb**

Chicken Pieces: Mild & Spicy with Skin

	C	F	Cb
Breast	380	20	16
Leg	160	9	5
Thigh	280	21	7
Wing	210	14	8
Nuggets: 6 pieces	225	14	15
9 Pieces	340	20	23
Tenders: Mild/Spicy, 3 pieces	445	21	29
5 pieces	740	34	48
Sandwiches & Wraps: Each			
Chicken Tender Po'Boy: Blackened	580	32	39
Spicy/Mild	600	33	55
Cajun Fish Po'Boy	750	52	75
Catfish Po'Boy	800	51	59
Popcorn Shrimp Po' Boy	660	41	61
Seafood: Catfish Fillets, 3 pieces	380	19	37
Butterfly Shrimp (8)	420	25	34
Popcorn Shrimp, 4 oz	390	25	28

Popeye's® cont... (Sept '18)

Sides:	C	F	Cb
Biscuit	205	13	20
Cajun Fries, regular	270	14	33
Cajun Rice, regular	185	6	24
Cole Slaw, regular	140	10	12
Corn on the Cob (1)	210	6	34
Mashed Potatoes, w/ Cajun Gravy	110	4	18
Onion Rings, regular	280	19	25
Red Beans & Rice, regular	245	16	22
Breakfast:			
Biscuits: Chicken	490	26	47
Egg	510	29	41
Egg & Sausage	690	45	43
Sausage	540	36	41
Sausage & Gravy	510	33	42
Grits	370	5	80
Hash Rounds	360	20	41
Desserts:			
Hot Sweet Potato Pie 3.4 oz	350	19	41
Mardi Gras Cheesecake, 3 oz	320	21	29
Mississippi Mud Pie, 3 oz	260	7	50
Sliced Pecan Pie, 3.4 oz	410	21	52

Port of Subs® (Sept '18)

Figures Based on West Coast Outlets **C** **F** **Cb**

Cold Submarine S'wiches: Per 5" White Sub with
Cheese, Lettuce, Tomato Vinegar, Oil, Salt & Oregano

	C	F	Cb
#1 Ham, Salami, Capicolla Pepperoni, Provolone	410	16	41
#2 Ham & Turkey, Provolone	360	8	40
#3 Salami & Turkey, Provolone	385	13	39
#4 Ham, Salami, Provolone	365	12	41
#5 Smoked Ham, Turkey, Cheddar	370	10	39
#6 Vegetarian, 3 Chse	430	22	43
#7 Roast Beef, Prov.	355	9	39
#8 Turkey, Provolone	380	8	39
#10 Rstd Chicken Breast, Provolone	340	9	39
#11 Ham, American Cheese	345	8	42
#12 Salami, Provolone	390	17	40
#13 Pepprd Pastrami Turkey, Swiss	375	9	39
#15 Salami, Pepperoni, Provolone	390	18	39
#16 Chkn, Pepperoni, Pepper Jack	375	15	39
#17 Tuna, Provolone	450	20	41
#18 Roast Beef, Turkey, Provolone	370	8	39

continued next page...

Updated Nutrition Data ~ www.CalorieKing.com
Persons with Diabetes ~ See Disclaimer (Page 22)

Port of Subs® cont... (Sept '18)

Figures Based on West Coast Outlets **C F Cb**
Hot Subs: Per 5" with White Bread

	C	F	Cb
BLT	305	11	38
Grilled Chicken, with Provolone	410	10	38
Hot Pastrami, with Provolone	545	28	41

Wraps: With 12" Wheat Tortilla, Cheese, Lettuce, Tomato, Onion, Vinegar, Oil, Salt & Oregano

	C	F	Cb
#2 Ham, Turkey, Provolone	565	18	55
# 8 Turkey Provolone	590	19	54
#11 Ham, with American Cheese	545	19	58

Fresh Salads: W/ Lettuce, Tomato, Onion, Cucumber & Olives, without Dressing

	C	F	Cb
Garden	70	3	10
Spinach	65	2.5	8
Tuna	445	28	15

Salad Dressings: Per 1 oz

	C	F	Cb
Creamy Italian	100	8	6
Honey Mustard	130	13	4
Ranch	110	12	1
Croutons, 1 package	30	1	5

Sides: Per Regular, 8 oz

	C	F	Cb
Caesar Bow Tie Pasta Salad	355	18	37
Cucumber Salad	125	11	4
Macaroni Salad	515	41	44
Potato Salad	325	13	52

Breakfast Sub: With American Cheese & Egg

5" Wheat Bread:	C	F	Cb
Peppered Bacon	410	19	38
Smoked Ham	390	15	38
Turkey Sausage	515	25	40
Flatbread: Peppered Bacon	415	20	35
Smoked Ham	400	17	35
Turkey Sausage	525	26	37

Desserts:

	C	F	Cb
Brownie	750	35	109
Chocolate Chunk Cookie, 4 oz	500	23	71
Oatmeal Raisin Cookie, 4 oz	480	20	69
White Choc. Macadamia Nut Cookie	520	26	66

Pret A Manger® (Sept '18)

Baguettes: **C F Cb**

	C	F	Cb
Chicken Mozzarella	550	20	57
Tuna & Cucumber	560	29	52
Roast Beef, Arugula & Parmesan	530	19	53

Hot Food: Per Pack

	C	F	Cb
Chicken Burrito	550	16	68
Falafel & Red Pepper Wrap	700	28	87
Spin. & Artichoke Gr. Chse on S'dough	590	28	57
Spinach & Tomato Mac & Cheese	440	21	47

Pret A Manger® cont (Sept '18)

Pots: **C F Cb**

	C	F	Cb
Banana & Honey	390	15	45
Blueberry & Granola	350	14	37
Egg & Quinoa	230	13	18
Seasonal Berries Yogurt	240	10	25

Sandwiches:

	C	F	Cb
Balsamic Chicken & Avocado	480	26	41
California Club	390	16	41
Chicken & Bacon	480	27	35
Classic Cheddar & Tomato	430	25	35
Egg Salad Toast	280	20	17
Tuna Salad	460	29	32

Soups: Per Container

	C	F	Cb
Green Chicken Pozole	240	7	27
Miso	50	1.5	6
Moroccan Lentil	380	17	45
Tomato Feta	230	14	23

Salads: Without Dressing

	C	F	Cb
Chef	290	15	14
Chicken Avocado	450	28	26
Chicken Caesar	270	10	8
Maine Lobster	200	9	4
Veggie Fiesta	440	27	32

Bakery: Per Pack

Croissants:	C	F	Cb
Almond	370	21	39
Pain au Chocolate	300	15	34
Pain au Raisin	390	20	46
Cookies: Carrot Cake, 2.5 oz	270	14	35
Chocolate Chunk, 2.5 oz	320	15	41
Harvest, 2.5 oz	280	12	40
Muffin, Blueberry, 4.5 oz	420	16	63

Pretzelmaker® (Sept '18)

Pretzels: Per Small Serving **C F Cb**

Bites:	C	F	Cb
Salted, 6 oz	500	14	85
Cinn. Sugar, 6 oz	530	14	90
Whole: Plain, 4 oz	310	3	66
Cinnamon Sugar, 5 oz	450	12	79
Garlic, 5 oz	430	12	74
Parmesan, 5 oz	450	15	66
Ranch, 5 oz	440	12	72
Pretzel Dogs: Regular	420	23	31
Mini (8)	430	29	33
Jalapeno (1), 6 oz	450	24	34

continued next page...

Pretzelmaker® cont... (Sept '18)

Sauces: Per 2 oz

	C	F	Cb
Caramel	100	1	22
Cheddar Cheese	80	6	6
Cream Cheese	200	20	2
Nacho Cheese	80	6	4
Pizza Sauce	30	1	6
Vanilla Glaze	170	0	42

Beverages: Per 20 oz Unless Indicated

Blended Drinks:

	C	F	Cb
Cool Cappuccino	430	22	58
Mango Madness	500	16	90
Mocha Mania	580	22	94
Power Pomegranate	490	16	86
Strawberry Bananza	500	16	85
Fresh Lemonade: Original, 20 oz	140	0	38
Strawberry; Raspberry, 20 oz, av.	210	0	52

Qdoba® (Sept '18)

Please Note: Nutritional Information is based on a single serving of each menu ingredient listed.

Burritos: Each with 12.5" Flour Tortilla, Cilantro-Lime Rice, Black Beans, Salsa Verde, Lite Sour Cream, Lettuce and Shredded Cheese

	C	F	Cb
Marinated Grilled Chkn	1035	37	124
Pulled Pork	1005	33	129
Seasoned Ground Beef	1055	40	124

Burritos: With 12.5" Flour Tortilla, 3-Cheese Queso Pinto Beans, Roasted Chili Corn Salsa, Guacamole & Lite Sour Cream

	C	F	Cb
Marinated Grilled Chicken	1020	47	104
Marinated Gr. Steak	1030	47	102
Pulled Pork	990	43	109
Seasoned Ground Beef	1040	50	104

Grilled Quesadillas: With 12.5" Flour Tortilla, Shredded Cheese, Pico de Gallo and Fajita Vegetables

	C	F	Cb
Grilled Chicken	685	30	64
Pulled Pork	655	26	60

3-Cheese Nachos: Per Serving, with Tortilla Chips, 3-Cheese Queso, Salsa Roja, Guacamole & Sour Cream

	C	F	Cb
Grilled Chicken	1120	64	98
Pulled Pork	1090	60	103

Qdoba® cont... (Sept '18)

Knock Out Tacos: Set Ingredients

	C	F	Cb
Bohemian Veg	230	9	28
Drunken Yardbird	220	8	25
Mad Rancher	230	10	21
Two Timer	290	13	28
Triple Threat	250	12	17
The Gladiator	280	17	16

Taco Salads: With Crunchy Flour Tortilla Bowl, Black Beans, Lettuce, Shredded Cheese, Brown Rice, Lite Sour Cream, Guacamole & Cilantro Lime Dressing

	C	F	Cb
Grilled Chicken	1270	66	116
Pulled Pork	1240	62	121
Seasoned Ground Beef	1290	69	116

Chips & Dip: Includes Tortilla Chips

	C	F	Cb
3- Cheese Queso	750	41	81
3-Cheese Queso, Guac. & Salsa Roja	900	51	92

Breakfast Burritos: With 12" Flour Tortilla

Chorizo & Seasoned Potato:

	C	F	Cb
with 3-Cheese Queso Sauce	820	40	80
with Shred. Cheese & Salsa Roja	820	38	79

Quiznos Subs® (Sept '18)

Subs: Per 8" Regular Japaleno Cheddar Sub, with Standard Menu Toppings Unless Indicated

Chicken:

	C	F	Cb
Apple Harvest	790	32	97
Baja; Mesquite	800	30	76
Carbonara	890	42	73
Honey Mustard	850	36	80
Southwest Chicken	860	45	73

Steak:

	C	F	Cb
Black Angus Steak, On Rosemary Parmesan	780	27	88
Chipotle Steak & Cheddar	840	44	73
French Dip	760	30	79
Peppercorn Steak	840	42	76

Deli Classic:

	C	F	Cb
Classic Italian	920	50	77
Spicy Monterey	600	15	81
Tuna Melt	660	22	76
Turkey Ranch & Swiss	670	25	73
Veggie Guacamole	810	44	81

Salads: Per Full Size, with Dressing Unless Indicated

	C	F	Cb
Apple Harvest Chicken	590	39	40
Carbonara, w/out dressing	700	51	15
Honey Mustard Chkn, w/out drsng	650	43	22
Turkey Bacon Guacamole	600	42	18

continued next page...

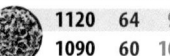

Updated Nutrition Data ~ www.CalorieKing.com
Persons with Diabetes ~ See Disclaimer (Page 22)

Quiznos Subs® cont... (Sept '18)

Savory Soups: *Reg., w/ 2 Crackers*

	C	F	Cb
Broccoli Cheese	245	15	22
Chicken Noodle	145	4.5	18

Breakfast:

	C	F	Cb
Subs: Bacon, Egg & Cheddar	370	17	34
Ham, Egg & Cheddar	340	16	29
Sausage, Egg & Cheddar	550	39	28

Desserts:

	C	F	Cb
Chocolate Chunk Cookie	390	19	54
Chocolate Brownie	310	16	40
Cinnamon Sugar Cookie	400	17	58
Oatmeal Raisin Cookie	360	12	58

Rally's/Checkers® (Sept '18)

Burgers/Sandwiches:

	C	F	Cb
Bacon Roadhouse	680	47	37
Baconzilla	910	62	43
Big Buford	660	39	39
Cheese Champ	430	21	39
Cheese Double	480	25	38
Classic Wings: Buffalo, 5 pieces	360	23	3
Honey BBQ, 5 pieces	430	23	19
Garlic Parmesan, 5 pieces	510	40	3

Fries:

	C	F	Cb
Fries, medium	500	24	63
Chili Cheese	590	30	72
Fully Loaded	870	56	72

Ranch One® (Sept '18)

Sandwiches:

	C	F	Cb
Chicken & Cheese	390	12	40
Chkn Philly, 9.3 oz	410	13	40
Grilled Classic Chicken, 9.4 oz	680	47	37
Original Crispy Chicken, 11.5 oz	640	31	60

Other Favorites:

	C	F	Cb
Chicken Fajitas, 10 oz	540	24	53
Chicken Platter, with Rice, 11.9 oz	270	6	28
Popcorn Chicken:			
Small, 5.5 oz	310	10	30
Large, 7.5 oz	420	14	40

Salads: *Completed*

	C	F	Cb
Grilled Chicken Caesar, 13.3 oz	430	30	14
Southwest Chicken, 17.5 oz	680	43	44

Fries:

	C	F	Cb
Medium, 5.8 oz	380	19	43
Large, 10.9 oz	530	27	58
Cheese Fries: Medium, 7.3 oz	490	27	46
Large, 11 oz	760	44	66

Red Hot & Blue® (Sept '18)

Starters:

	C	F	Cb
Catfish Fingers	590	19	75
Nachos, with Chili	1005	51	103
Shakin' Bacon Cheese Fries	2440	60	106

Burgers:

	C	F	Cb
ALL IN	915	52	46
Classic Blues	665	32	44

Ribs, Full Slab:

	C	F	Cb
Dry	1870	144	28
Sweet	1895	142	44
Favorite Entrees: Delta Catfish	835	42	57
Delta Surf & Turf	1025	68	38
Southern Fried Chicken Crispers	760	35	50
Rib & Crispers Platter	1060	68	39
BBQ Platters: Five Meat	935	63	15
Delta Double with Memphis Chkn	900	54	12
Pulled Pork	325	21	7
Smoked Sausage	965	68	36

Sandwiches:

	C	F	Cb
Fried Delta Catfish	655	25	71
Grilled Chicken	360	6	40
Pulled Pork	370	15	37
Sides: BBQ Beans	255	2	48
Collard Greens	50	2	7
Fried Ocra	190	8	29
Mashed Potatoes, with gravy	310	14	44
Memphis Fries, 6 oz	345	19	38
Potato Salad	405	28	33
Sweet Potato	495	0	114
Sweet Potato Fries	375	19	49
Salads: Grilled Chicken Caesar	770	46	47
Southern Fried Chicken	710	31	60

Red Lobster® (Sept '18)

Seaside Starters: *As Served*

	C	F	Cb
Fried Oysters	830	47	81
Lobster & Langostino Pizza	700	35	59
Mozzarella Cheesesticks	700	40	56
Oysters Half Shell (12), raw	530	11	85
Parrot Isle Jumbo Cocktail Shrimp	610	39	52
Seafood Stuffed Mushrooms	390	22	18
Signature Shrimp Cocktail	130	0	11
Sweet Chili Shrimp	1100	76	77

Land & Sea: *With Menu Set Sides*

	C	F	Cb
Cajun Chicken Linguini, full	1330	60	113
Maple Glazed Chicken Dinner	490	7	51
Rock Lobster & NY Strip (12 oz)	1250	83	27
Steak: Filet Mignon (6 oz)	460	23	26
Sirloin (7 oz)	500	23	26
Wood-Grilled Shrimp & Sirloin	580	26	27

continued on next page...

Red Lobster® cont... (Sept '18)

Lunch Classics: As Served

	C	F	Cb
Cajun Chicken Linguini, half order	680	30	60
Crab Linguini Alfredo, half order	620	29	57
Crunchy Popcorn Shrimp	430	19	49
Farm-Raised Catfish, Blackened	210	10	2
Garlic Shrimp Scampi	220	18	3
Hand Breaded Shrimp	240	11	23
Maple Glazed Chicken	360	5	50
Sailor's Platter	450	18	18
Wild Caught Flounder: Golden Fried	710	50	38
Oven Broiled	210	5	1

Savor The Sea:

Bar Harbour Lobster Bake	1250	55	108
Seafarer's Feast	1140	72	69
Seaside Shrimp Trio	1100	58	94
Ultimate Feast	1120	69	68

Side Dishes:

Baked Potato, Plain	210	2	45
Cheddar Bay Biscuit	160	10	16
Coleslaw	150	10	13
Creamy Lobster Mashed Potatoes	330	18	31
French Fries	290	12	42
Garden Salad, without dressing	110	5	11
Mashed Potatoes	190	9	24
Tomato Mozz. Caprese	160	11	9
Wild Rice Pilaf	160	3	30

Salads:

Caesar Salad: *With Dressing*

with Gr. Chicken	640	48	18
with Gr. Shrimp	610	15	18
With Salmon	830	65	18

Sauces: 100% Pure Melted Butter

	300	33	0
Blue Cheese Dressing	230	24	2
Caesar Dressing	300	32	0
Cocktail Sauce	45	0	11
Honey Mustard Dressing	200	18	9
Marinara Sauce	35	2	4

Desserts:

Brownie Overload	1020	57	121
Chocolate Wave	1110	62	134
Key Lime Pie	400	14	59
Warm Apple Crostada	590	30	74

For Complete Nutritional Data ~ see CalorieKing.com

Red Robin® (Sept '18)

Nutritional Information varies between restaurants. Please refer to Red Robin's website for further information.

Appetizers:

	C	F	Cb
Creamy Artichoke & Spinach Dip	820	44	71
Fried Pickle Nickels	750	52	61
Guacamole, Salsa & Chips	720	35	74
NachO M.G.	1390	74	115
Pretzel Bites	810	40	95
The O-Ring Shorty	920	58	93
Towering Onion Rings	1310	59	179
Voodoo Fries, with Ranch Sauce	1220	74	116

Jump Starters: Without Dressing

Cheese Sticks	550	30	43
Clamstrips	710	53	49
Fresh Fried Mshrms	420	23	53
Sweet Potato Fries	380	15	59
Wisconsin Cheese Curds	730	62	11

Entrées: With Menu Set Sides

Arctic Cod Fish & Steak Fries	1520	89	136
Clucks & Fries	1340	82	104
Ensenada Chicken Platter	480	18	27
Prime Rib Dip	600	25	57
Sear-ious Salmon	480	37	9
Shrimp & Cod Duo	1120	67	94

Burgers: Without Fries or other Options

Finest: Black & Bleu	920	55	51
Citrus Harissa Salmon	1000	69	61
The Marco Pollo	860	44	53
The Southern Charm	1210	68	88
Fire Grilled Burgers: A.1.	1170	73	73
Bleu Ribbon	1130	71	74
Burnin' Love	920	58	60
Chili Chili Chseburger	880	50	56
Grilled Turkey	660	36	53
Guacamole Bacon	1010	67	51
Keep It Simple, Beef	610	33	44
Prime Chophouse	1160	67	88
Red Robin Gourmet Cheeseburger	850	56	47
Royal Red Robin	1190	86	48
Sauteed 'Shroom	840	49	53
Whiskey River BBQ	1210	83	72

Tavern Menu Burgers: Big Ghost

Big Ghost	820	46	58
Big Pig Out	990	63	50
Four Cheese Melt	700	40	49
Red's Big Tavern	870	54	50
The Big Smoky Jack	860	49	59

Red Robin® cont... (Sept '18)

S'wiches & Wraps: W/out Sides

	C	F	Cb
BLTA Croissant	680	40	50
Caesars Chkn Wrap	840	50	61
Nacho Chicken Bacon Wrap	1130	67	82
Philly Cheesesteak Sandwich	910	61	53
Whiskey River BBQ Chicken Wrap	1050	59	81
Wrappin' California Club	990	64	64

Soups:
Baked Potato:

	C	F	Cb
1 Cup	260	15	23
1 Bowl	460	29	39

Clam Chowder: With Slice Garlic Toast

	C	F	Cb
1 Cup	230	13	19
1 Bowl	420	26	32

French Onion: With Slice Garlic Toast

	C	F	Cb
1 Cup	210	11	15
1 Bowl	380	22	23

Salads: Without Dressing

	C	F	Cb
Avo-Cobb-O	550	27	34
Crispy Chicken Tender	910	50	66
Mighty Caesar, with Caesar Dressing	670	51	24
Simply Grilled Chicken	320	9	29
Southwest	890	59	49

Sides: Chili Chili Cheese Fries

	C	F	Cb
	900	60	64
Coleslaw	240	17	19
Mac 'n' Cheese	290	16	25
Onion Rings	280	1	61
Steamed Broccoli	30	0	6
Steak Fries	350	16	48

Desserts:

	C	F	Cb
Gooey Chocolate Brownie Cake	950	37	150
Mountain High Mudd Pie	1360	59	193

Roly Poly® (Sept '18)

Wraps:
Per 6" White Tortilla Unless Indicated

	C	F	Cb
Chicken: Basil Cashew Chicken	300	10	30
Catalina Chicken	315	11	28
Chicken Caesar	310	11	30
Chicken Fajita	315	9	28
Cobb Salad	255	12	27
Oriental Chicken	230	4	29
Santa Fe Chicken	305	11	28
Beef/Ham: Philly Melt	280	11	25
Ranch Roast	320	15	28
Tuna: Classic Tuna Melt	340	17	26
Popeyes Tuna on Wheat	305	10	31
Texas/Thai Hot Tuna, average	300	11	30
Turkey: Applejack	320	12	30
California	330	12	30

Round Table Pizza® (Sept '18)

Appetizers:

	C	F	Cb
Boneless Wings, Oven Roasted:			
with BBQ Sauce (1)	100	2	13
with Buffalo Sauce (1)	90	3.5	8
Garlic Bread: 1 piece	70	3.5	9
with Cheese, 1 piece	110	6	9
Garlic Parmesan Twists, 1 twist	170	5	25

Pizzas: Per ½ of Large 14" Pizza

	C	F	Cb
Original Crust: Cheese	230	10	24
Chicken & Garlic Gourmet	240	10	24
Gourmet Veggie	230	10	25
Guinevere's Garden Delight	220	8	26
Hawaiian	220	8	27
Italian Garlic Supreme	270	14	24
King Arthur Supreme	270	13	26
Maui Zaui, with Polynesian Sce	260	10	29
Montague's All Meat Marvel	290	15	24
Smokehouse Combo, Pepperoni	290	14	27
Triple Play Pepperoni	250	12	24
Pan Crust: Cheese	280	10	35
Chicken & Garlic Gourmet	290	10	35
Gourmet Veggie	280	10	35
Guinevere's Garden Delight	270	9	36
Hawaiian	280	8	37
Italian Garlic Supreme	320	14	35
King Arthur Supreme	320	13	35
Maui Zaui w/ Polynesian Sauce	340	12	41
Montague's All Meat Marvel	340	16	35
Smokehouse Combo, Chicken	350	12	37
Triple Play Pepperoni	330	14	36
Skinny Crust: Cheese	210	10	19
Chicken & Garlic Gourmet	220	11	19
Gourmet Veggie	210	10	20
Guinevere's Garden Delight	200	9	21
Hawaiian	210	8	22
Italian Garlic Supreme	260	15	19
King Arthur Supreme	260	14	21
Maui Zaui w/ Polynesian Sauce	240	11	23
Montague's All Meat Marvel	290	17	20
Smokehouse Combo, Chicken	260	12	22
Triple Play Pepperoni	240	13	19

Sandwiches: Chicken Club

	C	F	Cb
	670	27	58
Ham Club	670	30	59
RT Pizza Veggie	550	21	62
Turkey Club	650	27	59
Tukey Pesto	710	37	56
Turkey Sante-Fe	730	40	57

For Complete Nutritional Data ~ see CalorieKing.com

233

Rubio's Mexican Grill® (Sept '18)

Burritos: Each with Flour Tortilla, with Chips

Beef:	C	F	Cb
Baja Grilled, with Steak	890	34	99
Especial, with Steak	1120	39	149
Chicken:			
Baja Grilled, with Chicken	850	31	100
Especial, with Chicken	1080	36	150
Seafood: Ancho Citrus Shrimp	1040	37	148
Beer Battered Fish	1090	57	119
Classic Grilled Shrimp	930	38	117
Grilled Wild Mahi Mahi	950	37	120
Shrimp & Bacon	1100	53	116
Wild Alaska Coho Salmon	950	38	122

Tacos: Each, with Corn Tortilla Unless Indicated

Original: Fish	330	20	27
Fish, Especial	390	25	29
Chicken, Grilled: Classic	250	13	20
Gourmet	330	19	21
Seafood, Grilled:			
Mango Wild Mahi Mahi, Flour Tortilla	280	15	24
Salsa Verde Shrimp, Flour Tortilla	220	17	24
Wild Alaskan Salmon	230	10	23
Wild Mahi Mahi	230	9	22

Sides:

Black Beans: Reg., 4 oz	120	1.5	19
Large, 9.4 oz	280	2.5	46
Citrus Rice: Reg., 2.3 oz	100	1.5	21
Large, 6 oz	270	4	53
Mexican Rice: Regular, 2.3 oz	100	1.5	20
Large, 6 oz	270	4	53
No Fried Pinto Beans: Reg., 4 oz	120	1	19
Large, 10.9 oz	300	2	51
Tortilla Chips: Regular, 1.8 oz	210	2.5	43
Large, 4 oz	460	5	96
Salsas, average all types	10	0	2

Salad & Bowls: Entrée Size, Includes Dressing

Calif. Bowl, w/ Chkn/Salsa verde	660	23	81
Chipotle Orange Salad, w/ Shrimp	430	26	36
Chopped Salad:			
with Blackened Coho	520	35	27
with Grilled Chicken	480	32	20
with Grilled Mahi Mahi	490	34	19
with Grilled Veggies	440	33	29
with Pan Seared Shrimp	440	33	19

Ruby Tuesday® (Sept '18)

Shareables: As Served

	C	F	Cb
Crispy B'milk Chicken Bites, classic	575	29	34
Shrimp Fondu, with Chips	1035	62	73
Spinach Artichoke Dip, with Chips	1115	68	98
Spicy Pork Rinds	295	12	14

Burgers: With Fries Unless Indicated

Bacon Cheeseburger, w/o fries	815	47	36
Classic Burger	1085	51	98
Classic Cheeseburger, w/o fries	720	39	36
Colossal Burger	1700	89	121
Hickory Bourbon Bacon Burger	1465	77	111
Smokehouse Burger	1395	68	123
Triple Prime Burger	1085	51	98
Triple Prime Cheeseburger	1140	55	98

Lunch/Dinner Entrees: Without Sides

Chicken: Asiago Bacon Chicken	495	28	9
Chicken Bella	290	10	4
Chicken Fresco	370	22	3
Hickory Bourbon	250	5	18
Pasta & More:			
Chicken & Broccoli	1405	83	101
Crispy Chicken Mac 'N Cheese	1310	67	91
Parmesan Shrimp Pasta	505	20	48
Primavera	1230	83	86
with Grilled Chicken	1410	87	87
with Grilled Shrimp	1290	83	86
Ribs & Chops:			
Hickory Boubon Pork Chop	570	22	23
Classic BBQ Ribs: Half Rack	470	22	21
Full Rack	940	47	42
Texas Dusted Ribs: Half Rack	590	33	24
Full Rack	1100	68	30
Seafood:			
Grilled Salmon	490	30	0
Blackened Tilapia	205	6	2
Hickory Bourbon Salmon	575	30	18
New Orleans Seafood	345	14	4
Steak: New York Strip, 10 oz	565	40	0
Hickory B'rbon Bacon Sirloin, 6 oz	285	7	12
Ribeye, 12 oz	760	55	1
Top Sirloin, 8 oz	420	22	2

Updated Nutrition Data ~ www.CalorieKing.com
Persons with Diabetes ~ See Disclaimer (Page 22)

Ruby Tuesday® cont... (Sept '18)

Sandwiches: With French Fries

	C	F	Cb
Avocado Grilled Chicken	1220	59	101
Avocado Turkey Burger	1265	67	102
Crispy Chicken: Original	1235	55	133
BBQ Ranch	1445	67	148
with Pimento	1655	96	137
Grilled Chicken	1045	44	99

Sides:

	C	F	Cb
Braised Greens	85	3	8
Caesar Salad, with Caesar Dressing	385	31	16
Dirty Rice	215	5	31
French Fries	505	24	63
Fresh: Baked Potato	250	3	51
Grilled Zucchini	15	0	2
Steamed Broccoli	45	2	5
Garden Salad, without Dressing	265	18	13
Lemon Pepper Coleslaw	255	23	7
Loaded Baked Potato	560	27	51
Mashed Potatoes	295	16	32
Onion Rings	350	19	37
Rice Pilaf	190	1	40
Southern Green Beans	130	6	10
Sweet Potato Fries	445	23	55
White Chedd. Bacon Mac 'N Chse	290	15	19

Salads: With Standard Components & Dressing

	C	F	Cb
BBQ Chicken Cobb	745	46	21
Kickin' Chicken Caesar	1255	90	52
Southern Fried Chicken	490	31	16

Soups:

	C	F	Cb
Broccoli & Cheese	260	18	17
Garden Vegetable	85	1	16
Roasted Tomato	270	14	24

Desserts: As Served

	C	F	Cb
Apple Crumble Skillet	875	46	103
Cake: Caramel Crunch	760	37	99
Chocolate Fall	1375	59	180
Key Lime	765	44	86
Oreo Cookies & Cream	725	32	95
New York Cheesecake	975	61	90
Peach Melba Tart	640	31	78

For Complete Menu ~ see CalorieKing.com

Runza® (Sept '18)

Burgers:

	C	F	Cb
¼ LB: BBQ Bacon & Swiss	530	32	26
Bacon Cheeseburger	510	31	23
Cheeseburger	400	22	23
French Onion	490	29	26
Hamburger	350	18	21
Spicy Jack	570	38	23
Swiss cheese Mushroom	480	29	24

Chicken Sandwiches:

	C	F	Cb
BBQ Grilled	400	11	40
Buffalo/Deluxe, av.	360	11	37
Spicy Jack Grilled	530	27	35
Wraps: Buffalo Jr. Chicken	320	16	31
Ranch Jr. Chicken	310	16	31

Chicken Strips, 2 pieces | 220 | 12 | 14 |

Runza Sandwiches: Original

	C	F	Cb
Runza Sandwiches: Original	530	20	67
BBQ Bacon Runza	730	34	72
BLT Runza	745	40	68
Cheese Runza	580	24	69
Original Runza	530	20	67
Spicy Jack Runza	750	41	69
Swiss Cheese Mushroom Runza	620	28	68

Sides:

	C	F	Cb
Chili	290	11	26
French Fries: Small	210	9	28
Medium	300	13	40
Large	440	19	59
French Onion Dip	70	5	3
Frings, Medium	320	17	39
Onion Rings: Medium	320	19	35
Large	550	31	58

Salads: Without Dressing

	C	F	Cb
Southwest Chicken Salad, w/ Salsa	310	15	26
Side Salad	20	0	4
Sweet Berry Chicken	370	19	21

Dressings:

	C	F	Cb
Honey Mustard	200	18	9
Ranch	180	18	3

Soups: Per Bowl

	C	F	Cb
Boston Clam Chowder	280	15	29
Broccoli Cheese	240	16	20
Chicken Tortilla	150	6	16
Potato Bacon	260	14	30

Kids:

	C	F	Cb
Junior: Cheeseburger, plain	250	13	18
Hamburger, plain	200	9	16
Swiss Cheese Mushroom Burger	300	17	17

Desserts:

	C	F	Cb
Choc. Chip Cookie	370	18	53
Ice Cream Cones, all flavors	210	6	32
Shake, Cappuccino, regular	490	12	82
Sundaes: Caramel; Chocolate	300	7	51
Turtle	360	13	53

7-Eleven® (Sept '18)

Breakfast Sandwiches:

	C	F	Cb
Biscuits:			
Sausage, 3.3 oz	330	22	28
Spicy Chicken, 4.5 oz	270	14	30
Croissants:			
Sausage, Egg & Cheese, 4.7 oz	450	32	23
English Muffin:			
Egg, Bacon & Chse, 4.5 oz	300	14	28
Egg, Cheese & Sausage, 5 oz	390	25	24
Salads: Per Container			
Balsamic Garden Salad,			
with Chicken, 6.5 oz	170	9	18
BLT, 8 oz	270	18	12
Caprese Salad, 4.5 oz	150	11	7
Chicken Caesar, 7.5 oz	390	28	17
Chicken Caesar Pasta Salad, 9 oz	540	24	61
Kale & Quinoa Salad, 6 oz	300	18	30
Mediterranean Pasta Salad, 8.5 oz	490	29	49
Side, 5 oz	30	0	7
Sandwiches/Melts:			
Chicken, Bacon Ranch Melt, 7.4 oz	560	22	56
Chicken Salad Sandwich, 6.6 oz	470	21	49
Double Cheeseburger,			
with American Cheese, 9.6 oz	800	54	35
Egg Salad Sandwich, 6.8 oz	480	24	50
Go!Smart Turkey Sandwich	300	2.5	48
Grilled Chicken Sandwich,			
with Honey Mustard BBQ Sauce, 6 oz	340	10	39
Italian Melt, 7.8 oz	610	39	38
Southwest Turkey Sandwich, 8 oz	560	28	48
Steak & Cheese Melt, 7.8 oz	680	35	57
Sides:			
Hash Browns (1), 2 oz	100	5	12
Potato Wedges (6), 0.7 oz	240	4.5	27
Taquitos:			
Chicken & Monterey Jack, (2), 5.3 oz	330	12	44
Drinks: Cappuccino, 8 fl.oz	180	4	36
Caramel Macchiato, 8 fl.oz	190	5	34
Cuban Coffee, with milk, 8 fl.oz	200	7	34
French Vanilla Cappuccino, 8 fl.oz	190	6	34
Skinny, 8 fl.oz	140	4.5	30
Hot Chocolate, 8 fl.oz	170	2.5	37
Peppermint Mocha, 8 fl.oz	180	4	36
Pumpkin Spice Late, 8 fl.oz	190	6	35
Slurpees, average all flavors:			
12 oz cup	95	0	26
22 oz cup	175	0	44
28 oz cup	220	0	56
Sugar Free, 12 oz cup	30	0	9

Saladworks® (Sept '18)

Salads: W/out Dressing or Bread	C	F	Cb
Bently	290	15	11
Buffalo Bleu	350	12	29
Chicken Caesar	370	15	29
Cobb	370	23	19
Farmhouse	270	12	28
Fire Roasted Cabo	350	17	25
Greek	200	11	17
Mandarin Chicken	230	4	25
Mediterranean	330	23	16
Sophie's Salad	310	13	35
Thai Chicken	200	6	20
Tivoli	470	21	41
Turkey Club	290	7	38
Paninis: Buffalo Chicken	870	36	85
Caprese	940	47	94
Chicken Parmesan	870	32	93
Turkey Melt	1020	49	90
Sandwiches: Avocado BLT	830	55	60
Loaded Chicken Salad	370	9	28
Tuna Salad	410	8	57
West Coast Turkey	580	30	51
Wraps: Bentley	550	21	63
Buffalo Bleu	660	20	82
Chicken Caesar	610	20	81
Cobb	690	33	71
Farmhouse	590	20	82
Fire Roasted Cabo	670	25	78
Madarin Chicken	530	12	83
Mediterranean	650	34	92
Sophie's Salad	550	17	81
Thai Chicken	410	9	70
Tivoli	610	27	63
Turkey Club	460	14	61
Soups: Per Medium Serve, without Bread Roll			
Baked Potato	345	23	28
Broccoli Cheddar	275	19	18
Chicken Dumpling	180	5.5	21
Chicken Noodle	180	5	18
Chicken Tortilla	260	14	19
Homestyle Tomato	300	21	25
Lasagna, with Turkey Sausage	235	11	21
Maine Lobster Bisque	470	39	21
New England Clam Chowder	370	26	22

Sandella's® (Sept '18)

Grilled Flatbread:

	C	F	Cb
Buffalo Chicken	420	10	47
Brazilian Bacon	560	17	79
Brazilian Chicken	510	10	73
El Paso	710	19	97
Hawaiian	610	17	89
Meatball	630	29	56
Pesto Chicken	610	28	56
Spinach & Bacon	660	39	52
Without Meat:			
Artichoke	570	23	65
Brazillian	440	9	71
Healthy Veggie	360	7	54
Italian Veggie	400	10	59
Pesto & Peppers	530	27	52

Paninis: With Standard Toppings

	C	F	Cb
Americana	580	25	54
Arizona Chicken	660	23	78
BBQ Chicken	490	2.5	92
Beef Fajita	640	28	59
Bistro Ham & Brie	560	19	70
Brazilian Beef, without cheese	500	6	86
Holiday Ham	770	21	110
Napoli Chicken	440	17	50
Pastrami Melt	500	15	52
Philly Cheese	590	25	55
Spinach, Ham & Swiss	550	20	61
Tuscan Chicken	540	21	55

Quesadillas: With Standard Toppings

	C	F	Cb
California	500	23	53
Mediterranean	400	16	53
Thai Veggie	570	27	59
Veggie & Mozzarella	340	7	53

Salads: Includes ½ Flatbread

	C	F	Cb
Fiesta, with Light Bals. Vinaigrette	360	8	54
Greek, with Light Bals. Vinaigrette	310	15	37
Santa Fe	420	24	35

Rice Bowls: Includes Flatbread & Standard Toppings

	C	F	Cb
Black Bean & Rice	840	20	130
Chicken Fajita	750	20	104
Roma Pesto	740	23	107
Thai Peanut Saute	680	16	116

Wraps: With Standard Toppings

	C	F	Cb
California Turkey	410	10	55
Chipotle Chicken	350	7	55
Pesto Turkey	460	15	54
Sweet & Spicy Chicken	400	7	64

Sarku Japan® (Sept '18)

Bento Box:

	C	F	Cb
Fried Rice: Beef	830	32	98
Chicken	820	35	95
Shrimp	750	27	96

D'Lite Meals:

	C	F	Cb
Vegetarian:			
Fried Rice	430	10	79
Noodles	640	14	109
Steamed Rice	410	6	83

Teriyaki Meals: With Steamed Rice

	C	F	Cb
Beef	580	16	80
Beef & Shrimp	690	21	85
Chicken	640	24	79
Chicken & Shrimp	750	29	85
Shrimp	530	12	80

Sushi Hand Rolls: Per Roll

	C	F	Cb
Salmon Skin	210	7	27
Seafood	170	1.5	29
Spicy Tuna	180	3.5	27
Sauce, Teriyaki, 1.5 oz	45	0	9
Sides: Chicken Egg Roll	160	6	21
Dumplings (6)	260	12	29
Edamame	170	7	11
Miso Soup	50	2	6
Seaweed Salad	70	2	13
Shrimp Tempura (3)	390	30	23
Vegetable Spring Roll	190	9	15

Schlotzsky's® (Sept '18)

Sandwiches:

Angus:

	C	F	Cb
Corned Beef Reuben	890	38	81
Pastrami & Swiss	830	33	79
Pastrami Reuben	900	40	84
Chipotle Chicken	530	9	78
Deluxe Original	980	47	81
Fiesta Chicken	810	31	78
Fresh Veggie	500	14	74
Ham & Cheese, Original	730	25	81
Roast Beef & Cheese	780	30	81
Smoked Turkey Breast	500	6	80
The Original	780	34	78
The Sicilian	730	43	42
The Tuscan	700	35	49
Traditional Brisket	780	30	82
Turkey Bacon Club	770	30	81
Turkey Original	820	33	81
Turkey & Guacamole	520	11	78

continued next page...

Schlotzsky's® cont... (Sept '18)

10" Pizzas: Per Pizza	C	F	Cb
BBQ Chkn & Jalapeno	920	21	148
Combination Special	960	38	119
Double Cheese	840	27	115
Fresh Veggie	920	35	118
Grilled Chicken & Pesto	910	29	114
Pepperoni & Double Cheese	980	42	115
Mac: Brisketeer	1090	49	69
Double Cheese	920	51	67
Poultry In Motion	1130	47	70
Shrimpy The Best	1070	45	71
Smokey Brisketeer	1120	50	74
Salads: Without Dressing or Breadsticks			
Chicken Caesar	680	17	29
Cranberry, Apple, Pecan & Chicken	640	27	68
Southwest Chicken	600	29	44
Turkey Avocado Cobb	610	33	42
Soup: Per 10 ozBowl			
Broccoli Cheese	185	12	14
Chicken & Wild Rice	280	14	25
Chicken Tortilla	315	16	27
Loaded Baked Potato	385	31	29
Timberline Chili	380	21	27
Tomato Basil	320	26	21
Chips:			
Baked: Regular; BBQ	130	3	25
Other varieties, average	230	14	24
Kidz Meals: Without Cookie or Drink			
Cheese Pizza	540	17	78
Ham Sandwich	220	2	40
Pepperoni Pizza	590	22	78
Turkey Sandwich	220	2	40
Desserts:			
Brownie (1)	370	19	49
Cookies: Chocolate Chip (1)	160	7	24
Oatmeal Raisin; Sugar, (1), av.	155	5	24
Breakfast: Per Whole Burrito/Sandwich			
Burritos: Bacon	460	22	41
Ham	490	21	4
Sausage	570	31	41
Veggie	430	19	44
Sandwiches: Bacon	500	21	51
Ham	530	22	50
Sausage	650	32	49
Veggie	500	21	51
Tacos: Bacon; Sausage, average	250	14	18
Ham	290	17	18
Veggie	220	10	21
Sides: Hash Brown, 1 piee	60	5	8
Mixed Fruit, 1 scoop	20	0	6

Second Cup® ~ see CalorieKing.com

Shakey's® (Sept '18)

Pizzas: Per Slice, 1/10 Medium Size	C	F	Cb
Big Island: Pan Crust	210	6	30
Thin Crust	160	6	19
California Pizzarito: Pan Crust	265	12	30
Thin Crust	215	11	19
Cheese: Pan Crust	190	5	30
Thin Crust	135	5	17
Firehouse: Pan Crust	280	13	30
Thin Crust	230	12	20
Garden Veggie: Pan Crust	205	6	30
Thin Crust	150	6	19
Rustic Garlic Chicken: Pan Crust	215	6	30
Thin Crust	160	6	18
Shakey's Special: Pan Crust	255	11	30
Thin Crust	200	10	18
Texas BBQ Chicken: Pan Crust	220	6	32
Thin Crust	165	5	20
Ultimate Meat: Pan Crust	310	15	30
Thin Crust	260	14	20
Rice: Mexican Rice, 1/2 cup	100	0	22
Pilaf, 1/2 cup	120	3	22
Sides & Extras: Enchilada (1)	80	2	37
Boneless Chicken Strip (1)	125	7	10
Garlic Bread, 1 piece	180	4	30
Macaroni & Cheese, 1 cup	350	17	33
Macaroni Salad, 1/2 cup	220	14	19
Mashed Potatoes, 1/2 cup	65	1	13
Mojo Potatoes, medium	430	23	51
Potato Salad, 1/2 cup	100	3	17
Golden Fried Chicken: Per Piece			
Breast	360	11	16
Leg	175	10	6
Thigh	350	24	9
Wing	130	9	4

Shari's® (Sept '18)

Breakfast: As Served	C	F	Cb
Bacon & Eggs without extras	290	22	2
BMP Omelette	850	71	7
Bone-In Hickory Ham & Potato P'cakes	880	38	75
Buttermilk Pancakes	420	10	73
Country Omelette without extras	670	52	8
Denver Omelette without extras	650	51	10
Eggs Benedict with Hashbrowns	830	47	66
French Toast	780	51	68
Fresh Caramel Pecan Cinn. Roll	1190	41	182
Meat Lover's Skillet	1240	98	39
Panini	980	61	70
Sausage & Eggs without extras	630	57	2

Updated Nutrition Data ~ www.CalorieKing.com
Persons with Diabetes ~ See Disclaimer (Page 22)

Shari's® cont... (Sept '18)

Breakfast (Cont): *As Served*

	C	F	Cb
Shari's Potato Pancakes	570	17	96
The Shari's Sampler	1100	76	60
Ultimate Country Fried Steak	1070	72	69
USDA Top Sirloin Steak	790	52	32
Waffle without extras	250	4	49

Lunch: *Without Side Choices*

	C	F	Cb
Burgers: Bavarian	970	43	60
Bleu Cheeseburger	630	34	41
Cheddar Cheesebuger	660	36	41
Hamburger	580	30	41
Pepperjack Cheese	680	38	41
Ranch Hand BBQ Bacon Chsebgr	1090	72	60
Swiss Cheeseburger	620	33	41
Flatbread Paninis, Pastrami	700	28	58
Quiche: BMP Trio	390	27	23
Ham & Cheese Trio	380	25	22

Salads: *Entrée Size, with Dressing*

	C	F	Cb
Northwest Steak	850	45	66
Rustic Tuscan Chicken	510	32	21
Salmon Caesar	940	66	43

Sandwiches: *Per Whole Sandwich*

	C	F	Cb
Crispy Chicken BLT	890	56	64
Cuban, on Ciabatta	540	23	47
Prime Rib Dip	540	21	52

Dinner: *With Menu Set Sides & Bread*

	C	F	Cb
Beer Battered Fish & Chips	1700	132	110
Cedar Plank Salmon	750	44	48
Chicken Mushroom Alfredo	1130	46	117
Country Fried Steak Dinner	1310	80	112
Gr. Chkn Mozzarella Bruschetta	610	28	48
Slow Cooked Pot Roast	1440	78	91
Slow Roasted Turkey	920	35	96

Sides, Add-Ons:

	C	F	Cb
Baked Potato, Plain	160	0	37
French Fries	370	24	36
Loaded Mashed Potatoes	410	21	42
Onion Rings (6)	390	24	39
Red Skin Mshd Potato	260	8	40
Rice Pilaf	90	5	10
Sauteed Button Mushrooms	220	23	1
Shrimp Scampi	360	30	2
Stuffed Hashbrowns	420	28	32

Shari's® cont... (Sept '18)

Sides, Add-Ons (Cont):

	C	F	Cb
Shrimp Skewers (2)	190	11	1
Steakhouse Mac 'n Cheese	510	27	45
Tater Tots: Plain	370	26	33
with Chipotle Mayo	650	56	36

Desserts: *Per Slice*

	C	F	Cb
Cheesecake	350	22	34
Chocolate Lava Cake	660	27	100

Classic Pies:

	C	F	Cb
Banana Cream Dream	460	24	53
Chocolate Cream Supreme	540	30	62

Gourmet Pies:

	C	F	Cb
Creamy Caramel Pecan Crunch	770	49	76
Peanut Butter Chocolate Silk	660	45	60
S'mores Galore	560	31	68
Velvet Chocolate Silk	580	38	56

Sheetz® (Sept '18)

Breakfast Sandwiches:

	C	F	Cb
Dreamy Bacon Croissant	400	22	33
Twisted BLT	710	42	53
Walker Breakfast Ranger	550	23	58
Burgerz: Big Mozz	600	27	48
Boss Bacon	710	50	26
Cowboy	650	33	46
Twisted Swiss	730	40	50

Hot Dogs: *With Standard Hot Dog*

	C	F	Cb
BLT Hot Dog	450	28	33
Firehouse	390	22	35
Junkyard	340	16	38
Philly	340	17	35
Shmokehouse	370	18	37

Mac & Cheese Platter:

	C	F	Cb
Boom Chicka	510	27	40
Meatball	610	37	35
Morning	480	28	35
Szechuan Fire	370	15	37

Sandwichez:

	C	F	Cb
Deli: Boom Boom BLT	820	46	52
Ciabatta Bing	620	34	53
Garden of Eatin	440	16	54
Grilled Chicken: Big Mozz	560	18	51
Carolina Slaw	440	16	37
Twisted Brunch	780	40	50

Subz: *Per Half*

	C	F	Cb
Big Philly Sub, on Pretzel Sub	640	25	66
Cali Turkey Flatbread Sub	720	43	44
Protein Parm, on Herb Sub	460	15	47
Southwest Veggie, on White Sub	440	18	56
Spring Chicken Flatbread Sub	450	19	39

continued next page...

Fast - Foods & *Restaurants*

Sheetz® cont... (Sept '18)

Sidez:

	C	F	Cb
Coleslaw	80	3.5	12
Crispy Chicken Stripz: 3 pieces	330	11	39
5 pieces	550	18	65
Fryz, w/out sauce, 1 cup	390	13	64
Hard Cooked Egg (1)	70	4.5	0
Jalapeno Poppers, w/out Sce	330	18	35
Loaded Fryz, plain	600	20	97
Mac & Cheese, plain, 1 order	190	7	25
Onion Rings, no sauce, 1 cup	470	27	52
Popcorn Chicken, without Sauce:			
Regular	300	14	28
Large	610	28	55

Sizzler® (Sept '18)

Burgers & Sandwiches:

	C	F	Cb
⅓ lb Burgers: Bacon Cheeseburger	950	67	44
Classic: Burger	830	57	44
Cheese Burger	920	64	45
Double Mega Bacon	1250	91	44
Malibu Melt	1840	155	69
Turkey Patty	510	30	39
Sandwiches: Double Hibachi Chkn	440	4	14
Grilled Chicken Club	580	19	39
Malibu Chicken	870	63	52

Hot Entrées: Small, without Sides, Condiments, Dipping Sauce or Optional Accompaniments

	C	F	Cb
Chicken: Grilled Hibachi Chicken	220	2	7
Italian-Herb Chicken, 7 oz	230	6	1
Malibu Chicken, Single	680	60	14
Pasta: Fettuccine Alfredo	960	51	85
Cajun Penne	1030	71	108
Ribs:			
BBQ: 6 bones	1870	145	32
9 Bones	2820	213	61
Seafood: Fish & Chips, 2 pieces	1410	102	93
Grilled Salmon, 6 oz	370	23	3
Ultimate Shrimp Trio	1230	62	85
Steaks:			
Burgundy Mushroom Sirloin Tips	480	16	38
Combos: Steak & Hibachi Chicken	500	14	20
Steak & Lobster Tail	720	51	2
Steak & Malibu Chicken	920	62	30
Porterhouse, 20 oz	1430	108	2
Tri Tip: Slow Roast BBQ, 5 oz	680	39	52
6 oz	790	44	54
Tri Tip Sirloin: 8 oz	340	16	0.5
10 oz	440	20	3
12 oz	530	24	3

Sizzler® cont... (Sept '18)

Sides:

	C	F	Cb
Baked Potato: Foil	350	13	54
Loaded Foil	530	32	54
Salted	510	30	55
Loaded	760	57	55
Baked Yam with Maple Topping	410	11	75
Balsamic Brussels Sprouts	150	7	20
Broccoli, steamed	40	0	7
with Butter	70	4.5	7
Button Mushroom Saute	180	17	5
Cilantro Lime Rice	150	7	20
Garlic Mashed Potatoes	150	2.5	9
Green Beans	80	5	8
Grilled Onions	80	6	7
Roasted Corn with Herb Butter	80	2.5	13
Roasted Red Potatoes	130	0	8
Spinach Saute	70	1.5	5
Street Fries, 5 oz	350	22	37
Sweet Potato Fries	610	48	39
Vegetable Medley	80	45	8
Zucchini Planks	20	0	3

For Complete Menu & Data ~ see CalorieKing.com

Skyline Chili® (Sept '18)

Burritos:

	C	F	Cb
Chili Deluxe	610	33	38
Original	610	31	54
Coneys/Sandwiches:			
Coneys: Cheese, w/ onions & mstrd	350	23	25
Coney, plain	220	13	22
Sandwiches: Chili Cheese,			
with onions & mustard	290	17	24
Plain, with onions & mustard, av.	180	8	23
Ways: Per Regular Serving			
Chili Spaghetti with Bean & Onion:			
Small	250	10	34
Regular	490	19	68
Large	670	26	94
Bowls: Chili	200	12	0
Loaded Chili	480	28	20
Vegetarian Black Beans & Rice	400	14	48
Steamed Potatoes: 3-Way Potato	620	26	65
Cheddar Potato	630	33	65
Sour Cream Potato	460	19	65
Salads: Without Dressing			
Buffalo Chicken	220	11	12
Greek	210	12	17
Fries: Chili Cheese	840	53	61
Regular	430	24	51

240

Updated Nutrition Data ~ www.CalorieKing.com
Persons with Diabetes ~ See Disclaimer (Page 22)

Smoothie King® (Sept '18)

Fruit Smoothies: Per 20 oz Cup **C** **F** **Cb**
Figures Include Turbinado. Without Turbinado, deduct 100 calories and 23 carbs.

Fitness Blends:

	C	F	Cb
Orig. High Protein: Banana	315	9	32
Chocolate	365	9	42
Pineapple	315	9	29
Peanut Power Plus:			
Chocolate	700	26	98
Strawberry	680	21	112
The Activator:			
Blueberry Strawberry	300	1.5	49
Chocolate	220	3	24
Strawberry Banana	270	1.5	42
The Hulk: Chocolate	770	27	110
Strawberry	910	27	145
Vanilla	770	27	110

Slim Blends:

	C	F	Cb
Slim-N-Trim: Chocolate	250	3	41
Strawberry	240	2	52
Vanilla	210	2.5	40

Take A Break Blends:

	C	F	Cb
Banana Boat	470	4	101
Caribbean Way	380	0	97
Muscle Punch	360	0.5	85
Pineapple Surf	420	1	98
Yogurt D-Lite	330	4	60
Wellness Blends: Acai Adventure	450	3	101
Carrot Kale Dream	290	1	67

32 fl.oz Cup: Multiply 20 fl.oz figures by 1.5
40 fl.oz Cup: Multiply 20 fl.oz figures by 2
Kids Cup Smoothies: *Per 12 fl.oz Cup*

	C	F	Cb
Apple Kiwi Bunga	180	0	45
Choc-A-Laka	200	2	41
Lil' Angel	190	0	49

Snappy Tomato® (Sept '18)

	C	F	Cb
Snappetizers: Bone In Wings(6)	460	34	4
Wedge Fries, plain	220	10	28
Pasta: Plain Spaghetti/Rigatoni, av.	350	1.5	71
Toppings: Bacon	120	8	0.5
Black or Green Olives	50	4.5	2
Cheese	90	7	1
Chicken	120	2.5	1
Onions	10	0	3
Pepperoni	140	10	0
Tomatoes	5	0	1
Sauce: Ranch	570	60	8
Snappy	80	2	8
Salads: Crispy Chicken, w/o dressing	280	9	24
Garden, withgout dressing	90	4.5	11
Grilled Chicken, without dressing	160	2.5	10
Dessert, Brownie Bites	500	30	60

Sonic Drive-In® (Sept '18)

Burgers: **C** **F** **Cb**

	C	F	Cb
Bacon Cheeseburger, with Mayo	770	46	53
Bacon Dble Cheeseburger, with Mayo	1030	65	54
Cheeseburger: w/ Mayo	680	39	54
with Ketchup	600	28	58
¼ lb Double Cheeseburger w/ Mayo	960	59	55
Jalapeno Dble Chseburger, w/ Mstrd	850	48	54
Jr. Burger	330	16	32
Jr. Deluxe Cheeseburger	440	27	32
Veggie Burger, with Mayo	530	22	69

Chicken:

	C	F	Cb
Sandwiches: Classic Crispy Chicken	570	31	51
Classic Grilled Chicken	490	22	42
Crispy Tender Chicken	460	24	41
Wings: Asian Sweet Chili (6)	470	24	32
Honey BBQ (6)	470	24	33
Buffalo (6)	440	28	17
Tenders: Crispy 3 piece Dinner	280	14	16
5 piece Dinner	470	24	26

Coneys & 6" Hot Dogs:

	C	F	Cb
All American Dog	410	21	41
Chicago Dog	400	20	41
Chili Cheese Coney	470	29	34
New York Dog	400	23	35
Original Pretzel Dog	320	20	23
Wraps: Crispy Chicken	510	22	56
Grilled Chicken	410	14	39
Natural Cut Fries: Small	250	12	33
Medium	290	13	38
Large	470	22	63

Sides: *Per Medium Serving*

	C	F	Cb
Ched 'R' Peppers	710	48	56
Chili Cheese Fries	450	26	42
Handmade Onion Rings	580	29	74
Mozzarella Sticks	590	29	61
Tots with Cheese	450	28	43

Breakfast:

	C	F	Cb
Breakfast Bacon Toaster	610	31	52
Breakfast Burrito: Bacon	470	25	35
Ham	440	20	38
Sausage	500	30	35
CroiSonic Sandwich: with Bacon	560	37	31
with Sausage	670	49	31
Cinnasnacks (3), without Frosting	340	15	44
French Toast Sticks, (4) w/out Syrup	480	25	54

continued next page...

Sonic Drive-In® cont... (Sept '18)

	C	F	Cb
Ice Cream Cone,			
Vanilla	250	12	30
Ice Cream Sundaes:			
Caramel; Chocolate, av.	505	22	69
Hot Fudge	520	26	65
Strawberry	440	21	55
Add Ons, Pecans	60	6	1
Classic Shakes: *Per Medium*			
Caramel	920	43	118
Chocolate	900	41	119
Fresh Banana	850	41	108
Hot Fudge	940	48	113
Peanut Butter	1110	72	96
Strawberry	830	41	104
Vanilla	820	45	89
Master Shakes: *Per Medium*			
Cheesecake	840	43	101
Oreo Cheesecake	1030	51	131
Oreo Chocolate	1090	49	148
Oreo Peanut Butter	1300	80	125
Strawberry Cheesecake	930	43	124
Sonic Blast: *Per Medium*			
Butterfingers Pieces	960	48	121
Choc. Chip Cookie Dough	990	57	111
M&M's Minis Choc. Candy	1060	54	127
Oreo Pieces	860	44	103
Reese's Peanut Butter Cups	990	55	110
Snickers Bars	890	46	103
Lemonade: Small	160	0	42
Medium	270	0	69
Large	400	0	105
Frozen Limeade: Small	190	0	53
Medium	280	0	74
Large	430	0	116
Iced Coffee: *Per Medium*			
Original, no add ins	100	6	11
French Vanilla add in	140	6	20
Praline Pecan add in	140	6	20

For Complete Nutritional Data ~ see CalorieKing.com

Souplantation® (Sept '18)

	C	F	Cb
Soups: *Per 3 fl.oz Cup*			
Asian Ginger Broth	10	0.5	2
Big Chunk Chicken Noodle	35	1	4
Deep Kettle Chili	90	3	11
Yankee Clipper Clam Chowder	265	19	19

Souplantation® cont... (Sept '18)

	C	F	Cb
Hot Bar: *Per Cup*			
Classic Macaroni & Cheese	340	13	44
Four Cheese Alfredo with Fettuccine	320	11	44
Garden Fresh Veggie Marinara w/ Spag.	250	5	41
Prepared Salads: *Per ½ Cup*			
Ancient Grains Quinoa Blend	40	0.5	7
Joan's Broccoli Madness	160	12	10
Fresh Herb Slaw	70	5	5
Picnic Macaroni, with Ham	190	11	18
Tuna Tarragon	210	11	21
Bakery:			
Bread: Buttermilk Cornbread,			
1 piece	140	5	21
Multigrain, East Coast, vegan	80	2	12
Sourdough: Californian, vegetarian	70	0	13
West Coast, vegan	110	0	22
Focaccia: Cheesy Garlic,	60	2	9
Quattro Formaggio	70	2	9
Muffins: Brownie Bite (1)	170	11	18
Lemon (1), gluten free	200	8	29
Wild Blueberry (1)	160	7	22
Desserts: *Per ½ Cup*			
Creamy Almond Rice Pudding	140	2.5	25
Chocolate Chip Cookie Bar (1)	90	4	12
Red Raspberry Gelatin	110	0	26
Soft Serve, Chocolate/Vanilla, av.	100	2	20
Tapioca Pudding	140	2.5	25

For Complete Nutritional Data ~ see CalorieKing.com

Southern Tsunami® (Sept '18)

	C	F	Cb
Rolls: *With White Rice*			
Hybrid:			
Berry: Eel, 6 oz	240	6	43
Immitation Crab	230	5	44
Blueberry: Salmon, 8 oz	360	16	45
Smoked Steelhead, 8 oz	340	13	45
Tuna, 8 oz	340	15	45
Crunchy Dragon Roll: Salmon, 8 oz	560	31	59
Steelhead, 8 oz	530	28	59
Done Deal, Tuna, 7 oz	330	12	41
Happy Mango, 8 oz	410	19	51
Jalapeno, Tuna, 8 oz	290	10	48
Mango Shrimp, 6 oz	360	19	42
Red Rock, 7 oz	360	14	44
Spicy Mango, Tuna, 8 oz	380	20	45
Ultimate Chili, Salmon, 6 oz	290	11	39

242

Southern Tsunami® cont... (Sept '18)

Rolls (Cont): With White Rice

	C	F	Cb
Chef Samplers:			
A, 5.5 oz	240	7	37
Premium, 5.5 oz	260	9	35
Plus Rolls: *Per 12 oz*			
California	450	8	88
Cream Cheese Plus: Eel	620	25	82
Salmon/Smoked	590	23	76
Seaside Plus: Eel	670	21	103
Salmon	620	18	91
Spicy Plus: Salmon	640	28	78
Yellowtail	670	29	78
Vegetable Plus Combo	430	8	89
Wraps: Berry, 4.6 oz	200	9	28
California, 6.6 oz	270	15	26
Cream Cheese & Tuna, 6.6 oz	230	14	39
Mango, 6.6 oz	130	4.5	22
Spicy Crm Chse & Salmon, 6.6 oz	320	23	15
Salads: Without Dressing			
Edamame, 8 oz	300	6	30
Hawaiian Poke, w/ Steelhead, 14 oz	790	38	94
Sea Breeze, 4 oz	90	2.5	17
Tropical Mango, 7.5 oz	290	25	14
Dressings/Sauces:			
Ginger Dressing, 2 Tbsp	50	1.5	8
Peanut Sauce, 1.4 oz	60	0	12
Sweet Chili Sauce, 1.4 oz	100	0	24
Wasabi Dressing, 2 Tbsp	35	2	2

Starbucks® (Sept '18)

Brewed Coffee: Per 16 fl.oz Grande without Whipped Cream

Caffe Misto (Au Lait):	C	F	Cb
with Coconut Milk	70	4.5	7
with Nonfat Milk	70	0	10
with Soy Milk	100	3	13
with Whole Milk	130	7	10

Chocolate: Per 16 fl.oz Grande without Whipped Cream

Hot Chocolate:			
with 2% Milk	320	9	47
with Coconut Milk	270	10	42
with Soy Milk	320	8	51
with Whole Milk	360	13	47
White Chocolate Mocha:			
with 2% Milk	360	11	53
with Nonfat Milk	310	5	53
with Soy Milk	360	9	57
with Whole Milk	400	15	53

Starbucks® cont... (Aug '18)

Hot Espresso Beverages:

Per 16 fl.oz Grande without Whipped Cream

	C	F	Cb
Caffe Latte: with Coconut Milk	140	8	14
with Nonfat Milk	130	0	20
with Soy Milk	190	6	24
with Whole Milk	230	12	19
Cappuccino: with Coconut Milk	140	8	14
with Nonfat Milk	80	0	12
with Soy Milk	120	3.5	16
with Whole Milk	140	7	12
Caramel Macchiato: Coconut Milk	200	8	32
with Nonfat Milk	200	1.5	36
with Soy Milk	250	6	39
with Whole Milk	280	11	35
Cinn. Dolce Latte: Coconut Milk	220	7	37
with Nonfat Milk	220	0	42
with Whole Milk	310	11	41
Espresso: 1 Doppio, 2 fl.oz	10	0	2
1 Solo, 1 fl.oz	5	0	1
Espresso Con Panna, 1 Solo, 1 fl.oz	30	2.5	2
Latte Macchiato: with 2% Milk	190	7	19
with Soy Milk	180	5	23
with Whole Milk	220	11	19

Iced Espresso: Per 16 fl.oz Grande w/out Whipped Cream

Caffe Latte: with Coconut Milk	90	5	10
with Nonfat Milk	90	0	13
with Soy Milk	130	3.5	17
with Whole Milk	150	7	13
Vanilla Latte: with 2% Milk	190	4	30
with Coconut Milk	160	4.5	28
with Nonfat Milk	160	0	31
with Whole Milk	210	6	30

Fizzios, Ginger Ale; Lemon Ale,

Orange Cream, 16 fl oz Grande, av.	100	0	26

Frappuccino Blended: Cold, Per 16 fl.oz Grande with Whole Milk without Whipped Cream

Caffe Vanilla	310	3	68
Caramel	280	3.5	60
Coffee	240	3	50
Java Chip	350	7	68
Mocha	300	4	51
White Chocolate Mocha	300	5	61

continued next page... ...

Starbucks® cont... (Sept '18)

Frappuccino Blended Creme:

	C	F	Cb
Per 16 fl.oz Grande with Whole Milk and Whipped Cream			
Double Chocolaty Chip	420	20	57
Red Velvet Cake Creme	480	18	75
Vanilla Bean Creme	400	16	60

Refreshers: Per 16 oz Grande

Cool Lime	110	0	27
Mango Dragonfruit Lemonade	140	0	33
Very Berry Hibiscus Lemonade	120	0	30

Teas: Per 16 fl.oz Grande, with Whole Milk

Hot Tea Latte:			
Classic Chai Tea	270	7	45
Green Tea, sweetened	280	11	34
Iced Tea Latte:			
Chai	260	7	44
Green Tea, sweetened	250	10	31

Drink Extras:

Caramel Drizzle, 1 teaspoon	15	0.5	2
Flavored Syrup: 1 Pump	20	0	5
Sugar-Free, 1 Pump	0	0	0
Mocha Syrup, 1 Pump	25	0.5	6
Sweetened Whipped Cream:			
Grande/Venti, cold drinks, av.	110	11	3
Grande/Venti, hot drinks	75	7	3

Breakfast, Hot:

Bacon, Gouda & Egg B'fast S'wich	370	19	32
Chicken Sausage & Bacon Biscuit	450	22	35
Ham & Cheese Croissant	320	17	28
Sausage, Cheddar & Egg Sandwich	500	28	41
Seared Steak & Egg Tomatillo Wrap	410	18	43
Smoked Shoulder Bacon Sandwich	570	22	35

Bistro Protein Boxes: As Prepared

Chicken BLT	580	23	58
Cheese & Fruit	450	27	34
PB & J	520	26	53
Smoked Turkey	570	23	54

Paninis:

Ancho Chipotle Chicken	500	19	57
Roasted Tomato & Mozzarella	350	13	42
Turkey Pesto	540	21	55

Sandwiches:

Chicken BLT Salad	470	25	35
Egg Salad	480	27	42
Turkey & Havarti	460	21	31

Starbucks® cont... (Sept '18)

Bakery: Each

	C	F	Cb
8-Grain Roll	380	6	70
Almond Croissant, 3.5 oz	410	22	45
Banana Nut Bread, 4.4 oz	420	22	52
Blueberry Muffin, w/ Yogurt & Honey, 4 oz	380	16	53
Blueberry Scone, 3.5 oz	380	17	54
Butter Croissant, 2.2 oz	260	15	27
Cheese Danish, 2.8 oz	290	14	33
Chewy Chocolate Cookie, 4.3 oz	570	29	75
Cinnamon Morning Bun, 3.9 oz	390	15	56
Classic Coffee Cake, 3.5 oz	390	16	57
Dble Choc. Chunk Brownie	490	28	55
Iced Lemon Pound Cake, 4.4 oz	470	20	68
Old-Fashioned Glazed D'nut, 4 oz	480	27	56
Summer Berry Swirl Croissant	360	13	54
Greek Yog. Parfait, w/ Blueberries, Honey & Granola	240	2.5	42

Bottled Drinks ~ See Page 37

Steak Escape® (Sept '18)

Cheesesteaks: Per Medium

Bourbon & Bacon	1100	64	89
Grand Escape	690	28	66
Original Philly Whiz	710	30	68
Sriracha	790	34	73
Steakhouse Sirloin	1040	64	74

Sandwiches:

Cajun Chicken	660	23	68
French Onion	830	33	75
Grand Escape	660	19	68
Turkey Club	550	14	65
Wild West BBQ	700	20	75

Wraps:

Crispy Bacon Club	890	57	53
Grandest Chicken	590	21	56
Grand Escape	600	27	57
Italian Hottie	770	43	57
Ragin' Cajun Chicken	610	26	54
Smokin' BBQ	700	32	68
Steakhouse Sirloin	950	63	65

Salads:

Bourbon & Bacon	720	54	33
Cubano	530	38	10
Hangover	630	29	50

Potatoes:

Bourbon & Bacon	1020	54	101
Delerious Dagwood	1100	66	74
Hangover	800	29	88
Simply Chicken	460	4	72
Triple Cheesesteak	910	45	78

For Complete Nutritional Data ~ see CalorieKing.com

Steak 'n Shake® (Sept '18)

	C	F	Cb
Steakburgers: *Without Fries*			
Bacon Lovers	840	57	34
Bacon 'n Cheese: Single	430	25	29
Double	570	37	29
Cajun Double	720	52	30
Chipotle Double	650	44	37
Guacamole: Single	540	37	36
Double	700	50	37
Jalapeno Crunch	790	53	42
Portobello & Swiss	740	50	36
Royale	780	55	32
Single Burger with Cheese	380	20	32
The Original: Double	460	26	33
With Cheese	530	32	33
Western BBQ 'N Bacon	720	41	52
Chili: 3-way	710	21	96
5-way	1160	57	103
Chili Deluxe: Bowl	1000	56	71
Cup	500	28	36
Chili Mac: Regular	1200	61	112
Supreme	1410	78	114
Melts: Frisco	960	66	52
Veggie, with Portobellos	620	45	44
Signature Steak Franks:			
Chili Cheese Frank	710	44	46
Steak Frank, footlong, with mustard	390	23	32
Salads: *Without Dressing*			
Beef Taco	950	73	43
Fried Chicken	600	36	34
Fries: *Per Regular*			
Reg.; Cajun; Parm. & Garlic Herb, av.	450	24	55
Cheese Fries	590	35	63
Chili Cheese Fries	760	39	83
Sides:			
Coleslaw	160	11	13
Onion Rings, Regular	330	17	39
Breakfast:			
Breakfast Bowl with Hash Browns	460	42	11
Bagel Sandwich: With Bacon	450	16	53
With Sausage	690	37	53
Banana Pancakes	970	16	189
Biscuits: Bacon	380	25	33
Bacon, Egg & Cheese	520	35	34
Sausage & Egg	690	50	34
Hash Browns, Shredded	300	28	15
Milk Shakes: Per Regular			
Banana	5700	17	126
Birthday Cake	840	26	136
Reese's Choc. Peanut Butter	900	47	98
Salted Caramel	730	20	124

Subway® (Sept '18)

	C	F	Cb
Fresh Fit Sandwiches on 6" 9-Grain Wheat Sub:			
Includes lettuce, tomatoes, onions, green peppers & cucumber. Oil or mayo not included			
Black Forest Ham	290	4.5	46
Oven Roasted Chicken	320	5	46
Roast Beef	320	5	45
Subway Club	310	4.5	46
Sweet Onion Chicken Teriyaki	370	4.5	58
Turkey Breast	280	3.5	46
Veggie Delite	230	2.5	44
Sandwiches on 6" 9-Grain Wheat Sub: Includes lettuce, tomatoes, onions, green peppers & cucumber. Oil or mayo not included			
Chicken & Bacon Ranch Melt	590	30	44
Cold Cut Combo	340	12	43
Italian B.M.T.	390	17	43
Meatball Marinara	460	18	53
Spicy Italian	470	9	43
Steak & Cheese	360	10	43
Kids Meal Sandwiches: Figures based on 9-grain wheat bread, lettuce, tomatoes, onions, green peppers and cucumbers. Oil or mayo not included.			
Black Forest Ham	180	2.5	30
Roast Beef	200	3	30
Turkey Breast	180	2	30
Veggie Delite	150	1.5	29
Sandwich Condiments & Extras: For 6" Sandwiches			
Bacon Strips (2)	80	5	1
Cheese: American, 2 triangles	40	3.5	1
Cheddar, 2 triangles, 0.3 oz	60	4.5	0
Swiss, 2 triangles, 0.3 oz	50	4.5	0
Chipotle Southwest Sauce, 0.8 oz	100	10	1
Honey Mustard Sce, Fat-Free, 0.8 oz	30	0	7
Mayonnaise: 1 Tbsp, 0.5 oz	110	12	0
Light, 1 Tbsp, 0.5 oz	50	5	1
Mustard, Yellow or Deli Brown, 2 tsp	5	0	1
Olive Oil Blend, 1 tsp	45	5	0
Ranch Dressing	110	11	1
Sweet Onion, Fat-Free, 0.8 oz	40	0	9

continued next page....

Subway® cont... (Sept '18)

Breakfast:

	C	F	Cb
Omelet Sandwiches on 6" 9 Grain Bread: *With Regular Egg*			
Bacon, Egg & cheese	450	18	44
Black Forest Ham, Egg & Cheese	400	14	45
Breakfast B.M.T.	500	23	47
Egg & Cheese	370	13	44
Mega Melt	590	29	45
Sausage, Egg & Cheese	510	24	45
Steak, Egg & Cheese	440	15	46
Sunrise Subway Melt	510	20	48
Omelet on 6" Flatbread: *With Regular Egg*			
Bacon, Egg & Cheese	460	21	43
Black Forest Ham, Egg & Cheese	410	16	44
Breakfast B.M.T.	520	25	46
Egg & Cheese	380	15	42
Mega Melt	600	31	44
Sausage, Egg & Cheese	520	26	44
Steak, Egg & Cheese	450	18	45
Sunrise Subway Melt	530	22	47

Egg White Omelets: *Deduct 40 cals and 5g fat from Regular Egg Omelet*

	C	F	Cb
8" Pizza: Bacon	840	31	98
Cheese	720	23	97
Meatball	860	33	100
Pepperoni	840	33	97
Sausage	860	35	98
Flatizza: *Includes 9 Grain Wheat Bread*			
Cheese	400	16	43
Pepperoni	500	26	44
Spicy Italian	500	25	44
Veggie	410	17	45
Side of Hash Browns, 3.6 oz	220	10	30

Salads (6g Fat or Less): *Figures based on lettuce, tomatoes, spinach, onions, green peppers, olives & cucumbers. Dressing or croutons not included.*

	C	F	Cb
Black Forest Ham	110	3	13
Oven Roasted Chicken	150	3.5	13
Roast Beef; Subway Club, average	140	3.5	12
Rotisserie Style Chicken	170	4.5	12
Turkey Breast	110	2	13
Veggie Delite	60	1	11

Soup: *Per 8 oz Bowl*

	C	F	Cb
Beef Chili, with Beans	360	22	20
Black Bean	210	1	39
Broccoli Cheddar	170	9	18
Creamy Chicken & Dumpling	150	4.5	20
Creamy Chicken & Wild Rice	190	11	16
Homestyle Chicken Noodle	110	3	14
Loaded Baked Potato, with Bacon	210	13	15
Mediterranean Vegetable	110	3	14
Spicy Chicken Tortilla	110	4.5	12
Tomato Basil	130	6	15

Subway® cont... (Sept '18)

Cookies & Desserts:

	C	F	Cb
Brownie, 3 oz	370	17	51
Chocolate Chip Cookie, 1.5 oz	210	10	29
Oatmeal Raisin Cookie, 1.5 oz	200	8	30
Raspberry Cheesecake, 1.6 oz	200	9	29

Sweet Tomatoes®

Same Menu & Data as Souplantation ~ See Page 242

Swiss Chalet® (Sept '18)

Canadian Outlets

	C	F	Cb
Starters: Chicken Spring Rolls (4)	340	16	31
Caesar Salad, without Dressing	90	3	13
Chalet Wings (10), w/out Sauce	560	34	13
Cheese Perogies (7)	420	10	69
Stuffed Garlic Cheese Loaf	860	57	63
Burgers: *Without Sides or Accompanying Sauce*			
Classic Hamburger, with Mayo	520	21	50
Ultimate Bacon Cheeseburger	730	42	46
Veggie Burger with Mayo	440	15	50
Poutine: Rotisserie Beef	1800	97	190
Shawarma	2170	135	178
Taco	1840	102	186
Ribs: *Without Add On Sauce or Sides*			
BBQ Side Ribs: ⅓ Rack	480	33	1
½ Rack	720	50	1
Full Rack	1440	100	2
BBQ Back Ribs: ½ Rack	460	30	0
Full Rack	920	61	1
Rotisserie Chicken: *Without Sides, Sauces or Bread*			
Chicken & Shrimp	940	35	88
Chicken Pot Pie, 1 pie	610	35	43
Double Leg: with skin	490	31	0
without skin	320	16	0
Half Chicken: with skin	530	27	0
without skin	380	14	0
Quarter Chicken:			
Dark Meat: with skin	240	16	0
without skin	160	8	0
White Meat: with skin	290	11	0
without skin	220	6	0
Sandwiches: *Without Sides or Accompanying Sauce*			
Chicken Kaiser: Dark Meat	570	18	47
White Meat	480	8	47
Classic Hot Chicken:			
Dark Meat	610	21	51
White Meat	520	11	51
Entree Salads: *Without Dressing*			
Rotisserie Chicken Caesar	420	11	38
Spinach & Mandarin Chicken	400	16	28
Sweet Heat Salad with Chicken	340	9	30

Updated Nutrition Data ~ www.CalorieKing.com
Persons with Diabetes ~ See Disclaimer (Page 22)

Swiss Chalet® cont... (Sept '18)

Sides:

	C	F	Cb
Caesar Salad without Dressing	50	1.5	8
Creamy Coleslaw	200	14	15
Fresh Cut Fries	720	37	86
Gravy	45	1.5	7
Loaded Baked Potato	380	13	54
Mashed Potatoes	170	5	27
Sauteed Mushrooms	140	1	30
Seasoned Rice	250	3.5	50
Multigrain Roll	110	1	22
White Roll	110	0	22

Dressings: Chalet, 1 oz

	C	F	Cb
Chalet, 1 oz	160	14	6
Caesar, 1 oz	180	18	2
Ranch, 1 oz	140	14	2

Sauce: Chalet Dipping, 1 oz

	C	F	Cb
Chalet Dipping, 1 oz	25	0.5	5
Cajun, 1 oz	50	4.5	2
Plum, 2 oz	100	0	26

Desserts/Pies: Slice

	C	F	Cb
Apple Pie, 6 oz	440	19	65
Classic Vanilla Cheesecake, 4.1 oz	380	25	32
Coconut Cream Pie, 6.1 oz	540	33	57
Lemon Meringue Pie, 6.5 oz	400	11	73
Pecan Pie, 5.15 oz	590	29	79

Taco Bell® (Sept '18)

Burritos: W/ Standard Components

	C	F	Cb
7-Layer, no meat	440	16	59
Beefy 5-Layer	500	19	64
Cheesy Potato, w/ Beef	480	21	55
Cheesy Potato Griller, no meat	340	13	50
Chili Cheese, no meat	370	17	40
Combo, with Beef	450	18	51
Shredded Chicken	420	20	47
Supreme: with Seasoned Beef	400	15	52
with Steak	390	12	50
XXL Grilled Stuft: Beef	870	40	97
Marinated Steak	840	35	94
Shredded Chicken	830	34	92
Nachos, Triple Layer, with Beef	320	15	41

Power Menu: With Standard Menu Component

	C	F	Cb
Power Bowls: Chicken, shredded	500	20	54
Steak	510	21	55
Veggie	480	19	65

Specialties:

	C	F	Cb
Chalupa Supreme: With Standard Menu Components			
Seasoned Beef	350	18	33
Shredded Chicken	330	16	31
Crunchwrap Supreme: W/ Standard Menu Components			
Seasoned Beef	530	21	71

Taco Bell® cont... (Sept '18)

Specialties (Cont):

	C	F	Cb
Gordita Supreme: With Standard Menu Component			
Seasoned Beef	280	12	31
Shredded Chicken	270	11	30
Steak	270	9	30
MexiMelt, Beef	250	13	19
Nachos BellGrande,			
Seasoned Beef	750	38	85
Quesadillas: Cheese	460	26	37
Fire Grilled Chicken	510	28	38
Steak	510	28	38

Tacos: With Standard Menu Components

	C	F	Cb
Crunchy: Seasoned Beef	170	9	13
Supreme. S'nd Beef	190	11	15
Double Decker:			
Regular, Seasoned Beef	320	13	36
Supreme, Beef	340	15	39
Soft: Seasoned Beef	180	9	18
Supreme, Seasoned Beef	210	10	20
Shredded Chicken	170	8	16
Spicy Potato	230	12	27

Taco Salads: With Standard Menu Components

	C	F	Cb
Express Fiesta, Seasoned Beef	580	26	65
Fiesta: Seasoned Beef	760	39	78
Shredded Chicken	720	33	73
Steak	730	34	75

Sides: Per Regular Size

	C	F	Cb
Black Beans & Rice	190	4	35
Cheesy Fiesta Potatoes	230	12	28
Chips & Guacamole	230	14	23
Pintos 'n Cheese	190	7	22
Seasoned Rice	120	2	23

Breakfast: With Standard Menu Components

	C	F	Cb
Crunchwrap: Bacon	660	42	51
Sausage	700	46	51
Grande Scrambler Burrito:			
Bacon	650	33	65
Sausage	640	34	65
Quesadillas: Bacon	510	28	37
Sausage	500	29	37
Steak	500	26	38
Sweets: Caramel Apple Empanada	280	13	38
Cinnabon Delights:			
4 Pack	310	18	35
12 Pack (serves 4)	930	53	104
Cinnamon Twist	170	6	27

Note: Nutritional data in New York outlets may vary slightly.
Please check Taco Bell website

Taco Cabana® (Sept '18)

Burritos: **C** **F** **Cb**

Includes Flour Tortilla, Rice, Refried Beans, Romaine, Meat, Shredded Cheese, Pico de Gallo & Sour Cream

	C	F	Cb
Beef Cabana	720	29	79
Brisket Canana	790	40	76
Chicken Cabana	770	30	81
Flame Grilled Chicken Fajita	730	26	79
Steak Fajita	990	44	107

Enchiladas:

Beef (1)	200	11	14
Cheese (1)	320	23	13
Chicken (1)	280	13	21

Quesadillas: *Small, with Guacamole & Sour Cream*

Brisket	920	63	51
Cheese	770	50	51
Flame-Gr. Chkn Fajita	840	52	52
Steak	850	55	52

Tacos:

Crispy: Beef	180	8	15
Shredded Chicken	200	9	16
Soft: Bean & Cheese	300	14	31
Beef, ground	210	9	21
Black Bean	220	5	38
Brisket	280	13	31
Carne Guisada	210	8	20
Chkn Breast Fajita, flame grilled	210	6	21
Shredded Chicken	240	9	23
Steak	220	9	21
Street, Beef (3)	460	25	40

Salads: *Includes Shell, Lettuce Meat, Shredded Cheese, Pico de Gallo & Sour Cream*

Beef, ground	570	34	37
Chicken, shredded	610	35	39
Chicken Fajita, flame grilled	570	31	36
Steak	600	36	36

Sides & Add-Ons:

Borracho Beans, 8 oz	290	6	40
Guacamole, 3 oz	110	9	7
Queso, 3 oz	110	8	5
Refried Beans with Cheese, 8 oz	530	29	49
Rice, 8 oz	310	6	58
Salsa, all flavors, 1 oz	5	0	1
Sour Cream, 1 fl.oz	50	5	1

Taco Del Mar® (Sept '18)

Burritos: *Includes Flour Tortilla,*   **C** **F** **Cb**
Rice, Refr. Beans, Meat, Cheese, Pico de Gallo & Sour Crm

Regular:	C	F	Cb
Chicken	910	31	115
Ground Beef	950	37	116
Pork	900	31	115
Shredded Beef	910	31	116
Steak	870	27	117

Burrito Bowls: *Per Regular Bowl, with Rice, Refried Beans, Meat, Cheese & Pico de Gallo & Sour Cream*

Beef, shredded	600	24	64
Chicken	600	24	63
Ground Beef	640	30	64
Pork	590	24	63
Steak	560	20	65

Nachos: *Includes Chips , Refried Beans, Meat, Cheese, Pico de Gallo, Guacamole & Sour Cream*

Beef:			
Ground	1210	78	90
Shredded	1160	71	90
Cheese	1040	66	88
Chicken	1170	72	89
Fish	1200	74	100
Pork	1150	71	89
Shrimp	1110	66	90

Platters: *Includes Meat, Cheese, Rice, Refried Beans, Lettuce, Pico, Guacamole, Sour Cream & Enchilada Sauce*

Enchilada: *Per 2 Soft Corn Tortillas*

Beef:			
Ground	890	37	106
Shredded	710	34	59
Cheese	810	32	105
Chicken	850	31	105
Fish	880	33	116
Pork	830	30	104
Shrimp	660	29	59
Steak	680	31	60

Quesadillas: *Includes Flour Tortilla, Meat, Cheese & Pico*

Beef:			
Ground	760	41	59
Shredded	710	34	59
Cheese	590	29	57
Chicken	720	35	58
Fish	750	37	69
Pork	700	34	58
Shrimp	660	29	59
Steak	680	31	60

Updated Nutrition Data ~ www.CalorieKing.com
Persons with Diabetes ~ See Disclaimer (Page 22)

Taco Del Mar® cont... (Sept '18)

Taco Salads: Includes Shell, Cheese **C** **F** **Cb**
Refried Beans, Lettuce, Meat & Pico de Gallo

	C	F	Cb
Beef: Ground	750	45	60
Shredded	700	38	59
Chicken	710	38	59
Fish	730	41	70
Pork	690	38	58
Shrimp	650	33	60
Steak	670	35	61

Note: Nutritional Information varies from state to state.
Please refer to Taco Del Mar Website

Taco John's® (Sept '18)

Burritos:	C	F	Cb
Bean Burrito	360	10	54
Beef Grilled Burrito	590	31	54
Chicken Grilled Burrito	580	28	53
Meat & Potato: Beef Burrito	510	24	59
Crunchy Chicken Burrito	580	25	8
Steak	520	23	58
Chips:			
& Queso, 6.7 oz	430	25	43
Mexi Rolls: Without Nacho Cheese			
4 Pieces, 8 oz	370	21	30
6 Pieces, 10 oz	550	32	45
Nachos:			
Super Nachos:			
Regular, 12.6 oz	790	47	72
Potato Oles: Per Serving			
Small, 5 oz	480	27	52
Medium, 7 oz	670	38	73
Large, 9 oz	860	49	94
Super Potato Oles:			
Small, 9.7 oz	650	40	59
Regular, 16.8 oz	1090	67	98
Quesadillas:			
Cheesy, 5.5 oz	450	24	40
Chicken, 8.6 oz	530	25	48
Tacos:			
Crispy Taco	170	10	11
Softshell Taco: Beef	210	10	21
Chicken	180	5	20
Stuffed Grilled Taco	540	25	58
Taco Bravo	320	13	36

Taco John's® (Sept '18)

Salads: Without Dressing	C	F	Cb
Beef Taco Salad	540	33	40
Chicken Taco Salad	500	27	44
Side Salad, 3.25 oz	40	2.5	3
Sides: Per Serving			
Nachos, 5 oz	380	23	39
Refried Beans, 9.5 oz	320	17	46
Condiments:			
Bacon Ranch, 1.5 oz	120	9	10
House Dressing, 1.5 oz	70	7	2
Nacho Cheese Sce, 3 oz	110	9	5
Salsa, 2 oz	10	0	2
Sour Cream, 2.5 oz	140	13	4
Breakfast:			
Burritos: Bacon & Potato, 7.7 oz	540	25	57
Potato & Bacon Oles Scrambler	1080	68	86
Spicy Chorizo, 8.2 oz	500	27	45
Sausage Scrambler, 8.7 oz	650	33	60
Desserts:			
Churro, 2 oz	200	9	29
Mexican Donut Bites, 3.2 oz	290	12	47

Taco Mayo® (Sept '18)

Burritos:	C	F	Cb
Bean	450	14	63
Double Smothered Double Queso			
Chicken	850	39	83
Fajita: Grilled Chicken	485	25	42
Grilled Steak	525	28	43
Super, Beef	525	21	56
Supreme, Chicken	420	19	40
Mexicali Bowls: Chicken	1225	71	91
Steak	1245	73	92
Queso: Chicken	1035	48	92
Steak	1055	50	93
Quesadilla Platter:			
Chicken	690	40	45
Steak	730	43	47
Tacos:			
Crispy Taco, Beef	160	9	10
Soft Taco: Beef	230	10	19
Chicken	185	8	16
Taco Burger	360	15	32
Salads: As Per Menu Description			
Beef	650	33	55
Chicken	445	26	31
Steak	465	28	33
Sides:			
Mexicali Rice	175	9	17
Potato Locos, Small	400	25	27
Queso-N-Chips	575	35	63
Refried Beans	225	4	34
Tostada	295	13	37

Fast - Foods & *Restaurants*

Taco Time® (Sept '18)

Burritos:	C	F	Cb
5 Alarm	420	15	58
Chicken B.L.T.	600	31	46
Sweet Pork	550	18	72
Big Juan: Chicken	590	16	79
Seasoned Beef	650	22	83
Casita: Chicken	450	16	44
Seasoned Beef	510	22	48
Crisp Burrito:			
Chicken	380	17	39
Meat	390	17	43
Pinto Bean	380	13	53
Soft Burrito: Pinto Bean	380	10	56
Seasoned Beef	420	16	46
Veggie	440	17	60
Nachos: Original	900	39	91
Chicken	970	39	92
Seasoned Beef	1020	45	96
Optionals:			
Green Chili Pork: Burrito	460	18	43
Chimichanga	590	21	65
Enchiladas	340	12	26
Tacos:			
Soft Tacos: Chicken	360	10	42
Junior	300	13	29
Pork	440	16	43
Seasoned Beef	410	16	45
Super Soft Tacos: Chicken	500	16	61
Pork	590	21	62
Seasoned Beef	560	21	65
Fries:			
Mexi: Small, 3.2 oz	190	12	19
Regular, 4.7 oz	300	19	29
Stuffed: Small, 4.5 oz	320	20	29
Regular, 6.6 oz	460	28	42
Salads:			
Fiesta, Chicken,12.3 oz	340	11	37
Taco: Chicken, 8 oz	310	14	26
Seasn'd Beef , 7.5 oz	360	19	28
Soup, Enchilada, 8 oz	130	0.5	20
Breakfast:			
Burritos: *Regular Size*			
Bacon & Egg	450	20	48
Egg & Cheese	370	16	40
Sausage & Egg	560	30	48
Quesadilla	300	17	18
Taters & Gravy, regular	410	27	36
Desserts:			
Churro: Plain	210	16	15
Bavarian Cream	320	8	54
Cinnamon Crustos	320	5	64

TCBY® (Sept '18)

Soft Serve Frozen Yogurt: 4 fl.oz	C	F	Cb
Super Fro Yo: Bananas Foster	90	0	23
Cake Batter; Golden Vanilla	105	2	22
Cheesecake	105	2	22
Chocolate	110	1.5	23
Dutch Chocolate	95	0	23
Greek Honey Vanilla	100	0	20
Old Fashioned Vanilla	90	0	23
White Chocolate Macadamia	70	0	18
White Chocolate Mousse	120	1.5	24
Dairy Free/Sorbet:			
Chocoalte Almond	100	1	28
Kiwi Strawberry Sorbet	90	0	22
Limeade Sorbet	110	0	28
Mango Sorbet	95	0	24
Watermelon Sorbet	100	0	25
Vanilla Almond	100	1	28
No Sugar Added: Chocolate	65	0	18
Mountain Blackberry	65	0	18
Salted Caramel	70	0	18
Hand-Scooped Frozen Yogurt:			
Butter Pecan: Kid's, 4 fl.oz	220	10	27
Small, 6.4 fl.oz	350	16	43
Regular, 12.8 fl.oz	705	32	86
Chunky Choc. Cookie Dough:			
Kid's, 4 fl.oz	220	7	33
Small, 6.4 fl.oz	350	11	53
Regular,12.8 fl.oz	705	22	106
Cookies & Cream:			
Kid's, 4 fl.oz	200	6	32
Small, 6.4 fl.oz	320	10	51
Regular, 12.8 fl.oz	640	19	102
Peanut Butter Delight:			
Kid's, 4 fl.oz	250	13	30
Small, 6.4 fl.oz	400	21	48
Regular, 12.8 fl.oz	800	42	96
Pralines & Cream: Kid's 4 fl.oz	210	6	27
Small, 6.4 fl.oz	335	10	43
Regular, 12.8 fl oz	670	19	86
Vanilla Bean: Kid's,4 fl.oz	170	4.5	27
Small, 6.4 fl.oz	270	7	43
Regular, 12.8 fl.oz	545	14	86

Updated Nutrition Data ~ www.CalorieKing.com
Persons with Diabetes ~ See Disclaimer (Page 22)

TGI Friday's® (Sept '18)

Appetizers/Snacks:

	C	F	Cb
BBQ Chicken Flatbread	650	32	66
Bucket of Bones	1570	82	120
Cheeseburger Sliders (2)	620	37	45
Chips & Salsa	290	13	31
Chkn Quesadilla, w/ Guacamole	1250	87	58
Crispy Brussels Sprouts	670	54	38
Loaded Potato Skins,			
with Ranch Sour Cream	1620	91	167
Mozzarella Sticks, w/ Marinara	820	50	54
Pan Seared P'stickers, w/ Szech. Sce	590	25	72
Spinach Queso Dip	770	54	66
Warm Pretzels, w/ Beer-Cheese Sce	1190	60	125

Burgers: Without Sides

	C	F	Cb
Bacon Cheeseburger	840	54	47
Buffalo Wingman's	920	60	45
Philly Cheesesteak	1000	65	58
Signature Whiskey-Glazed	1110	55	110
Turkey Burger	520	22	48

Chicken & Seafood:

	C	F	Cb
Crispy Chkn Fngrs, Fries & Hon Msrd	1030	59	87
Gr. Salmon, Jasmine Rice & Veggies	820	38	85

Pasta,

	C	F	Cb
Chicken Parmesan	1560	92	116

Ribs: With Coleslaw & Seasoned Fries

	C	F	Cb
BBQ: Half Rack	830	49	77
Full Rack	1190	73	93
Whiskey Glazed: Half Rack	1030	49	126
Full Rack	1520	74	177

Sandwiches: W/out Sides

	C	F	Cb
French Dip	950	49	74
Southern Fried Chicken	930	57	67
Turkey & Avocado BLT	770	42	51
Whiskey Glazed Chicken	1110	57	100

Steaks: With Mashed Potatoes & Lemon Butter Broccoli

	C	F	Cb
Centre Cut Sirloin: w/ Parm. Butter	640	41	34
w/ Shrimp & Whiskey Glaze	910	38	98
New York Strip: with Parm Butter	985	56	37
with Whiskey Glaze	1100	46	91

Salads: Includes Menu Set Dressing

	C	F	Cb
BBQ Chicken	920	48	73
Caesar, with Grilled Salmon	910	70	32
Pecan-Crusted Chicken	1220	84	82
Strawberry Fields Salad	700	55	39

TGI Friday's® cont... (Sept '18)

Salad Dressing: Per 1.25 oz

	C	F	Cb
Balsamic Vinaigrette	190	19	4
Bleu Cheese	200	21	1
Caesar	190	20	1
Honey Mustard	200	18	8
Ranch	130	14	1

Signature Sides: Coleslaw

	C	F	Cb
Coleslaw	100	8	5
Giant Onion Rings	510	26	61
Jasmine Rice Pilaf	420	11	72
Lemon Butter Broccoli	150	11	11
Mashed Potatoes	220	11	21
Seasoned Fries	320	16	40
Sweet Potato Fries	390	20	50

Soups: French Onion

	C	F	Cb
French Onion	590	18	84
White Chedd. Brocc. Chse	280	20	18

Soup Of The Day:

	C	F	Cb
New England Clam Chowder	500	30	45
Tomato Basil	300	24	20

Desserts: Per Whole Dish

	C	F	Cb
Brownie Obsession	1200	60	153
Oreo Madness	500	21	76
Tennessee Whiskey Cake	1110	52	151

Signature Slushes:

	C	F	Cb
Blue Raspberry	170	0	42
Mango Peach Lemonade	170	0	44
Red Bull Passion, regular	210	0	54
Strawberry Lemonade	150	0	38

Thundercloud Subs® (Sept '18)

Subs: Small, with Standard Toppings

	C	F	Cb
Classic: BLT	365	17	35
Smoked Chicken	270	4	35
Turkey	255	4	36
Low Fat: Genoa Salami	265	6	35
Roast Beef	290	4	35

Signature Subs:

	C	F	Cb
Club	445	19	38
California Club	475	23	40
NY Italian	540	30	37
Office Favorite	790	39	71
Texas Tuna	675	44	39
Veggie Delite, with Hummus	385	19	52

T.J. Cinnamons® (Sept '18)

Bakery:

	C	F	Cb
Orig. Gourmet Cinn. Roll, 7.8 oz	840	42	106
Pecan Stick Bun, 8.3 oz	940	49	111

Tim Hortons® (Sept '18)

	C	F	Cb
Breakfast:			
Biscuit Sandwich:			
Sausage, Egg & Cheese	500	33	33
Steak, Egg & Cheese	390	20	33
English Muffin Sandwich:			
Bacon, Egg & Cheese	330	15	28
Sausage, Egg & Cheese	440	26	28
Grilled B'Fast Wraps:			
Bacon	420	23	37
Sausage	530	34	37
Oatmeal, with Mixed Berries, reg.	220	2.5	29
Hash Brown, regular	130	7	16
Hot Bowls: Per 10 fl.oz			
Chili	290	16	20
Chicken Noodle Soup	120	1.5	21
Clam Chowder	190	7	23
Harvest Vegetable Soup			
Sandwiches: BLT	420	15	56
Chicken Salad Croissant	430	23	35
Cold Cut Trio	540	28	48
Crispy Chicken	460	16	57
Turkey Bacon Club	400	11	51
Wraps, Grilled Chipotle Steak	460	22	40
Donuts: Apple Fritter	310	8	53
Boston Creme Filled	220	6	37
Chocolate, Glazed	280	14	37
Chocolate Dip	200	6	34
Double Chocolate	260	14	32
Honey Cruller	280	18	27
Old Fashioned, Plain	210	10	25
Timbits: Chocolate, Glazed	90	3	14
Apple Fritter; Honey Dip, average	50	1.5	9
Old Fashion, Plain	50	2.5	7
Bagels: 12 Grain	330	9	55
Other varieties, av., 4 oz	300	3	59
Cream Cheese Spread, Light, 1.5 oz	100	8	2
Cinnamon Roll, Frosted	370	14	56
Cookies, Peanut Butter, 1.83 oz	280	17	27
Croissants, Cheese	260	14	29
Danish, Maple Pecan	370	21	43
Greek Yogurt, Vanilla, 7 oz	270	5	40
Muffins: Choc. Chip, 4 oz	420	16	66
Fruit Explosion, 4.3 oz	340	10	58
Raisin Bran, 4 oz	370	12	63
Wild Blueberry, 4 oz	340	11	57
Beverages: Without Sugar			
Cappuccino, 10 oz	70	0	11
Hot Chocolate, 10 oz	240	6	45
Latte, 9.6 fl.oz	150	6	3
Mocha Latte, 9.6 fl.oz	240	6	37
Cold: Frozen Lemonade, Orig., 12 oz	120	0	20
Iced Capp®, w/ Lt Milk, 12.8 fl.oz oz	180	1.5	39
Iced Coffee, with Milk, 12.8 fl.oz	70	1	12

Togo's® (Sept '18)

California Outlet ~ Please check local outlet for menu items and nutritional information

	C	F	Cb
Cold Sandwiches: Per Regular 6", with Menu Set Components on White Bread			
Albacore Tuna	670	27	72
California Club	710	34	70
Chicken Salad	620	22	70
Greek Veggie	800	42	90
Ham & Swiss	690	28	70
Hummus	670	26	93
Salami & Provolone	1020	61	68
The Italian	880	47	70
Turkey & Avocado	700	32	74
Turkey & Cranberry	650	18	86
Hot Sandwiches: Per Regular 6", with Menu Set Components on White Bread			
Meatball	890	40	81
Pastrami	740	34	73
Pepperjack Pastrami Melt	1010	59	73
Roast Beef	710	21	67
Sandwich Dressings: Mayo, reg.	150	16	0.5
Sriracha Sauce, regular	240	24	4
Sweet Baby Ray's BBQ, regular	50	0	13
Wraps: Per Whole 12" Spinach Tortilla Wrap, with Menu Set Components			
Asian Chicken	650	28	70
Chicken Caesar	570	21	62
Santa Fe Chicken	720	34	70
Salads: Per Full Salad, with Dressing			
Asian chicken	670	43	44
Chicken Caesar	450	26	22
Santa Fe Chicken	800	57	40
Salad Dressings: Caesar, 2.5 oz	150	12	8
Italian Vinaigrette, 2.5 oz	310	33	2
Ranch, 2.5 oz	270	29	2
Thousand Island, 2.5 oz	310	28	12
Zesty Pepitas, 2.5 oz	340	35	3
Soups: Per Regular, 10 fl.oz			
Broccoli Cheese	380	24	31
Chicken Noodle	125	3	23
Chicken Tortilla	155	6	21
Garden Vegetable	90	0.5	18
Brownie, Choc. Chunk, 3 oz	430	22	57
Cookies: Dark Choc. Chunk, 3 oz	410	21	53
Oatmeal Raisin, 3 oz	360	13	57
Peanut Butter Chip, 3 oz	410	23	48

Updated Nutrition Data ~ www.CalorieKing.com
Persons with Diabetes ~ See Disclaimer (Page 22)

Tropical Smoothie Cafe® (Sept '18)

Menu & Nutrition Differ from Outlets to **C** **F** **Cb**
Outlet. Please Check Instore. Figures below Based On Irvine, CA

Breakfast:

All American Omelet Wrap	430	20	37
Peanut Butter Crunch Flatbread	590	24	77
Southwest Omelet Wrap	580	36	38

***Toasted Sandwiches:** Per Whole Ciabatta Sandwich*

Turkey Apple Dijon	640	31	52
Turkey Bacon Ranch	560	20	59
Tropical Chicken Salad	610	33	52

***Toasted Wraps:** In Flour Tortilla*

Baja Chicken	640	24	67
Buffalo Chicken	510	21	44
Caribbean Jerk Chicken	590	17	74
Hummus Veggie	690	39	68
Supergreen Caesar Chicken	610	31	42
Thai Chicken	500	15	62

***Classic Smoothies:** Per 24 oz with Turbinado*

Bahama Mama	500	4.5	117
Beach Bum	550	5	129
Blimey Limey	440	0	111
Blueberry Bliss	340	5	86
Health Nut, with Soy	530	4.5	101
Jetty Punch	370	0	94
Lean Machine	490	0	124
Mocha Madness	660	5	152
Muscle Blaster, with Whey	470	2	96
Peaches 'N Silk	360	0	91
Peanut Paradise, with Whey	690	17	105
Peanut Butter Cup	710	20	127
Sunrise Sunset	360	0	89
Sunshine	390	0	98

Tubby's® (Sept '18)

***Subs:** Per Regular 8" Sub, w/ Standard Igredients, w/out Added Sauce or Dressing* **C** **F** **Cb**

Deli-Subs:

Ham & Cheese	540	11	78
Turkey Breast & Cheese	550	11	77

Grilled Burger Subs: Big Tub

Big Tub	790	35	78
Cheeseburger Italiano	790	35	78
Loaded Burger	820	36	83
Pizza Burger	810	36	81

Tubby's® cont.... (Sept '18)

***Subs (Cont):** Per Reg. 8" Sub, with* **C** **F** **Cb**
Standard Ingredients, w/out Added Sauce or Dressing

Grilled Chicken Subs: Gr. Chicken

Gr. Chicken	450	4.5	75
Chicken & Broccoli	550	11	78
Chicken & Cheddar	540	11	75
Chicken Fajita	550	11	79

Grilled Steak Subs:

Loaded Steak	650	18	81
Pepper Steak & Cheese	630	17	77
Portabella Mushroom Steak	580	13	77
Steak & Cheese	630	17	78

Specialty Subs: BLT

BLT	570	21	72
Cold Veggie	490	10	86
Italian Sausage	600	22	78
Meatball	790	33	83
Tuna	570	11	76

Uno Pizzeria & Grill® (Sept '18)

***Appetizers:** Per Whole Dish* **C** **F** **Cb**

Mozzarella Sticks	1100	57	108
Muchos Nacos	1700	71	199
Shrimp & Crab Dip	1120	81	64

***Burgers:** With Fries*

Bacon Cheddar	1860	136	70
Wild Wild West	1740	120	96
Uno Burger	1500	108	70

***Entrees:** With Housemade Bread*

Chicken:

Baked Stuffed Spinoccoli	450	19	24
Herb Rubbed Chiken	590	41	19
Romano Crusted Chicken Parm.	1240	46	146

Pasta: With Housemade Bread

Chicken Spinoccoli	1380	66	123
Deep Dish Mac & Cheese	1860	107	158
Shrimp Scampi	1310	58	146

Steak & Seafood: Without Sides or Breadstick

Grilled Shrimp & Sirloin	880	56	19
Sirloin, 10 oz	680	41	18
Sirloin Steak Tips	590	24	22
Stockyard Strip Steak	520	14	19

***Deep Dish Individual Pizza:** Per Slice, ¼ Pizza*

Chicago Classic	560	39	28
Numero Uno	460	31	30
Prima Pepperoni	430	30	28

***Sides:** French Fries, 7.5 oz*

French Fries, 7.5 oz	450	33	35
Housemade Bread	120	1	18
Jumbo Onion Rings, 7.5 oz	370	7	68
Red Bliss Mashed Potatoes	280	14	36
Roasted Seasonal Veggies, 7.2 oz	70	4	8

***Dessert:** All American*

All American	640	28	90
Uno Deep Dish Sundae	1520	74	206

Villa Fresh Italian® (Sept '18)

Pizzas: Per Slice

	C	F	Cb
Neapolitan: Buffalo	770	46	52
Deluxe	530	22	55
Sausage & Pepperoni	550	25	53
Stuffed: Baked Ziti	845	33	97
Spinach & Mushroom	735	33	79

Entrees:

	C	F	Cb
Chicken Pasta Primavera, 16 oz	505	20	58
Fettuccini Alfredo, 14 oz	765	38	85
Mac & Cheese, 14 oz	725	54	39
Pasta Primavera, 16 oz	495	21	66
Spaghetti & Meatballs, 18 oz	840	28	112
Sides: Caesar Salad, 4 oz	90	5	9
Garlic Roll,	260	10	34
Garden Salad, 3 oz	15	1	3
Greek Salad, 6 oz	125	10	7
Roasted Potatoes, 6 oz	210	12	24
Sauteed Vegetables, 6oz	85	6	6

Vocelli Pizza® (Sept '18)

Pizzas:

Artisan: Per $^1/_8$ of Medium Pizza, with Menu Set Components

	C	F	Cb
BBQ Chicken	290	10	35
Chicken Carbonara	270	11	27
Chicken Pesto	260	10	27
Chicken Spinaci	250	9	28
Deluxe	260	11	29
Hawaiian	280	11	29
Meat Magnifico	290	13	28
Philly Steak	270	12	28
Quattro Cheese	260	10	27

Pasta: Single Serving

	C	F	Cb
Chicken Alfredo	1200	54	129
Chicken Parmesan	960	26	144
Chicken Pesto	1230	57	128

House Baked Subs: On Italian Bread

	C	F	Cb
Buffalo Chicken	950	39	86
Chkn Parmesan	990	39	105
Meatball	1170	55	103

Salads: Per Regular Size, without Dressing

	C	F	Cb
Chicken Caesar	180	4	14
Mediterranean	230	11	22
Tuscan Grilled Chicken	320	13	22

Stromboli: With Marinara Sauce

	C	F	Cb
Pepperoni, w/o veggie toppings	1410	62	149
Spicy Italian	1430	56	156
Steak	1350	48	156

Wahoo's Fish Taco® (Sept '18)

Bowls: W/ White Rice & Black Beans

	C	F	Cb
Chicken, Blackened/Charbroiled	920	23	133
Carne Asada	995	32	132
Carnitas	1090	34	134
Fish, Blackened	875	18	133
Salmon, Charbroiled	905	22	132

Burritos: With Brown Rice & White Beans

Banzai Blackened or Charbroiled:

	C	F	Cb
Chicken	585	19	6
Fish, average	540	14	75
Carne Asada	650	27	75
Carnitas	735	29	77
Shrimp	530	15	77
Tofu	535	17	78
Vegetarian	485	14	82
Side Kicks, Corn Tortillas, each	145	2	29

Shredder Sandwiches:

Blackened or Charbroiled:

	C	F	Cb
Chicken, average	360	17	29
Fish	385	21	29
Carne Asada	350	18	30

Wahoo Salads:

	C	F	Cb
Banzai Veggie	295	18	24

Blackened or Charbroiled:

	C	F	Cb
Chicken, average	415	22	14
Fish, average	470	28	14
Carne Asada	400	23	16
Soup, Chicken Tortilla	55	1	5

For Complete Nutritional Data ~ see CalorieKing.com

WAWA® (Sept '18)

Breakfast Sizzlis:

	C	F	Cb
Bagels: Bacon, Egg & Cheese	410	18	42
Pork Roll, Egg & Cheese	420	19	42
Sausage, Egg & Cheese	510	29	42
Turkey Ssg, Egg White & Cheese	360	10	42
Biscuit, Sausage, Egg & Cheese	670	45	47

Croissants:

	C	F	Cb
Bacon, Egg & Cheese	370	21	27
Chorizo	480	35	28
Sausage, Egg & Cheese	510	38	27
Muffin, Sausage, Egg & Cheese	450	30	28

Cold Hoagies: On Shorti Roll w/out Toppings

	C	F	Cb
Egg Salad	590	35	55
Italian	410	13	51
Roast Beef	390	4.5	51
Tuna Salad	630	37	57
Veggie	290	9	55

WAWA® cont... (Sept '18)

Hot Hoagies: On Shorti Roll	C	F	Cb
Beefsteak Burger	680	36	65
Chicken Steak	370	8	51
Meatball Parmesan	540	38	24

Quesadillas: Without Toppings			
Beef & Cheddar Cheese	560	28	46
Cheddar Cheese	440	21	45
Chicken & Cheddar Cheese	500	21	46

Soups: Per Medium Serving			
Baked Potato w/ Cheddar & Bacon	400	27	26
Broccoli Cheddar Soup	300	22	15
Chicken Noodle	190	7	20
New Eng. Clam Chowder	320	20	24
Tomato Soup	320	22	27

Sides: Per Medium without Toppings			
Chili	330	15	32
Macaroni & Cheese	450	22	45
Mashed Potatoes	450	26	45
Meatballs in a Cup	320	21	18
Rice	270	0	59

Bakery:			
Apple Fritter	510	19	79
Brownie	490	22	72
Muffins: Banana Walnut	610	33	74
Blueberry	570	28	72
Chocolate Chip	680	34	86

Hot Beverages: Per 16 oz, without Extras			
Hot Cappuccino, with 2% milk	130	5	13
Mocha Latte, with 2% milk	330	7	59

Milkshake, Chocolate,			
with whipped Cream, 16 oz	970	50	117

Wendy's® (Sept '18)

Breakfast:	C	F	Cb
Artisan Egg & Bacon Sandwich	320	17	25
Bacon Breakfast Bowl	510	28	44
Honey Butter Chicken Biscuit	500	26	48
Homestyle Potatoes, medium	250	9	39
Sausage & Egg Burrito	360	20	29
Sausage Breakfast Bowl	640	42	46
Two Sausage Biscuits	960	65	70

Hamburgers:			
Daves: Single	570	34	40
Double	810	51	41
Triple	1090	72	43

Wendy's® cont... (Sept '18)

Hamburgers (Cont):	C	F	Cb
Baconator	950	62	40
Double Stack	390	21	26
Jr. Bacon Cheeseburger	380	22	25
Jr. Cheeseburger	280	13	26
Jr. Cheeseburger Deluxe	340	19	27
Son of Baconator	630	39	37

Sandwiches: With Standard Toppings			
Crispy Chicken	330	16	33
Grilled Chicken	370	10	38
Homestyle Asiago Club	660	34	52
Spicy Asiago Ranch Chicken Club	670	32	55
Spicy Chicken	510	20	54
Wraps: Grilled Chicken	270	10	24
Spicy Chicken	370	20	30

Chicken: Nuggets:			
Nuggets: 4 pieces	170	11	10
6 pieces	250	16	14
10 pieces	420	27	24
Tenders: 3 piece	330	6	22
4 piece	430	21	29

Dipping Sauces: Per 1 oz			
Barbecue	45	0	11
Buttermilk Ranch	120	12	2
Creamy Sriracha	120	12	3
Honey Mustard	90	7	7
Sweet & Sour	45	0	12

Fresh-Made Salads: Full Size w/ Menu Set Dressing			
Apple Pecan Grilled Chicken	560	24	52
Berry Burst Chicken	460	17	41
Spicy Chkn Caesar	720	42	44

Sides:			
Baconator Fries	490	28	45

Baked Potatoes:			
Bacon Cheese	440	14	64
Cheese	430	13	65
Sour Cream & Chives	310	2.5	63

Natural Cut Fries: Jr.	230	10	30
Small, 4 oz	320	15	43
Medium, 5 oz	420	19	56
Large, 6.5 oz	530	24	70

Rich Meaty Chili: Small	170	5	16
Large	250	7	23

Frosty:			
Chocolate; Vanilla, average:			
Small	345	9	57
Medium	460	12	77
Large	580	15	96

For Complete Nutritional Data ~ see CalorieKing.com

Whataburger® (Sept '18)

Burgers & Sandwiches:

	C	F	Cb
Whataburger:			
#1 Original	590	25	62
#2 Double Meat	830	44	62
#3 Triple Meat	1080	63	62
#4 Jalapeno & Cheese	680	32	63
#5 Bacon & Cheese	750	37	62
#6 Double Meat Jr.	420	20	37
#7 Whataburger Jr.	310	11	37
Other Burgers & Sandwiches:			
Avocado Bacon Burger	820	52	51
Chop House Cheddar Burger	1110	69	61
Green Chili Double	980	57	61
Monterey Melt	1090	68	62
Sweet & Spicy Bacon Burger	1080	62	69
Whatachick'n:			
Bites: 6 pieces, without sauce	450	22	33
9 pieces without sauce	640	31	45
Sandwich	530	20	55
Strips, 3 pieces, w/out sce	530	28	42
Taco, Chicken Fajita, soft	340	11	31
French Fries: Small, 3 oz	280	14	35
Medium, 4.5 oz	420	21	52
Large, 6 oz	560	28	70
Onion Rings: Medium, 3.2 oz	300	17	32
Large, 4.8 oz	450	25	49
Salad: Without Dressing			
Garden:			
w/ Grilled Chicken	290	12	12
with Whatachick'n	400	20	21
without Chicken	160	9	9
Breakfast:			
Biscuits: Plain	290	16	32
with Gravy	470	29	46
Honey Butter Chicken	560	33	51
Biscuit Sandwiches:			
with Bacon	470	29	32
with Sausage	630	45	32
Cinnamon Roll	430	10	79
On A Bun: with Bacon	350	15	34
with Sausage	520	31	34
Platters: with Bacon	580	36	36
with Sausage	740	52	36
Taquitos: with Cheese	350	19	28
with Bacon, Egg & Cheese	400	22	28
with Potato, Egg & Cheese	440	25	38
Desserts:			
Chocolate Chunk Cookie	230	11	31
Hot Apple Pie, 3 oz	270	14	34
Malts: Chocolate, 20 oz	570	11	109
Vanilla, 20 oz	520	12	93
Shake, Chocolate, 20 oz	550	12	101

White Castle® (Sept '18)

Note: Nutritional Information varies from state to state. Please check instore

	C	F	Cb
Sliders: Original	140	6	13
Double	240	12	21
Bacon & Cheddar:			
Crispy Chicken	290	16	21
Grilled Chicken	270	15	14
Bacon Cheese	220	14	13
Cheddar Cheese	170	9	14
Cheese	160	9	14
Double	300	17	21
Chicken & Waffles: Crispy	350	18	36
Savory Grilled	340	18	30
Chicken: Breast	220	10	20
Ring	200	10	16
Savory Grilled	180	7	13
Fish	340	24	18
Surf & Turf	540	38	27
Veggie: with Ranch	270	18	21
with Sweet Thai Sauce	160	5	23
Sides: Clam Strips, medium	410	34	9
Cheese Fries, 7 oz	400	27	35
Chicken Rings: 3 piece	160	10	6
9 piece	320	20	12
Fish Nibblers: Small	320	16	28
Medium	590	29	51
Mozzarella Cheese Sticks, 3 sticks	460	33	26
Onion Chips, medium	930	65	73
Onion Rings, Small	480	33	40
French Fries: Kids	250	16	24
Small, 5.2 oz	330	21	32
Medium, 9.4 oz	600	39	57
Breakfast:			
Sliders: Bacon, Egg & Cheese	210	12	13
Egg & Cheese	160	7	13
Original, w/- Egg & Cheese	220	13	13
Ssg, Egg & Cheese	310	22	13
Waffle:			
with Bacon, Egg & Chedd. Cheese	350	22	27
with Sausage, Egg & Ched. Chse	450	32	28
Toasted Sandwiches:			
Bacon, Egg & Cheese	340	19	29
Egg & Cheese	230	9	29
Ssg, Egg & Cheese	380	23	29
Hash Round Nibblers: Small	360	28	25
Medium	600	46	42
Dessert:			
On A Stick: Fudge Dipped Brownie	250	12	33
Fudge Dipped Cheesecake	180	10	21
Gooey Butter Cake	220	10	32

Updated Nutrition Data ~ www.CalorieKing.com
Persons with Diabetes ~ See Disclaimer (Page 22)

Wienerschnitzel® (Sept '18)

Hot Dogs: On Hot Dog Bun

	C	F	Cb
Original: Bacon Street Dog	350	20	30
Chicago Dog	330	15	37
Chili Dog	300	15	30
Chili Cheese Dog	350	20	30
Deluxe Dog	290	14	30
Junkyard Dog	430	24	42
Kraut Dog	280	14	29
Mustard Dog	280	14	28
Relish Dog	290	14	31
Pretzel Bun Substitute, Add	80	1	15

Burgers:

	C	F	Cb
Chili	320	14	28
Chili Cheeseburger	370	18	28

Specialties:

	C	F	Cb
Corn Dogs: Regular (1)	230	13	21
Mini (6 pack)	300	18	24
Jalapeno Poppers, (6 pack)	300	16	31
Ranch Dressing	150	16	1
Polish Ssg S'wich	490	32	38

Sides:

	C	F	Cb
Chili Cheese Fries: Regular	560	31	58
Bacon Ranch, regular	900	66	60
Triple Cheese, Double Bacon, reg.	900	66	39
French Fries: Small	310	16	38
Medium	440	23	54
Large	750	39	92
Po'taters: Small	390	27	33
Medium	670	47	56
Large	1110	78	94

Breakfast:

	C	F	Cb
Biscuits: Egg, Bacon, Cheese	490	30	36
Egg, Sausage, Cheese	540	34	40
Burritos: Egg, Bacon, Cheese	370	19	29
Egg, Sausage, Cheese	460	28	33
French Toast Sticks	530	28	61
Syrup, 1 oz	120	0	31

Desserts:

	C	F	Cb
Classic Banana Split	760	24	131
Cones: Regular, Plain, 5 oz	250	9	41
Chocolate Dipped, 5 oz	450	27	50
Freezees,			
Oreo; M&M, Reese's, av.	630	25	99
Shakes, Chocolate with Oreo	950	35	155
Sundaes:			
Caramel; Choc; Hot Fudge, av.	400	15	64
Strawberry	370	14	59

Winchell's® (Sept '18)

Donuts: Per Donut

	C	F	Cb
Buttermillk Bars, Choc Iced/Glazed	420	19	61
Jelly Filled:			
Apple with Cinnamon Crumb	370	15	53
Raspberry with Glaze	390	13	61
Strawberry with Sugar	380	13	60
Old Fashioned, Glazed; Maple Iced	410	17	60
Raised Ring: Chocolate Iced	270	10	41
Sugared	230	9	34

WingStreet (Sept '18)

Chicken: Without Dipping Sauce

Bone Out Wings: Per Wing	C	F	Cb
Buffalo, Mild	90	4	10
Garlic Parmesan	130	9	6
Honey BBQ	100	4	11
Ranch Rub	80	4	6
Traditional Bone In Wings: Per Wing			
Buffalo, Medium/Hot	100	4.5	5
Garlic Parmesan	140	11	0.5
Spicy Garlic	120	8	3
Sides: Baked	60	2	4
Breadstick (1)	140	4.5	19
Straight Cut Fries, with Ketchup	500	24	67
Stuffed Garlic Knot	80	2.5	10

Woody's Bar-B-Q® (Sept '18)

Starters:

	C	F	Cb
Breaded Wings (10)	700	47	13
Beef Chili Cheese Fries	805	38	63

Dinner Entrees: Without Sides

	C	F	Cb
½ Chicken	840	56	0
Baby Back Combo	680	48	1
Baby Back Ribs	520	40	2
Beef Prime Rib	760	62	1
New York Strip	490	36	2
Pork Sampler	1010	62	4
Ribeye Steak	735	54	2

Sandwiches: Per Regular, without Sides

	C	F	Cb
Beef	390	14	28
Pork	490	26	29

Wraps: Without Sides

	C	F	Cb
Beef BBQ	380	13	31
Pork BBQ	440	21	31
Extras: BBQ Beans	170	8	20
Cobettes	80	1	18
French Fries	185	7	28
Garlic Toast	120	6	14
Green Beans	50	2.5	6
Okra	95	1	21
Squash	140	1	28

Yard House® (Sept '18)

Appetizers: With Sides & Sauce	C	F	Cb
Buffalo Wings, Traditional	1020	68	10
California Roll	1000	56	97
Chicken Nachos	2380	148	155
Fried Mac & Cheese	1520	103	109
Poke Nachos	870	59	51
Spinach Cheese Dip	1280	98	73
Snacks: Asado Taco (1)	240	13	16
Guacamole & Chips	760	49	75
Hot Spicy Edamame	500	41	19
Sweet Potato Fries	660	35	78
Grilled Burgers: Without Fries			
BBQ Bacon Cheddar Burger	1170	78	51
Black Truffle Cheeseburger	920	57	49
Kurobuta Pork Burger	930	52	63
Fries, 1 Serving	360	16	51
House Favorites: With Sides & Sauce			
Fish & Chips	1720	128	101
Mac & Cheese, w/ Chicken, full	1860	124	113
Parmesan Crusted Pork Loin	1130	45	81
Sesame Chicken Noodles	1580	96	71
Spicy Jambalaya Pasta, full	1310	67	103
Pizza: Margherita	840	28	110
The Carnivore	1400	75	101
Seafood: With Sides & Sauce			
Ginger Crusted Salmon	1070	63	65
Lobster Garlic Noodles	1030	57	76
Soups:			
Chicken Tortilla, bowl	980	75	45
Clam Chowder, bowl	360	23	26
Salads: Full Entree Size, with Dressing			
Cobb Chicken	1000	68	31
Kale, Grilled Shrimp Caesar	710	46	34

For Complete Nutritional Data ~ see CalorieKing.com

Yoshinoya® (Sept '18)

Entrees: As Served			
Grilled Steak Bowl: Regular	570	11	97
Large	850	17	144
Beef Bowl: Regular	730	27	91
Large	1040	38	131
With Vegetables: Regular	650	20	95
Large	960	29	141
Teriyaki Chicken Bowl:			
Regular, without Skin	740	15	110
Large, without Skin	1090	21	166
Grilled Tilapia: with Rice & Slaw	570	13	91
with Rice, Veggies & Teriyaki Sce	590	12	100
Sides, Clam Chowder Soup	210	7	34
Kid's Meals: Beef	350	11	48
Teriyaki Chicken without skin	340	6	53

For Complete Nutritional Data ~ see CalorieKing.com

Zaxby's® (Sept '18)

Zappertizers: With Menu Set Sauce	C	F	Cb
Buffalo Dip & Tater Chips	1020	70	77
Cheddar Bites, with Marinara Sauce	690	42	58
Fried Mushrooms, with Zestable Sce	590	46	39
Tater Chips, with Ranch Sauce	880	64	70
Zalads: With Texas Toast, Without Dressing			
Blackened Blue	540	27	32
Buffalo Blue	690	37	43
Fried Cobb Zalad	820	46	42
Fried House Zalad	700	38	41
Garden House Zalad	400	24	31
Grilled Cobb Zalad	680	35	34
Grilled House Zalad	560	28	33
Dressings: Per 1.2 oz Serving			
Blue Cheese	180	19	2
Caesar	90	8	2
Honey French	150	12	9
Mediterranean	140	14	4
Ranch	160	16	2
Sandwich Meals: With Menu Set Components			
Cajun Club	1040	49	92
Chicken Finger	1190	64	106
Chicken Salad	990	58	90
Grilled Chicken	900	38	97
Kickin' Chicken	1130	57	102
Nibblerz	1340	69	131
Zaxby's Club	1300	75	101
Wings & Fingers: With Sweet & Spicy Sauce			
Boneless: 5 Wings	410	19	37
10 Wings	810	37	73
20 Wings	1620	74	146
Traditional: 5 Wings	340	20	10
10 Wings	670	39	20
20 Wings	1340	78	40
Chicken Finger: 1 Finger	120	5	8
5 Fingers	600	23	42
10 Fingers	1210	47	85
20 Fingers	2420	93	180
Sides:			
Crinkle Fries: Regular, 5 oz	370	16	50
Large, 8 oz	590	36	86
Texas Toast:			
1 Slice, 1.5 oz	150	7	19
Basket, 4.5 oz	460	22	56
Kidz Meals:			
Kiddie Finger, 8.5 oz	720	41	63
Kidz Nibbler, 7.5 oz	670	31	78
Kiddie Cheese, 8.5 oz	840	46	91

Zero Sub's® ~ see CalorieKing.com

Updated Nutrition Data ~ www.CalorieKing.com
Persons with Diabetes ~ See Disclaimer (Page 22)

Notes on Cholesterol

- **Cholesterol** is a white waxy substance produced mainly by our liver. It is also found in animal food products. Plant foods have no cholesterol.

- **Cholesterol is essential to life.** It is a structural part of every body cell wall and is the building block for vitamin D, sex hormones, and bile acids which help in the digestion of dietary fats. **Cholesterol is also vital for a healthy brain** (which contains some 20% of total body cholesterol).

- **The body makes sufficient cholesterol** for its needs and does not rely on cholesterol in the diet. Dietary fats have a major influence on blood cholesterol levels. (See next page)

- **A high blood cholesterol level increases** the risk of atherosclerosis - the thickening of arteries that can reduce or block blood flow to the heart, brain, eyes, kidneys, sex organs and other body parts.

  This in turn increases the risk of heart attack, stroke, blindness, kidney failure, impotence and other blood circulatory problems.

  Other risk factors which increase the risk of atherosclerosis include high blood pressure, smoking, obesity and uncontrolled diabetes.

HEART ATTACK WARNING SIGNALS

Many victims die before reaching the hospital by ignoring warning signals and delaying medical help. Symptoms vary and commonly include:

- **Chest pain,** vice-like squeezing or burning sensation in center of the chest or between the shoulder blades, or in the mid-back. Pain may even feel like severe indigestion.

- **Pain** may be felt in the arms, shoulders, neck or jaw.

- **Shortness of breath** often occurs with or before chest discomfort.

- **Other signs,** with or without pain, include a cold sweat, nausea or light-headedness.

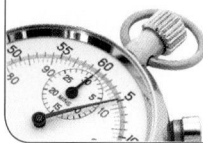

If you experience any of the above symptoms call IMMEDIATELY for medical help. Every minute counts.

Call 9-1-1 *or your emergency number*

BLOOD CHOLESTEROL

CHECK YOUR RISK!

Total Cholesterol Level (mg/dl) ▼	Risk of Heart Attack ▼
240 and above	~ **High Risk**
200 - 239	~ **Borderline/High**
Below 200	~ **Desirable**

❤ **Know your cholesterol level, particularly if there is a family history of heart disease or stroke. If your level is high, see your doctor.**

❤ **All adults should have their cholesterol, HDL and triglycerides tested at least every 5 years.**

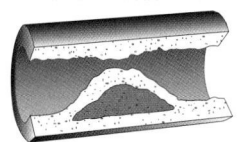

▲ **Atherosclerosis can clog arteries and impede blood flow to the heart or other body organs.**

▼ **A thrombus (blood clot) can form on unstable, festering athero-sclerotic plaque and rapidly block blood flow. A heart attack or stroke can result.**

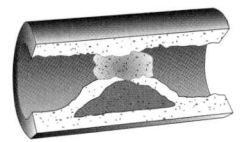

Fats & Cholesterol Guide

The amount and type of dietary fat has the greatest influence on blood cholesterol levels.

Fats in food are a mixture of 3 basic types: saturated, monounsaturated, and polyunsaturated. Animal fats are mainly saturated while plant oils and fish oils are mainly mono- and polyunsaturated.

Saturated fats have subgroups known as long-chain, medium-chain, and short-chain fats. Most of the long chain fats raise blood cholesterol, and increase the risk of blood clots and thrombosis leading to artery blockage.

Long-chain saturated fats are found mainly in full-cream milk, cheese, butter, cream, fatty meats and sausages, and processed foods.

Medium-chain fats (MCT) have little effect on LDL-cholesterol but may raise "good" HDL. *Note: Coconut oil has some MCT but is mainly saturated fat – so limit use.*

Monounsaturated fats tend to more selectively lower 'bad' LDL cholesterol and maintain the protective 'good' HDL cholesterol in the bloodstream – but only if they replace saturated fats in the diet. Foods rich in monounsaturates include canola and olive oils, canola margarine, peanuts, and avocados.

Polyunsaturated fats consist of two main classes. **Omega-6** polyunsaturates tend to lower blood cholesterol. Rich sources include safflower, sunflower and corn oils.

Omega-3 polyunsaturated fats can lower blood cholesterol; significantly lower blood triglycerides; and reduce the rise of thrombosis, heart arrythmmia, and artery spasm.

Best practical omega-3 sources include canola oil and margarine, soybean oil and fish.

A balanced intake of the two omega classes is important for optimal health. For most Americans, slightly increasing omega-3 intake would help attain a more ideal balance.

Trans fats from hydrogenated vegetable oils and shortenings should also be avoided. They are common in commercial baked and fried food products such as cakes, muffins, pastries, doughnuts, fried snacks and french fries.

DIETARY FATS COMPARISON

■ Saturated Fat   ▨ Monounsaturated Fat
Polyunsaturated Fats:
□ Linoleic (Omega-6) ■ Alpha-Linolenic (Omega-3)

OILS — PERCENTAGE CONTENT

OILS	Saturated	Monounsaturated	Linoleic (Omega-6)	Alpha-Linolenic (Omega-3)
CANOLA OIL	7	63	20	10
LINSEED/FLAX OIL	9	19	17	55
SAFFLOWER OIL	9	14	77	
GRAPESEED OIL	10	22	68	
SUNFLOWER OIL	11	23	66	
CORN OIL	14	32	52	2
OLIVE OIL	14	76	10	
SOYBEAN OIL	15	23	54	8
PEANUT OIL	19	45	34	2
COTTONSEED OIL	26	16	58	
PALM OIL	51	39	10	

SPREADS & FATS
Saturated Fat includes 'Trans Fats'   □ WATER CONTENT

	Saturated	Monounsaturated	Omega-6	Omega-3	Water
LIGHT MARGARINE	14	14	21	51	
CANOLA MARGARINE	18	45	12	6	19
POLYUNSATURATED MARG	24	20	36	20	
BUTTER	57	18	2		24
LARD	41	47			12
BEEF FAT	44	37	4		15

GOOD SOURCES OF OMEGA-3 FATS

Plant Sources	Omega-3 Fats (Grams)
Canola Oil, 1 Tbsp, ½ fl.oz	1.5g
Flaxseed Oil, 1 Tbsp	8g
Soybean Oil, 1 Tbsp	1.2g
Canola Margarine, 1 Tbsp, ½ oz	1g
Soybeans, cooked, ½ cup, 4 oz	0.5g
Walnuts, ½ oz	0.5g

FISH - *Per 4 oz Serving*

High Content: Salmon (Chinook), Tuna, Trout (Lake), Sardines, Herring, Mackerel — 3g, 3g

Medium Content:
Salmon, (Pink/Red/Coho), 4 oz — 2g

Fair Content: *Per 4 oz Serving*
Bass, Catfish, Cod, Grouper, Hake, Halibut, Kingfish, Perch, Pollock, Shark, Trout (Rainbow), Tuna, Crab, Oysters, Blue Mussels, Shrimp, Squid — 0.5-1g

How Much Is Needed?

As little as 1-2 grams daily of omega-3 fats may benefit general health. High doses of fish-oil supplements should only be taken as directed by your Healthcare provider.

Dietary Cholesterol

Cholesterol in food varies in its effect on blood cholesterol level (BCL) from person to person. Much depends on the amount and type of fat and fiber eaten at the same meal.

Any elevating effect of dietary cholesterol on BCL is more likely to occur when the diet is high in saturated fat. Little elevation, if any, generally occurs when dietary fats are balanced in favor of mono- and poly-unsaturated fats (including omega-3 fats).

Example: While fish does contain cholesterol, the omega-3 fats can prevent any increase in BCL. Conversely, a meal containing no cholesterol but rich in saturated fat may result in a significant increase in BCL - as well as impairing artery wall functions.

Consequently, the need to be overly concerned about dietary cholesterol is being de-emphasized in favor of simply limiting total fat, saturated fat, and trans fat in particular – and substituting unsaturated fats (including omega-3 fats).

Note: Persons with familial (genetic) hyper-cholesterolemia should limit cholesterol; and ideally follow a plant-based diet.

The liver usually cuts back its own cholesterol production in response to cholesterol in the diet. Many people can consume high-cholesterol foods without concern.

However, it is difficult to identify just who is at risk - the so-called 'hyper-responders'. Because over 50% of Americans have a BCL above ideal levels, it may be prudent to limit cholesterol intake to less than 300mg daily, as well as to adopt a heart-healthy diet.

This limitation still allows the inclusion of most foods that are regularly eaten – even the overly maligned egg.

Avocados (like all plant foods) contain no cholesterol. Their fats are mainly monounsaturated and can lower blood cholesterol.

CHOLESTEROL COUNTER

Cholesterol is found only in foods of animal origin. Plant foods contain no cholesterol.

	Cholesterol mg
Meat - Average all types:	
Lean Meat, cooked, 120g	100
Fatty Meat, cooked, 120g	100
Fat, thick strip, 60g	40

Note: While lean meat and fat have similar amounts of cholesterol, choose lean meat to limit fat intake.

	Cholesterol mg
Chicken/Turkey, average, 120g	100
Organ Meats: Liver, fried, 4 oz	500
Brains, beef, pan fried, 3 oz	1700
Sausages: Frankfurter, 40g	25
Salami, 2 slices, 55g	40
Bacon: 3 slices, cooked, 30g	20
Fish: Fish fillets, average, ckd, 120g	70
Tuna/Salmon, canned, 100g	50
Scallops, 9 medium, 3 oz	30
Prawns, raw, 100g	110
Oysters, raw, 6 medium, 85g	45
Crayfish, Crab, cooked, 100g	70
Eggs (Chicken), 1 large	210
1 medium	180
Egg White, *Scramblers*	0
Milk/Yoghurt: Whole, 1 cup, 250ml	30
Light/low-fat Milk (1%), 1 cup	10
Skim/Non-fat, 1 cup	10
Soy Milk, Tofu, Tempeh	0
Cheese: Natural/Hard/Cream, 30g	30
Cottage, low-fat, 2 Tbsp, 40g	5
Cream Cheese, 30g	25
Fats: Butter, 1 Tbsp, 20g	45
Margarine, Oils (vegetable)	0
Mayonnaise, 1 Tbsp	10
Cream: Heavy, whipping, 2 Tbsp, 40g	40
Light/Sour, 2 Tbsp	10
Ice Cream: Full-fat (10-11%), 100ml/50g	20
Low-fat (less than 4%), 50g	5
Fruit, Vegetables, Avocados	0
Nuts, Seeds, Grains	0
Coffee, Tea, Beer, Wine	0

For Comprehensive Food Listings ~ see www.CalorieKing.com

Blood Cholesterol ~ Diet Hints

DIETARY HINTS TO LOWER BLOOD CHOLESTEROL

1. **Maintain a healthy weight.**
   If overweight, lose weight with a sensible, low-fat meal plan and daily exercise.

2. **Reduce saturated fat intake by:**

   (a) eating less dairy fat. Choose low-fat or fat-reduced varieties of milk, yogurt, soy drinks, cheese, and ice cream.

   (b) replacing saturated fats with fats and oils rich in monounsaturated and polyunsaturated fats. Choose vegetable oils such as extra-virgin olive, canola and soybean. Avoid solid frying fats.

   Note: *Promise Active* and *Benecol* spreads contain plant stanol esters which can lower total and LDL cholesterol.

   (c) eating less fat from meat and poultry. Choose lean cuts of meat and skinless chicken. Go easy on lunch meats, salami and fatty sausages. Enjoy fish.

   (d) eating less saturated and trans fats from baked and fried fast-foods. Avoid deep-fried foods. Avoid donuts, cakes, pastries and cookies unless made with healthier fats and oils.

3. **Increase your soluble fiber intake.**
   Foods rich in soluble fiber include beans, lentils, chickpeas, hummus, nuts, seeds, psyllium-seed husks and psyllium-fiber supplements. Oat bran, rice bran and barley are also good sources, as are fruit, vegetables and avocados.
   (See Fiber Guide - Page 264-269).

4. **Eat more soy bean products such as:**
   soy drinks, tofu, tempeh (cultured soy beans), soy flour, soy vegetarian foods and edamame (fresh green soybeans).
   Soy protein in place of animal protein can significantly decrease high blood cholesterol levels as well as 'bad' LDL cholesterol and blood triglycerides while 'good' HDL cholesterol is maintained. For best results, eat at least 25g of soy protein per day (from 3-4 servings).

5. **Eat more fruit, vegetables, and whole grains** in place of high-fat foods. Aim for 2 fruits and 5 servings of vegetables per day. They also contain valuable antioxidants. The fat of avocados (and most nuts) is mainly unsaturated and can lower blood cholesterol levels.

6. **Limit cholesterol to 300mg per day.** (Extra Notes ~ See Previous Page)

7. **Avoid brewed unfiltered coffee** (espresso; plunger-style). Several cups per day may raise blood cholesterol. Filtered coffee is fine.

8. **Spread your food intake over the day.** Have 5-6 small meals per day rather than just 2-3 large meals. Nibbling, versus gorging, favors lower blood cholesterol.

ALCOHOL – WINE

Alcohol is a mixed bag. Moderate amounts of 1-2 drinks daily appear to reduce the risk of heart attack and ischemic stroke in older persons.

However, larger amounts increase the risk of high blood pressure, obesity, heart failure and hemorrhagic stroke, and can aggravate hypertriglyceridemia: as well as many other health hazards. (See Alcohol Guide – Page 23)

The speculative benefits of moderate alcohol intake have been overstated in the media. The overriding harmful effects of excess alcohol do not allow its recommendation for any aspects of health promotion.

Fruit, Vegetables & Tea Also Protect:

Red wine and red grapes (more so than white) contain antioxidants which may help protect cholesterol in the blood from becoming oxidized. Many fruits, vegetables, grains, nuts and tea also contain protective antioxidants.

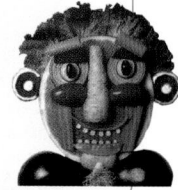

Fats in the diet affect more than blood cholesterol levels. They can also strongly influence blood clot formation and thrombosis, as well as blood flow and ultimate oxygen delivery to body parts and organs. While advanced atherosclerosis can impede blood flow to the heart and other organs, it is thrombosis (complete blockage by blood clots) or arterial spasm which commonly results in a heart attack or stroke.

Plant and fish oils rich in omega-3 fats lessen the risk of blood clots, thrombus formation, and artery spasm by reducing platelet stickiness and adhesion to artery walls. This also reduces inflammation of the artery wall lining. This in turn reduces the risk of atherosclerotic plaque becoming unstable and reactive.

Omega-3 fats also improve blood flow by reducing blood viscosity and increasing the flexibility of red blood cells that need to flex and twist on themselves in order to squeeze through tiny narrow capillaries often half their diameter.

A diet high in saturated fats (longer chain) has the opposite effect by stiffening red blood cell membranes and increasing blood viscosity, thereby hindering blood flow.

Stiff red blood cells may also form aggregates that resemble coin stacks. In narrow blood vessels, this further impedes blood flow and impairs oxygen release through the much-lessened surface area of red blood cell membranes exposed to blood.

Note: Smoking, lack of exercise, and stress can have similar adverse effects on thrombosis, red blood cell flexibility, and blood flow.

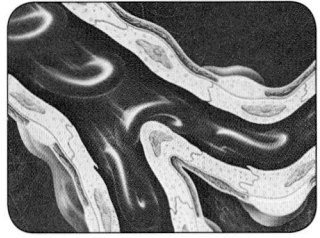

▲ *Picture of Healthy Blood Flow*

Flexible red blood cells twist and slide through tiny capillaries - often half the diameter of red blood cells.

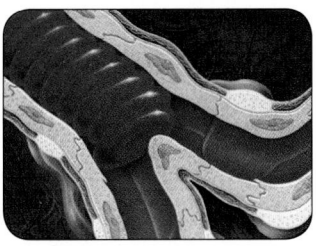

▲ *A Not-So-Healthy Picture!*

Red blood cells have lost their flexibility and ability to twist and slip through capillaries. They are stacked up, thereby impeding blood flow.

A diet high in saturated fats can contribute to this picture - as can smoking, lack of exercise, and stress.

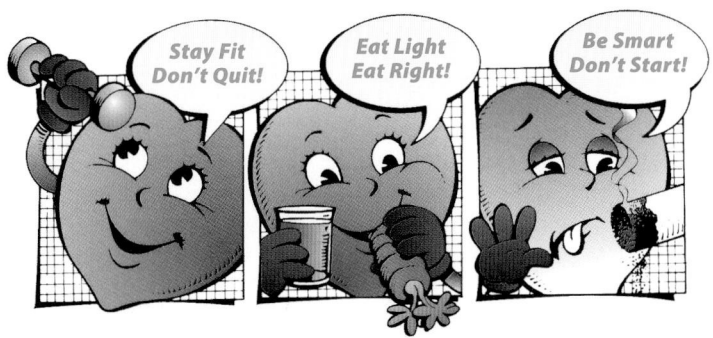

Fiber Guide

Introduction

`Fiber`

Fiber is the general term for those parts of plant food that we cannot digest (although bacteria in the large bowel partly digests fiber through fermentation). It is not found in foods of animal origin (meats, dairy products).

Fiber promotes intestinal health, bowel regularity, can benefit diabetes and blood cholesterol levels, and may help prevent colon cancer. High-fiber foods also assist weight control.

Most Americans don't eat enough fiber – less than 20 grams/day – instead of a healthier 25 to 35 grams/day.

Types of Fiber

Plant foods contain a mixture of different fibers in varying proportions. Insoluble and soluble fiber categories are based on their solubility in water. All types of fiber are beneficial to the body.

♦ Insoluble fibers (cellulose, hemi-celluloses, lignin) make up the structural parts of plant cell walls.

> **Best food sources** are wheat bran, corn bran, rice bran, wholegrain cereals and breads, beans and peas, nuts, seeds, and the skins of fruits and vegetables.

These fibers absorb many times their own weight in water. They create a soft bulk and hasten the passage of waste products through the intestines.

They promote bowel regularity, and aid in the prevention and treatment of uncomplicated forms of **constipation, diverticulosis and hemorrhoids.**

The risk of colon cancer may also be reduced by fiber's diluting effect on potentially harmful substances.

♦ Soluble fibers **(pectin, gums, mucilages)** are found mainly within plant cells, soy milk (whole bean) and products.

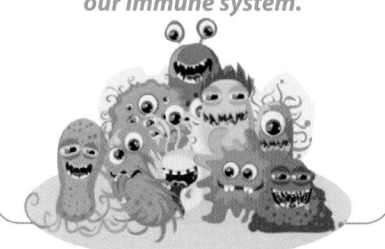

A fiber-rich diet assists the growth of friendly gut microbes that can benefit our metabolism, weight and blood glucose levels – as well as hunger, mood and our immune system.

Best Sources of Soluble Fiber:

Fruits and vegetables, oat bran, barley, beans and peas, prunes, psyllium and flax seed.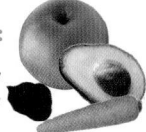

These fibers form a gel which slows both stomach emptying and the absorption of sugars from the intestines. **This helps to control blood sugar levels.**

Weight control is also aided by the slower emptying of the stomach and the feeling of **fullness provided by soluble fiber.**

Soluble fiber can also lower blood cholesterol by binding bile acids and excreting them. More body cholesterol must then be broken down to supply bile acids for emulsification of dietary fats. **Rice bran, while not high in soluble fiber, can also lower blood cholesterol.**

♦ Resistant starch is that part of starchy foods (approx. 10%) which is tightly bound by fiber and resists normal digestion. Friendly bacteria in the large bowel ferment and change the resistant starch into short-chain fatty acids, which are important to bowel health and may protect against colon cancer.

Starchy foods include bread, cereals, rice, pasta, potatoes and legumes.

Fiber & Weight Control

Fiber can assist weight control in several ways. Fiber-rich foods such as fresh fruit and vegetables, potatoes and wholegrain bread contain few calories for their large volume (due to their low-fat, high-water content).

Their bulk fills the stomach and satisfies the appetite much sooner than fiber-depleted foods. The extra chewing time also contributes to satiety, and gives the stomach time to register a feeling of fullness. Excessive calories are less likely to be consumed.

Fiber-depleted foods and drinks are more concentrated in calories; e.g. fats, sugar, candy, soft drinks, fruit juices, alcohol. They require little or no chewing. Large amounts with excessive calories can be consumed before the appetite is satisfied.

Example: Whereas one fresh apple might satisfy the appetite, an apple juice drink with the equivalent sugars and calories of 2-3 apples only minimally satisfies the appetite. (See illustration below.)

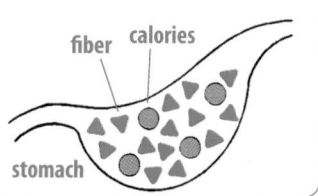

High-fiber foods fill the stomach. Fewer calories are consumed.

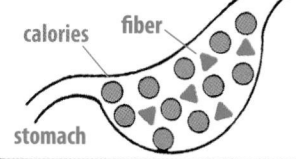

Low-fiber foods are more concentrated in calories. More food must be eaten to fill the stomach.

EFFECTS OF REMOVING FIBER FROM FOOD

2-3 pieces of fresh fruit produces 1 glass of fruit juice. The removal of fiber concentrates the sugar and calories.

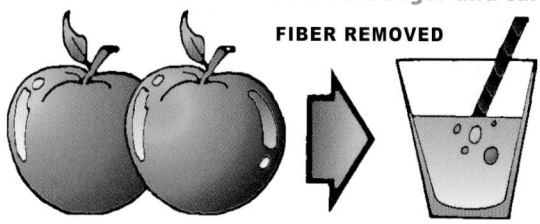

FIBER REMOVED

FRESH FRUIT	(Comparison)	FRUIT JUICE
High Fiber	←	Negligible Fiber
Low Calorie Density	←	High Calorie Density
Long Eating Time	←	No Eating Time (Drink)
Satisfies Hunger	←	Does Not Satisfy Hunger
Sugar Slowly Absorbed	←	Sugar More Quickly Absorbed
Less Insulin Required	←	More Insulin Required
Supports Gut Microbes	←	Few Benefits to Microbes

Fiber Guide ~ Constipation

Constipation

Constipation can reasonably be defined as a failure to have a bowel movement at least every second day – and just as importantly, without straining or pain.

Typically, constipated stools are too hard, too narrow and too small.

The **main cause** is simply a lack of dietary fiber. Other contributing factors include insufficient fluids, too little exercise, emotional stress, gastrointestinal disease, lack of proper dentition to chew high-fiber foods, and some medications (e.g. some antacids, antidepressants, pain medications).

Note: Check with your doctor to rule out any underlying medical problem – especially if you have a change in bowel habits in middle-age or later years.

DESIRABLE FIBER INTAKE

Adults: 25-35gm per day
Children (under 18): Age + 5gm
Example: 6-year old (6 + 5)= 11gm

SAMPLE FOOD QUANTITIES
For 35 Grams of Fiber/Day

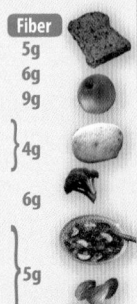

	Fiber
Breakfast Cereal (higher-fiber)	5g
plus 4 slices wholegrain Bread	6g
plus 3 servings fresh Fruit	9g
plus 1 medium Potato (w. skin)	}4g
or 1 cup Brown Rice	
or ½ cup wholegrain Pasta	
plus 3-4 servings Veggies/Salad	6g
plus 1 cup Bean Soup	
or ¼ cup Baked/Soy Beans	}5g
or ½ cup Corn/Peas/Lentils	
or 1¼ oz Almonds (natural)	
or 3 medium Figs	

HINTS TO INCREASE FIBER AND AVOID CONSTIPATION

① **Breakfast is an important** contributor to daily fiber intake. Eat high-fiber breakfast cereals (bran-based cereals, oatmeal etc.). Add 1-2 tablespoons of unprocessed bran. Dried fruits, chopped nuts, soy grits, and seeds are also excellent additions to cereals.

Note: A gradual increase in fiber will prevent bloating, gas or pain. People intolerant to bran may benefit from psyllium-based fiber supplements and cereals.

② **Drink adequate water daily.** Fiber works by absorbing many times its own weight in water.

③ **Eat wholegrain breads,** or fiber-enriched breads. They have over double the fiber of regular white bread.

④ **Enjoy fruit as fresh fruit** with skin rather than as fruit juice. Enjoy wholegrain pasta, barley, brown rice, nuts and seeds.

⑤ **Eat more vegetables,** salads and legumes – especially cooked beans, lentils, potatoes with skins, avocado, broccoli, brussels sprouts, cabbage, carrots, celery, and peas.

⑥ **Add bran** (barley/rice/wheat) or soy grits to soups, casseroles, yogurt, desserts, cookies, cakes. Also use whole-meal flour or soy flour in place of white flour. Use nuts, seeds, and ground linseed.

⑦ **Snack** on fresh or dried fruits, carrot or celery sticks, popcorn, nuts or seeds, wholegrain crackers, high-fiber bars (low-fat). Limit amounts if overweight.

⑧ **Exercise regularly** to strengthen abdominal muscles and stimulate the gut. Keep up water intake, especially in warm weather.

⑨ **Avoid** indiscriminate and regular use of harsh laxatives. They can overstimulate the intestinal muscles and may make normal bowel activity impossible. It may take several weeks to restore normal bowel function.

FOODS WITH ZERO FIBER
- **Dairy Products (Milk, Cheese, etc)**
- **Meats, Poultry, Fish, Eggs**
- **Fats/Oils, Sugar/Syrups**
  (Only foods of plant origin contain fiber.)

Breakfast Cereals   `Fiber`
General Mills:
Basic 4, 1 cup, 2 oz	3
Cheerios (Honey Nut; Multigrain), 1 c., 1 oz	2
Fiber One, 1/2 cup, 1.1 oz	14
Multi-Bran Chex, 1 cup, 2 oz	7
Oatmeal Crisp Almond, 1 cup, 2 oz	4
Raisin Nut Bran, 1 1/4 cup, 2 oz	6
Total, average all types, 3/4 cup, 1 oz	3
Wheat Chex, 1 cup, 2 oz	6
Wheaties 3/4 cup, 1 oz	3

Health Valley:
Amaranth Flakes, 3/4 cup, 1 oz	3
Crunches & Flakes, 3/4 cup, 1.9 oz	4
Fiber 7 Flakes, 3/4 cup, 1 oz	7
Golden Flax, 3/4 cup, 1.9 oz	6
Granola (Low-Fat), 3/4 cup, 2 oz	6
Healthy Fiber Flakes, 3/4 cup, 1.1 oz	4
Oat Bran Flakes, all types, 3/4 cup, 1 oz	2
Oat Bran O's, 3/4 cup, 1 oz	3
Real Oat Bran, 1/2 cup, 1.7 oz	5

Kellogg's:
All-Bran, 1/2 cup, 1.1 oz	10
All-Bran w. Extra Fiber, 1/2 cup, 1 oz	13
All-Bran Bran Buds, 1/3 cup, 1.1 oz	13
Corn Flakes, Fruit Loops, Smacks 1 cup, 1 oz	1
Cocoa/Rice Krispies Treats, 1 1/4 cup, 1 oz	0
Complete: Wheat Flakes, 3/4 c., 1 oz	5
Oat Bran Flakes, 3/4 cup, 1.1 oz	4
Corn Pops, 1 cup, 1.1 oz	0
Cracklin' Oat Bran, 3/4 cup, 1.7oz	6
FiberPlus Antioxidants:	
Berry Yogurt Crunch, 1 c., 1.9 oz	10
Cinnamon Oat Crunch 3/4 c., 1.1 oz	9
Frosted Mini Wheats, 24 bisc., 2 oz	5
Granola w. Raisins, 2/3 cup, 2.1 oz	3
Raisin Bran, 1 cup, 2.1 oz	7
Smart Start, Strong Heart,	
Cinnamon Raisin, 1 cup, 1.8 oz	4
Special K, 1 cup, 1.1 oz	0.5

`Fiber` ~ Fiber (grams)

Breakfast Cereals (Cont)   `Fiber`
Kashi:
GoLEAN Cereal, 1 cup, 1.8 oz	10
GoLEAN Crunch!, 1 cup, 1.9 oz	8
GoLEAN Bars, avg. (1)	6
Good Friends: Original, 1 cup, 1.9 oz	12
Cinna-Raisin Crunch, 1 cup, 1.8 oz	8
Heart to Heart, 3/4 cup, 1.2 oz	5
7 Whole Grain Pilaf, 1/2 cup, cooked, 5 oz	7
7 Whole Grain Puffs, 1 cup, 0.7 oz	1

Quaker:
Cap'n Crunch, 3/4 cup, 1 oz	1
100% Natural Granola,	
avg., 1/2 cup, 1.8 oz	3
Crunchy Corn Bran, 1 cup, 1 oz	5
Life Cereal, 3/4 cup, 1.1 oz	2
Oat Bran, 1/2 cup, 1.4 oz	6
Oatmeal, average, 1 packet	3

Post:
100% Bran, 1/3 cup, 1 oz	9
Alpha Bits, 1 cup, 1 oz	2
Blueberry Morning, 1 cup, 1.9 oz	5
Cranberry Almond Crunch, 1 cup, 1.8 oz	3
Fruit & Bran, 1 cup, 1.9 oz	6
Grape-Nuts, 1/2 cup, 2 oz	7
Great Grains, 2/3 cup, 1.9 oz	5
Honey Bunches of Oats, 3/4 cup, 1.1 oz	2
Shredded Wheat & Bran, 1/2 cup, 2 oz	8

Brans & Supplements, Metamucil
Oat Bran: 1 Tbsp (level)	1
1/3 cup, (5 1/3 Tbsp), 1 oz	5
Rice Bran, raw. 1/3 cup, 1 oz	6
Wheat Bran, Unprocessed:	
Raw, 1 Tbsp	1.5
2 Tbsp (level), 1/4 oz	3
1/4 cup, (4 Tbsp), 1/2 oz	6
Wheat Germ, Raw, 1/4 cup, 1 oz	4
Psyllium Seed Husks, 2 Tbsp	8
Fibersure, 1 heaping tsp	5
Metamucil: Orange, 1 rnd Tbsp, 11g	3
Fiber Wafers (2)	6

Hot Cereals, Oatmeal
Bulgur (cracked Wheat), ckd, 1 cup	8
Corn/Hominy Grits, dry, 3 Tbsp, 1 oz	0.5
Cream of Wheat, cooked, 3/4 cup	1
Oatmeal (uncooked 1/3 cup), ckd, 2/3 cup	3

Fiber Counter

Breads & Crackers | Fiber

Bread: White, 1 slice, 1 oz — 0.6
Whole-wheat, 1 slice, 1 oz — 1.5
Wholegrain, 1 slice, 1 oz — 2
Rye, Pumpernickel, 1 oz — 1.5
Bagel/Roll/Bun, 1 medium, 2 oz — 1.5
Pita, whole wheat, 6.5" pocket — 4.5
Crackers: Graham, average, 2 — 0.4
Saltine, 4 crackers — 0.4
Crispbreads, average, 2 — 4
Matzo, 1 board, 1 oz — 1
Rice Cakes, average, 1 cake — 0.3
Tortilla: Regular, 6" — 0.5
Whole-wheat, 6" — 1.3

Barley, Pasta, Rice & Flours

Barley, pearled, raw, 1/4 cup, 1.7 oz — 8
Rice:
White, cooked, 1 cup — 0.6
Brown, cooked, 1 cup — 3.5
Rice-A-Roni, average, 1 cup, prepared — 1.5
Spaghetti/Noodles: Cooked, 1 cup — 2
Whole-Wheat, cooked, 1 cup — 4
Flour: Wheat, All-purpose, 1 cup, 4.5 oz — 3.5
Whole-Wheat, 1 cup, 4.5 oz — 15
Cornmeal, stone ground, 1 cup, 4.5 oz — 13
Carob Flour, 1 cup, 3.5 oz — 41
Rye Flour, 1 cup, 3.5 oz — 15
Soy Flour: Defatted, 1 cup, 3.5 oz — 17
Full-fat, raw, 1 cup, 3 oz — 8
Soy Meal, defatted, 1 cup, 4.5 oz — 14

Frozen Entrees & Dinners

Average All Brands: Per Serving
Beans/Chili base, average — 6-10
Potato/Pasta base, average — 4-6
Vegetable base, average — 3
Meat/Chicken base, average — 2-3
Pizzas, 1/4 large, average — 3
Vegetarian Soy Burgers, 1 pattie — 4

Soups

Chicken Noodle, 1 cup — 0.5
Tomato Soup, average, 1 cup — 0.5
Vegetable Soup, average, 1 cup — 3
Health Valley: Per 1 Cup
Black Bean; Minestrone — 8
Tomato — 1
5 Bean Vegetable; Lentil & Carrots — 10
Mushroom Barley; Vegetable — 4
Split Pea — 8
Progresso, High Fiber, all flavors, 1 cup — 7

Fast Foods & Restaurants | Fiber

Hamburgers: Small, average — 1.5
Large/Whopper, average — 2.5
Hot Dog, Regular — 1.5
French Fries: Small serving, 2.5 oz — 2.5
Regular/Medium, 3.5 oz — 3.5
Chicken Nuggets, 6 pack — 0.5
Chicken Sandwich, average — 2
Taco, average — 4
Sundaes, Shakes, Soft Drinks — 0
Arby's, Classic Roast Beef Sandwich — 1
Denny's: Grilled Chicken Salad, no bread — 4
Classic Burger, no fries — 4
Club Sandwich, no fries — 2
Grilled Chicken Sandwich, no fries — 4
Domino's: 12", Classic/Thin, 1 slice — 1
Deep Dish, 1 slice — 3
Feast Pizza, Classic/Thin, 1 slice — 2
McDonald's: Big Mac — 3
Hamburger; Quarter Pounder — 3
Egg McMuffin — 2
Grilled Chicken Caesar Salad — 4
Pizza Hut: Per 1 Slice, Medium
Pan Pizza: Cheese, Pepperoni — 1
Supreme — 2
Thin 'n Crispy, Supreme — 2
Hand-Tossed, average all varieties — 2
Subway: Sandwich, white roll, av. — 4
With Honey Wheat Roll, average — 3
Salads, average — 4

Cakes, Cookies, Snack Bars

Apple/Fruit Pie, 1 serving, 4 oz — 2
Cake: With plain flour, 1 serving, 3.4 oz — 1.5
With whole-wheat flour, 1 serving — 4
Carrot Cake, 4 oz — 4
Cookies, oatmeal, (3 small/1 large) — 1
Donuts, medium, 1.7 oz — 0.7
Fruit Cake, 1 serving, 1.5 oz — 2
Fig Bars, 1 cookie, 0.5 oz — 0.7
Muffins, Oat Bran (2 small, 1 large), 4 oz — 5
Granola Bars, average, 1 bar — 2
Atkins Advantage Bars, average — 7
Clif Bars, 2.5 oz — 5
Curves, Chocolate Peanut Bar, 1 oz — 5
Fi-Bar Chewy & Nutty, 1 bar — 1
Fiber One (Gen. Mills), 1.4 oz bar — 9
FiberPlus, all bars, 1.2 oz — 9
Health Valley: Fruit/Granola Bars — 3
Cereal Bars — 1
Luna Bars, avg., 1.7 oz — 3
Special K, Protein Meal Bar, 1.6 oz — 5

Fiber Counter

Chocolate, Chips, Popcorn | Fiber
Cheese Balls/Curls/Twists	1
Chocolate, Hard Candy, 1 oz	0
Chocolate with nuts/fruit, 2 oz bar	1.5
Mars Bar, 1.8 oz	1
Potato Chips; corn chips, 1 oz	1
Popcorn, 3 cups	3
Pretzels, Twists (6)	1

Nuts, Seeds
Almonds: Natural, 25 nuts, 1 oz	3.5
Blanched (skins removed), 1 oz	3
Cashews, Filberts, Pecans, 1 oz	1.7
Peanuts, Mixed Nuts, Coconut, 1 oz	2.5
Peanut Butter, 2 Tbsp, 1 oz	2
Pistachio Nuts, dried, shelled, 1 oz	3
Walnuts, Black/English, dried, 1 oz	2
Seeds: Amaranth, 2¹/₂ Tbsp, 1 oz	3.5
Flax Seeds, 3 Tbsp, 1 oz	7
Psyllium Seed Husks, 5 Tbsp, 1 oz	20
Quinoa Seeds, 3 Tbsp, 1 oz	1.7
Sesame Seeds, whole, 1 oz	3.4
Sesame Butter/Tahini, 2 Tbsp, 1.1 oz	1.4
Sunflower kernels,¹/₄ cup, 1 oz	3.8
Teff Seeds, 1 oz	3.8

Fruit – Fresh
Apples: 1 medium, 5¹/₂ oz (whole)	
with skin + core	3.7
with skin, no core	3.2
without skin, no core	1.7
Apricots, 2 medium, 4 oz	1.5
Avocado, average, ¹/₂ medium	6
Banana, 1 medium, 6 oz (w. skin)	3
Blueberries, raw, ¹/₂ cup, 2.5 oz	1.7
Cherries, sweet, raw, 8 fruits, 1.6 oz	1
Grapefruit, average, ¹/₂ fruit, 10 oz	1.4
Grapes, 1 medium bunch, seedless, 7 oz	2
Kiwifruit, 1 medium, 2.7 oz	2.3
Mango, 1 medium, 11 oz (whole)	1.6
Melons, Cantaloupe, 4 oz (edible)	1
Nectarine, 1 medium, 4 oz	1.9
Olives, average all types, 7 jumbo, 2 oz	1.5
Oranges, 1 medium (7-8 oz w. skin)	
5¹/₂ oz (peeled)	3.8
Passionfruit, 2 medium, 2.5 oz	5
Peaches, 1 large, 6 oz	2
Pears, raw, 1 medium, 6 oz	4.5
Pineapple, 1 slice, 3 oz	1.2
Plums, 2 medium, 6 oz	1.8
Strawberries, 6 medium/3 large, 2 oz	1
Watermelon, 4 oz (edible)	0.5

Fruit – Dried, Juice | Fiber
Dried Fruit: Apricots, 8 halves, 1 oz	2.2
Dates (3 med); Raisins (2 Tbsp), 1 oz	1.5
Figs, 3 medium,1¹/₂ oz	5
Prunes, 4 medium, 1 oz	2
Fruit Juice: Orange/Apple etc, 1 glass	<0.5
Prune Juice, 5 oz	1.4
Carrot Juice, 8 oz	1.8

Vegetables
Asparagus, 4 medium spears	1.3
Bean Sprouts, ¹/₂ cup, 2 oz	1
Beans: Snap/Green, ¹/₂ cup, 2 oz	2
Baked Beans in Tom Sce, ¹/₂ c, 4.5 oz	5
Dried Beans, ckd, average, ¹/₂ cup	7
Beets, ckd, slices, ¹/₂ cup, 3 oz	1.7
Broccoli, cooked, ¹/₂ cup, 3 oz	2.4
Brussels Sprouts, ckd, ¹/₂ cup, 3 oz	3.5
Cabbage: White, ckd, ¹/₂ cup, 2.5 oz	1
Red, ckd, ¹/₂ cup,2.5 oz	2
Carrots, 1 medium (7¹/₂"), ¹/₂ cup, 3 oz	2.5
Cauliflower, cooked, 3 flowerets, 2 oz	1.5
Celery, raw, diced, 1 cup, 3.5 oz	1.6
Chickpeas (Garbanzos), ckd, ¹/₂ c., 3 oz	6.5
Corn: Kernels, cooked, ¹/₂ cup, 2¹/₂ oz	2.5
Corn on the Cob, 1 ear, 5 oz	4
Cucumber/Lettuce/Mushrooms, 2 oz	0.5
Eggplant, raw, sliced, ¹/₂ cup , 1.5 oz	2
Lentils, cooked, ¹/₂ cup, 3.5 oz	8
Mixed Vegetables, frozen, cooked, ¹/₂ cup	3
Onions: Raw, 1 medium, 4 oz	1.5
Spring Onions, chop., ¹/₄ cup, 1 oz	0.7
Peas: Green, raw, ¹/₂ cup, 2.5 oz	3.7
Cowpeas (Black-eyed), ckd, ¹/₂ cup	10
Split Peas, cooked, ¹/₂ cup, 3.5 oz	8
Peppers, sweet, raw, 1 large, 6 oz	3
Potatoes: 1 medium, with skin, 5 oz	4
1 medium, without skin	2.5
¹/₂ cup mashed, 3.5 oz	1.5
French Fries, small, 2.6 oz	3
Spinach, cooked, ¹/₂ cup, 3 oz	2.2
Squash: Summer, cooked, ¹/₂ cup, 3 oz	2.5
Winter, cooked, ¹/₂ cup, 3.5 oz	2.4
Tomatoes: 1 medium, 4.5 oz	1.5
Tomato Sauce, 1 cup	0.3
Soybean Products: Miso, ¹/₂ c., 5 oz	7.4
Tempeh, cooked, 1 piece, 3 oz	3
Tofu, ¹/₂ cup, 4.4 oz	0.4

Salads:
Side Salad, average	1
Bean Salad, ¹/₂ cup	5
Coleslaw, ¹/₂ cup	1
Potato Salad, ¹/₂ cup	2

Protein Guide

General Notes

- **Protein has many important body functions.** It builds and repairs muscle, and is the basis of our body's organs, hormones, enzymes, and antibodies to fight infection.

- **Protein is also an emergency fuel** in the absence of sufficient carbohydrate and fats. For this reason, weight loss should be gradual so as to preserve protein levels in muscle, the heart and other body organs.

- **It is easy to obtain sufficient protein,** even if vegetarian. **Plant proteins are not inferior to animal proteins.** In fact, eating more soy and other plant proteins, and less animal protein, may help to build stronger bones and prevent osteoporosis, and may help to control blood cholesterol levels.

- **When changing to a vegetarian diet,** include soybeans, and other beans, soy milk drinks (calcium-enriched), lentils, tofu, tempeh, nuts and wholegrain breads and cereals. Milk, yogurt, cheese and eggs can enhance nutrient intake.

Protein & Muscle

- Although muscles are built of protein, protein is not a special fuel for working muscle cells – carbohydrates and fats are.

- In fact, a diet high in protein (and fat) and low in carbohydrate can significantly reduce the performance of endurance sports athletes. **Carbohydrates** are the best fuel for muscles exercised for long periods.

- Any **extra protein** required by athletes and body-builders can easily be obtained from the extra food eaten to satisfy hunger and energy needs.

- Remember, **excessive protein** intake will not build bigger muscles. Any excess is converted and stored as fat. Excess protein can also strain the kidneys, which excrete the waste products of protein metabolism.

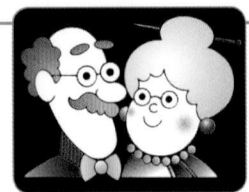

Elderly people (and dieters) must eat sufficient food to ensure adequate protein intake.

Inadequate protein leads to a drop in immune response with greater susceptibility to illness and infections. Muscle strength and muscle mass also drop.

Protein needs are easily met with sensible eating. Athletes who eat enough food for their energy needs can obtain sufficient protein.

RECOMMENDED DAILY PROTEIN INTAKE
~ HEALTHY RANGE ~
(Lower figure is RDA)

		PROTEIN
Children:	1-3 yrs	13g-26g
	4-8 yrs	19g-38g
	9-13 yrs	34g-64g
Males:	14-18 yrs	52g-120g
	19+	56g-120g
Females:	14+	46g-110g
Pregnancy:		71g-120g
Breastfeeding:		71g-120g

Note: On lower-calorie diets, aim for higher amounts of protein within the Healthy Range.

Pro ~ Protein (grams)

Meat | **Pro**

Bacon, 3 medium slices	6
Ground Beef Patty, lean, cooked, 3 oz	21
Ham: Luncheon, 2 slices, 1$\frac{1}{2}$ oz	7
Roasted, 2 pieces, 3 oz	18
Lamb chop, broiled, 3 oz	22
Liver, cooked, 3 oz	23
Pastrami, 3 slices, 1$\frac{3}{4}$ oz	10
Pork, cooked, lean, 3 oz	24
Roast Beef, lean, 2 slices, 3 oz	24
Sausages: Bologna, 2 sl., 2 oz	7
Braunschweiger, 2 sl., 2 oz	8
Pork link, thick, 2 oz	6
Frankfurter, 1$\frac{1}{3}$ oz	5
Salami, hard, 3 slices, 1 oz	7
Steak: Average all cuts, lean (no fat)	
Small (4 oz raw/3 oz cooked)	23
Medium (6 oz raw/4$\frac{1}{4}$ oz cooked)	34
Large (10 oz raw/7$\frac{1}{2}$ oz cooked)	57
Veal cutlet, 1 medium	23
Vegetarian, 1 pattie	13

Chicken/Turkey: *Without Skin*

Chicken, cooked: Breast, Roasted, 4 oz	36
Leg/Thigh,Roasted, 2 oz	14
$\frac{1}{2}$ Whole Chicken	60
Drumstick, Rstd, 1 med., 3 oz	13
Turkey: Light meat, cooked, 3 oz	28
Dark meat, lean, 3 oz	24

Fish

Fresh Fish: *Per 4 oz, cooked*	
Cod, Flounder/Sole, Pollock	28
Catfish, Haddock, Halibut, M/Mahi	28
Ocean Perch, Swordf., Orange Roughy	28
Canned Fish: Tuna, Light, 3 oz	25
White, 3 oz	23
Salmon, pink, 3 oz	17
Salmon, red, 3 oz	17
Sardines, 3 whole (3"), 1$\frac{1}{4}$ oz	9
Anchovies, 1 can, 1$\frac{1}{2}$ oz	13
Shellfish: Crabmeat, 3 oz	17.5
Clams, raw, 4 large/9 sml, 3 oz	11
Crayfish, cooked, 3 oz	20
Lobster, cooked, 3 oz	17
Oysters, raw, 6 medium, 3 oz	7
Scallops, 2 lge/5 small, 1 oz	5
Shrimp, raw, 6 large, 1$\frac{1}{2}$ oz	8.5
Fish Products: Fish Sticks, 4 sticks	10
Fish Portions, in batter, 4 oz	13
Gefilte Fish, 1 medium ball, 2 oz	8

Eggs | **Pro**

1 Large Egg, whole	6
Egg Yolk	3
Egg White	3
Omelet: Plain, 2 eggs	13
Ham & cheese	17
Egg Substitutes, (liquid):	
Egg Beaters, $\frac{1}{4}$ cup, 2 oz	4.5
Better 'n Eggs/Scramblers, $\frac{1}{4}$ cup, 2 oz	6

Milk, Yogurt, Ice Cream

Milk: Whole: 2%, 1 cup	8
Low-Fat (1%); Fat-Free, 1 cup	8.5
Chocolate Milk, 1 cup	8
Thick Shake: Chocolate, 10 oz	9
Vanilla, 10 oz	11
Soymilk, (fortified), average, 1 cup	7
Soy Dream, Enriched, shelf-stable, 1 cup	7
Yogurt, average all brands:	
Plain, 6 oz	8
Fruit flavors, 6 oz	7
Chobani, Greek, Plain, 6 oz	14
Soy, fruit flavors, 6 oz	7
Ice Cream: Rich, $\frac{1}{2}$ cup	2
Regular, Vanilla, $\frac{1}{2}$ cup	2.5
Sherbet, $\frac{1}{2}$ cup	1
Custard, baked, $\frac{1}{2}$ cup	7

Cheese

Hard Cheeses, average, 1 oz	7
Cottage Cheese, $\frac{1}{2}$ cup	13
Cream Cheese, avg., 1 oz	2
Ricotta, part skim, $\frac{1}{2}$ cup	14

Bread, Bagels, Biscuits

Bread: *With enriched flour*	
1 slice, 1 oz	2
4 thin slices, 4 oz	8
4 thick slices, 6 oz	1.2
Bagel, plain 2 oz	6
Biscuits, 1 oz	2
Pita Bread, 1 pita, 1$\frac{1}{2}$ oz	4
Pumpernickel, 1 slice, 1 oz	3

Infant/Baby Foods | **Pro**

Infant Formula Milk:	
Enfamil/Gerber/Similac,	
Regular/Low Iron , 5 fl.oz	2.2
Isomil/Nursoy/ProSobee,	
Baby Cereals: *Average all brands*	
Dry, 4 Tbsp, $\frac{1}{2}$ oz	1
Jars, with fruit, 4$\frac{1}{2}$ oz	1

Protein Counter

Breakfast Cereals **Pro**

Hot Cereals ~ *Cooked:*

Bulgur, cooked, 1 cup, 5 oz	9
Oatmeal: Reg., non-fortified, 1 cup	6
Instant, fortified, avg., 1 pkt	4
Quaker, all flavors, $^1/_2$ cup	5
Corn/Hominy Grits: 1 cup	3
Quaker: Reg., 3 Tbsp, 1 oz	2
Instant White, 1 packet	2
Cream of Wheat, 1 cup	4

Brands ~ *Ready-To-Eat*

General Mills:

Cheerios, Original, 1 cup, 1 oz	3
Chex, Corn, 1 cup, 1.1 oz	2
Kix, Original, $1^1/_4$ cups, 1 oz	2
Lucky Charms, Original, $^3/_4$ cup, 1 oz	2
Total, Raisin Bran, 1 cup, 1.8 oz	3
Wheaties, $^3/_4$ cup, 1 oz	2

Health Valley:

Amaranth Flakes, $1^1/_4$ cups, 2 oz	6
Bran Flakes, with Raisins, 1 cup, 1.8 oz	5
Corn Crunch-Ems, 1 cup, 1 oz	2
Oat Bran Flakes, with Raisins, 1 cup, 1.9 oz	5
Rice Crunch-Ems, $1^1/_4$ cups, 1 oz	2

Kashi:

Good Friends, 1 cup, 1.9 oz	5
GoLean Crunch!, 1 cup, 1.9 oz	9
7 Whole Grain Flakes, 1 cup, 1.75 oz	6

Kellogg's:

All-Bran, Original, $^1/_2$ cup, 1 oz	4
Apple Jacks, 1 cup, 1 oz	1
Corn Flakes, 1 cup, 1 oz	2
Low-fat Granola with Raisins $^2/_3$ cup, 2.1 oz	5
Product 19, 1 cup, 1 oz	3
Rice Krispies, $1^1/_4$ cup, 1.2 oz	2
Smart-Start Strong Heart, 1 c., 1.75 oz	4
Special K: All flavors, 1 c., 1.1 oz	2
Protein, $^3/_4$ cup, 1.1 oz	10

Post:

Grape Nuts, Original, $^1/_2$ cup, 2 oz	8
Raisin Bran, 1 cup, 2 oz	5

Quaker:

Corn Bran Crunch, $^3/_4$ cup, 1 oz	2
Granola, $^1/_2$ cup, 1.7 oz	5
Honey Graham Oh's, $^3/_4$ cup, 1 oz	1
Life, Original, $^3/_4$ cup, 1.1 oz	3

Brans & Wheatgerm **Pro**

Oat Bran, raw, 1 Tbsp	2
Rice Bran, raw, 2 Tbsp	1
Wheat Bran, unprocessed, 2 T.	1
Wheat Germ, 2 Tbsp, $^1/_2$ oz	4

Grains & Flours, Yeast

Amaranth, $^1/_2$ cup, 3.4 oz	14
Barley, $^1/_2$ cup, 3.2 oz	12
Buckwheat Flour, Whole-groat, 1 cup	15
Carob Flour, 1 cup, 3.6 oz	5
Corn Flour, 1 cup, 4 oz	11
Corn Meal, 1 cup, $4^1/_2$ oz	8
Flour: White, 1 cup, 5.6 oz	9
Wholegrain, 1 cup, $4^1/_4$ oz	16
Millet, wholegrain, 1 cup, $3^1/_2$ oz	12
Rye Flour: Dark, 1 cup, $4^1/_2$ oz	18
Light, 1 cup, $3^1/_2$ oz	9
Soy Flour, full fat, 1 cup, 3 oz	29
Yeast: Brewers, 2 Tbsp, $^1/_2$ oz	8
Nutritional Yeast Flakes *(Red Star)*, 1 heaping Tbsp, $^1/_2$ oz	8

Rice, Spaghetti, Macaroni

Rice: Brown/White, average 1 cup cooked, $6^1/_2$ oz	5

Spaghetti/Macaroni/Noodles (enriched):

Cooked, 1 cup, $4^1/_2$ oz	7
Canned: in Tomato Sce, $^1/_2$ cup	2
with Meatballs, 1 cup, 8 oz	10
Macaroni & Cheese, 1 cup, 9 oz	8

Soups

With Noodles/Vegetables, 1 cup	3
With Meat/Beans/Peas, 1 cup	8

Fruit

Fresh/Canned:

Average, all types, 1 medium/2 small fruit	1
Avocado, $^1/_2$ medium	2
Dried Fruit: Apricots, 8 halves, 1 oz	1
Dates, 6 dates, 2 oz	1.5
Figs, 4 medium figs, 2 oz	2
Prunes, 5 medium, $1^1/_2$ oz	1
Raisins, 1 oz	1
Fruit Juice: Average, 1 cup	0.5
Prune Juice, 6 fl.oz	1
Tomato Juice, 1 cup, 8 fl.oz	1.5

Vegetables | Pro

	Pro
Beans: Snap/green, $^1/_2$ cup, 2 oz	1
Dried: Average all types, cooked, $^1/_2$ cup	7
Baked Beans, $^1/_2$ cup 4$^1/_2$ oz	5
Bean Sprouts, mung, 1 c., 4 oz	3
Broccoli, 3raw, $^1/_2$ cup, 1$^1/_2$ oz	1.5
Cabbage; Cauliflower, raw, 1 c. 3 oz	1.5
Corn: Raw, $^1/_2$ cup kernels, 3 oz	2.5
1 ear trimmed to 3$^1/_2$"	2
Lentils, cooked, $^1/_2$ cup 3$^1/_2$ oz	9
Mushrooms, raw, $^1/_2$ c., sliced	1
Peas: Green, raw, $^1/_2$ c., 2$^1/_2$ oz	4
Split Peas, cooked, 1 cup, 7 oz	16
Potatoes: *Cooked:*	
1 medium, with skin, 5 oz	3.3
without skin, 4 oz	2.3
French Fries, small, 2.6 oz	2
Potato Salad, $^1/_2$ cup, 4 oz	3.5
Pumpkin, $^1/_2$ cup mashed, 4.3 oz	1
Seaweed, kelp, 1 oz	<1
Spinach, cooked, $^1/_2$ cup, 3 oz	2.7
Squash, ckd, all types, $^1/_2$ cup	1
Tomatoes, 1 medium, 4$^1/_2$ oz	1
Vegetables, mixed, ckd, 1 cup	2.5
Soybeans, cooked, $^1/_2$ cup, 3 oz	14

Tofu, Tempeh, Miso

	Pro
Tofu, raw, firm, $^1/_2$ cup, 4$^1/_2$ oz	10
Tempeh, $^1/_2$ cup, 3 oz	16
Miso, $^1/_2$ cup, 5 oz	16
Miso Soup, 1 cup	3
Soybean Protein *(TVP),* 1 oz	18

Cakes, Pastries, Pies

	Pro
(Made with enriched flour)	
Carrot w. cream cheese frosting, 4 oz	4
Cheesecake, 1 piece, 4 oz	6
Chocolate, 1 piece, 2 oz	2
Fruitcake, 1 piece, 3 oz	4
Plain, 1 piece, 3 oz	4
Croissant, plain, 2 oz	5
Danish Pastry, 1 pastry, 2$^1/_4$ oz	4
Donuts, average, 2 oz	4
Muffins, average, 1 med., 1$^1/_2$ oz	3
Pancakes, 4" diam., two, 2 oz	4
Pies: Fruit, 1 piece, 5$^1/_2$ oz	4
Pecan, 1 piece, 5 oz	7
Puddings, average, $^1/_2$ cup, 4$^1/_2$ oz	4
Waffles, 1 large, 2$^1/_2$ oz	7

Peanut Butter | Pro

	Pro
Regular: 2 Tbsp, 1.1 oz	8
Peter Pan Plus, 2 Tbsp, 1.1 oz	8

Sugar, Honey, Jam

	Pro
Sugar: White	0
Brown, 1 Tbsp	0
Molasses: Light/Med., 1 Tbsp	0
Blackstrap, 1 Tbsp, $^3/_4$ oz	0
Corn Syrup, 1 Tbsp, $^3/_4$ oz	0
Honey, Jams, Jelly	0

Candy, Chocolate, Carob

	Pro
Candy, sugar-based	0
Chocolate: Plain, 2 oz bar	4
with nuts, 2 oz bar	6
Carob, plain, 2 oz	6

Cookies, Crackers, Chips

	Pro
Cookies, average, 4 cookies	2
Crackers, Graham, 2$^1/_2$" sq., (2)	1
Rice Cakes, average, one	1
Corn/Potato Chips, 1 oz	2

Nuts:

	Pro
Almonds, shelled, 20-25 nuts	6
Brazil Nuts, 7-8 medium nuts, 1 oz	4
Cashews, 12-16 nuts, 1 oz	5
Macadamias, 1 oz	2
Peanuts, dry rsted, 40 nuts, 1 oz	6
Pecans, 24 halves, 1 oz	2
Walnuts, 15 halves, 1 oz	4

Seeds:

	Pro
Sesame Seeds, dry, 1 Tbsp	2
Pumpkin Kernels, dry, hulled, 1 oz	7
Sunflower Seeds, dried, hulled, 1 oz	6
Tahini, 1 Tbsp, $^1/_2$ oz	2.5

Granola & Food/Protein Bars

	Pro
Granola Bars, average, 1 bar, 2 oz	2
Anytime Health,	
Meal Repl. Bars, 80g	20
Snack Bars, 50g	12
Balance Bars, Original, average all, 1.76 oz	14
Bariatrix, Proti-Bars (1), 1.4 oz	15
Dr Soy, Protein Bars, 1.76 oz	10
GeniSoy, Protein Bar, 1.6 oz	15
Jenny Craig, Bars, av., 1.8 oz	5
Met-Rx, "Big 100", av. 3.5 oz	27
Myoplex 30, all flavors, 3 oz	30
Optifast 800, all flavors, 2 oz	14
PowerBar, Energize, 2 oz	6
Slim-Fast, Protein Meal Bars, 1.7 oz	10
Special K: Protein Meal, 1.6 oz	10
Protein Snack, 0.9 oz	4

Protein Counter

High Protein Drinks	Pro
Anytime, Health,	
Whey Prot. Isolate, all flav., 1 oz	25
Atkins, Shakes, 11 fl.oz	18
Boost, High Protein, 8 fl.oz bottle	15
Carnation, B'fast Essentials, 11 fl.oz	10
Curves, Protein Drink, 2 scoops, dry	15
dotFIT, First String,	
Choc., 2 scps, 2.65 oz	21
Ensure, Plus, 8 fl.oz bottle	13
Gatorade, Protein Recovery Shake, 11 oz	20
GeniSoy, Protein Shake, 1 scoop, 1.2 oz	14
Met-Rx, Meal Replacement, RTD	40
Myoplex, Original Nutrition Shake, 1 pkt	42
Optifast 800, prepared, 8 fl.oz	14
Slim-Fast Shakes: Meal, 10 oz can	10
High Protein Meal, 10 fl.oz bottle	20
Special K20, Protein Water, 16 fl.oz	5
Weider, Mass 1000, 4 scoops, 7 oz	34

Coffee, Tea, Soda

Coffee, Coffee Substitutes, 1 cup, 8 fl.oz	0
Coffee, with 2 oz milk, 1 cup, 8 fl.oz	2
Caffe latte, large, 16 fl.oz	12
Cappuccino, large, 16 fl.oz	8
Frappuccino, average, 16 fl.oz	6
Hot Chocolate, with milk, 1 cup, 8 fl.oz	8
Soft Drinks/Soda	0
Tea, all types	0

Beer, Wine, Spirits

Beer, 12 fl.oz	1
Wines, red/white, 1 glass	0
Spirits/Liquor	0

Fast-Foods/Burgers

Pancakes, average all outlets, 3	8
Shakes, Chocolate, 16 fl.oz	12
Sundaes, Average all outlets	7
Arby's:	
Chopped Farmhouse Salad, Crispy Chicken	28
Roast Beef Sandwich: Classic	23
Double	38
Burger King: Big Fish Sandwich	16
Double Bacon Cheeseburger	25
Whopper Sandwich	28

Fast Foods/Burgers (Cont)	Pro
Carl's Jr:	
Charbroiled Chicken Club Sandwich	42
Famous Star Hamburger with Cheese	28
Super Star Hamburger with Cheese	48
Domino's Pizza: Hand Tossed (12")	
Buffalo Chicken, 1 slice	13
Honolulu Hawaiian, 1 slice	11
Ultimate Pepperoni, 1 slice	12
KFC: Original Breast	39
Extra Crispy Chicken Tenders	10
Grilled, Breast	38
McDonald's: Big Mac	25
Buttermilk Crispy Chicken S'wch	28
Cheeseburger	15
Chicken McNuggets (4)	10
Filet-O-Fish	18
Hamburger	13
Quarter Pounder with Cheese	31
French Fries: Small, 2.5 oz	3
Large, 5.4 oz	
Salad, Bacon Ranch	33
Shakes, medium	14
Breakfast: Egg McMuffin	18
Bacon, Egg & Cheese McGriddles	18
Sausage Burrito	12
Sausage McMuffin with Egg	21
Pizza Hut: Per Medium, 1 slice, 1/8 Pizza	
Thin 'n Crispy, Supreme	9
Pan Pizzas, average	10
Hand Tossed: Pepperoni Lover's	11
Ultimate Cheese Lover's	10
Subway : 6" Subs with standard toppings, no oil	
Black Forest Ham	18
Meatball Marinara	21
Spicy Italian	20
Subway Melt	26
Turkey Breast	18
Taco Bell: Bean Burrito	14
Cheesy Gordita Crunch	20
Chicken Quesadilla	27
Chicken/Steak Chalupas	16
Grilled Soft Steak Taco	12
Steak Burrito Supreme	20
Wendy's:	
Asiago Ranch Chicken Club	38
Dave's Double Cheeseburger	49
Jr Hamburger	14

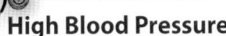

High Blood Pressure

Many American adults have hypertension (high blood pressure), and are unaware of it. It is generally symptomless, so **have your blood pressure checked annually** – particularly if it runs in the family.

Untreated hypertension overworks the heart, damages arteries and promotes atherosclerosis. This in turn greatly increases the risk of heart disease, stroke, blindness, kidney disease and impotence. The earlier hypertension is detected, the sooner it can be brought under control.

BLOOD PRESSURE CLASSIFICATION

For Adults Age 18 & Older ~ Not Acutely ill or on Medication (American Heart Association)

	DIASTOLIC		**SYSTOLIC**
Normal ➤	Below 80	and	Below 120
Prehypertension ➤	80-89	or	120-139
Hypertension:			
Stage 1 ➤	90-99	or	140-159
Stage 2 ➤	100 or more	or	160 or more

Treating Hypertension

Prehypertension (in the chart above) means you don't have high blood pressure now but are likely to develop it in the future.

You can take steps to lessen the risk by adopting healthy lifestyle habits such as:
- reducing sodium intake
- eating adequate fruit and vegetables
- losing weight if overweight
- limiting alcohol to 2 drinks or less daily
- quitting smoking
- exercising regularly, managing stress.

Stage 1 hypertension can often be treated with the above lifestyle changes.

Stage 2 hypertension usually requires drug therapy. However, salt restriction, abstaining from alcohol, and the above lifestyle changes will improve the success of drug therapy, and enable smaller drug doses to be prescribed.

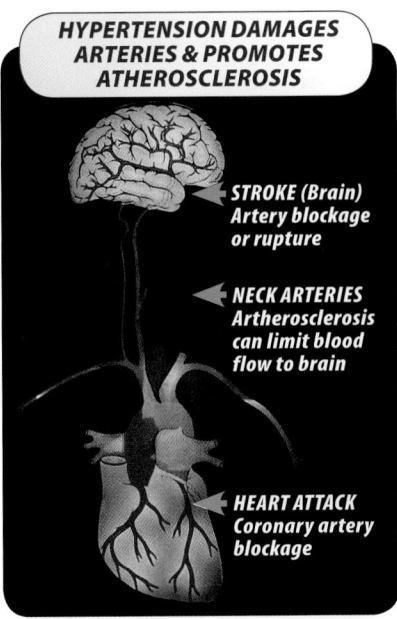

HYPERTENSION DAMAGES ARTERIES & PROMOTES ATHEROSCLEROSIS

STROKE (Brain)
Artery blockage or rupture

NECK ARTERIES
Artherosclerosis can limit blood flow to brain

HEART ATTACK
Coronary artery blockage

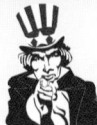

STROKE
KNOW THE WARNING SIGNS

Stroke is a medical emergency! If you notice one or more of these signs, call 9-1-1 or your doctor immediately.

These signs may be signalling a possible stroke or transient ischemic attack:

- **Sudden weakness** or numbness in your face, arm, or leg on one side of your body.
- **Sudden confusion,** trouble speaking or understanding. Slurred speech.
- **Sudden trouble seeing,** in one or both eyes.
- **Sudden trouble walking,** dizziness, loss of balance or coordination.
- **Sudden severe headache** - 'a bolt out of the blue' - with no apparent cause.

Extra Info: www.stroke.org

Salt & Sodium Guide

Salt & Sodium

- **Sodium is a mineral element** most commonly found in salt (sodium chloride). It also occurs naturally in much smaller amounts in animal and plant foods, and water – normally sufficient for our needs without having to add salt to our diet.

- **Sodium is required** for nerve and muscle function, as well as to balance the amount of fluid in our tissues and blood. Sodium acts like a sponge to attract and hold fluids in body tissues.

- **Excess sodium** can cause water retention, and increase the risk of developing hypertension. Very high salt intake may also increase the risk of stomach cancer.

- **Too little sodium** may cause low blood pressure (hypotension), and decrease blood flow to the heart, brain and kidneys – especially during exercise. (A certain blood volume is required to sustain the blood pressure needed for adequate blood flow in the capillaries).

Salt-Sensitive Persons

- **Normally, our kidneys** excrete excess dietary sodium. The thirst we feel after a salty meal is the body calling for water to dilute the sodium, and enable the kidneys to flush out excess sodium.

- **However, 'salt - sensitive'** persons (up to 70% of adults) tend to retain excess sodium (above approximately 3000mg daily) instead of excreting it. Such persons are more likely to develop hypertension and would benefit most from sodium restriction. Assume you are susceptible if there is a family history of hypertension.

- **Although not everyone will benefit, all Americans are being asked to moderate their salt and sodium intake** as a public health measure – particularly because so many do not know whether or not they have hypertension, and also because we do not know just who is salt-sensitive.

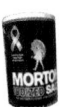

The American Heart Association recommends a **maximum sodium intake of 1500mg per day** for adults with normal blood pressure.

Persons with hypertension and kidney ailments are usually restricted to as little as **1000mg sodium per day**. Your doctor will discuss the correct sodium level for you.

FINDING HIDDEN SODIUM

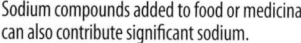

On average, **less than one third of our sodium intake comes from the salt shaker.** The rest is hidden in processed foods that have salt added during manufacture.

Sodium compounds added to food or medicinals can also contribute significant sodium.

Sodium bicarbonate in particular is widely used in antacid tablets (such as *Alka Seltzer*) and powders. Sodium bicarbonate contains 27% sodium by weight. Each gram has 270mg of sodium. Large amounts of sodium can be unwittingly consumed – up to 600mg per tablet. (See Antacids ~ Page 280)

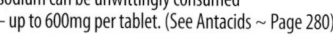

Example: 2 *Alka-Seltzer* Tablets = 1000mg sodium

Other sodium compounds include monosodium glutamate (MSG), sodium ascorbate, sodium nitrite, and sodium citrate.

POTASSIUM BALANCES SODIUM

Potassium helps to balance sodium by helping the kidneys to excrete excess sodium. Fruit and vegetables are rich sources of potassium - another reason to ensure you have your 5-7 servings every day.

Nuts also provide potassium as well as magnesium and other heart-healthy nutrients and anti-oxidants. Eat them unsalted.

Note: This info is only for people with normal kidney function. Also not for persons on potassium-sparing diuretics.

ALCOHOL DANGER

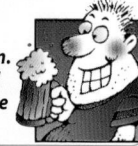

Excessive alcohol intake contributes to hypertension. Susceptible persons should avoid or limit alcohol intake to 1-2 drinks per day.

Salt Sodium Guide

Sodium accounts for only 40% of the weight of salt (sodium chloride). Examples:

1 gram (1000mg) Salt has 400mg Sodium

1 teaspoon (5g) Salt has 2000mg Sodium

HINTS TO REDUCE SODIUM

- **Cut down use of the salt shaker.** Start with an easy 50% cut in sodium by using Lite Salt (*Morton*) or *Cardia* Salt. Then gradually cut back until you can leave the salt shaker off the table. Sea salt is still high in sodium.

- **Use fresh herbs,** and salt-free seasonings to add flavor to food.

- **Choose low-sodium,** sodium-free, and reduced-sodium products in place of regular, salted products.

- **Check food labels for sodium levels.** FDA Guidelines for sodium descriptors are:
  - **Reduced Sodium:** At least 25% less sodium than the original product
  - **Low Sodium:** 140 mg or less/serving
  - **Very Low Sodium:** 35mg or less/serving
  - **Sodium Free:** Less than 5mg/serving
  - **No Salt Added:** Made without the salt normally added, but still contains the sodium that is a natural part of the food

- **Use reduced-sodium breads,** butter and margarine. Regular varieties are considered high in sodium in view of their significant contribution to our diet.

- **Go easy on salty condiments and sauces** such as ketchup, mustard, soy sauce, spaghetti sauces, and salad dressings. Use low-sodium varieties.

- **Limit pizzas and salty fast-foods.** Check the *CalorieKing.com* food database.

- **Avoid salty snack foods** such as potato chips, corn chips, salted nuts, pretzels and cheesy-flavored snacks. **Choose unsalted** popcorn, nuts or seeds. Eat more fruit.

- **Don't salt children's food** to your taste.

- **Avoid antacids with** sodium bicarbonate (such as *Alka-Seltzer*). They are high in sodium. Look for low-sodium alternatives.

FOODS HIGH IN SODIUM

- Bread (4 slices/day), Bagels, Biscuits
- Cheese, Butter, Margarine
- Pickles, Sauerkraut, Olives
- Condiments, Sauces
- Salad Dressings
- Canned vegetables/salads/beans
- Deli Salads (with dressing)
- Frozen/Packaged Meals/Entrees
- Soups: Canned/dry; bouillon cubes
- Meats: Ham, bacon, sausage, luncheon meats, smoked meats
- Canned Fish (in brine/salt)
- Sea Salt, Garlic/Celery Salt
- Snack Foods (potato chips, pretzels)
- Tomato Juice (Canned), V8 Vegetable Juice
- Fast Foods: Pizza, Burgers, Chicken
- *Alka-Seltzer* Antacid

MODERATE SODIUM

- Meat, Fish, Poultry - Unprocessed
- Milk, Yogurt, Soy Drinks, Eggs
- Peanut Butter
- Breakfast Cereals (less than 200mg/serving)
- Chocolate Candy, Fruit/Nut Bars
- *Reduced Sodium & Low Sodium* Products

FOODS LOW IN SODIUM

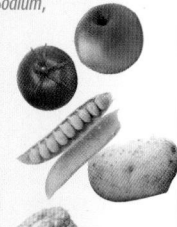

- Products labelled *Very Low Sodium*, or *Sodium Free*
- Bread (No Salt Added)
- Fresh fruits and vegetables
- Canned and Dried Fruits
- Potatoes, Rice, Pasta
- Dried Beans & Lentils, Tofu
- Nuts & Seeds (unsalted)
- Corn & Popcorn (unsalted)
- Pepper, Spices, Herbs
- Jam, Honey, Syrup
- Candy, Gum
- Hard & Jelly Candy
- Coffee, Tea, Alcohol
- Fresh Fruit Juices, Water

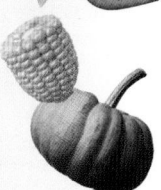

Sodium Counter

Milk & Dairy Products

Sodium ~ Sodium (mg)

	Sodium
Milk: Whole/lowfat/skim, average 1 glass, 8 fl.oz	120
Whole, low sodium, 1 cup	5
Choc Milk, 1 cup	130
Soy Milk, 8 fl.oz	30
Buttermilk, cultured, 8 fl.oz	250
Dry/Powder, skim, 1/4 cup, 1 oz	110
Yogurt, with fruit average, 8 oz	130
Cheese: Bleu, 1 oz	330
Cottage Cheese, Creamed, 1/2 cup, 4 oz	450
Kraft: American, 2% milk, 1 sl., 0.7 oz	230
Philadelphia Cream Cheese Brick, Orig.,1 oz	105
Parmesan, 1 oz	425
Process Cheese., average,1 oz	430
Ricotta Cheese, 1/2 cup, 4 oz	110
Swiss, Deli Deluxe, 1 slice	40

Ice Cream, Frozen Yogurt

Icecream, average, 1/2 cup	50
Frozen Yogurt, 1/2 cup	50

Fats/Oils

Butter/Margarine:	
Regular, 2 Tbsp, 1 oz	230
Unsalted, reg., 2 Tbsp, 1 oz	5
Mayonnaise, avg., 2 Tbsp, 1 oz	160
Oils/Lard/Drippings	0
Cream, average, 1 Tbsp	5
Coffee-Mate: Powdered, 1 tsp	2
Liquid, 1 Tbsp	5

Eggs

Whole, 1 large	70
Omelet: 2 egg, plain	220
With 1 oz Cheddar Cheese	400
Egg Beaters: Original, 3 Tbsp	90
Flavors, average, 3 Tbsp	140

Meats

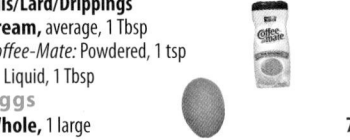

Meat, average all types, cooked Beef/Lamb/Veal/Pork, 4 oz	80
Corned Beef, cooked, 3 oz	800
Bacon, cooked, 2 slices, 0.5 oz	270
Ham, 3 oz	1100

Chicken & Turkey

Chicken/Turkey, cooked, unsalted, 4 oz	80
Stuffing Mixes, average., 1/2 cup	500

Sausages & Meats

	Sodium
Bologna, 1 oz	280
Frankfurter, 2 oz	640
Ham, chopped, 0.8 oz slice	290
Liverwurst (Braunschweiger), 1 oz	320
Pepperoni, 5 slices, 1 oz	570
Salami: Cooked, 1 oz	350
dry/hard, 1 oz	600
Sausage, 1 oz link	220
Pork, 2 oz patty	260
Spam: Classic, 2 oz	790
25% Less Sodium, 2 oz	580
Turkey Roll, 1 oz	160

Fish:

Fresh Fish: average, plain	
Cooked, 4 oz, without bone	60
Broiled w. butter, 4 oz	150
Breaded & fried, 4 oz	320
Fish fillets, batter-dipped 3 oz	350
Fish sticks, 1 oz stick	160
Gefilte Fish, with broth, 1 pce, 1.5 oz	220
Herring, pickled, 2 pces, 1 oz	260
Lobster, meat only, 4 oz	180
Oysters, fresh, 6 med., 3 oz	95
Salmon: Canned, 3 oz	460
No Salt Added, 3 oz	65
Smoked fish, average, 3 oz	650
Tuna: Canned, drained, 3 oz	160
Light, drained, 3 oz	200
No Added Salt, 3 oz	40
Spicy Flavored, 5 oz	260

Entrees & Meals

Frozen Meals, average	600-1300
Lean Cuisine, average	700
Stouffer's, For One, Beef Pot Roast	1570
Dinners, average	900-1300
Side Dishes, average	400-600
Pizza, frozen, 1/4 large, 6 oz	800-1200
Microwave, Cup Meals	900-1200
Cup O'Noodles, average	1500

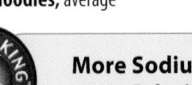

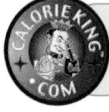

**More Sodium Counts:
www.CalorieKing.com**

Soups

	Sodium
Condensed: Average, 1 cup, 8 oz	800-1000
Low Sodium, average	70
Chicken Noodle, average, 1 cup	900
Bouillon Cube, average	950
Ramen Noodle Soup, av., 3 oz pkg	1500
Soup Cups, average	850
Soup Mixes, average, 1 cup	900

Condiments, Sauces, Dressings

A-1 Sauce, 1 Tbsp	280
Barbecue Sauce, 1 Tbsp	130
Bragg's Liquid Aminos, 1 tsp	220
Chili Sauce, 1 Tbsp	230
Ketchup: Tomato, 1 Tbsp	180
Low Sodium, 1 Tbsp	20
Mayonnaise, 1 Tbsp	80
Mustard, 1 tsp	70
Pizza Sauce, 1/2 cup	700
Salad Dressings, 2 Tbsp, 1 oz	160-400
Spaghetti Sauce, 1/2 cup	500
Soy Sauce: 1 Tbsp	900
Lite, 1 Tbsp	600
Sweet & Sour, 1/2 cup	250
Tabasco, 1 tsp	25
Vinegar, Lemon Juice	0
Worcestershire, 1 Tbsp	65
Tomato: Sauce, 1 cup	1200
Paste/Puree (salted), 1/2 cup	1000
No Salt Added, 1/2 cup	75

Salt & Salt Substitutes

Table Salt: 1 teaspoon, 6g	2400
Single Serve package, 1 g	400
Cardia Salt, 1 teaspoon	1080
Lite Salt, 1 teaspoon, 6g	1200
Morton, No Salt Substitute, 1 tsp	5
Garlic/Onion/Seasoned Salt, 1 tsp, 4g	1350
Garlic/Seasoned Salt 1 teaspoon, 4g	1300
Sea Salt, 1 teaspoon, 5g	2250

Seasonings, Herbs & Spices

Baking Powder, 1 tsp, 3g	340
Baking Soda (Sodium bicarb), 1 tsp, 3g	810
Accent, Flavor Enhancer, 1 tsp	680
Chili Powder, 1 tsp, 3g	25
Curry Powder	0
Lemon Pepper 1 tsp	340
Meat Tenderizer, 1 tsp, 5g	1750
MSG (Monosodium Glutamate), 5g	500
Mrs Dash, Blends/Marinades	0
Old Bay: Seasoning, 1 tsp, 2.4 oz	640
Seasoning, Less Sodium, 1 tsp, 2.4 oz	380
Pepper, Mustard (dry), 1 tsp	1
Yeast, Nutritional, 1 Tbsp	10

Breakfast Cereals

	Sodium
Kellogg's:	
All-Bran, Original, 1/2 cup, 1 oz	80
Special K, Original, 1¼ cups, 1.4 oz	270
Corn Flakes, 1 cup, 1 oz	200
Raisin Bran, with Banana, 1 cup, 2 oz	105
Quaker:	
Corn Crunch, 1 cup, 1.3 oz	220
Multigrain Flakes, av., 3/4 c., 2.2 oz	40
Puffed Rice/Wheat, 2 cups, 1 oz	0
Simply Granola, average, 1/2 cup	30
General Mills, Total, 3/4 cup, 1 oz	140
Oatmeal: Regular, 3/4 cup	1
Quaker, Instant Maple & Brown Sugar (1 pkt)	260

Breads, Bagels, Crackers

Bread: Thin Slice, average 1 oz	140
Thick Slice, 1.5 oz	210
Low Sodium, 1 oz	10
Bagels: Plain, medium, 2 oz	200
Large, take-out, average, 4 oz	550
Panera Bread, 3.8 oz	460
Biscuits, average, 1 oz	180
Bun/Roll: 1 medium, 1.5 oz	200
Large, 4 oz	560
Crackers: Saltine, 2 crackers	70
Low Salt, 2	25
Graham, 2 regular	50
Croissant, Plain, average, 2 oz	280
Rice Cakes, average	25
Ritz Crackers, Hint of Salt, 1 oz	60
Ry-Krisp, Crispbread, Sesame, 0.7 oz	70

Cookies, Cakes, Desserts

Cookies: Average, 2-3 cookies, 1 oz	100
Average, 1 cookie, 2.5 oz	180
Baked Custard, 1/2 cup	100
Brownie, 1.5 oz	130
Carrot Cake, 8 oz	650
Cheesecake, 7 oz	350
Cinnamon Sweet Roll, 2 oz	250
Danish, Apple/Fruit	250
Donut, average	150
Muffins: 1 medium, 2 oz	150
1 extra large, 4 oz	300
Pancakes, (4"), x 3	360
Fruit Pies, average, 7 oz	600
Pudding: Average, 1/2 cup	160
Jell-O Instant Pudding Mix, 1/4 pkg	360
Waffles: Home-made, 7", 2.5 oz	350
Frozen: Average, 1.2 oz	260
Aunt Jemima, Homestyle, av., 2.5 oz	480

Sodium Counter

Fruit & Juices
	Sodium
Fresh Fruit, average all types, 1 serving	1
Dried/Canned Fruit, 1/2 cup	1
Fruit Juice: Fresh, squeezed, 6 fl.oz	1
Commercial, aver., 6 fl.oz	20
Tomato Juice *(Campbell's),* 8 fl.oz	680
Low Sodium (No Salt Added), 8 fl.oz	140
V8 Vegetable *(Campbell's):*	
11.5 fl.oz bottle	880
Low Sodium, 5.5 fl.oz can	80

Vegetables
Fresh/Frozen (No Salt Added): Per 1/2 Cup
Asparagus, Bean Sprouts, Corn	3
Beets, Carrots, Celery, 1/2 cup	40
Broccoli, Cabbage, Cauliflower	10
Cucumber, Green Beans, Mushroom, Okra	3
Onions, Peas, Potato, Pumpkin, Squash	3
Peppers, Hot Chili, raw, each	3
Spinach, Turnips, 1/2 cup, cooked	40
Tomato, 1 medium, 5 oz	10
Canned: Asparagus, 4 spears	300
Beans, baked in tomato sauce	450
Beets, 1/2 cup, 3 oz	240
Corn Kernels, 1/2 cup, 3 oz	190
Creamed, 1/2 cup, 4.5 oz	330
Mushrooms w. butter sce, 2oz	550
Peas, 1/2 cup, 3 oz	250
Sauerkraut, 1/2 cup, 4 oz	750

Pickles, Olives
Olives: pickled: Green, 1 large	90
Ripe/black, 1 large	40
Pickles: Bread & Butter, 4 slices, 1 oz	200
Dill, 1 pickle, 2.5oz	900
Sweet, 1 gherkin, 0.5 oz	130

Soybean Products
Miso (Soy Paste), 1/4 c., 2.5 oz	2500
Soybean Protein Isolate, 1 oz	280
Tempeh, Natural, 1/2 cup, 3 oz	5
Tofu, average, 1/2 cup, 4 oz	5

Jam, Honey, Syrups
Jam/Jelly, 1 Tbsp	2
Honey/Maple Syrup, 1 Tbsp	1
Log Cabin, Syrup, 1 fl.oz	35
Lite, 1 fl.oz	90

Peanut Butter
Peanut Butter: Regular, 2 Tbsp, 0.5 oz	190
Jif, Low Sodium, 2 Tbsp	65
Trader Joe's, Unsalted, 2 Tbsp	5

Snacks, Nuts
	Sodium
Cheese Balls/Curls, 1 oz	280
Cheetos, 1 oz	290
Corn/Tortilla Chips: average, 1 oz	220
Fritos, Lightly Salted, 1 oz	80
Granola bars, average, 1 bar	80
Nuts: Plain, unsalted, 1 oz	1
Lightly salted, 1 oz	80
Salted or Honey Roasted, 1 oz	160
Popcorn: Plain (unsalted), 1 cup	1
Flavored, average, 1 cup	60
Salt added, 1 cup	180
Potato Chips: Plain, 1 oz	160
Lay's, Lightly Salted, 1 oz	85
Flavored, average, 1 oz	200
Pretzels: Regular, 3, 1 oz	450
Soft, salted, large	1000

Candy, Chocolate
Chocolate, milk, 1 oz	30
Fudge, chocolate, 1 oz	55
Candy Bars, average, 1.5 oz	60
Hard Candy, 1 oz	10
Licorice, 1 oz	30

Beverages, Alcohol
Coffee or Tea, 1 cup	1
Cocoa: Dry, plain, 1 Tbsp	0
Mix, average, 1 envelope	120
Quik, 2 tsp	35
Soft Drinks, average, 8 fl.oz	20
Mineral Water: Perrier, 8 fl.oz	5
Gatorade, Thirst Quencher, 8 fl.oz	110
Red Bull: 8.4 fl.oz can	105
Sugar Free, 8.4 fl.oz	200
Water, Average, 1 cup, 8 fl.oz	5
Alcohol: Beer, average, 12 fl.oz	15
Wines, average, 4 fl.oz	10
Spirits (distilled), 1.5 fl.oz	1

Antacids ~ Alka-Seltzer
Alka-Seltzer: *Per Tablet*	Sodium
Original; Heartburn	570
Extra Strength	590
Lemon Lime	500
Gold	310
Alka-Mints, chewable	0
Bromo Seltzer, 3/4 capful	760
Picot, 1 packet, 5g	670
Rolaids, All types	0
Tums, Regular/Extra Strength	0

Cold & Flu ~ Alka-Seltzer Plus
Effervescents, average, 1 tablet	480
Fast Crystal Packs; Liquid Gels	0

Fast-Foods & Restaurants — Sodium

Burger King:
	Sodium
Bacon Double Cheeseburger	740
Cheeseburger	560
Hamburger	380
Whoppers: Original	980
With Cheese	1540
Whopper Jr.	390
Chicken Sandwich, Original	1170
Sides: French Fries, medium, salted	570
Onion Rings, medium	1080
Breakfast, Ham, Egg & Cheese Croissan'wich	1030

Denny's:
	Sodium
Burgers: Bacon Avocado Cheeseburger	1830
Spicy Sriracha	2210
Sandwiches: Club	2180
Prime Rib Philly Melt	2340
Dinner: Brooklyn Spaghetti & M'balls w/ Bread	2480
Sirloin Steak, with Bread	1260
Sides: Broccoli	20
French Fries, salted, 6 oz	110
Red-Skinned Potatoes	590
Soup: Loaded Baked Potato, 12 oz bowl	1770
Vegetable Beef, 12 oz bowl	3420
Breakfast: Buttermilk Pancakes (2), w/ Marg.	1390
Moons Over My Hammy Omelette, w/ Hash	2560
Supreme Skillet, 10 oz	1180
Sides: Hash Browns, 1 serving	360
Hearty Breakfast Sausage	840
Dessert, Arml Apple Pie Crisp, 1 slice, 13 oz	620

Jack In The Box:
	Sodium
Burgers: Bacon Ultimate Cheeseburger	1590
Hamburger	570
Jumbo Jack Cheeseburger	990
Sandwiches: H'style Ranch Chicken Club	1880
Sourdough Grilled Chicken Club	1500

KFC:
	Sodium
Chicken Breast: Original	1190
Extra Crispy	1150
Georgia Gold, Grilled	760
Popcorn Nuggets, Large	1820
Sandwich, Crispy Twister	1260
Tenders, Extra Crispy Tenders, each	610
Wings, HBBQ Hot (1)	160
Sides: Macaroni & Cheese	660
Mashed Potatoes with Gravy	510
Potato Wedges	700

Fast-Foods & Restaurants — Sodium

McDonalds:
	Sodium
Burgers: Big Mac	950
Cheeseburger	680
Double	1040
Hamburger	480
Quarter Pounder with Cheese	1090
Chicken McNuggets: 6 pieces	510
Spicy Buffalo Sauce, 1 package, 0.8 oz	510
Sandwich, Buttermilk Crispy Chicken	1050
French Fries: Small, 2.6 oz	160
Medium, 3.9 oz	230
Large, 5.9 oz	350
Ketchup, 1 package, 10g	90
Breakfast: Egg McMuffin	730
Big Breakfast, reg. size Biscuit	1490
Hash Browns, 2 oz	320
Hotcakes, with Syrup & Whipped Margarine	610
Sausage McGriddle	990
Southern Style Chicken Biscuit, regular	1140
Desserts/Shakes: Hot Fudge Sundae	170
Strawberry McCafe Shake, medium	230

Pizza Hut:
	Sodium
Original Pan Pizza: *Per Slice, Medium 12"*	
Meat Lovers	660
Cheese	440
Pepperoni Lover's	600
Supreme	500

Subway: *On 9 Grain Wheat Bread*
	Sodium
6" Sandwiches: *With Set Menu Toppings, no oil*	
Chicken Bacon Ranch Melt	1290
Meatball Marinara	1000
Spicy Italian	1490
6" Breakfast S'wich: *With Set Menu Toppings,no oil*	
Bacon, Egg & Cheese Omelet	1310
BMT Egg & Cheese Omelet	1630
Mega Melt Egg White & Cheese Omelet	1830
Sausage, Egg & Cheese Omelet	1400

Taco Bell:
	Sodium
Burritos: Beefy 5-Layer	1000
Supreme, Chicken	1110
Chalupa Supreme, Chicken/Steak, av	515
Gordita Supreme, Steak	550
Nachos: BellGrande	1310
Supreme	850
Specialties, Cheese Quesadillas	980
Tacos: Soft Chicken	450
Crunchy Supreme	340

Index A - C

FAST-FOODS INDEX
~ PAGE 175 ~

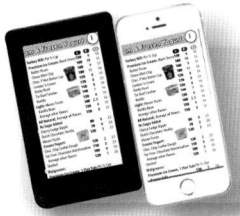

i-BOOK EDITIONS

NOW AVAILABLE FOR
• iPHONE • iPAD

Fully Searchable & Enhanced

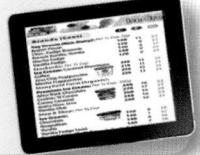

Index D - I

FAST-FOODS INDEX
~ PAGE 175 ~

Index P - S

FAST-FOODS INDEX
~ PAGE 175 ~

Notes

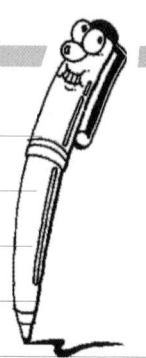

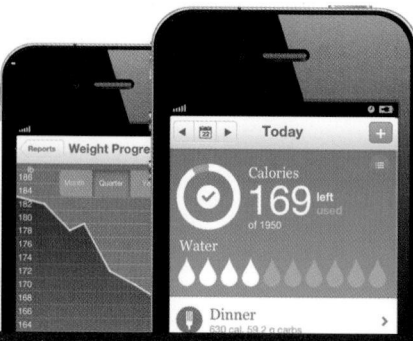
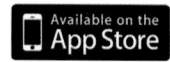